CORONARY ARTERY DISEASE IN WOMEN

For a catalogue of publications available from ACP–ASIM, contact:

Customer Service Center
American College of Physicians–American Society of Internal Medicine
190 N. Independence Mall West
Philadelphia, PA 19106-1572
215-351-2600
800-523-1546, ext. 2600

Visit our Web site at www. acponline.org

CORONARY ARTERY DISEASE IN WOMEN

WHAT ALL PHYSICIANS NEED TO KNOW

EDITED BY PAMELA CHARNEY, MD, FACP

ASSOCIATE PROFESSOR OF MEDICINE
ASSISTANT PROFESSOR OF OBSTETRICS & GYNECOLOGY
AND WOMEN'S HEALTH
JACOBI MEDICAL CENTER
ALBERT EINSTEIN COLLEGE OF MEDICINE
BRONX, NY

AMERICAN COLLEGE OF PHYSICIANS
PHILADELPHIA

Clinical Consultant: David R. Goldmann, MD, FACP
Acquisitions Editor: Mary K. Ruff
Manager, Book Publishing: David Myers
Administrator, Book Publishing: Diane McCabe
Production Supervisor: Allan S. Kleinberg
Production Editors: Scott Thomas Hurd and Karen Nolan
Interior Designer: Patrick Whelan
Cover Designer: Jeanette Jacobs

Printed in the United States of America
Composition by Fulcrum Data Services, Inc.
Printing/binding by Versa Press

American College of Physicians (ACP) became an imprint of the American College of Physicians—American Society of Internal Medicine in July 1998.

Library of Congress Cataloging-in-Publication Data

Coronary Artery Disease in Women: What All Physicans Need To Know / edited by Pamela Charney.
      p.   cm. — (Women's Health series)
    Includes bibliographical references and index.
    ISBN 0-943126-68-1 (alk. paper)
    1. Coronary heart disease. 2. Women — diseases. 3. Coronary heart disease — sex factors. 4. Coronary heart disease — Risk factors. I. Charney, Pamela, 1954–. II. Series: Women's health series (Philadelphia, Pa.)
    [DNLM: 1. Coronary Diseas. 2. Women.
WD 300C8194 1999]
RC685.C6C6315 1999
616.1'23'0082—dc21
DNLM/DLC
for Library of Congress   98-28030
                                          CIP

The authors and publisher have exerted every effort to ensure that drug selection and dosage set forth in this manual are in accord with current recommendations and practice at the time of publication. In view of ongoing research, occasional changes in government regulations, and the constant flow of information relating to drug therapy and drug reactions, the reader is urged to check the package insert for each drug for any change in indications and dosage and for added warnings and precautions. This care is particularly important when the recommended agent is a new or infrequently used drug.

99 00 01 02 03/9 8 7 6 5 4 3 2 1

THERE IS SOMETHING ABOUT THE WOMEN...
WITH LOVE FOR SUSAN AND ASHLEY

Contributors

Abigail Adams, MD
Assistant Professor of Medicine
General Medicine/Primary Care
University of Massachusetts Medical School
Worcester, MA

Christine M. Albert, MD, MPH
Brigham and Women's Hospital
Division of Preventive Medicine
Harvard Medical School
Boston, MA

Weihang Bao, PhD
Tulane Center for Cardiovascular Health
Tulane School of Public Health and
  Tropical Medicine
New Orleans, LA

Malcolm R. Bell, MB, BS, FRACP
Consultant, Division of Cardiovascular
  Diseases and Internal Medicine
Associate Professor of Medicine
Mayo Medical School
Rochester, MN

Ainat Beniaminovitz, MD
Assistant Attending Physician
Columbia Presbyterian Hospital
New York, NY

Gerald Sanders Berenson, MD, FACP
Tulane Center for Cardiovascular Health
Tulane University Medical Center
New Orleans, LA

Kathleen Berra, MSN, ANP
Clinical Coordinator
Stanford Center for Research in
  Disease Prevention
Stanford University School of Medicine
Palo Alto, CA

Roger S. Blumenthal, MD, FACC
Assistant Professor of Medicine
Division of Cardiology
Director of Henry Ciccarone Center for
  the Prevention of Heart Disease
Johns Hopkins University School of
  Medicine
Baltimore, MD

Debra Perkins Bonollo, BA
Research Coordinator
Division of Preventive and Behavioral
  Medicine
University of Massachusetts Medical
  School
Worcester, MA

Trudy L. Bush, PhD, MHS
Professor of Epidemiology
Department of Epidemiology and
  Preventive Medicine
Women's Health Research Group
University of Maryland School of
  Medicine
Baltimore, MD

Pamela Charney, MD, FACP
Associate Professor of Medicine
Assistant Professor of Obstetrics &
  Gynecology and Women's Health
Jacobi Medical Center
Albert Einstein College of Medicine
Bronx, NY

Ellen Cohen, MD
Associate Professor of Internal
  Medicine
Albert Einstein College of
  Medicine
Montefiore Medical Center
Bronx, NY

Laura J. Collins, MD, FACC
Assistant Professor of Medicine
Division of Cardiology
University of Texas Health Science Center
San Antonio, TX

Michelle Del Valle, MD
Instructor of Clinical Medicine
Albert Einstein College of Medicine
Bronx, NY

Pamela S. Douglas, MD, FACC, FACSM
Associate Professor of Medicine
Harvard Medical School;
Director, Non-Invasive Cardiology
Beth Israel Deaconess Medical Center
Boston, MA

Jonathan M. Evans, MD
Community Internal Medicine
Section of Geriatrics, Department of
  Internal Medicine
Mayo Clinic
Rochester, MN

Mary P. Evans, MD
Assistant Professor of Obstetrics and
  Gynecology
Mayo Clinic
Rochester, MN

Joan M. Fair, RN, NP, PhD
Research Project Director
Stanford Center for Research in Disease
  Prevention
Stanford University School of Medicine
Palo Alto, CA

Kevin C. Fleming, MD
Community Internal Medicine
Section of Geriatrics, Department of
  Internal Medicine
Mayo Clinic
Rochester, MN

William H. Frishman, MD, FACP
Professor of Medicine and Pharmacology
Chairman, Department of Medicine
New York Medical College;
Chief of Medicine
Westchester Medical Center
Valhalla, NY

Henry N. Ginsberg, MD
Professor of Medicine
Director, Irving Center for Clinical
  Research
Columbia University College of
  Physicians and Surgeons
New York, NY

Kurt Joseph Greenlund, PhD
Assistant Professor
Department of Community Health
  Sciences
Tulane Center for Cardiovascular Health
Tulane School of Public Health and
  Tropical Medicine
New Orleans, LA

Renee S. Hartz, MD
Professor of Surgery
Tulane University Medical Center
New Orleans, LA

David R. Holmes, Jr., MD
Professor of Medicine
Director of Cardiac Catheterization
  Laboratory
Mayo Medical School;
Consultant in Cardiovascular Diseases
  and Internal Medicine
Rochester, MN

Sue C. Jacobs, PhD
Associate Professor
Director, Counseling Psychology
  Training Program
Department of Counseling
University of North Dakota
Grand Forks, ND

Lynne L. Johnson, MD
Professor of Medicine
Director of Nuclear Cardiology
Brown University
Rhode Island Hospital
Providence, RI

Paula A. Johnson, MD, MPH
Assistant Professor of Medicine
Divisions of General Medicine and
  Cardiology
Harvard Medical School;
Medical Director, Quality Improvement
Brigham and Women's Hospital
Boston, MA

Wahida Karmally, MS, RD, CDE
Associate Research Scientist
Director of Nutrition
Irving Center for Clinical Research
Columbia University
New York, NY

Abby C. King, PhD
Associate Professor of Health Research
  and Policy
Stanford University School of Medicine
Stanford, CA

Ami Laws, MD
Assistant Professor of Medicine
Division of Endocrinology
Stanford University School of Medicine
Stanford, CA

Eva M. Lonn, MD, FRCPC, FACC
Associate Professor of Medicine
Division of Cardiology
McMaster University
Hamilton, Ontario, Canada

Donna M. Mancini, MD
Associate Professor of Medicine
Division of Cardiology
Columbia Presbyterian Hospital
New York, NY

JoAnn E. Manson, MD, DRPH, FACP
Associate Professor of Medicine
Harvard Medical School
Boston, MA

Thomas H. Marwick, MD, PHD
Professor of Medicine
University of Queensland
Princess Alexandria Hospital
Brisbane, Queensland,
Australia

D. Douglas Miller, MD
Professor and Associate Chairman
Department of Internal Medicine
St. Louis University Health Center
St. Louis, MO

Theresa Ann Nicklas, DRPH
Associate Professor of Community
  Health Sciences
Tulane Center for Cardiovascular
  Health
Tulane School of Public Health and
  Tropical Medicine
New Orleans, LA

Judith Keller Ockene, PHD, MED
Professor of Medicine
Director, Division of Preventive and
  Behavioral Medicine
Department of Medicine
University of Massachusetts Medical
  School
Worcester, MA

Steve R. Ommen, MD
Division of Cardiovascular Diseases and
  Internal Medicine
Mayo Clinic
Rochester, MN

Eric D. Peterson, MD, MPH
Assistant Professor of Medicine
Division of Cardiology
Duke University Medical Center
Durham, NC

Leslee J. Shaw, PHD
Associate Professor of Medicine
Division of Cardiology
Associate Director
Emory Center for Outcomes Research
Emory University
Atlanta, GA

**Sathanur Ramachandaran
  Srinivasan, PHD**
Research Professor
Department of Community Health
  Sciences
Tulane Center for Cardiovascular Health
Tulane School of Public Health and
  Tropical Medicine
New Orleans, LA

Peter H. Stone, MD
Associate Professor of Medicine
Division of Cardiology
Co-Director, Samuel A. Levin Cardiac Unit
Director, Clinical Trials Program
Brigham & Women's Hospital
Harvard Medical School
Boston, MA

Deborah M. Swiderski, MD
Assistant Professor of Medicine
Albert Einstein College of Medicine
Montefiore Medical Center
Bronx, NY

Judith M. E. Walsh, MD, MPH
Clinical Assistant Professor of Medicine,
  Epidemiology, and Biostatistics
University of California–San Francisco
San Francisco, CA

Wendy Ann Wattigney, MS
Associate Scientist
Tulane Center for Cardiovascular Health
New Orleans, LA

Nanette K. Wenger, MD, MACP
Professor of Medicine (Cardiology)
Emory University School of Medicine;
Chief of Cardiology
Grady Memorial Hospital;
Consultant, Emory Heart Center
Atlanta, GA

Mary E. Wheat, MD
Assistant Clinical Professor
  of Medicine
Albert Einstein College of
  Medicine
Bronx, NY;
Director, Student Health Services
Barnard College
Columbia University
New York, NY

**Salim Yusuf, MBBS, DPHIL, FRCPC,
  FRCP(UK), FACC**
Professor of Medicine
McMaster University;
Director, Division of Cardiology
Hamilton General Hospital
Hamilton, Ontario, Canada

Preface

The management of coronary artery disease is rapidly evolving. Increased attention is being paid to patient characteristics that may affect outcome. Although there is an expanding literature about the relation of gender to coronary artery disease, the data have not yet been translated into the practice patterns of most clinicians. *Coronary Artery Disease in Women: What All Physicians Need To Know* reviews all important aspects of coronary artery disease, with an emphasis on gender differences, age, and race. Although the authors are from various parts of the United States and are experts in several specialities, they reach consensus on many issues.

Over the past 10 years, there has been increasing public and professional attention focused on gender differences in the diagnosis and management of common medical conditions. Federal legislation has required funding agencies to include previously under-represented groups, such as female, African-American, and Hispanic populations, in proposed clinical trials (1). Within the medical profession, the emergence of evidence-based medicine has fostered critical re-examination of the older literature. Physicians are increasingly individualizing risk factors and therapeutic options. And, as the number of women clinicians and academicians has increased, many have become interested in reconsidering how gender affects health. The few isolated solo voices have now reached choral proportions.

My personal interest in how coronary artery disease may differ in women and men is long-standing. As a primary care internist, first as a Kaiser physician and then at Jacobi Medical Center, a New York City public hospital, I have cared for many special women and men with coronary artery disease. Since the mid-1980s, I have been involved with a Society of General Internal Medicine group re-examining large hypertension treatment trials for information about women (2).

Subsequently, as part of the planning of the core curriculum for the General Internal Medicine–Women's Health Residency track, I conceptualized a month-long intensive course for residents and senior medical students entitled "Coronary Artery Disease and Gender" (3). That course, and eventually this book, became a reality with the aid of my colleague and friend Dr. Paul Marantz. Participants have repeatedly been surprised how much has been studied but how difficult it can be to locate literature that addresses common questions in clinical practice. Therefore, this book reviews what we currently know about women and coronary artery disease and attempts to provide a framework for integrating future knowledge. While preparing this book, I learned much more than I expected to; I hope as you read you have a similar experience.

Many thanks are due patients and colleagues, including Joanne Ciuti, our administrator, and the first General Internal Medicine–Women's Health Track residents: Drs. Dwight Matthias, Annmarie Baldanti, Anshu Taneju, and Brenda Vozza-Zeid.

Pamela Charney, MD, FACP

REFERENCES

1. **National Institutes of Health**. NIH Guide 20:1. 8 Feb. 1991.
2. **Anastos K, Charney P, Charon RA, et al.** Hypertension in women: what is really known? The Women's Caucus, Working Group on Women's Health, Society of General Internal Medicine. Ann Intern Med. 1991;115:287-93.
3. **Lemberg L, Marantz P, Love M, Charney P**: General Internal Medicine–Women's Health Track. SGIM Forum. 1997;20(5).

Contents

DIAGNOSIS

MANAGEMENT

CONCLUSION

Introduction

CHAPTER 1

The Natural History of Coronary Artery Disease in Women

Epidemiology, Coronary Risk Factors, and Clinical Characteristics

NANETTE K. WENGER, MD

Epidemiology

Coronary artery disease (CAD) is the leading cause of mortality for adult women in the United States, accounting for more than 250,000 deaths annually (Fig. 1-1) (1)—i.e., one-third of all deaths in women. Among the gender-specific characteristics of CAD in women is its greater age dependency than for men. One in nine U.S. women aged 45 to 64 years has clinical manifestations of CAD in contrast to one in three women 65 years of age or older (Fig. 1-2). Stated otherwise, whereas by age 60 one in five U.S. men has had a coronary event, this has occurred in only 1 of 17 U.S. women. About one quarter of all deaths in the United States are caused by CAD, but a substantially greater percentage of these coronary deaths occurs in men than in women until the eighth decade of life. Nonetheless, owing to the aging of the U.S. population and a greater representation of women in the elderly age group, more women than men die from CAD annually. Importantly, almost 20,000 women in the United States younger than 65 years of age die of myocardial infarction each year, and more than one third of these women are younger than 55 years of age.

Highlighting the difference between facts and perceptions, a 1995 Gallup poll showed that four of five women and one of three primary care physicians in the United States were unaware that heart disease was the leading cause of death for women. The widespread misconception is that breast cancer is the major health problem for women in the United States. Data confirm the prominence of CAD in the spectrum of etiologies for mortality of postmenopausal women. Their lifetime mortality risk from CAD is 31% compared with 2.8% for both hip fracture (as a surrogate for osteoporosis) and breast cancer. Stated otherwise, a postmenopausal woman is ten times as likely to die from CAD as from breast cancer (Fig. 1-3).

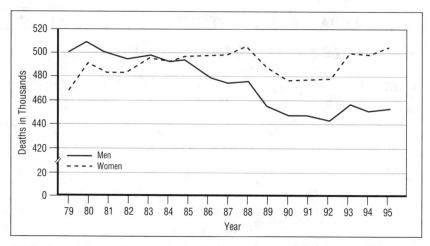

Figure 1-1 Cardiovascular disease mortality trends for men and women, 1979-95. Data from: National Center for Health Statistics and the American Heart Association. (Reprinted from 1999 Heart and Stroke Statistical Update. Dallas: American Heart Association; 1998:2; with permission.)

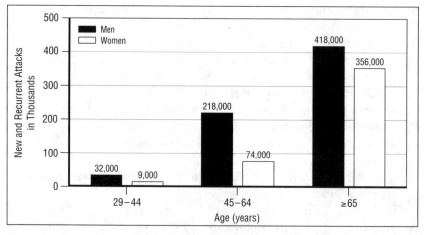

Figure 1-2 Estimated annual number of men and women experiencing heart attack by age and sex. Extrapolated from rates in the ARIC community surveillance study of the NHLBI, 1987-94. Data do not include silent myocardial infarctions. (Reprinted from 1999 Heart and Stroke Statistical Update. Dallas: American Heart Association; 1998:11; with permission.)

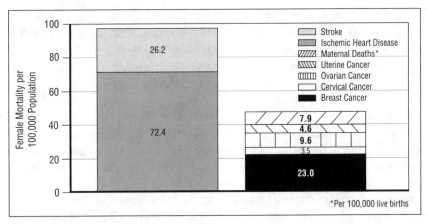

Figure 1-3 Etiologies of mortality in women. According to 1989 data from the National Center for Health Statistics, deaths from CAD and stroke in women increased to a combined annual rate of 98.6 per 100,000 population. The cardiovascular death rate in women was thus more than double the cumulative total for maternal mortality and deaths from breast, uterine, ovarian, and cervical cancer (48.6/100,000). (Reprinted from Wenger NK. Coronary heart disease in women: a "new" problem. Hosp Pract. 1992;27: 59-74; with permission.)

Coronary artery disease is a major contributor to hospitalizations and physician visits for women as well. Further, the symptoms of CAD are a prominent cause of disability. Thirty-six percent of women aged 55 to 64 years of age known to have CAD are disabled by the symptoms of their illness, this percentage increasing to 55% among women older than 75 years of age (2).

The clinical onset of CAD in U.S. women who undergo natural menopause is, on average, 10 years later than that for men, with myocardial infarction occurring as much as 20 years later. Convincing explanations for the gender-age disparities in the occurrence of CAD remain elusive. Nonetheless, women following bilateral oophorectomy or with early natural menopause develop CAD at younger age.

The age-adjusted death rate for CAD is 25% to 30% higher for U.S. black women than for white women, and the death rate from myocardial infarction for black women is double that for white women. Age-adjusted death rates from heart disease are four times higher in white women and six times higher in black women than their death rates for breast cancer.

Coronary Risk Factors and Their Reduction

Coronary risk factors are highly prevalent in women of all racial and ethnic groups in the United States (3,4). Indeed, recent data from the National Center for Health Statistics delineate that only 30% of U.S. women are free of at least one major coronary risk factor, with even this small percentage declining in women of older age. Based on 1991 information from the National Center for Health Statistics, encompassing women from 20 to 74 years of age, more than one third had hypertension, more than one quarter had hypercholesterolemia and were cigarette smokers and were overweight, and six of ten U.S. women had a sedentary lifestyle, rendering this the most prevalent risk attribute for women. Worthy of emphasis is the female-male crossover in risk characteristics with aging, such that hypertension and hypercholesterolemia are more prevalent in men than in women at young to middle age but become more prevalent in women than in men at older age (Fig. 1-4). Further, during the past two to three decades women have had less reduction in coronary risk factors than have men, likely owing to the major attention to coronary risk reduction in men.

Traditional coronary risk factors are shared by women and men, although, based on follow-up data from the National Health and Nutritional Examination Survey (NHANES I), risk factor epidemiology differs between the sexes (5). Specifically, hypertension imparts a comparable relative risk for women as for men (1.5), with hypercholesterolemia associated with somewhat greater relative risk for men than women, 1.4 versus 1.1. Diabetes is a far more serious risk attribute for women, with a relative risk of 2.4 compared with 1.9 for men. Overweight imparts comparable relative risk by gender, 1.4 for women

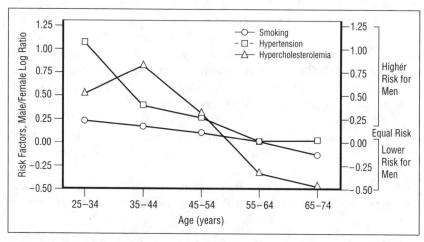

Figure 1-4 Male/female risk factor prevalence log ratios by age; pooled data from four independent surveys (1979-86); treatment and control cities combined; Stanford Five-City Project. (Reprinted from Williams EL, Winkleby MA, Fortmann SP. Changes in coronary heart disease risk factors in the 1980s: evidence of a male/female crossover effect with age. Am J Epidemiol. 1993;137:1056-67; with permission.)

versus 1.3 for men; and smoking a somewhat greater relative risk for women than men, 1.8 and 1.6 respectively (Fig. 1-5). Based on limited data, control of risk factors appears to confer comparable relative benefit for women and men. Coronary risk factors are more prevalent and tend to cluster among women with less favorable socioeconomic and educational status, mandating intensive attention to coronary risk reduction in these underserved populations. Socioeconomic circumstances are particularly relevant for elderly U.S. women; almost twice as many women aged 65 years and older are likely to be at the poverty level (15.4%) than are comparably aged men (7.6%), with poverty rates particularly high among black, Hispanic, and Native American women. Additionally, some risk factors unique to women contribute to coronary risk.

Cigarette Smoking

Currently, equal numbers of U.S. women and men smoke cigarettes, mostly because of far more effective smoking cessation among men than women. Further, women's smoking behavior has changed, being characterized by an earlier onset of cigarette smoking and a greater intensity of smoking. More than 3000 young people begin smoking daily in the United States, half of them girls; among high school senior girls, the highest cigarette smoking rates exist for white girls owing to a major decrease in the smoking behavior of black girls.

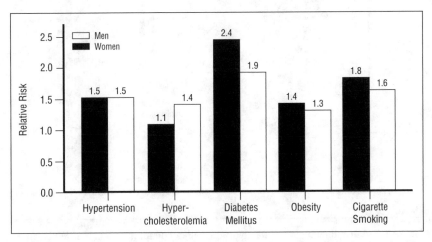

Figure 1-5 Coronary risk factors for men and women. (Reprinted from Centers for Disease Control. Coronary heart disease incidence by sex—United States, 1971-1987. MMWR Morb Mortal Wkly Rep. 1992;41:526-9; with permission.)

Cigarette smoking triples the risk for myocardial infarction, even among premenopausal women, and is an important contributor to sudden cardiac death in young women as well. The cardiovascular risk is accentuated in oral contraceptive users who smoke. Additionally, smoking lowers the age at menopause, on average $1\frac{1}{2}$ to 2 years, with the longer duration of menopausal status potentially augmenting coronary risk. Cigarette smoking lowers the age at initial myocardial infarction more for women than for men (Fig. 1-6) (6).

In reports from the Nurses Health Study, the number of cigarettes smoked correlated with the risk of angina pectoris, nonfatal myocardial infarction, and fatal CAD (7), but even women who smoked fewer than five cigarettes daily more than doubled their coronary risk. There is no evidence that smoking cigarettes with reduced nicotine or tar levels lowers the coronary risk of smoking.

Nonetheless, within 2 years of smoking cessation, former smokers decreased their cardiovascular mortality risk by 24% (8), with the risk approaching that of nonsmoking women within 3 to 5 years of smoking cessation. Benefit occurred regardless of the duration or intensity of smoking or the age at which smoking cessation occurred, reinforcing recommendations for smoking cessation even for older women (9,10). Benefit occurred even in the presence of defined CAD, following both myocardial infarction and coronary artery bypass graft surgery (9); smoking cessation was associ-

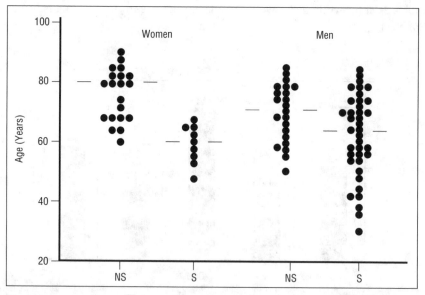

Figure 1-6 Age at time of first acute myocardial infarction for male and female nonsmokers (NS) and smokers (S). Bars denote median values. (Reprinted from Hansen EF, Andersen LT, Von Eyben FE. Cigarette smoking and age at first acute myocardial infarction, and influence of gender and extent of smoking. Am J Cardiol. 1993;171:1439-42; with permission.)

ated with an increase in survival and a decrease in the reinfarction rate. (Techniques for smoking cessation are discussed in Chapter 2.)

Diabetes Mellitus

Diabetes is a considerably more powerful coronary risk factor for women than for men, essentially negating the gender-protective effect even for pre-menopausal women (11). Although diabetes is a less frequent risk attribute for women than many other major risk factors for CAD, women older than 45 years of age are twice as likely as men to develop diabetes. Based on data from the Nurses Health Study, maturity-onset diabetes mellitus confers a three- to seven-fold excess of cardiovascular events (12). Because the incidence of diabetes was less among women who exercised regularly (13), a regular exercise regimen should be recommended as a preventive strategy, particularly for women at high risk for diabetes (i.e., those who have had gestational diabetes or those with a strong family history of diabetes). Additionally, control of other coronary risk factors is associated with a greater reduction in the risk of myocardial infarction in diabetic than in nondiabetic women, emphasizing the importance of multifactorial risk reduction in this high-risk population. Further, precise blood glucose control appears to lessen coronary events.

Diabetes is associated with a less favorable outcome of clinical coronary events as well (14–16). Both the hospital and long-term prognosis of myocardial infarction are less favorable for diabetic than nondiabetic patients, with this prognosis substantially worsened for diabetic women than for diabetic men compared with their nondiabetic counterparts. In the Framingham cohort, the risk of a coronary event for a diabetic versus a nondiabetic woman was 5.4-fold increased compared with a 2.4-fold increase for a diabetic versus a nondiabetic man. Diabetic women who have a myocardial infarction incur a doubled risk of reinfarction and a fourfold increase in the risk of development of heart failure. Additionally, among patients who undergo myocardial revascularization procedures, both coronary artery bypass graft surgery and percutaneous transluminal coronary angioplasty, more women than men are diabetic; diabetes likely contributes to their less favorable outcome from such procedures.

Hypercholesterolemia and Other Lipid Abnormalities

Attention to hypercholesterolemia derives from a large number of population studies which show that cholesterol levels continue to predict coronary risk both in middle-aged and older women (17). Low levels of high-density lipoprotein (HDL) cholesterol place women at particularly high risk. Women have higher levels of HDL cholesterol, about 10 mg/dL, than men across the life span; HDL concentrations decrease only minimally in the menopausal years and beyond. Based on Framingham data, an increase of 10 mg/dL in HDL cholesterol confers a 40% to 50% decrease in coronary risk for women. At young to middle age, women have lower levels of low-density lipoprotein (LDL) cholesterol than do men; nonetheless, LDL levels in women rise progressively with age, particularly in the postmenopausal years, and at least to age 70, so that elderly women have higher levels of LDL cholesterol than do elderly men (18). The contribution to this disparity of the early deaths of men with high levels of LDL cholesterol has not been well examined. Of interest is that the age-related risk in total cholesterol levels is far less prominent in black than in white women, and indeed the cholesterol-CAD relationship is less prominent for black than for white women (19,20). However, once clinical CAD becomes evident, black women have less favorable outcomes than do their white counterparts.

Recent clinical trials have documented the efficacy of pharmacologic risk reduction of hypercholesterolemia in women. Cholesterol lowering in the Scandinavian Simvastatin Survival Study (4S) in patients following myocardial infarction and with angina decreased the occurrence of major coronary events by 35% for women and 34% for men, with women constituting 19% of the study cohort (21). Benefit was maintained at older age and in diabetic patients. Cholesterol lowering with pravastatin in postinfarction patients with average cholesterol levels in the Cholesterol and Recurrent Events (CARE) trial reduced death or recurrent infarction by 46% in women compared with 26% in men, a statistically significant difference; women represented 14% of the study cohort (22). Additionally, in the Asymptomatic Carotid Artery Progression Study (ACAPS) symptomatic women and men without clinical evidence of CAD but with elevated levels of LDL cholesterol had decreased progression of early carotid atherosclerosis associated with lipid-lowering with lovastatin. Estrogen had little added benefit in women assigned to lovastatin, but this nonrandomized estrogen use decreased atherosclerosis progression in women assigned to placebo (23). In a primary prevention trial, AFCAPS/TexCAPS, women and men with average cholesterol levels but low HDL cholesterol levels experienced fewer coronary events with lovastatin versus placebo in addition to a low saturated fat, low cholesterol diet (24).

Most women with defined CAD enrolled in the Heart and Estrogen/Progestin Replacement Study (HERS) during 1993-94, 47% of whom were taking a lipid-lowering drug, had levels of LDL cholesterol that exceeded NCEP treatment goals (25). The more intensive pharmacotherapy for women clearly has the potential to provide benefit.

The role of lipoprotein(a) levels in predicting coronary risk for women remains controversial, as is the role of elevated triglyceride levels. Although triglyceride levels do not appear to confer independent coronary risk for men, some studies suggest that such is the case for women (26–28), particularly when associated with low levels of HDL cholesterol. Data on the role of dense LDL particles are also conflicting.

Hypertension

In the United States more than 50% of white women and 79% of black women older than 45 years of age have hypertension, with the racial discrepancy being more pronounced for women than for men. In the population older than 65 years of age, 71% of U.S. women have hypertension, and more women than men in this population are hypertensive. The greater prevalence of hypertension in U.S. women than men largely reflects their increased longevity and high prevalence of hypertension at elderly age. Based on the U.S. National Health Examination Follow-up Survey (NHEFS), obesity appears a more important contributor to hypertension for women than for men; central obesity and its associated hyperinsulinemia and insulin resistance are particularly implicated.

More men than women have hypertension at young to middle age, but this pattern changes with aging. Levels of systolic blood pressure continue to rise among women, at least to age 80, such that isolated systolic hypertension is more prominent in elderly women than in elderly men (Fig. 1-7) (4). Blood pressure should be measured annually, even among older women, because a woman who is normotensive in the early menopause may develop hypertension at older age. The control of isolated systolic hypertension in persons aged 60 years of age and older in the Systolic Hypertension in the Elderly Program (SHEP) reduced the occurrence of stroke, fatal cardiovascular events, and nonfatal cardiovascular events in both genders, with women comprising 57% of the study population (29). Therapy with a diuretic and the addition of low-dose beta-blockade, when needed, reduced stroke by 36% and CAD by 25%.

Because only limited numbers of women have been included in most clinical trials of antihypertensive therapies, there is conflicting information regarding gender-specific outcomes, particularly whether women respond differently to specific antihypertensive therapies than do men; racial differences may also be important.

When electrocardiographic evidence of left ventricular hypertrophy is present, it increases cardiovascular risk for women and for men, but with greater risk rates for women, highlighting the importance of blood pressure control for women to avert left ventricular hypertrophy (30).

Obesity

Obesity has increased in prevalence in the United States in both genders (4) but is particularly prominent in populations with lower educational and income levels; among women, obesity predominates in blacks, Hispanics, and

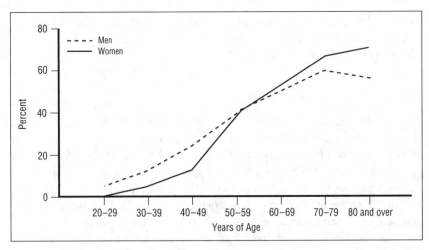

Figure 1-7 Prevalence of hypertension among persons 20 years of age and older by sex and age—United States, 1988-91. A *person with hypertension* is defined as either having elevated blood pressure (systolic pressure of at least 140 mm Hg or diastolic pressure of at least 90 mm Hg) or taking antihypertensive medication. Percents are based on an average of six measurements of blood pressure. (Reprinted from Centers for Disease Control and Prevention, National Center for Health Statistics, National Health and Nutrition Examination Survey III (Phase I). Health—United States, 1995. Hyattsville, Maryland: Public Health Service; 1996:34; with permission.)

Native Americans (Fig. 1-8). The U.S. National Center for Health Statistics 1991 report defines 50% of black women and more than 33% of white women as being at least 20% greater than desirable weight. Increased body weight appears directly related to increased all-cause mortality, but this association is particularly prominent for younger women. The pattern of body fat distribution also warrants attention; a waist-to-hip ratio in excess of 0.8 is associated with a substantial increase in coronary risk (31,32). This pattern of central obesity is often associated with insulin resistance, non–insulin-dependent diabetes mellitus, hypercholesterolemia, and hypertension (i.e., multiple mechanisms whereby obesity can impart risk). This syndrome is often characterized by low levels of HDL cholesterol and elevated triglyceride levels as well.

Weight control improves the cardiovascular risk profile, although the optimal mode or modes for weight reduction in women—diet, exercise, or combinations thereof—has not been well examined. However, frequent substantial fluctuations in weight are also associated with increased coronary risk. Fifteen-year follow-up data from the Nurses Health Study confirm the direct relationship between increased body weight and all-cause mortality; when smokers were excluded there was no excess mortality rate for lean women.

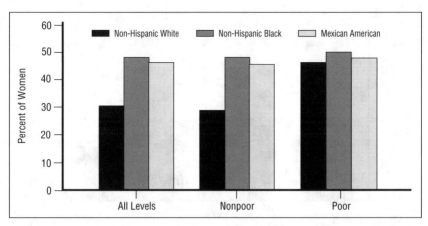

Figure 1-8 Prevalence of overweight among women 20 years of age and older by race, Hispanic origin, and poverty status—United States, 1988-91. Data are age adjusted. All levels include persons of unknown poverty status. *Overweight* is defined for women as body mass index greater than or equal to 27.3 kg/m². These cut points were used because they represent 85th percentiles for women 20 to 29 years of age in the 1976-80 National Health and Nutrition Examination Survey. Excludes pregnant women. (Reprinted from Centers for Disease Control and Prevention, National Center for Health Statistics, National Health and Nutrition Examination Survey III [Phase I]. Health—United States, 1995. Public Health Service: Hyattsville, Maryland; 1996:39; with permission.)

Physical Inactivity

Physical inactivity, an independent risk factor for CAD in women, is the most prevalent coronary risk factor (33), with physical inactivity predominating in populations with lower educational and income levels (Fig. 1-9).

Objectively measured physical fitness is associated with a more favorable coronary risk profile for women than it is for men (34), with the associations being particularly prominent for higher levels of HDL cholesterol, lower levels of triglycerides, and improved insulin utilization.

In the studies of physical activity for coronary prevention that included women, and where data were analyzed separately by gender, at least a 50% reduction in coronary risk was evident in physically active versus inactive women. Based on questionnaire responses, a graded inverse association between physical activity and all-cause mortality was evident in postmenopausal women as well (35). This confirms the epidemiologic studies suggesting that exercise decreases coronary risk even in older age women. Even at older age, a decrease in myocardial infarction risk by 50% was evident with modest habitual leisure-time activities, equivalent to 30 to 45 minutes of walking three times weekly (36).

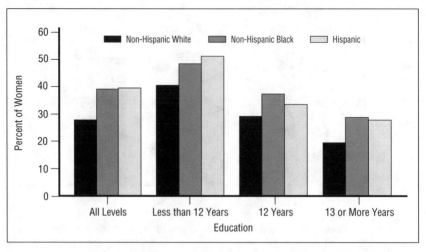

Figure 1-9 Prevalence of sedentary lifestyle among women 25 years of age and older by race, Hispanic origin, and years of education—United States, 1991. Percentages are age adjusted. The category "All Levels" includes persons with unknown education level. (Reprinted from Centers for Disease Control and Prevention, National Center for Health Statistics, National Health Interview Survey. Health—United States, 1995. Public Health Service: Hyattsville, Maryland; 1996:40; with permission.)

High-intensity, high-impact exercise is more frequently associated with musculoskeletal injuries for elderly women than for elderly men. An exercise regimen for these women should consist of low-impact aerobic activity at low-to-moderate intensity (37).

Review of the literature related to exercise rehabilitation in *Clinical Practice Guideline: Cardiac Rehabilitation* of the U.S. Agency for Health Care Policy and Research identifies that fewer women than men following a coronary event are referred to exercise rehabilitation by their treating physicians; this discrepancy is particularly prominent for elderly women (38). These under-referral data raise concern, given the documented benefits of physical activity in improving exercise tolerance for women and the potential for coronary risk reduction in the cardiac rehabilitation setting.

Fibrinogen

In the Framingham Heart Study, elevated levels of fibrinogen predisposed men to both initial and recurrent coronary events but were associated only with initial coronary events in women. In a number of epidemiologic studies, fibrinogen independently predicts total coronary disease, myocardial infarction, and sudden death in patients with angina. Fibrinogen levels appear to be favorably influenced by estrogen in a number of epidemiologic investigations.

Aspirin and Antioxidants

Although men older than 40 years of age derive preventive benefit by routine use of aspirin in preventing myocardial infarction, the observational data for women are conflicting. Despite the suggestion in the Nurses Health Study that regular aspirin protected against initial myocardial infarction, the potential benefit may not be worth the risk since the rate of myocardial infarction is low in women and there is an increased risk of hemorrhagic stroke with aspirin use (39). Risk reduction with aspirin in the Nurses Health Study was evident for women using one to six tablets of aspirin weekly but not for those taking larger amounts. Benefit was greatest for women at high coronary risk because of cigarette smoking, hypercholesterolemia, and hypertension. (For discussion of the evidence regarding aspirin for secondary prevention in women, see Chapter 9.)

Data for both women and men are limited and conflicting regarding the role of antioxidant therapies and interventions designed to alter homocysteine levels (40,41).

Psychosocial Factors

Psychosocial factors likely constitute important coronary risk characteristics for women. Risk factor prevalence is greater and risk factors tend to cluster among socioeconomically and educationally disadvantaged women, with socioeconomic circumstances being particularly relevant for elderly women. The poverty level (15.4%) for women 65 years of age and older in the United States is twice as high as that for men of comparable age (7.6%); poverty rates are particularly high among black, Hispanic, and Native American women. A recent Commonwealth Fund population survey identified a substantial decrease in the attention to exercise, diet, and the use of preventive services among U.S. women older than 65 years of age (42). This further highlights the need for intensive efforts at risk reduction to disadvantaged subsets of women, including elderly women.

Psychosocial predictors of CAD in women in the Framingham population included low educational level, infrequent vacations, and tension (43). In the Nurses Health Study, shift work was associated with an increased risk of CAD. Potential explanations for this association include psychosocial job strain and social isolation (44); an alternative explanation is that this work pattern is a surrogate for other coronary risk attributes.

Postmenopausal Hormone Therapy

Increasing attention is currently directed towards the role of postmenopausal hormone therapy as a coronary risk intervention unique to women. The basis for this interest includes four key points: 1) coronary disease predominates in postmenopausal women; 2) there are a number of biologically plausible mechanisms of estrogen benefit (45,46); 3) there is consistent evidence in a large number of observational studies (47) (predominantly of oral estrogen use); and 4) meta-analysis of these studies suggests a 30% to 50% reduction in coronary risk among women who use such therapy.

Observational studies further depict a greater benefit of hormone therapy for women at high coronary risk or with defined coronary disease, particularly those with angiographically severe coronary disease. Observational data also suggest survival benefit in estrogen users after coronary artery bypass graft surgery (48) and survival and reinfarction benefit after coronary angioplasty (49). Among the biologically plausible mechanisms of estrogen benefit are favorable effects on the lipid profile, with a decrease of LDL cholesterol and an increase of HDL cholesterol levels, averaging 10% to 15% each. Estrogen therapy, however, uniformly elevates triglyceride levels. Fibrinogen levels are reduced, as are levels of PAI-1 and adhesion molecules, with a resultant improved coagulation profile. Additionally, estrogen has a favorable effect on the vascular endothelium, presumably mediated by hormone receptors in the endothelium, with resultant promotion of coronary vasodilatation and prevention or reversal of paradoxic vasoconstriction, even in atherosclerotic coronary arteries. Estrogen lowers endothelin levels, increases prostacyclin biosynthesis, is associated with modulating of ion channels with calcium antagonist effects in opening of potassium channels and resultant vasodilatation, and may further provide benefit by antioxidant effects.

Despite the substantial benefit attributed to hormone use in a large number of observational studies, an inherent weakness of these studies is the likelihood of a selection bias, given the healthy cohort of women that is typically prescribed estrogen. A further limitation is the virtual absence of data on the nonoral routes of estrogen administration and, until very recently, on the effects of combined estrogen/progestin use (50). Observational data on cardioprotection from hormone use were derived predominantly from middle-to-upper socioeconomic class white women, with minimal or absent information regarding the effect of hormone therapy on nonwhite women and those of lower socioeconomic status; data are also limited for elderly women. Nonetheless, in the Cardiovascular Health Study (51), an observational study of community-dwelling elderly individuals, women who were current postmenopausal hormone users had a more favorable cardiovascular risk profile and a more favorable spectrum of preclinical cardiovascular characteristics, well into the eighth decade of life. By contrast, a recent retrospective case-control study showed no significant decrease in the odds ratio for myocardial infarction associated with current hormone use after adjustment for confounding variables (52). Randomized clinical trial data are requisite to define the role of estrogen and estrogen/progestin combinations as coronary preventive therapy for women.

A randomized controlled trial, the Postmenopausal Estrogen/Progestin Interventions (PEPI) study (53), examined the effect of unopposed estrogen and several estrogen/progestin combinations on the coronary risk profile; the hypothesis of the PEPI trial was that hormones decreased coronary risk by favorably altering coronary risk factors. Although the PEPI data provide intermediate end points (i.e., the effect of hormone use on coronary risk attributes), the study was not designed to ascertain the effect of hormone use on coronary events. All hormone regimens significantly decreased LDL cholesterol and increased HDL cholesterol and fibrinogen levels compared with placebo (Fig. 1-10). Although all hormone regimens increased triglyceride levels, none increased blood pressure or body weight. Thus hormone therapy resulted in a more favorable coronary risk profile. However, because women in the PEPI trial who had not had a hysterectomy sustained a 33% three-year occurrence of adenomatous or atypical endometrial hyperplasia, a precursor of endometrial cancer, with the use of unopposed estrogen, such women should receive estrogen plus a progestin. Unopposed estrogen remains appropriate for women who have undergone a hysterectomy.

Noncoronary benefits of estrogen use include a marked reduction in osteoporosis and osteoporotic fractures, a reduction in menopausal symptoms, and a decrease in the urogenital symptoms of estrogen deficiency. Other benefits under investigation are the potential lessened risk of Alzheimer disease (54) and of colon cancer with estrogen use. Adverse features of hormone therapy of greatest concern among women and their physicians include the increased risk for breast cancer with hormone use, particularly with long-term use, and the increased risk of venous thromboembolism. In the Nurses Health Study, the relative risk of breast cancer with hormone use was greatest for women older than 60 years of age (RR 1.71) and for women who had used hormones for more than 5 years (RR 1.45) (55,56), both of which are characteristics of women who use hormones for coronary and osteoporosis protection. Coronary risk was lessened most prominently in the Nurses Health Study among high-risk women, with benefit becoming attenuated after about 10 years owing to the increased incidence of breast cancer (56). The U.S. Office of Technology Assessment, the European Position Paper on HRT in the Menopause, and a 1996 WHO Statement all define a breast cancer risk of 1.2 to 2.4 for 10 or more years of hormone use. Additionally, there is a small absolute, but significant relative, risk of venous thromboembolism with hormone use. In the Oxford study, the relative risk for spontaneous deep vein thrombosis and pulmonary embolism was 3.5 (57), with comparable documentation from the Puget Sound study (58); only the risk for pulmonary embolism, a relative risk of 2.1, was delineated in the Nurses Health Study (59). Similar data continue to be reported by others (60,61).

The Heart and Estrogen/Progestin Replacement Study (HERS) was the first prospective, randomized, controlled, secondary prevention trial of daily estrogen/progestin in women with established CAD (50). At an average of 4 years of follow-up, there were no overall significant differences in primary and secondary cardiac outcomes, although HDL cholesterol levels increased by 10% and LDL cholesterol levels decreased by 11%. An increased risk of coronary events was associated with hormone use in the first year, and a trend of decreasing coronary events was noted by the fourth and fifth years. There

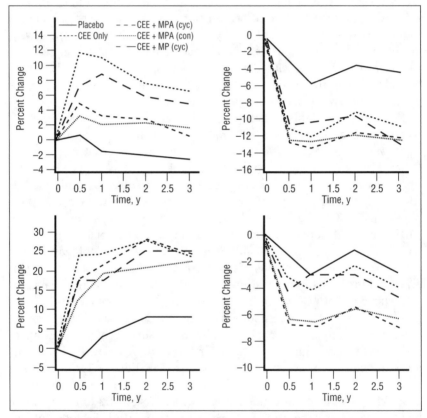

Figure 1-10 Effects of unopposed estrogen and several estrogen/progestin regimens on coronary risk profile. Mean percent change from baseline by treatment arm for high-density lipoprotein cholesterol (*top left*), low-density lipoprotein cholesterol (*top right*), triglycerides (*bottom left*), and total cholesterol (*bottom right*). Abbreviations: CEE = conjugated equine estrogen; MPA = medroxyprogesterone acetate; MP = micronized progesterone. (Reprinted from The Writing Group for the PEPI Trial. Effects of estrogen or estrogen/progestin regimens on heart disease risk factors in postmenopausal women: the Postmenopausal Estrogen/Progestin Interventions (PEPI) trial. JAMA. 1995;273:199-208; with permission.)

was an increase in venous thromboembolic events and gallbladder disease in women on daily estrogen/progestin. The HERS recommendations are that women with CAD do not initiate use of this estrogen/progestin regimen for secondary prevention but that such women already receiving this hormone therapy could continue for potential late benefit. Primary prevention was not addressed by HERS.

Based on currently available data, and pending the results of randomized controlled trials with clinical outcomes, hormone use is likely to most benefit women with established coronary disease or at high risk for its occurrence, and to benefit least those with a personal or family history of breast cancer and those at increased risk for venous thromboembolism.

Clinical Characteristics

Angina Pectoris

Angina pectoris, both stable and unstable, is the predominant initial and subsequent clinical presentation of CAD in women; this contrasts with myocardial infarction and sudden death as the most common presentations for men (62). Nonetheless, until recent years, women with chest pain had far less aggressive diagnosis and management than did their male counterparts. This likely reflected misinterpretation of data from the Framingham Heart Study suggesting that angina is a benign problem for women. In the Framingham cohort, 25% of men considered to have angina pectoris incurred a myocardial infarction within the subsequent 5 years, whereas 86% of women in the study considered to have angina pectoris never developed myocardial infarction (62).

The difference between a history of chest pain, the sole basis for the diagnosis of angina pectoris in the Framingham cohort, and documented coronary obstruction resulting in the pain of myocardial ischemia in women become evident with publication of data from the Coronary Artery Surgery Study (CASS) registry. In this report, 50% of women, as contrasted with 17% of men, referred by their treating physician for coronary arteriography based on chest pain considered of sufficient severity to warrant evaluation for coronary artery bypass graft surgery, had minimal or no coronary artery atherosclerotic obstruction (63–65). Two important points can be derived from the CASS Registry data. First, many women with chest pain clinically indistinguishable from angina pectoris have no significant atherosclerotic obstruction of their coronary arteries. The clinical history alone is inadequate to make this differentiation, and objective confirmatory testing is required. Second, defining an atherosclerotic etiology for chest pain is important, because the clinical diagnosis of CAD has more adverse prognostic implications for women than for men.

Interestingly, re-review of the Framingham data identified that the oldest of the women considered to have angina, those aged 60 to 69 years, had the same adverse outcome as did the men, reinforcing the important influence of age on CAD in women.

Descriptors of chest pain by women become important in defining their pretest likelihood of coronary disease, yet this description is often determined by a woman's perception of her symptoms. Unless women consider coronary disease to be a part of their illness experience, they are unlikely to appropriately recognize or interpret chest pain symptoms as being of cardiac origin. Women who present with angina tend to be older than men and more frequently have associated hypertension, diabetes, and heart failure; in contrast, they are less likely to have had either a prior myocardial infarction or a myocardial revascularization procedure (66). In patients older than 65 years of age, exertional chest pain is associated with a gender-neutral risk of coronary death, a 2.7 relative risk for women versus 2.4 for men, with this association independent of other coronary risk factors (67). In the Established Populations for Epidemiologic Studies of the Elderly (EPESE) population as well, exertional angina was equally predictive of coronary death for women and for men.

As information has expanded about the lethality of CAD in women, this appreciation of the adverse prognosis of women with CAD has occasioned a major change in clinical practice, such that objective testing is more likely to be undertaken earlier in women who present with chest pain syndromes. Nonetheless, in a recent evaluation of the emergency room care of patients presenting with new onset chest pain, women with similar symptoms were diagnosed and treated less aggressively than were men (68). The predictive accuracy of noninvasive diagnostic tests in women presents a challenge, and the optimal test or test selection algorithm has yet to be determined (69). (Diagnostic testing is discussed in Chapter 13.)

In recent years, however, abnormal noninvasive test results in women are far more likely to occasion referral to coronary arteriography than was the case a decade ago (70). Gender-related differences in referral to coronary arteriography after exercise thallium testing in several series were related only to a higher rate of abnormal test results in men (71). Further, in this population, women were less likely to have severe disease at coronary arteriography. Among patients in another study not referred for invasive test procedures or myocardial revascularization following abnormal noninvasive testing, the long-term outcomes for nonrevascularized women were less favorable than for their male counterparts (72). Most contemporary reports from cardiovascular centers suggest a comparable approach to myocardial revascularization in both genders based on the results of coronary arteriography (73,74).

Important data regarding coronary morbidity in women are available from the Survival and Ventricular Enlargement (SAVE) trial. Prior to the index infarction that determined eligibility for enrollment in this study, an infarction that resulted in an ejection fraction of less than 40%, men were twice as likely as women to have been referred for coronary arteriography and coronary artery bypass graft surgery (75). This gender gap occurred despite similar histories of angina pectoris for women and men and despite the fact that women reported significantly greater physical activity limitation owing to anginal symptoms than did men, 50% versus 31% (64). This burden of functional impairment owing to anginal symptoms warrants consideration as a compelling indication for myocardial revascularization in that the medical management of the women subsequently enrolled in the SAVE trial had been unable to prevent preinfarction functional disability in one half of the women.

Myocardial Infarction

Despite the less common initial presentation of CAD as myocardial infarction for women than for men in the Framingham Heart Study (35% versus 50%), initial episodes of myocardial infarction were more likely fatal for women, 39% versus 31% (76); 30-day mortality rates were comparably increased in women, 28% versus 16% (77); and early reinfarction was more common in women, 25% versus 22% (77). Women were also more likely than men to have silent and unrecognized myocardial infarction. As was the case in the Framingham cohort, women today are more likely than men to have silent and unrecognized myocardial infarction, potentially related to their older age or to their complicating comorbidities, particularly diabetes and hypertension. Despite these findings, it remains uncertain whether gender differences exist in the occurrence of silent myocardial ischemia. As in Framingham, women today uniformly have higher hospital mortality rates following myocardial infarction than do men (78,79).

Even with the contemporary reduction in mortality from acute myocardial infarction, data from the Myocardial Infarction Triage and Intervention Registry depict a higher hospital mortality for women than for men, 16% versus 11% (80,81). The presentation of myocardial infarction as regards symptoms, delayed arrival to hospital, and hemodynamic and electrocardiographic findings in this study was comparable for women and men. Despite this comparability, women were not as aggressively treated and were less likely to be triaged to acute interventions, including coronary thrombolysis, coronary angiography, and acute percutaneous transluminal coronary angioplasty (PTCA) (Fig. 1-11). Women in this Registry also had a greater one-year mortality following myocardial infarction and an earlier and more frequent recurrence of

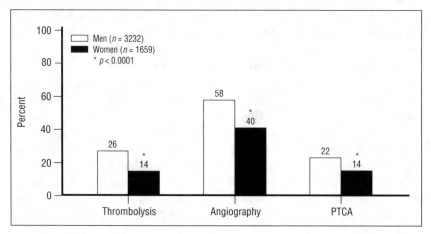

Figure 1-11 Unadjusted frequencies of utilization of thrombolytics, angiography, and angioplasty in the MITI registry. (Reprinted from Roger VL, Gersh BJ. Myocardial infarction. In: Julian DG, Wenger NK (eds). Women and Heart Disease. London: Martin Dunitz; 1997: 135-50; with permission.)

infarction among survivors. These gender differences lessened, but did not disappear, after controlling for older age and comorbidity.

At presentation to hospital, women with myocardial infarction are more likely to have a higher Killip class, and more frequently have tachycardia, atrioventricular block, and pulmonary rales. Women are also more likely to have their myocardial infarction complicated by shock, heart failure, recurrent chest pain, cardiac rupture (82), and stroke, although these gender differences lessen with correction for comorbidity and for older age (83–85). Because antecedent stable angina is more common among women than men who present with an initial myocardial infarction, question has been raised as to whether earlier diagnostic testing to identify a high-risk subset of women may avert the initial myocardial infarction. More women than men in the Worcester Heart Study had a history of angina pectoris before their initial myocardial infarction (86). Pre-existing angina in patients admitted for myocardial infarction in the Israel SPRINT study was associated with an increased risk of both inhospital mortality and posthospital mortality. In the Danish TRACE study, both short- and long-term mortality after myocardial infarction were also less favorable for women. Although there appeared to be comparable recognition and management of acute coronary events in middle-aged men and women in the Scottish MONICA population, more men died before hospitalization, but fatality rates in women were higher after admission to hospital. Comparable data derive from the MILIS study (87); in addition to an excess of posthospital deaths, the poorer postinfarction prognosis for women was characterized by more frequent angina and heart failure, with a particularly adverse prognosis for black women. In the Israeli SPRINT study (88) women were twice as likely as men to die in the early weeks following myocardial infarction and to have earlier and more frequent reinfarction. Diabetes contributed substantially to the unfavorable prognosis with myocardial infarction for women in the Multicenter Postinfarction Study (89), independent of ventricular ejection fraction.

In patients with unstable angina or non–Q-wave myocardial infarction in the TIMI III Registry study, women had less severe coronary disease than did men and, in addition to being less likely to receive intensive anti-ischemic medical therapies, had less frequent coronary arteriography and fewer myocardial revascularization procedures (90). Nonetheless, women and men had similar outcomes, raising concern that a similar outcome with less severe disease may actually constitute a less favorable result for women than for men. Additionally, women in this Registry database were less likely to be treated with beta-blocking drugs, aspirin, heparin, and nitroglycerin. Comparable data were derived from a recent study of drug treatment for suspected acute myocardial infarction, identifying a consistently lower use of thrombolytic agents, beta-blocking agents, and aspirin, as recommended in U.S. national guidelines, for women than for men (91). In the Medicare database, physician specialty and geographic factors best predict beta-blocker treatment for elderly patients after myocardial infarction (92). Based on randomized controlled trial data, there is strong evidence of a substantial reduction in mortality conferred by the use of these therapies. The reduction in mortality with beta-blocker use in the ISIS-I and MIAMI trials was greater for women than for men and for older than for younger patients.

Coronary thrombolysis has significantly decreased the mortality from acute myocardial infarction. In the Western Washington Trial, 16% of women versus 25% of men were considered eligible for coronary thrombolysis; 55% of eligible women versus 78% of eligible men actually received thrombolytic therapy (93). In the Survival and Ventricular Enlargement (SAVE) Study, fewer women than men received thrombolytic therapy (94). Although women in the GUSTO-I trial had comparable survival benefit to men from the application of coronary thrombolysis, despite their excess occurrence of bleeding complications and particularly of intracranial hemorrhage, the unadjusted 30-day mortality rates for women remained more than twice those for men, 13% versus 4.8% (95). Women were also at increased risk for shock, heart failure, and reinfarction (96,97). However, even among randomized patients in GUSTO, the median time from the onset of chest pain to admission and treatment was longer for women than for men (96). The comparative contributions of gender, older age, and comorbidities must be evaluated in that women in the study were older than the men; had more hypertension, diabetes, and hypercholesterolemia; and were more likely to have their myocardial infarction associated with heart failure and shock. Because comparable infarct-related artery patency resulted from coronary thrombolysis and there was comparable response of the ventricular myocardium to ischemia and reperfusion for women and for men, these features do not account for the difference in 30-day mortality (Fig. 1-12) (97). In the Thrombolysis in Myocardial Ischemia II (TIMI-II) study, women with acute myocardial infarction treated with thrombolytic therapy had higher rates of six-week morbidity and mortality than did men (98). The one-year gender ratio of myocardial infarction death was not altered by coronary thrombolysis in the GISSI trial (99), with one-year mortality rates for women being twice those for men, 29.8% versus 15.2% respectively.

Primary angioplasty may be an attractive option for women with acute myocardial infarction. Women in the Primary Angioplasty and Myocardial Infarction (PAMI) trial were more likely than men to have early mortality and life-threatening hemorrhagic complications from coronary thrombolysis. Primary PTCA compared with coronary thrombolysis decreased the risk of intracranial bleeding and improved survival for women; the inhospital prognosis of women and men was equally favorable following primary PTCA (100).

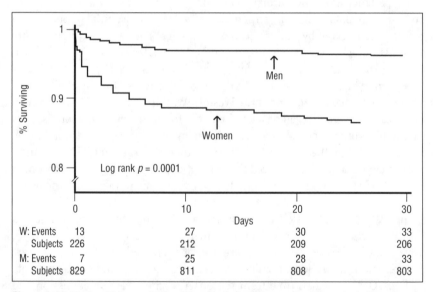

Figure 1-12 Kaplan-Meier analysis of the effect of gender on 1-year survival after myocardial infarction (W = women; M = men). (Reprinted from Woodfield SL, et al. Gender and acute myocardial infarction: is there a different response to thrombolysis? J Am Coll Cardiol. 1997;29:35-42; with permission.)

Potential contributors to the less favorable outcome for women with myocardial infarction, in addition to their older average age and comorbidity, includes their lesser eligibility for thrombolytic therapy. This in great part reflects their substantially later arrival to hospital but may also relate to the greater frequency of unrecognized infarction owing to atypical clinical presentations such as painless dyspnea, abdominal pain, neck and shoulder pain, and extreme fatigue. It remains conjectural whether the potential suboptimal use of medical therapies may also contribute, because few of the standard antianginal drugs have been systemically or comparatively evaluated in women. As noted, there is prominent underutilization of U.S. guideline-based medical therapies. Finally, until recent years, there was less intensive postinfarction risk stratification for women, limiting their referral for myocardial revascularization procedures when appropriate. Women are more likely than men to be treated by a primary care physician (101) and to be admitted to a general ward rather than a coronary care unit (84,102); the impact of these variables requires ascertainment. Psychosocial complications of infarction are also more common among women, particularly anxiety, depression, sexual dysfunction, and guilt about illness. Women are less likely to return to remunerative work following myocardial infarction and, if they do so, their return to work is more delayed, despite their earlier resumption of moderate- to high-intensity household tasks during convalescence (103).

Myocardial Revascularization: Coronary Artery Bypass Graft Surgery and Transcatheter Revascularization Procedures

Myocardial revascularization procedures are also associated with less favorable results for women, with the hospital mortality and perioperative complication rates after coronary artery bypass grafting (CABG) surgery double that for men. In all reported series, female gender best predicted higher surgical and hospital mortality rates from coronary artery bypass graft surgery, with an excess of surgical complications among survivors. Female gender imparted a far more unfavorable prognosis than did left ventricular dysfunction. Case series or registry data, rather than randomized controlled clinical trials, provide most of the gender comparisons for myocardial revascularization procedures. Given the paucity of randomized trial data, baseline gender differences assume major importance. Uniformly, in the reported series, women are older than men; have more frequent comorbidity, particularly diabetes and hypertension; and describe greater functional impairment and more advanced symptomatic classes of chest pain (104,105). In the Bypass Angioplasty Revascularization Investigation (BARI) trial, women undergoing revascularization were older than men, had more coronary risk factors, and were more likely to have unstable angina (106). The more severe and unstable angina among women has as a consequence the greater likelihood of requiring urgent or emergency myocardial revascularization. It has not been well ascertained whether the more frequent severe and unstable angina in women referred for myocardial revascularization reflects gender-related differences in clinical presentation; delayed presentation of women to their physicians following symptom onset; or delayed recognition of the disease and referral of women, and in particular older women, by their physicians for myocardial revascularization procedures. Also unclear is whether more women than men refuse revascularization procedures when they are recommended.

In the Coronary Artery Surgery Study (CASS), an important randomized surgical trial, perioperative CABG mortality was 4.5% for women compared with 1.9% for men (63). The hospital mortality rate remained double for women in the more recent Myocardial Infarction Triage and Intervention Registry data, 13% for women compared with 6% for men (107). Following CABG surgery, women have a greater perioperative occurrence of heart failure symptoms; given their preserved ventricular systolic function, these symptoms likely represent ventricular diastolic dysfunction (108). In addition, women have lower rates of graft patency than men, are less likely to receive an internal mammary artery graft, have less symptomatic relief from surgery, more frequent perioperative infarction and heart failure, and are more likely to require reoperation within the initial 5 years following CABG surgery. Nonetheless, the excess CABG mortality described for women is solely a perioperative phenomenon in that women who survive the operative hospitalization have a comparable 15-year survival to that described for men (109). However, in a prospective study, at 6 months after CABG surgery, hypertension and hypercholesterolemia were inadequately controlled in women, although smoking cessation improved (110). Less favorable psychosocial outcomes following CABG surgery are also described for women (111), including more frequent depression, delayed resumption of preoperative activities, and a lesser and later return to remunerative employment. The potential contributors of older age, greater comorbidity, lesser social support, widowhood, limited financial resources, etc., to the adverse social outcomes of women following CABG surgery have yet to be completely evaluated. However, recent questionnaire survey data suggest gender-neutral physical and psychosocial functioning by 6 months postoperatively, when adjusted for age and severity of disease (112).

Women referred for PTCA are more likely to be older than their male counterparts, to have a history of heart failure and unstable angina, and to have hypertension, hypercholesterolemia, and diabetes. They are less likely to have had previous myocardial infarction (113,114). In the 1985 NHLBI PTCA Registry (115), twice as many women as men referred for coronary angioplasty were considered either inoperable or at high surgical risk, and more women than men had unstable angina. Four-year follow-up Registry data indicated that more women had died in the interval following PTCA but that myocardial infarction and the need for CABG surgery were comparable by gender. However, Registry women were more likely to have not only residual angina but more severe angina, and, not surprisingly, were receiving more maintenance antianginal medications.

Currently, the procedural success and safety of PTCA is comparable for women and men (113,114,116,117). Despite these initially favorable results, women have less long-term symptomatic relief and decreased long-term survival following PTCA, the latter predominantly related to their older age (118). Women are also less likely to have subsequent surgical revascularization. The newer transcatheter revascularization procedures are associated with lower success rates and higher complication rates in women, predominantly related to the larger size of these devices relative to the smaller coronary artery size of women. Little is known about gender differences, if any, in restenosis rates after coronary intravascular procedures, and data regarding gender differences with coronary intravascular stenting are at best preliminary. Similar rates of restenosis were described for women and men in the CAVEAT trial, both with directional atherectomy and with balloon angioplasty (119).

During the past decade, there has been a doubling of the performance of coronary arteriography among women and an almost threefold increase in the rates of both CABG surgery and PTCA and other transcatheter revascularization procedures. Among the variables likely to have a deleterious impact on the outcome of myocardial revascularization are that women are generally older than men, describe greater preprocedural functional impairment, are more likely to have severe and unstable angina, and owing to their unstable presentation are more likely to require urgent or emergency surgery. Are women, therefore, not referred earlier owing to their increased risk, completing the vicious circle of late referral, urgent or emergency revascularization, and resultant excess risk? Their increased serious comorbidity, particularly diabetes and hypertension, is also likely contributory. As is the case with myocardial infarction, fewer women than men, and particularly older women, following myocardial revascularization procedures are referred to cardiac rehabilitation for exercise training and coronary risk reduction (38).

Summary

Only in recent years has the magnitude and lethality of CAD in women been widely appreciated. Women with symptomatic CAD also sustain greater morbidity, have more functional limitations, and consequently have substantially greater impairment of their quality of life (75). As was the case in the Framingham Heart Study, women today are more likely than men to die with an episode of myocardial infarction; this less favorable outcome is now also evident after coronary angioplasty. Subsequent to the delineation of these data in the Framingham cohort, the prognosis of CAD is also influenced by access to diagnostic procedures and to subsequent therapy. These, in turn, are influenced by physician decisions, patient decisions, reimbursement issues, and societal perceptions of the importance of CAD as a health problem of women, among others.

High priority must be accorded to educating women, across the life span, that CAD is their pre-eminent health problem. Additionally, optimal methods for encouragement of adoption of healthy lifestyles and of coronary risk reduction, again across the life span, must be ascertained for women, with continued investigation of the role of the risk intervention unique to women, postmenopausal hormone therapy.

The past decade has witnessed enormously favorable responses of the clinical and research communities to the diagnostic and therapeutic challenge of CAD in women. In addition to ascertainment of the optimal noninvasive test or tests for the evaluation of chest pain syndromes in women, evaluation of pharmacotherapy for CAD in women must be intensified, so as to define the optimal drugs and drug dosages. Appropriate use of guideline-based pharmacotherapy offers major opportunities for improving the coronary care of women. Critical is the ascertainment whether and which of the current more prompt and vigorous invasive diagnostic and therapeutic procedures offer benefit for women, so as to enable the selection among the approaches likely to be associated with the most favorable outcome.

REFERENCES

1. **Wenger NK.** Coronary heart disease in women: evolving knowledge is dramatically changing clinical care. In: Julian DG, Wenger NK (eds). Women and Heart Disease. London: Martin Dunitz; 1997:21.
2. **Pensky JL, Jette AM, Branch LG, et al.** The Framingham Disability Study: relationship of various coronary heart disease manifestations to disability in older persons living in the community. Am J Public Health. 1990;80:1363.
3. **Eaker ED, Chesebro JH, Sacks FM, et al.** Cardiovascular disease in women. Circulation. 1993;88(part 1):1999.
4. **National Center for Health Statistics.** Health: United States—1990. U.S. Public Health Services, Centers for Disease Control: Hyattsville, MD; 1991.
5. **Centers for Disease Control.** Coronary heart disease incidence, by sex—United States, 1971-1987. MMWR Morb Mortal Wkly Rep. 1992;41(SS-2):526.
6. **Hansen EF, Andersen LT, Von Eyben FE.** Cigarette smoking and age at first acute myocardial infarction and influence of gender and extent of smoking. Am J Cardiol. 1993;71:1439.
7. **Willett WC, Green A, Stampfer MJ, et al.** Relative and absolute excess risks of coronary heart disease among women who smoke cigarettes. N Engl J Med. 1987;317:1303.

8. **Kawachi I, Colditz GA, Stampfer MJ, et al.** Smoking cessation in relation to total mortality rates in women: a prospective cohort study. Ann Intern Med. 1993;119:992.

9. **Hermanson B, Omenn GS, Kronmal RA, et al, and participants in the Coronary Artery Surgery Study.** Beneficial six-year outcome of smoking cessation in older men and women with coronary artery disease: results from the CASS Registry. N Engl J Med. 1988;319:1365.

10. **Prescott E, Hippe M, Schnohr P, et al.** Smoking and risk of myocardial infarction in women and men: longitudinal population study. BMJ. 1998;316:1043.

11. **Barrett-Connor EL, Cohn BA, Wingard DL, et al.** Why is diabetes mellitus a stronger risk factor for fatal ischemic heart disease in women than in men? The Rancho Bernardo Study. JAMA. 1991;265:627.

12. **Manson JE, Colditz GA, Stampfer MJ, et al.** A prospective study of maturity-onset diabetes mellitus and risk of coronary heart disease and stroke in women. Arch Intern Med. 1991;151:1141.

13. **Manson JE, Rimm EB, Stampfer MJ, et al.** Physical activity and incidence of non–insulin-dependent diabetes mellitus in women. Lancet. 1991;338:774.

14. **Donahue RP, Goldberg RJ, Chen Z, et al.** The influence of sex and diabetes mellitus on survival following acute myocardial infarction: a community-wide perspective. J Clin Epidemiol. 1993;46:245.

15. **Liao Y, Cooper RS, Ghali JK, et al.** Sex differences in the impact of coexistent diabetes on survival in patients with coronary heart disease. Diabetes Care. 1993;16:708.

16. **Miettinen H, Lehto S, Salomaa V, et al, for the FINMONICA Myocardial Infarction Register Study Group.** Impact of diabetes on mortality after the first myocardial infarction. Diabetes Care. 1998;21:69.

17. **Manolio TA, Pearson TA, Wenger NK, et al.** Cholesterol and heart disease in older persons and women: review of an NHLBI Workshop. Ann Epidemiol. 1992;2:161.

18. **Kannel WB.** Nutrition and the occurrence of prevention of cardiovascular disease in the elderly. Nutr Rev. 1988;46:68.

19. **Demirovic J, Sprafka JM, Folsom AR, et al.** Menopause and serum cholesterol: differences between blacks and whites—the Minnesota Heart Survey. Am J Epidemiol. 1992;136:155.

20. **Knapp RG, Sutherland SE, Keil JE, et al.** A comparison of the effects of cholesterol on CHD mortality in black and white women: twenty-eight years of follow-up in the Charleston Heart Study. J Clin Epidemiol. 1992;45:1119.

21. **Scandinavian Simvastatin Survival Study Group.** Randomised trial of cholesterol lowering in 4444 patients with coronary heart disease: the Scandinavian Simvastatin Survival Study (4S). Lancet. 1994;344:1383.

22. **Sacks FM, Pfeffer MA, Moyé LA, et al, for the Cholesterol and Recurrent Events Trial Investigators.** The effect of pravastatin on coronary events after myocardial infarction in patients with average cholesterol levels. N Engl J Med. 1996;335:1001.

23. **Espeland MA, Applegate W, Furberg CD, et al, for the ACAPS Investigators.** Estrogen replacement therapy and progression of intimal-medial thickness in the carotid arteries of postmenopausal women. Am J Epidemiol. 1995;142:1011.

24. **Downs JR, Clearfield M, Weis S, et al.** Primary prevention of acute coronary events with lovastatin in men and women with average cholesterol levels: results of AFCAPS/TexCAPS. JAMA. 1998;279:1615.

25. **Schrott HG, Bittner V, Vittinghoff E, et al, for the HERS Research Group.** Adherence to National Cholesterol Education Program treatment goals in postmenopausal

women with heart disease: the Heart and Estrogen/Progestin Replacement Study (HERS). JAMA. 1997;277:1281.

26. **Bass KM, Newschaffer CJ, Klag MJ, et al.** Plasma lipoprotein levels as predictors of cardiovascular death in women. Arch Intern Med. 1993;153:2209.

27. **Castelli WP.** The triglyceride issue: a view from Framingham. Am Heart J. 1986;112: 432.

28. **Criqui MH, Heiss G, Cohn R, et al.** Plasma triglyceride level and mortality from coronary heart disease. N Engl J Med. 1993;328:1220.

29. **SHEP Cooperative Research Group.** Prevention of stroke by antihypertensive drug treatment in older persons with isolated systolic hypertension: final results of the Systolic Hypertension in the Elderly Program (SHEP). JAMA. 1991;265:3255.

30. **Kannel WB, Wilson PWF.** Risk factors that attenuate the female coronary disease advantage. Arch Intern Med. 1995;155:57.

31. **Hartz A, Grubb B, Wild R, et al.** The association of waist hip ratio and angiographically determined coronary artery disease. Int J Obes. 1990;14:657.

32. **Kaplan NM.** The deadly quartet: upper-body obesity, glucose intolerance, hypertriglyceridemia, and hypertension. Arch Intern Med. 1989;149:1514.

33. **Anda RF, Waller NM, Wooten KG, et al.** Behavioral risk factor surveillance, 1988. MMWR Morb Mortal Wkly Rep. 1990;39(SS-2):1.

34. **Blair SN, Kohn HW III, Paffenbarger RS Jr, et al.** Physical fitness and all-cause mortality: a prospective study of healthy men and women. JAMA. 1989;262:2395.

35. **Kushi LH, Fee RM, Folsom AR, et al.** Physical activity and mortality in postmenopausal women. JAMA. 1997;277:1287.

36. **Lemaitre RN, Heckbert SR, Psaty BM, et al.** Leisure-time physical activity and the risk of nonfatal myocardial infarction in postmenopausal women. Arch Intern Med. 1995;155:2302.

37. **Pollock MJ, Carroll JF, Graves JE, et al.** Injuries and adherence to walk/jog and resistance training programs in the elderly. Med Sci Sports Exerc. 1991;23:1194.

38. **Wenger NK, Froelicher ES, Smith LK, et al.** Cardiac Rehabilitation. Clinical Practice Guideline No. 17. Rockville, MD: U.S. Department of Health and Human Services, Public Health Service, Agency for Health Care Policy and Research and the National Heart, Lung, and Blood Institute. AHCPR Publication No. 96-0672, October 1995.

39. **Manson JE, Stampfer MJ, Colditz GA, et al.** A prospective study of aspirin use and primary prevention of cardiovascular disease in women. JAMA. 1991;266:521.

40. **Folsam AR, Nieto FJ, McGovern PG, et al.** Prospective study of coronary heart disease incidence in relation to fasting total homocysteine, related genetic polymorphisms, and B vitamins: the Atherosclerosis Risk in Communities (ARIC) Study. Circulation. 1998;98:204.

41. **Robinson K, Arheart K, Refsum H, et al., for the European COMAC Group.** Low circulating folate and vitamin B_6 concentrations: risk factors for stroke, peripheral vascular disease and coronary artery disease. Circulation. 1998;97:437.

42. **Commonwealth Fund.** National Survey of Women's Health. New York: The Commonwealth Fund; 1993.

43. **Eaker ED, Pinsky J, Castelli WP.** Myocardial infarction and coronary death among women: psychosocial predictors from a 20-year follow-up of women in the Framingham study. Am J Epidemiol 1992;135:854.

44. **Kawachi I, Colditz GA, Stampfer MJ, et al.** Prospective study of shift work and risk of coronary heart disease in women. Circulation. 1995;92:3178.

45. **Samaan SA, Crawford MH.** Estrogen and cardiovascular function after menopause. J Am Coll Cardiol. 1995;26:1403.

46. **Vogel RA, Corretti MC.** Estrogens, progestins, and heart disease: can endothelial function divine the benefit? Circulation. 1998;97:1223.

47. **Ettinger B, Friedman GD, Bush T, et al.** Reduced mortality associated with long-term postmenopausal estrogen therapy. Obstet Gynecol. 1996;87:6.

48. **Sullivan JM, El-Zeky F, Vander Zwaag R, et al.** Estrogen replacement therapy after coronary artery bypass surgery: effect on survival. J Am Coll Cardiol. 1994;23:7A.

49. **O'Keefe JH Jr, Kim SC, Hall RR, et al.** Estrogen replacement therapy after coronary angioplasty in women. J Am Coll Cardiol. 1997;29:1.

50. **Hulley S, Grady D, Bush T, et al., for the Heart Estrogen/Progestin Replacement Study (HERS) Research Group.** Randomized trial of estrogen plus progestin for secondary prevention of coronary heart disease in postmenopausal women. JAMA. 1998;280:605.

51. **Manolio TA, Furberg CD, Shemanski L, et al, for the CHS Collaborative Research Group.** Associations of postmenopausal estrogen use with cardiovascular disease and its risk factors in older women. Circulation. 1993;188(part 1):2163.

52. **Sidney S, Petitti DB, Quesenberry CP Jr.** Myocardial infarction and the use of estrogen and estrogen-progestogen in postmenopausal women. Ann Intern Med. 1997;127:501.

53. **Writing Group for the PEPI Trial.** Effects of estrogen or estrogen/progestin regimens on heart disease risk factors in postmenopausal women: the Postmenopausal Estrogen/Progestin Interventions (PEPI) trial. JAMA. 1995;273:199.

54. **Kawas C, Resnick S, Morrison A, et al.** A prospective study of estrogen replacement therapy and the risk of developing Alzheimer's disease: the Baltimore Longitudinal Study of Aging. Neurology. 1997;48:1517.

55. **Colditz GA, Hankinson SE, Hunter DJ, et al.** The use of estrogens and progestins and the risk of breast cancer in postmenopausal women. N Engl J Med. 1995;332:1589.

56. **Grodstein F, Stampfer MJ, Colditz GA, et al.** Postmenopausal hormone therapy and mortality. N Engl J Med. 1997;336:1769.

57. **Daly E, Vessey MP, Hawkins MM, et al.** Risk of venous thromboembolism in users of hormone replacement therapy. Lancet. 1996;348:977.

58. **Jick H, Derby LE, Myers MW, et al.** Risk of hospital admission for idiopathic venous thromboembolism among users of postmenopausal oestrogens. Lancet. 1996;348:981.

59. **Grodstein F, Stampfer MJ, Goldhaber SZ, et al.** Prospective study of exogenous hormones and risk of pulmonary embolism in women. Lancet. 1996;348:983.

60. **Grady D, Hulley SB, Furberg C.** Venous thromboembolic events associated with hormone replacement therapy. JAMA. 1997;278:477.

61. **Gutthann SP, Rodriguez LAG, Castellsague J, et al.** Hormone replacement therapy and risk of venous thromboembolism: population based case-control study. BMJ. 1997;314:796.

62. **Lerner DJ, Kannel WB.** Patterns of coronary heart disease morbidity and mortality in the sexes: a 26-year follow-up of the Framingham population. Am Heart J. 1986;111:383.

63. **Kennedy JW, Killip T, Fisher LD, et al.** The clinical spectrum of coronary artery disease and its surgical and medical management, 1974-1979: the Coronary Artery Surgery Study. Circulation. 1982;66(suppl III):III-16.

64. **Principal Investigators of CASS and Their Associates.** The National Heart, Lung, and Blood Institute Coronary Artery Surgery Study (CASS). Circulation. 1981;63(suppl I):I-1.

65. **Thomas JL, Braus PA.** Coronary artery disease in women: a historical perspective. Arch Intern Med. 1998;158:333.

66. **Pepine CJ, Abrams J, Marks RG, et al, for the TIDES Investigators.** Characteristics of a contemporary population with angina pectoris. Am J Cardiol. 1994;74:226.

67. **LaCroix AZ, Guralnik JM, Curb JD, et al.** Chest pain and coronary heart disease mortality among older men and women in three communities. Circulation. 1990;81:437.

68. **Lehmann JB, Wehner PS, Lehmann CU, et al.** Gender bias in the evaluation of chest pain in the emergency department. Am J Cardiol. 1996;77:641.

69. **Wenger NK (guest ed).** Symposium: gender differences in cardiac imaging. Am J Card Imaging. 1996;10:42.

70. **Mark DB, Shaw LK, DeLong ER, et al.** Absence of sex bias in the referral of patients for cardiac catheterization. N Engl J Med. 1994;330:1101.

71. **Lauer MS, Pashkow FJ, Snader CE, et al.** Gender and referral for coronary angiography after treadmill thallium testing. Am J Cardiol. 1996;78:278.

72. **Shaw LJ, Miller DD, Romeis JC, et al.** Gender differences in the noninvasive evaluation and management of patients with suspected coronary artery disease. Ann Intern Med. 1994;120:559.

73. **Sullivan AK, Holdright DR, Wright CA, et al.** Chest pain in women: clinical, investigative, and prognostic features. BMJ. 1994;308:883.

74. **Weintraub WS, Kosinski AS, Wenger NK.** Is there a bias against performing coronary revascularization in women? Am J Cardiol. 1996;78:1154.

75. **Steingart RM, Packer M, Hamm P, et al, for the Survival and Ventricular Enlargement Investigators.** Sex differences in the management of coronary artery disease. N Engl J Med. 1991;325:226.

76. **Kannel WB, Abbott RD.** Incidence and prognosis of myocardial infarction in women: the Framingham Study. In: Eaker ED, Packard B, Wenger NK, et al (eds). Coronary Heart Disease in Women. New York: Haymarket Doyma; 1987:208.

77. **Kannel WB, Sorlie P, McNamara PM.** Prognosis after initial myocardial infarction: the Framingham study. Am J Cardiol. 1979;44:53.

78. **Kostis JB, Wilson AC, O'Dowd K, et al, for the MIDAS Study Group.** Sex differences in the management and long-term outcome of acute myocardial infarction: a statewide study. Circulation. 1994;90:1715.

79. **Chandra NC, Ziegelstein RC, Rogers WJ, et al., for the National Registry of Myocardial Infarction-I.** Observations of the treatment of woman in the United States with myocardial infarction: a report from the National Registry of Myocardial Infarction–I. Arch Intern Med. 1998;158:981.

80. **Kudenchuck PJ, Maynard C, Martin JS, et al, for the MITI Project Investigators.** Comparison of presentation, treatment, and outcome of acute myocardial infarction in men versus women (The Myocardial Infarction Triage and Intervention Registry). Am J Cardiol. 1996;78:9.

81. **Maynard C, Litwin PE, Martin JS, et al.** Gender differences in the treatment and outcome of acute myocardial infarction: results from the Myocardial Infarction Triage and Intervention Registry. Arch Intern Med. 1992;152:972.

82. **Radford MJ, Johnson RA, Daggett WM Jr, et al.** Ventricular septal rupture: a review of clinical and physiological features and an analysis of survival. Circulation. 1981;64:545.

83. **Adams JN, Jamieson M, Rawles JM, et al.** Women and myocardial infarction: agism rather than sexism? Br Heart J. 1995;73:87.

84. **Clarke KW, Gray D, Keating NA, et al.** Do women with acute myocardial infarction receive the same treatment as men? BMJ. 1994;309:563.

85. **Jenkins JS, Flaker GC, Nolte B, et al.** Causes of higher in-hospital mortality in women than in men after acute myocardial infarction. Am J Cardiol. 1994;73:319.

86. **Goldberg RJ, Gorak EJ, Yarzebski J, et al.** A community-wide perspective of sex differences and temporal trends in the incidence and survival rates after acute myocardial infarction and out-of-hospital deaths caused by coronary heart disease. Circulation. 1993;87:1947.

87. **Tofler GH, Stone PH, Muller JE, et al, and the MILIS Study Group.** Effects of gender and race on prognosis after myocardial infarction: adverse prognosis for women, particularly black women. J Am Coll Cardiol. 1987;9:473.

88. **Greenland P, Reicher-Reiss H, Goldbourt U, et al, and the Israeli SPRINT Investigators.** In-hospital and 1-year mortality in 1,524 women after myocardial infarction: comparison with 4,315 men. Circulation. 1991;83:484.

89. **Smith JW, Marcus FI, Serokman R, with the Multicenter Postinfarction Research Group.** Prognosis of patients with diabetes mellitus after acute myocardial infarction. Am J Cardiol. 1984;54:718.

90. **Stone PH, Thompson B, Anderson HV, et al, for the TIMI III Registry Study Group.** Influence of race, sex, and age on management of unstable angina and non–Q-wave myocardial infarction: the TIMI III Registry. JAMA. 1996;275:1104.

91. **McLaughlin TJ, Soumerai SB, Willison DJ, et al.** Adherence to national guidelines for drug treatment of suspected acute myocardial infarction: evidence for undertreatment in women and the elderly. Arch Intern Med. 1996;156:799.

92. **Krumholz HM, Radford MJ, Wang Y, et al.** National use and effectiveness of β-blockers for the treatment of elderly patients after acute myocardial infarction: National Cooperative Cardiovascular Project. JAMA. 1998;280:623.

93. **Maynard C, Althouse R, Cerqueira M, et al.** Underutilization of thrombolytic therapy in eligible women with acute myocardial infarction. Am J Cardiol. 1991;68:529.

94. **Pfeffer MA, Moyé LA, Braunwald E, et al, for the SAVE Investigators.** Selection bias in the use of thrombolytic therapy in acute myocardial infarction. JAMA. 1991;266:528.

95. **Lee KL, Woodlief LH, Topol EJ, et al.** Predictors of 30-day mortality in the era of reperfusion for acute myocardial infarction. Circulation. 1995;91:1659.

96. **Weaver WD, White HD, Wilcox RG, et al, for the GUSTO-I Investigators.** Comparisons of characteristics and outcomes among women and men with acute myocardial infarction treated with thrombolytic therapy. JAMA. 1996;275:777.

97. **Woodfield SL, Lundergan CF, Reiner JS, et al.** Gender and acute myocardial infarction: is there a different response to thrombolysis? J Am Coll Cardiol. 1997;29:35.

98. **Becker RC, Terrin M, Ross R, et al, and the Thrombolysis in Myocardial Infarction Investigators.** Comparison of clinical outcomes for women and men after acute myocardial infarction. Ann Intern Med. 1994;120:638.

99. **Gruppo Italiano per lo Studio della Streptochinasi nell'Infarto Miocardico (GISSI).** Long-term effects of intravenous thrombolysis in acute myocardial infarction: final report of the GISSI study. Lancet. 1987;2:871.

100. **Stone GW, Grines CL, Browne KF, et al.** Comparison of in-hospital outcome in men versus women treated by either thrombolytic therapy or primary coronary angioplasty for acute myocardial infarction. Am J Cardiol. 1995;75:987.

101. **Jollis JG, DeLong ER, Peterson ED, et al.** Outcome of acute myocardial infarction according to the specialty of the admitting physician. N Engl J Med. 1996;335:1880.

102. **Tunstall-Pedoe H, Morrison C, Woodward M, et al.** Sex differences in myocardial infarction and coronary deaths in the Scottish MONICA population of Glasgow 1985 to 1991: presentation, diagnosis, treatment, and 28-day case fatality of 3991 events in men and 1551 events in women. Circulation. 1996;93:1981.

103. **Boogaard MAK, Briody ME.** Comparison of the rehabilitation of men and women post-myocardial infarction. J Cardpulm Rehabil. 1985;5:379.

104. **O'Connor GT, Morton JR, Diehl MJ, et al, for the Northern New England Cardiovascular Disease Study Group.** Differences between men and women in hospital mortality associated with coronary artery bypass graft surgery. Circulation. 1993;88(part 1):2104.

105. **Weintraub WS, Wenger NK, Jones EL, et al.** Changing clinical characteristics of coronary surgery patients: differences between men and women. Circulation. 1993;88(part 2):79.

106. **Jacobs AK, Kelsey S, Rosen A, et al, and the BARI Investigators.** Gender differences in patients undergoing coronary revascularization: a report from the Bypass Angioplasty Revascularization Investigation (BARI) trial [Abstract]. J Am Coll Cardiol. 1993; 21:272A.

107. **Maynard C, Weaver WD.** Treatment of women with acute MI: new findings from the MITI Registry. J Myocard Ischemia. 1992;4:27.

108. **Judge KW, Pawitan Y, Caldwell J, et al.** Congestive heart failure symptoms in patients with preserved left ventricular systolic function: analysis of the CASS Registry. J Am Coll Cardiol. 1991;18:377.

109. **Loop FD, Golding LR, MacMillan JP, et al.** Coronary artery surgery in women compared with men: analyses of risks and long-term results. J Am Coll Cardiol. 1983; 1:383.

110. **Allen JK, Blumenthal RS.** Coronary risk factors in women six months after coronary artery bypass grafting. Am J Cardiol. 1995;75:1092.

111. **King KB, Porter LA, Rowe MA.** Functional, social, and emotional outcomes in women and men in the first year following coronary artery bypass surgery. J Womens Health. 1994;3:347.

112. **Ayanian JZ, Guadagnoli E, Cleary PD.** Physical and psychosocial functioning of women and men after coronary artery bypass surgery. JAMA. 1995;274:1767.

113. **Weintraub WS, Wenger NK, Kosinski AS, et al.** Percutaneous transluminal coronary angioplasty in women compared with men. J Am Coll Cardiol. 1994;24:81.

114. **Welty FK, Mittleman MA, Healy RW, et al.** Similar results of percutaneous transluminal coronary angioplasty for women and men with postmyocardial infarction ischemia. J Am Coll Cardiol. 1994;23:35.

115. **Kelsey SF, James M, Holubkov AL, et al, and the Investigators from the National Heart, Lung, and Blood Institute Percutaneous Transluminal Coronary Angioplasty Registry.** Results of percutaneous transluminal coronary angioplasty in women: 1985-1986 National Heart, Lung, and Blood Institute's Coronary Angioplasty Registry. Circulation. 1993;87:720.

116. **Bell MR, Grill DE, Garratt KN, et al.** Long-term outcome of women compared with men after successful coronary angioplasty. Circulation. 1995;91:2876.

117. **Holmes DR Jr., Holubkov R, Vlietstra RE, et al, and the Co-investigators of the National Heart, Lung, and Blood Institute Percutaneous Transluminal Coronary Angioplasty Registry.** Comparison of complications during percutaneous transluminal coronary angioplasty from 1977 to 1981 and from 1985 to 1986: The National Heart, Lung, and Blood Institute Percutaneous Transluminal Coronary Angioplasty Registry. J Am Coll Cardiol. 1988;12:1149.

118. **Weintraub WS, Wenger NK, Delafontaine P, et al.** PTCA in women compared to men: is there a difference in risk [Abstract]? Circulation. 1992;86(suppl I):I-253.

119. **Jacobs AK, Faxon DP, Pinkerton CA, et al.** Impact of gender on outcome following percutaneous coronary revascularization: the CAVEAT experience [Abstract]. Circulation. 1993;88(part 2):I-448.

Prevention

Chapter 2

Smoking

Judith Keller Ockene, PhD, MEd
Debra Perkins Bonollo, BA
Abigail Adams, MD

Tobacco use is a major risk factor for the development of coronary artery disease (CAD) among women and also for many other serious illnesses, including cancer, lung disease, and complications of pregnancy. Women who smoke as few as one to four cigarettes per day have a 2.5-fold increased risk of fatal CAD and nonfatal myocardial infarction (MI) (1).

Most smokers want to quit, and the methodologies described in this chapter can be applied successfully to help them do it. Health care providers are often discouraged by what they perceive to be a lack of success in helping patients to stop smoking, yet there is good evidence that brief interventions are effective. At the very least, advice should be provided to every woman who smokes (2,3); "It is essential that clinicians determine and document the tobacco-use status of every patient (female) treated in a health care setting" (3).

This chapter provides an overview of the effects of smoking and benefits of cessation for women as compared with men. We review the prevalence of smoking and cessation, the factors that affect women's smoking, and practical and effective smoking intervention strategies that can be used with the smoking woman.

Effects of Smoking

Heart disease is the leading cause of death for women 35 years of age or older in the United States (4), and cigarette smoking has been strongly established as the major cause of heart disease (5,6). For example, over 60% of MI cases can be attributed to cigarette smoking among women who had their first MI before 50 years of age.

Cigarette smoking is a risk factor for sudden cardiac death (7). In a longitudinal population study (8), as in other studies (7), cigarette use increases the risk of coronary events more for women than men. Women seem to develop CAD a decade later in life than men. Cigarette smoking remains an important risk factor for CAD among women 65 years of age and older (9). In the Systolic Hypertension in the Elderly Program study, both women and men over 60 years of age who smoked had 73% more CAD-related events (e.g., MI, coronary artery bypass surgery, or angioplasty) than did nonsmokers (10).

For women during their reproductive years, epidemiologic data indicate the synergistic effect of smoking and the use of oral contraceptive pills (OCP) on CAD (11). Risk was significantly increased in early studies evaluating current usage of OCP containing more than 50 µg of estrogen. These early studies reported the highest rates of MI in women over 35 years of age who smoked. Even with the lower-dose OCP, smoking significantly increased the risk of CAD, and current recommendations limit pill use beyond 35 years of age to nonsmokers (12,13).

Both clinical and epidemiologic studies have consistently demonstrated that cigarette smokers are at increased risk for cerebrovascular and peripheral vascular disease as well as for cancers of many sites, chronic lung disease, and other chronic diseases (6,14). Passive exposure to tobacco is also deleterious (15). Of special concern to women is the demonstrated relationship of smoking to complications in pregnancy and low birth rate (6,16). The relationship of smoking to wrinkling of the skin in white women also can be an effective motivator for smoking cessation (14).

Benefits of Smoking Cessation

Smoking cessation benefits women of all ages. Although most data on these benefits come from studies of white men, the information about women is sufficient enough to indicate that the benefits of quitting are similar for both sexes (14). Most of the increased risk of suffering an initial MI dissipates within 2 to 3 years of stopping smoking for both women and men (17). For example, the Nurses Health Study (18) reports that women who stop smoking reduce their excess risk of developing CAD by one third within 2 years of cessation. After 2 years, their risk level falls to levels consistent with those who have never smoked (18).

Smokers who have already developed smoking-related diseases or symptoms will still benefit from cessation. Those with previous MI have reduced risks of reinfarction, sudden cardiac death, and total mortality if they quit

(14,19,20). Significant benefits accrue in pregnant women if they stop smoking before conception or even during their first 3 months of pregnancy—the risk of low birth weight can be decreased to that of people who have never smoked (14), and other complications of pregnancy are reduced.

In addition to medical benefits, many ex-smokers have better psychosocial functioning and are more likely to practice health-promoting and disease-preventing behaviors than continuing smokers (21). Most nicotine withdrawal symptoms disappear, but for some former smokers increased appetite and continual urges to smoke remain problematic. These problems (especially increased appetite) are of particular concern for women and are addressed later in this chapter.

Prevalence of Cigarette Smoking and Cessation Among Women

Estimates of the prevalence of smoking among specific populations of female smokers are presented in this section. Interventions targeted at these populations are warranted if we are to have the greatest impact on the health of women.

Women in General

The prevalence of smoking among women in the United States (i.e., the percentage of women who have smoked at least 100 cigarettes in their lifetime and who were smoking at the time they were interviewed) has declined over the last three decades (Fig. 2-1) (22). Data suggest, however, that smoking rates among young women are on the increase (23). White women in all childbearing age groups smoked more in 1992 than in 1991, as did Hispanic women, women below the poverty level, and those with more than 13 years of education.

Although smoking rates are slightly lower among women than men, men have decreased more dramatically over time their tobacco use (see Fig. 2-1). It is not certain whether the higher rate of cessation among men compared with women presents an accurate picture, because it may not reflect the proportion of men who switch to other forms of smoking (24). Data from the 1987 National Health Interview Survey's (NHIS) Cancer Epidemiology and Control supplement (25) were analyzed to update the previous calculations. By reclassifying former smokers who were using any tobacco products (e.g., cigars, pipes, chewing tobacco, snuff) as smokers, the difference in the quit ratio between women and men was reduced from 8.6 to 2.2 percentage points. However, studies of both unaided quitters and smokers in treatment suggest that women experience more difficulty in quitting, especially in the initial quit period, and are slightly more prone to relapse than men (26).

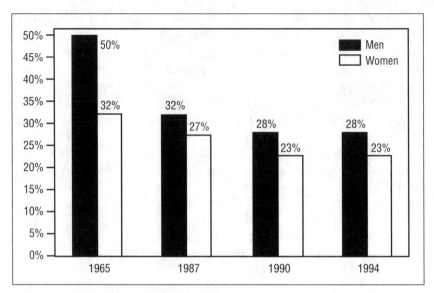

FIGURE 2-1 Prevalence of smoking among men and women in the United States. Data from U.S. Department of Health and Human Services, Centers for Disease Control and Prevention, Office of Smoking and Health (22).

Adolescent and Young Adults

The percentage of high school seniors who smoke every day declined in the years between 1976 and 1981 from 29% to 20%. Among adolescents, cigarette smoking rates were generally higher for women than for men in the 1980s (27), but today women and men are equally likely to smoke. Smoking (defined as having smoked one or more cigarettes per day during the previous 30 days) is highest among white, non-Hispanic high school girls (22% in 1991–92); however, only 4% of black, non-Hispanic high school senior girls were current smokers from 1991 to 1992 (28). Women have started smoking at younger ages; 84% of female smokers born between 1960 and 1964 started smoking before 20 years of age as compared with only 75% of those born between 1935 and 1939 (6). The greater rate of decline in male smoking rates from 1965 to the present (compared with female smoking rates) reflects both higher rates of smoking cessation and lower rates of smoking initiation for men.

Pregnant and Postpartum Women

Pregnant women present a unique opportunity for the prevention of CAD. Women who smoke are under social pressure not to smoke while pregnant. Spontaneous cessation is more likely during pregnancy than at any other time, with 40% of pregnant women stopping. Unmarried women, women with less than 12 years of education, and women who smoke more than one pack of cigarettes per day before pregnancy are significantly less likely to quit (~20% of women in each group stop smoking) than married women, women with more education, and women smoking less (29–31). National data from 1994 indicate that 27% of low-education and low-income women continue to smoke during pregnancy (32). Visits to health care providers during pregnancy are excellent opportunities for smoking intervention.

Although many women quit spontaneously during pregnancy, relapse rates are greater than 50% within 3 months after delivery, and are 70% by 6 months (29–31). Rates of postpartum relapse among women who stop smoking during pregnancy are also high in randomized studies of special interventions directed at pregnant smokers (33,34).

Physicians who encounter women who either have stopped smoking or continue to smoke during pregnancy should reinforce cessation or emphasize the need to stop, reminding the smoker of the importance of staying off cigarettes after delivery. Assistance or a referral can also be useful. The smoking cessation efforts of women who have recently delivered a child should be reinforced, because staying abstinent may require additional assistance. Methods for assisting smokers or former smokers are discussed later in this chapter.

Racial and Ethnic Minorities

In 1993, the smoking rate among black women was 21%; among white women, it was 24%. The lowest rates were seen in the female Hispanic (13%) and Asian and Pacific Islander populations (10%) (35), whereas the highest rates were in American Indian and Alaskan Native women (41%). Between 1980 and 1993, the proportion of women who were heavy smokers declined from 23% to 14%; a similar decline was seen among men. White women were more likely to be heavy smokers (17%) than were black (5%) or Hispanic women (4%) during 1992 to 1993.

In the Third National Health and Nutrition Examination Survey (36), completed between 1988 and 1994, current cigarette smokers comprised 33% of the 1762 black American women, 30% of the 2023 American women, and 15.7% of the 1481 Mexican-American women. Furthermore, the more years of formal education a woman had, the lower the rate of current tobacco use. Black and Mexican-American women had similar rates of tobacco use across all age groups, whereas white women were most likely to smoke between the ages of 25 and 34 years.

Racial and ethnic differences in serum cotinine, a nicotine metabolite, were also observed in the Third National Health and Nutrition Examination Survey (37). Black smokers had higher cotinine concentrations at all levels of tobacco consumption than Mexican-American or white smokers. The higher cotinine levels in black smokers have been found to be related to lower cotinine clearance rates, resulting in greater cotinine levels and a longer cotinine half-life after tobacco exposure (38). These studies provide a biologic rationale for the observation that black smokers are less successful in tobacco cessation efforts than white smokers (37).

Low-Income Women

Many women of low income are unemployed outside of the home, unmarried, and caring for children (39). Data on rates of smoking among women of low income are scarce, because low education is often used as the only measure for low income. For low-income pregnant women enrolled in the Women, Infants, and Children (WIC) supplemental nutrition program the smoking rate was 42% (40,41). In a small sample of British mothers of low-income households, 54% were smokers (39).

The high smoking rates found in this population suggest that for these women smoking cessation is especially difficult. "In a lifestyle stripped of new clothes, make-up, hair dressing, and evenings out, smoking can become an important symbol of one's participation in an adult, consumer society" (39). Interventions with low-income women need to address the complicated relationship between smoking and cultural norms. More research is desperately needed to understand how to work best with this population of women.

Older Women

In 1994, women aged 65 years and older had the lowest prevalence of smoking (11%), a statistic that has not changed since 1965 (28,42a). Although older smokers report similar smoking patterns, their motives for quitting are more numerous and the barriers against quitting are more difficult for them to overcome as compared with younger smokers aged 21 to 49 years (42b). Older smokers are less likely to accept that smoking is harmful to their health, and they are more likely to view smoking as a beneficial coping and weight-control tactic (43). Programs tailored to address these differences have been found to be successful in reaching older smokers (43,44).

Characteristics of Smokers
and Implications for Interventions

Cigarette smoking is a complex behavior pattern that, like most behavior patterns, is affected by multiple, interacting factors, including physiologic factors, personal characteristics (e.g., cognitive factors, information, personality, and demographic factors), environmental influences (e.g., social, cultural, economic), and other behaviors (e.g., drinking a beer triggers the craving for a cigarette). It goes through a sequence of phases from initiation to regular smoking to possible cessation and maintenance of cessation or relapse. During the initiation phase, individuals start experimenting with cigarettes, generally before they are 20 years old. They then move into the transition phase, in which environmental, psychological, and physiologic factors influence them to become smokers or nonsmokers. The sequence then proceeds through the phases of regular smoking, possible cessation, and maintenance of cessation. Relapse occurs at very high rates among those individuals who have stopped smoking. Often as many as 70% to 80% return to smoking within 1 year (6); thus, maintenance of cessation is often a difficult phase, and the physician must be aware of the importance of reinforcing maintenance among patients who have stopped smoking.

In each phase, different motives, needs, and environmental factors operate to determine whether an individual will move into the next phase (6). Initiation of smoking is strongly associated with social influences extrinsic to the individual (e.g., peer pressure) as well as with psychological variables (e.g., self-esteem, desire for status, and other personal needs). The sociologic variables that are so important during the formation of the behavior play a minor role in its maintenance. It becomes more and more tied to psychological and physiologic needs, thereby developing into a habit that is an intrinsic part of the person's life, serving many functions.

"We cannot rely on the 'sameness' of women but must address the complexities and differences of educational levels, income, culture, ethnicity, and race as we address ways to intervene with female smokers.... Not to address these diversities is to mistake 'some' women's health for 'all' women's health" (45).

Although physicians are not expected to become experts in psychological and behavioral theories, a general understanding of behavioral development and change can enhance a physician's ability to help patients alter harmful behaviors. Specific physiologic and social factors affect women smokers and the success of strategies for smoking cessation.

In this chapter, our focus is on interventions for cessation and maintenance of cessation; therefore, determinants of the phases of smoking are discussed. Examples of these determinants include potential differences in nicotine dependence and withdrawal, women as caregivers, negative affect, and weight concerns.

Nicotine Dependence and Withdrawal

Nicotine dependence is classified as a substance use disorder in DSM-IV (46), and the DSM-IV diagnostic criteria for nicotine withdrawal are presented in

Box 2-1. Smokers with more intense withdrawal symptoms have a more difficult time stopping smoking (47). The symptoms begin within 24 hours of cessation (or significant reduction of tobacco use), increase over 3 to 4 days, and gradually decrease over 1 to 3 weeks (48,49). Changes in appetite and problems with concentration seem to persist longer than do feelings of restlessness and irritability. Smokers who take in more nicotine (i.e., heavy smokers) typically have stronger withdrawal symptoms, but considerable variability does occur. Not all smokers are physiologically dependent on nicotine. Strategies for intervention must take into account nicotine dependence (discussed in the section on Interventions).

A number of physiologic factors may differentially affect the nicotine dependence and smoking cessation behavior of women and men. Differences in nicotine sensitivity and tolerance may account for variations in habitual smoking patterns following early exposure to nicotine (50). For example, women report more dependence on nicotine and a higher number and intensity of withdrawal symptoms than do men; this is because women may be more sensitive to nicotine even though they are generally lighter smokers (51). The data are not conclusive, however, and more research is needed.

Box 2-1 DSM-IV Diagnostic Criteria for Nicotine Withdrawal

A. Daily use of nicotine for at least several weeks

B. Abrupt cessation or reduction of nicotine use, followed by four (or more) of the following signs within 24 hours:

    Dysphoric or depressed mood

    Insomnia

    Irritability, frustration, or anger

    Anxiety

    Difficulty concentrating

    Restlessness

    Decreased heart rate

    Increased appetite or weight gain

C. Symptoms in criterion B cause clinically significant distress or impairment in social, occupational, or other important areas of functioning

D. Symptoms are not caused by a general medical condition and are not better accounted for by another mental disorder

Reprinted from Diagnostic and Statistical Manual of Mental Disorders. 4th ed. Washington, DC: American Psychiatric Associations, 1994; with permission.

Women as Caregivers and Social Supporters

With the exception of a few important studies (52–56), little research has systematically explored women's smoking experiences in the context of their domestic responsibilities. Marsh and Matheson (55) found that having children had no significant effect on smoking; rates of smoking were similar among married women with and without children. A relationship was detected, however, between full-time child care and smoking; mothers without paid employment were more likely to smoke than mothers with full- or part-time jobs. Furthermore, married women who had children and looked after the home full time had higher rates of smoking than all other categories of married women and higher rates than single women without children. One study of British mothers of low-income households found smokers reported a lower proportion of friends in whom they could confide as compared with nonsmokers (68% vs. 96%) (39), which suggest that female smokers may have less social support for quitting.

Data from 20 U.S. sites in the National Cancer Institute–funded Community Intervention Trial for Smoking Cessation revealed that women at all smoking levels were twice as likely as men to report feeling pressure from others to quit (after adjusting for education, income, ethnic group, age, and other factors) (56). The source of pressure was different for men compared with women; more women reported pressure from their children, whereas more men reported pressure from friends and coworkers. Interventions aimed at female smokers need to take into account women's perceived pressure from their children to quit smoking and available social supports for quitting smoking.

Negative Affect and Stress

Negative affect is a broad term referring to negative mood states (57) that are characterized as either high-arousal negative emotions (e.g., anxiety, anger, fear) or low-arousal negative emotions (e.g., feelings of sadness, depression, low energy, loneliness) (58). Women more than men tend to use smoking in high-arousal situations as a means of reducing tension, emotional discomfort, or feelings of stress (6,59). Situations involving negative affect or stress are considered key triggers for relapse (6,60) yet have been found to increase the likelihood of cessation for older women as compared with men in one prospective study (61). Therefore, learning more about how women cope with negative affect or stress during cessation and maintenance is necessary to identify healthy alternatives to smoking for women.

Women and men with more negative affect were found to have the best outcomes with supportive counseling interventions, whereas individuals with less pretreatment negative affect benefited most from skills training. In addition, the role of social support in buffering stress (62) suggests that women may benefit from interpersonal support in their cessation efforts more than men (63). Identifying individuals' levels of negative affect, stress, and support can be helpful in guiding the approach to intervention for individual women.

Weight Concerns

Many women report weight gain as a deterrent to smoking cessation and that weight concerns or actual gains in weight are related to their return to smoking. Studies suggest that 80% of all quitters will gain at least some weight and that the average amount is 5 to 8 lb (14,26,64–66); however, when female smokers are asked how much weight they would be willing to gain if they quit smoking, 75% answered 5 lb or less (40% answered 0 lb) (67). Intolerance to weight gain is so endemic among women that it constitutes a serious obstacle to quitting, remaining abstinent, and even contemplating quitting (26). The physician must acknowledge the concern over weight gain and help the smoker use strategies to prevent or decrease the likelihood of its occurrence. Strategies such as the use of nicotine gum (68a) or bupropion (68b) for delaying or decreasing weight gain are discussed later in this chapter.

Effect of Illness

A physician's effect on a patient's smoking also has been demonstrated to vary greatly with the context for change. The patient who is symptomatic or already ill is more likely to respond to the physician's advice than the patient who feels well and has few if any symptoms or abnormal findings (69,70). Randomized trials have shown high biochemically verified, sustained quit rates (50%–63%) at 6 months for patients who were advised to quit smoking by their physician after having an MI or after having been told they have CAD; also, significantly higher rates (65%–75%) were seen in patients who received additional counseling by health educators or nurses either by telephone or in person (70,71). These cessation rates are directly related to the severity of disease (70,72). Cessation rates are lower (30%–40%) when intervention is directed at those smokers who are not ill but who are at high risk for infarction (73). This relationship between cessation and disease status is consistent with the principles of the Health-Belief Model (74,75), which state that people are more likely to stop smoking if they 1) perceive themselves to be vulnerable to the actual effects of a particular behavior (e.g., smoking), and 2) determine that the benefits of change outweigh the costs.

Literature on the relationship of gender to smoking cessation in the face of CAD is scant. One study of patients with evidence of CAD demonstrated that women were less likely to stop smoking than were men ($p < 0.01$) (70). This is an area that still requires a substantial amount of research.

Summary of Factors Affecting Women's Smoking

Women's reasons for smoking and factors that affect their smoking are somewhat different than those for men. Some preliminary research suggests that women may be more sensitive to nicotine and therefore report greater dependency, even though they are lighter smokers. Women who are at home with children full time have higher rates of smoking than other categories of women. Women also report feeling more pressure from others to quit; this pressure is most often from their children and other family members. Stress and negative affect seem to be important factors influencing smoking cessation in women; they often smoke to relieve high levels of depression, anger, anxiety, or emotional discomfort, which often triggers relapse. Weight gain is a deterrent to smoking cessation in women and relates to their risk of relapse as well. Each of the noted factors must be taken into account if the physician is to be successful in treating female smokers.

Interventions for Smoking Among Women

Importance of the Health Care Provider

Several reasons exist as to why physicians and other members of the health care team can and should play a major role in helping women make behavioral changes. First, physicians are perceived by the general public as the most reliable and credible source of health information and advice (76), and physicians can significantly affect patient behaviors, such as smoking (2), diet (77), and adherence to medical regimens (78,79). Patients generally prefer to receive as much information as possible from physicians, who often do not appreciate this desire and underestimate how much information patients actually want (80,81). Second, physicians and the health care system have contact with at least 80% of the adults in the United States each year (82) and are thus an immediately available and potent source of information about the prevention of CAD for over 120 million individuals. Data from NHIS indicate that Americans visit a physician an average of 6 times per year (82), with the figure being higher for women. In addition, women visit pediatricians with their young children, making this another potential opportunity for lifestyle intervention to occur. Third, people think more seriously about their health and the impact of their lifestyle on it when they are in a physician's office or a hospital than at any other time. This window of opportunity can be used by physicians to reinforce smoking cessation messages to patients and their families. Furthermore, physicians who provide a continuity of care can repeatedly educate, intervene, and follow up with women who need to alter their lifestyle behaviors (83).

Finally, patients generally do not want to go to special programs for help in altering unhealthy behaviors. More than 90% of smokers who have quit smoking have done so on their own without formal smoking intervention programs (84), and most current smokers would prefer to stop without such a program. Physicians and other providers in the health care setting are not perceived as special programs; they are part of the natural environment of individuals who may require help for reduction of risk for CAD (85).

Evidence from both observational studies and clinical trials indicates that physicians who intervene with their smoking patients, no matter how briefly, have a significant impact on cigarette smoking behavior (3). In April 1996, the Agency for Health Care Practice Research issued the Smoking Cessation Guideline for Health Care Providers (3). In the development of this guideline, the smoking intervention literature was summarized, and the following conclusion was drawn: "Simple advice by one's physician to stop smoking is more effective than no advice at all, and as the physician-delivered smoking intervention becomes more intensive, the effects are greater" (3). Another conclusion was that the success of an intervention increases with the number of intervention modalities used, the number of health care professionals involved in the intervention, and the number of follow-up assessments conducted.

Studies also have demonstrated an increase in the likelihood that physicians will intervene with smokers and that they will have a favorable impact on patients' smoking behavior if 1) physicians are trained to deliver brief interventions and 2) general office procedures are in place that cue the physician to intervene with smokers and provide follow-up (3). To keep the interventions brief and to meet the special needs of patients, physicians can also refer patients to special programs or have someone in their office provide intervention and follow-up. Women making attempts to quit are more likely than men to use cessation programs (e.g., from mental health professionals) to provide some type of assistance and tend to prefer formal smoking cessation groups or help from health professionals (84,86).

Overcoming Barriers to Provider Interventions

Although physicians are generally aware of the benefits of implementing preventive interventions, a large percentage of physicians often do not intervene with lifestyle behaviors (83). Physicians report several barriers to providing such intervention, including time constraints, poor intervention skills, and the beliefs that they are not effective in their health behavior interventions and that patients do not want to talk about lifestyle behaviors when being seen for other problems. Other factors include reimbursement issues and the limited integration of prevention activities into office practice.

Barriers to physicians' implementation of interventions can be overcome. Physicians can achieve the skill level necessary for effective interventions with very little training. These interventions can be relatively brief (3–4 min) if they are focused and use the services of office staff, consultants, special programs, and supportive aids such as self-help materials. They also can be integrated easily into the outpatient encounter with office systems that are set up to facilitate integration with other services. Surveys have demonstrated that patients welcome their physicians' input for health behavior change; in fact, even patients who do not alter their behavior are more satisfied with (87) and more likely to refer other patients to those physicians who do intervene than to those who do not (2).

Many patients and physicians understandably are concerned about the lack of reimbursement for prevention-oriented visits; however, physicians can use legitimate billable diagnoses to receive reimbursement. For example, in most cases, physicians can receive reimbursement from third-party payers for patients with smoking-related problems (e.g., bronchitis). Reimbursement policies vary from state to state and among different insurers and types of policies.

Finally, physicians must have realistic expectations about the possibilities of health behavior change and adopt a new (or at least modified) mindset when dealing with behavioral change for risk-factor reduction. Change often comes slowly, and sometimes it seems as though little is accomplished. For example, smokers often quit three or four times over a period of approximately 5 years before they are successful in the long term (6). From a population perspective, there have been remarkable changes in smoking in the United States over the past 30 years, and the health professions have played an important role.

Although physicians and other providers in the health care system have a major role in the prevention of CAD, their intervention efforts do not exist in a vacuum; rather, these efforts occur simultaneously with other health promotion activities (88). Education is available through the media, worksites, and schools. Voluntary organizations and legislation have impacted on public knowledge and smoking in public places. Physicians, other health care providers, and the health care system as a whole are integral and important parts of these combined efforts (89).

Smoking Intervention Strategies for the Physician

Given that a large percentage of female smokers visit a physician or clinical setting each year, the clinician's role in facilitating smoking cessation, providing educational materials, or referring patients to additional services is important from both a clinical and public health perspective. Smoking cessation advice should be regarded as the minimal standard of practice, and when possible physicians should go beyond providing advice (3,90).

A brief intervention strategy that can be used by physicians to help female smokers stop smoking or maintain cessation is discussed below. This strategy can be accomplished in 3 to 10 minutes, depending on how ready the smoker is to stop smoking and how much assistance the physician is willing to provide. The strategy is based on the following assumptions:

1. Physicians have little time to spend counseling; therefore, interventions need to be brief.

2. Women are interested in stopping smoking.

3. Smokers who quit return to smoking several times before achieving long-term abstinence.

4. A return to smoking is not a failure; it can be used as a learning experience to help patients prepare for the next time.

5. Smoking cessation is a process, not a one-time event; it progresses from becoming aware of the need to stop smoking, to taking action, to maintaining cessation.

6. Women who are stopping smoking often have special needs to which attention must be paid (e.g., low confidence, the need for self-management and stress reduction skills, and concerns about weight management).

7. Pharmacologic therapies should be used when appropriate.

8. Other types of health care providers can assist the physician with interventions.

Three basic models for physician involvement can be used: 1) brief physician-delivered counseling, 2) brief physician-delivered counseling plus physician assistance, and 3) brief physician-delivered counseling with referral for comprehensive individual or group intervention (either one or multiple sessions) (91). An algorithm that incorporates all three models (Fig. 2-2) has been created over 15 years of research and development by Ockene and colleagues (91–93) at the University of Massachusetts Medical School as part of their provider-delivered smoking-intervention training program. This algorithm is similar to, but more extensive than, the one developed by the National Cancer Institute (94). It has been tested in several settings and found to be efficacious (2); i.e., when physicians deliver the 3- to 10-minute intervention, they have a significantly greater effect on their patients' smoking than

SMOKING INTERVENTION MODEL

ASK About Smoking at Every Opportunity

A. SMOKING STATUS:
    1. "Do you smoke?"
    2. "How much do you smoke?"
B. MOTIVATION:
    1. "Are you interested in stopping smoking?"
    2. "What are your reasons for wanting to stop smoking?"
C. PAST EXPERIENCE WITH QUITTING:
    1. "Have you ever tried to stop smoking before?"
    2. If so, "What happened?" "Why did you start smoking again?"
D. NICOTINE DEPENDENCY:
    1. "How soon after waking do you have your first cigarette?"
    2. "Did you experience symptoms of withdrawal when you stopped before?"
       (e.g., craving nicotine, irritability, anxiety, difficulty concentrating,
       restlessness, increased appetite)

ADVISE All Smokers to Stop

A. EXPRESS CONCERN: "I am concerned about your health and your family's
    health if you continue to smoke."
B. PERSONALIZE ADVICE TO QUIT: Refer to smoker's personal health concerns
    or clinical condition, reasons for cessation, smoking history, family history,
    personal interests, or social roles. Include benefits of quitting for smoker.

ASSIST Smoker in Stopping

A. IDENTIFY PERSONAL TRIGGERS for smoking and BRAINSTORM
    STRATEGIES for handling major triggers/urges.
B. PROVIDE SELF-HELP MATERIALS: Tailor materials and introduction of
    materials to smoker's needs. Provide list of referral resources.
C. DEVELOP PLAN FOR STOPPING:
    1. For the smoker who is READY TO QUIT: Set a quit date; help the smoker
       pick a date within the next 4 weeks, acknowledging that no time is ideal.
    2. For the HIGHLY NICOTINE-DEPENDENT SMOKER: a) Develop a tapering program;
       or b) consider prescribing nicotine replacement therapy (patch or nicotine gum).
    3. For the smoker who is NOT WILLING TO QUIT NOW: Provide motivational
       literature; encourage smoker to consider quitting; and ask about smoking
       again at the next visit/contact.

ARRANGE Follow-up Visit

A. SET FOLLOW-UP VISIT:
    1. For the smoker who SET A QUIT DATE: Set visit on or within 1–2 weeks
       after the quit date. For the smoker who DID NOT SET A QUIT DATE: Set
       visit within 4–6 weeks after initial contact.
    2. First follow-up visit: a) Assess smoking status and address problem
       areas; and b) develop relapse prevention strategies.
    3. Set a second follow-up visit for 1–2 months after first. Continue to set
       follow-up visits as appropriate.
B. FOLLOW-UP WITH SMOKER ON REFERRALS made to other cessation services.

FIGURE 2-2 Smoking intervention model.

physicians who provide advice only. The following overview of what the physician can do in the smoking cessation process must be adapted to the individual physician's needs and situation.

Brief Counseling (3–5 min)

The four basic brief counseling steps are as follows:

1. Ask about/assess smoking
2. Advise cessation
3. Assist (minimal)
4. Arrange for follow-up visit

The first step assesses whether the patient is interested in stopping and whether she is nicotine dependent (*see* Assessing Nicotine Dependency). The second step is advise cessation in a personalized way, ideally including the patient's reasons for wanting to quit. The third step includes providing self-help materials (Box 2-2) and nicotine-replacement therapy (NRT) or bupropion if appropriate (*see* Pharmacotherapy). During the fourth step, it is productive to convey that this issue is important enough to warrant close follow-up. Because the effectiveness of smoking cessation interventions are related to their intensity, it is beneficial to expand beyond this model when possible. Remember, even limited counseling is better than none.

Brief Behavioral Counseling with Physician Assistance (5–10 min)

Brief patient-centered behavioral counseling that is focused to provide assistance in developing specific strategies for cessation has been demonstrated to be significantly more effective in tobacco cessation than advice alone (2). It emphasizes the importance of the patient's input in developing an effective plan for change and can be accomplished using an additional 3 to 5 minutes of the physician's time (*see* Fig. 2-2). Of course, more time can be spent if desired or if available. A dose-response relationship exists between the intensity and duration of intervention and its effectiveness. The sequence of patient-centered counseling steps presented here is interchangeable and should be adapted to the physician's style and the patient's needs. The following topics help in the development of a plan for change.

Assessing Motivation—The patient's reasons for wanting to stop may be different from the physician's reasons for wanting her to do so. A patient may be more concerned about the impact of her smoking on her children than on her risk for disease. For some patients, lack of motivation may be related to a lack of confidence in their ability to stop smoking.

Box 2-2 Self-Help Materials for Smoking Cessation

For Physicians

   Clinical Practice Guideline: Smoking Cessation
   Agency for Healthcare Policy and Research
   To order: (202) 512-1800

   *How To Help Your Patients Stop Smoking: A National Cancer Institute
      Manual for Physicians*
   To order: (800) 4-CANCER

   *Clinical Opportunities for Smoking Intervention: A Guide for the Busy
      Physician*
   To order: (301) 592-8573

   AAFP Stop Smoking Kit
   American Academy of Family Physicians
   To order: (800) 944-0000

For Patients

   Clearing the Air
   National Cancer Institute
   To order: (800) 4-CANCER

   Smart Move
   American Cancer Society
   To order: Contact local ACS Chapter

   Freedom from Smoking for You and Your Baby
   American Lung Association
   To order: Contact local ALA Chapter

   Quitting Times: A Magazine for Women Who Smoke
   Fox Chase Cancer Center
   To order: Contact Massachusetts Tobacco Education Clearinghouse
      (617) 482-9485

Asking About Past Experiences (Including Resources Used and Problems Encountered)—Exploration of past experiences with cessation helps patients focus on possible past successes, no matter how small, and encourages them to believe that they are capable of cessation. Eighty percent of all smokers have stopped some time in the past (6). The physician can help patients focus on the resources they used and the positive feelings they had about themselves when they were nonsmokers.

Past experiences with cessation help prepare for potential problems and can reveal coping strategies that were successful in the past and can be used for the current cessation effort. For women, past problems often include difficulties with weight gain, depression, or anxiety. Once the problem is identified, possible coping strategies can be identified. For example, increasing exercise may prevent increases in appetite and weight. A patient can be asked open-ended questions about substitute behaviors, such as "What might you do instead of smoking?" If the individual cannot think of anything, ask more focused questions such as "Have you ever tried using exercise when you have had the urge to smoke?" or "Have you ever used deep breathing as a relaxation approach?"

Assessing Nicotine Dependency—It is important to determine whether the smoker is physiologically addicted to nicotine. Assessment of the patient's past experiences with cessation can determine whether she had experienced symptoms of nicotine withdrawal. The more intense the withdrawal symptoms were in previous quit attempts, the more likely they are to be a problem again. Assessment of withdrawal and the use of a specially developed scale for measuring addiction, the Fagerstrom Addiction Scale (Box 2-3) (95), can help the physician to decide whether to suggest the use of pharmacologic therapy in addition to educational and behavioral interventions, including tapering of cigarette usage (*see* Addressing Physiologic Dependency). Another sensitive indicator of possible difficulty in quitting is the length of previous quit attempts. On the average, withdrawal symptoms peak at 3 to 4 days, so a pattern of multiple attempts to quit with return to smoking after only a few days suggests that nicotine dependency is highly related to relapse for that individual. The smoker should 1) be alerted to the symptoms associated with withdrawal, 2) be aware that these symptoms decrease quickly, and 3) be offered a variety of approaches (e.g., NRT, bupropion, tapering nicotine intake before stopping "cold turkey") for handling them. With NRT, the smoker is able to attend to the psychological and behavioral factors of cessation while the drug is gradually discontinued (96).

Develop a Plan and Arrange Follow-up—The counseling sequence leads to a plan for change. The plan may focus on immediate goals, such as not staying at the table after completing dinner, changing cigarette brands, or learning a relaxation technique. It also can focus on goals closer to the endpoint, such as using pharmacologic therapies, relaxation techniques, or physical exercise in place of cigarettes. A written plan often indicates commitment from both the

---

Box 2-3 Fagerstrom Tolerance Questionnaire*

1. How many cigarettes a day do you smoke?
   0-15 [0]   16-25 [1]   25+ [3]
2. What is the nicotine yield per cigarette of your usual brand?
   0.3-0.8 g [0]   0.9-1.5 g [1]   1.6-2.2 g [2]
3. Do you inhale?
   Never [0]   Sometimes [1]   Always [2]
4. Do you smoke more during the morning than during the rest of the day?
   No [0]   Yes [1]
5. How soon after you wake up do you smoke your first cigarette?
   More than 30 min [0]   Less than 30 min [1]
6. Of all the cigarettes you smoke during the day, which would you most hate to give up?
   The first cigarette of the day [1]   All other answers [0]
7. Do you find it difficult to refrain from smoking in places where it is forbidden (e.g., in church, at the library, in a no-smoking cinema)?
   No [0]   Yes [1]
8. Do you smoke even if you are so ill that you are in bed most of the day?
   No [0]   Yes [1]

---

*This questionnaire measures the degree of physical dependence on the nicotine in cigarettes (scores for each answer are in brackets). A score of 0–3 indicates a light dependence; 4–7, medium dependence; 8–11, full dependence. Recommended revisions to the questionnaire include eliminating items 2 and 3 and adding additional categories to items 1 and 5 (97).
Adapted from Fagerstrom K. Measuring degree of physical dependency to tobacco smoking with reference to individualization of treatment. Addict Behav. 1978;3:235–41.

physician and patient and can include referral for some intensive assistance. Finally, end with an arrangement for a follow-up visit.

Brief Counseling with Referral to Group or Individual Counseling

The physician may refer patients for additional assistance to nurses, psychologists, social workers, and health educators for individual counseling or group intervention. When making a referral, it is important to spend a few minutes to ensure that the patient understands the reason for the referral and the process she needs to follow to meet with the specialist. Optimally, physicians should become familiar with referral resources in their own institution or community and develop a list of places or people to whom referrals can be made.

Addressing Physiologic Dependency—A formal evaluation of nicotine dependency can be made with the Fagerstrom Tolerance Questionnaire (FTQ) (*see*

Box 2-3) (95) or the revised FTQ (97). People who smoke more than a pack per day, those who smoke within 30 minutes of waking, and those who have difficulty refraining from smoking in public areas are likely to have the greatest difficulty with withdrawal symptoms. If the smoker reports having had intense withdrawal symptoms in the past, has a pattern of relapsing within a few hours or days, and scores high on the FTQ, then nicotine dependence probably plays an important role in maintaining the behavior. If the smoker is ready to quit but is highly dependent, either nicotine fading or pharmacologic interventions should be considered; for other patients, nicotine fading may serve as an intermediate goal.

Nicotine Fading

Nicotine fading has two components: 1) brand switching to a lower-nicotine-level cigarette, and 2) gradual reduction of number of cigarettes (i.e., tapering) (98). Switching brands one or more times over several weeks, in combination with reducing the number of cigarettes smoked by approximately one half per week, can reduce withdrawal symptoms in the person who smokes heavily; it also can help wean a smoker off a favorite brand. When tapering, it is important to remind the smoker not to inhale more deeply or smoke more of the cigarette than she did in the past. In addition, the smoker should be made aware that she should not cover the vents in the filter of lower-nicotine cigarettes because that increases nicotine availability. Decreasing the number of cigarettes per day by eliminating the "lower need" cigarettes, as defined by the patient, increases the smoker's sense of self-confidence. Tapering to fewer than 15 cigarettes per day is a realistic goal before quitting completely.

Pharmacotherapy

Pharmacotherapy includes the nicotine replacement products of nicotine-containing gum, transdermal nicotine patch, nicotine nasal spray, nicotine inhaler, and the non-nicotine product bupropion. It is strongly recommended that each of these products be used with two behavioral treatments. None are "magic" bullets. Table 2-1 lists the different products and their dosages and recommendations. The gum, approved in 1984, has been shown to be effective in aiding cessation when used in combination with behavioral treatment (99); however, certain side effects do exist, and the high rate of improper use of the gum has limited its effectiveness. Errors in use include: 1) chewing the gum too vigorously, rather than primarily "parking" it (i.e., letting the gum sit between the check and teeth for proper absorption; 2) using too few pieces per day (the recommended number is approximately half the number of ciga-

Table 2-1 Comparison of Currently Available Forms of Pharmacotherapy

Pharmacotherapy	Brand Name	Strength	Dose	Duration	Cost*
Transdermal nicotine (patches)					
Over the counter	Nicotrol	15 mg	1 patch for 16 h	6 wk	$155
	Nicoderm	7, 14, 21 mg	1 patch for 16 or 24 h	10 wk	$265
Prescription	Pro-Step	11, 21 mg	1 patch for 24 h	6–12 wk	$45.99 (box of 10) $42.69 (box of 7)
Nicotine polacrilex (gum)					
Over the counter	Nicorette	2, 4 mg	1 piece every 1–2 h	12 wk	$300 (full duration)
Nicotine nasal spray					$37 per
Prescription	Nicotrol NS	10 mg/mL (1 mg/dose delivered)	1–2 doses/h (maximum, 5 doses/h)	12 wk	bottle (100 doses)
Nicotine inhaler	Nicotrol	10 mg/cartridge			
Prescription	inhaler	(4 mg delivered)	6–16 cartridges/ day	12 wk initial treatment; 6–12 wk gradual reduction	$45 (box of 42 cartridges)
Bupropion hydrochloride SR	Zyban	150, 300 mg	150 mg/day for 3 days; increase to 300 mg/day (150 mg bid)	7–12 wk	$21 or less per week
Prescription					

*Prices as of December 1998.

rettes smoked); and 3) using it for too short a period of time (the recommended period is 3 to 6 months with tapered use).

The transdermal nicotine patch, marketed in slightly different formulations and delivery systems, also has been shown to be effective in aiding cessation of smoking (3). It provides a more passive delivery system (thereby improving compliance), allows for a more continuous delivery of nicotine, and avoids the gastrointestinal and oral side effects of the gum. Proper use is important for preventing relapse. Physicians should be clear on proper use by reading the insert materials provided.

Nicotine nasal spray has been approved for use in the United States. One study that tested the safety and efficacy of nicotine nasal spray found that it significantly enhanced success rates of continuous abstinence over placebo (100a). Reported side effects included throat irritation, coughing, sneezing, runny eyes and nose, palpitations, and nausea.

The nicotine inhaler is the newest NRT, being made available by prescription in June 1998. It addresses the pharmacologic, behavioral, and sensory stimuli aspects of smoking. The nicotine is absorbed through the lining of the mouth. Significantly more participants who had used the nicotine inhalers were continuously abstinent compared with those who had used the placebo inhalers (100b).

The most common problem is for the smoker to perceive NRT as a "magic" solution; a more appropriate way to present any formulation is as an aid to "take the edge off" the physical craving while the person "learns" to become a nonsmoker. Both the nicotine gum and patch are now available over the counter.

A sustained-release form of bupropion has also become available for treating smokers. It has been demonstrated to be effective for smoking cessation and was accompanied by reduced weight gain and minimal side effects (68b). Buproprion approximately doubles 6- to 12-month abstinence rates compared with those of the placebo. It may be a good choice for women who prefer an alternative to nicotine replacement and who do not have a history of seizures.

There is limited evidence that combining patch and gum or patch and bupropion may slightly increase quit rates over monotherapy. Combination therapy may be considered in persons who have failed on monotherapy.

Physiologic Feedback

Physiologic feedback with exhaled carbon monoxide (CO) levels, using small handheld devices, can provide a powerful motivator to people who are stopping smoking. The CO test can provide a baseline for the patient before tapering or cessation and can be used as feedback during the cessation process, because exhaled CO varies directly with the amount of tobacco smoked. Also, patients often perceive such changes as directly related to health benefits.

Addressing Smoking Cessation and Weight Gain

The Lung Health Study determined that although some weight gain can be delayed minimally through the use of the 2-mg nicotine gum, weight gain is a natural consequence of smoking cessation (68a). The average weight gain of 2 to 3 kg (101) cannot be equated to the medical risk of smoking a pack of cigarettes every day, but it is still an issue that is important to many women, providing a common excuse for returning to smoking. Several factors have been implicated, including an increase in metabolism from nicotine intake (102,103) and a change in preference for sweets after cessation (104). These biological factors, in combination with the use of food as a behavioral substitute, make it important to address weight management explicitly in most treatment programs (101,105).

When talking with a woman on the subject of potential weight gain, it is important to do the following: 1) acknowledge her concern, 2) discuss her perceptions of the cost/benefit of weight gain and smoking cessation, 3) discuss the importance of exercise and relaxation techniques as alternatives to smoking and food, 4) discuss the importance of monitoring food use and the need for healthful snacks, and 5) help her plan for how she will deal with difficult situations.

Addressing Psychological Dependency: Assessment of Behavioral Patterns Associated with Smoking

Assessment of behavioral patterns associated with smoking is helpful. Which cigarettes does the patient identify as "high-need"? Which are "low-need" cigarettes? Asking the smoker to use a scale of one to five for degree of need is often helpful. Self-monitoring or recording of cigarette use often reveals to both the smoker and the physician specific areas that need further attention. The following three general strategies for managing high-need or high-risk situations without smoking are useful: 1) avoidance of specific situations that bring on an urge to smoke; 2) substitution of alternative behaviors incompatible with smoking cigarettes when urges arise; and 3) use of cognitive restructuring to reshape positive beliefs about smoking or to counteract irrational thinking. Initially, avoidance of high-risk situations (e.g., going drinking with friends who smoke) may be most useful; however, this usually must be followed by developing alternative coping strategies.

A particularly valuable adjunct to smoking intervention is relaxation training. One of the most common reasons given for relapse is the inability to handle stressful situations (60). Habitual smokers may report having few, if any, alternative ways to manage stress. Certain types of relaxation training (e.g., deep breathing, brief meditation, visualization exercises) can be used as effective functional equivalents to smoking, because they can be used for a few moments at a time under almost any circumstances and may provide two of the benefits associated with smoking (i.e., a brief break from ongoing activity and a physiologically active relaxation effect). Relaxation training is also an important technique for weight management.

Preventing Relapse

A major difficulty in smoking cessation, as with other substance abuse behaviors, is maintenance of the changed behavior. As many as 70% of people who stop smoking relapse within a year. Up to 65% of people who quit smoking by themselves relapse within the first week after cessation (49). Women are slightly more prone to relapse than men.

Relapse prevention as a treatment technique was originally developed by Marlatt and Gordon (106) to help prevent the relapse of alcohol abuse and has been extrapolated for use in the treatment of nicotine abuse. Smokers and ex-smokers who learn relapse prevention skills maintain cessation longer and, if they relapse, smoke fewer cigarettes than do their counterparts who do not receive such training (107). An excellent discussion of relapse prevention from a self-management perspective is presented by Shiffman and colleagues (108). Many of the behavioral strategies mentioned above also are directed toward relapse prevention. Most people are susceptible to the abstinence violation effect, which is what happens when a person who has vowed to avoid a certain behavior "slips" and experiences feelings of guilt, shame, and loss of confidence that often lead quickly to re-engaging in the behavior (106). Recognizing in advance the possibility of the abstinence violation effect often protects the individual from having a highly charged emotional reaction to a slip and, thus, a full-blown relapse.

Setting Up the Office Practice To Support Interventions

If physicians are to implement smoking intervention, then learning intervention strategies and developing skills is not enough. Office systems need to be set up to remind the physician to intervene and provide the materials needed for intervention. If possible, office staff can assess and document smoking status for every patient at each clinical visit to ensure that all smokers are identified before they see a physician. Smoking status (i.e., current, former, never) can be easily added to the list of other vital signs (e.g., blood pressure, pulse, temperature, respiratory rate) that are routinely documented in a patient's chart during an office visit. This alone has been found to increase cessation rates among patients seen by a physician (109). Educational materials and referral lists should be easily available in the office for quick access and routine distribution to patients.

Summary

To stop smoking, a smoker must perceive this change as being beneficial and must believe that she can stop smoking. From the behavioral perspective, the smoker must learn new skills or enhance old skills that can be used in place of cigarettes to deal with problems as they arise. A smoker who demonstrates a high physiologic dependency on nicotine would benefit from pharmacologic intervention or tapering. This would allow her to work on the behavioral aspects, without needing to deal with the physiologic withdrawal at the same time. Finally, the physician and patient must be aware of the potential for relapse and understand the process that smokers go through when stopping long term. Follow-up is important. An important point is that brief advice or counseling can be effective. For the physician who wishes to go further, there are some very effective strategies; alternatively, the more complicated smoker can be referred to other providers.

REFERENCES

1. **Willett W, Greene A, Stampfer M, et al.** Relative and absolute excess risks of coronary heart disease among women who smoke cigarettes. N Engl J Med. 1987;317: 1303–9.

2. **Ockene J, Kristeller J, Goldberg R, et al.** Increasing the efficacy of physician-delivered smoking intervention: a randomized clinical trial. J Gen Intern Med. 1991;6: 1–8.

3. **Fiore M, Bailey W, Cohen S, et al.** Smoking Cessation: Clinical Practice Guideline No. 18. Rockville, MD: USDHHS, PHS, AHCPR Publication 96-0692; 1996.

4. **Parker S, Tong T, Bolden S, Wingo P.** Cancer Statistics. CA Cancer J Clin. 1996; 46:5–27.

5. **Bartecchi C, MacKenzie T, Schrier R.** The human costs of tobacco use. N Engl J Med. 1994;330:907–12.

6. **U.S. Department of Health and Human Services.** Reducing the health consequences of smoking: 25 years of progress: a report of the Surgeon General. PHS, Centers for Disease Control, Center for Chronic Disease Prevention and Health Promotion, Office of Smoking and Health. USDHHS Publication CDC 89-8411; 1989.

7. **Oparil S.** Pathophysiology of sudden coronary death in women: implications for prevention. Circulation. 1998;97:2103–5.

8. **Prescott E, Hippe M, Schnohr P, et al.** Smoking and risk of mycardial infarction in women and men: longitudinal population study. BMJ. 1998;316:1043–7.

9. **LaCroix A, Lang J, Scherr P, et al.** Smoking and mortality among older men and women in three communities. N Engl J Med. 1991;324:1619–25.

10. **Frost P, Davis B, Burlando A, et al.** Coronary heart disease risk factors in men and women aged 60 years and older: findings from the Systolic Hypertension in the Elderly Program (SHEP). Circulation. 1996;94:26–34.

11. **Stadel B.** Oral contraceptives and cardiovascular disease. N Engl J Med. 1981;305: 672–7.

12. **Thorogood M, Mann J, Murphy M, Vessey M.** Is oral contraceptive use still associated with an increased risk of fatal myocardial infarction? Report of a case control study. Br J Obstet Gynaecol. 1991;98:1245–53.

13. **Jonas M, Oates J, Ockene J, Hennekens C.** Statement on smoking and cardiovascular disease for health care professionals [Position Statement]. Circulation. 1992;86:1664–9.

14. **U.S. Department of Health and Human Services.** The Health Benefits of Smoking Cessation: A Report of the Surgeon General. Washington, DC: U.S. Govt Printing Office. USDHHS Publication CDC 90-8416; 1990.

15. **U.S. Department of Health and Human Services.** The Surgeon General's Report on the Health Consequences of Smoking for Women. USDHHS Publication; 1980.

16. **Barnes DE, Bero LA.** Why review articles on the health effects of passive smoking reach different conclusions. JAMA. 1998;279:1566–70.

17. **Rosenberg L, Palmer J, Shapiro S.** Decline in risk of myocardial infarction among women who stop smoking. N Engl J Med. 1990;322:213–7.

18. **Kawachi I, Colditz G, Stampfer M, et al.** Smoking cessation and time course of decreased risks of coronary heart disease in middle-aged women. Arch Intern Med. 1994;154:169–76.

19. **Sparrow D, Dawber T, Colton T.** The influence of cigarette smoking on prognosis after a first myocardial infarction: a report from the Framingham Study Group. J Chronic Dis. 1978;31:425–32.

20. **Salonen J.** Stopping smoking and long-term mortality after acute myocardial infarction. Br Heart J. 1980;43:463–9.

21. **Gerace T, Hollis J, Ockene J, Svendsen K.** Cigarette Smoking in the Multiple Risk Factor Intervention Trial (MRFIT) (Monograph). In: Ockene JK, Shaten J, Neaton J (eds). Smoking Cessation and Change in Diastolic Blood Pressure, Body Weight, Plasma Lipids. Prev Med. 1991;20:602–28.

22. **Centers for Disease Control and Prevention.** Cigarette smoking among adults: United States, 1994. MMWR Morb Mortal Wkly Rep. 1995;45:588–90.

23. **Centers for Disease Control and Prevention.** Cigarette smoking among women of reproductive age: United States, 1987–92. MMWR Morb Mortal Wkly Rep. 1994;43: 789–97.

24. **Jarvis M.** Gender and smoking: Do women really find it harder to give up? Br J Addiction. 1984;79:383–7.

25. **Schoenborn C, Boyd G.** Smoking and other tobacco use: United States, 1987. National Center for Health Statistics (NCHS). Vital Health Stat. 1989;10:169.

26. **Pomerleau C.** Smoking and nicotine-replacement treatment issues specific to women. Am J Health Behav. 1996;20:291–9.

27. **Centers for Disease Control and Prevention, National Center for Chronic Disease Prevention and Health Promotion, Office of Smoking and Health.** Preventing Tobacco Use Among Young People: A Report of the Surgeon General. Atlanta. USDHHS, PHS Publication; 1994.

28. **Husten C, Chrismon J, Reddy M.** Trends and effects of cigarette smoking among girls and women in the United States, 1965–1993. J Am Med Wom Assoc. 1996;51: 11–8.

29. **National Center for Health Statistics.** Health promotion and disease prevention: United States, 1985. In: Schoenborn C (ed). Atlanta, GA: USDHHS, PHS Publication 88-1591; 1988.

30. **Fingerhut L, Kleinman J, Kendrick J.** Smoking before, during, and after pregnancy. Am J Public Health. 1990;80:541–4.

31. **Williamson D, Serdula M, Kendrick J, Binkin N.** Comparing the prevalence of smoking in pregnant and nonpregnant women, 1985–1986. JAMA. 1989;261:70–4.

32. **Ventura S, Martin J, Mathews T, Clarke S.** Advance Report of Final Mortality Statistics, 1994. MMWR Morb Mortal Wkly Rep. 1996;44(Suppl).

33. **Sexton M, Hebel J.** A clinical trial of change in maternal smoking and its effect on birth weight. JAMA. 1984;251:911–5.

34. **Ershoff D, Mullen P, Quinn V.** A randomized trial of a serialized self-help smoking cessation program for pregnant women in an HMO. Am J Public Health. 1989;79:182–7.

35. **Centers for Disease Control and Prevention.** Cigarette smoking among adults: United States, 1993. MMWR Morb Mortal Wkly Rep. 1994;43:925–30.

36. **Winkleby MA, Kraemer HC, Ahn DK, Varady AN.** Ethnic and socioeconomic differences in cardiovascular disease risk factors: findings for women from the Third National Health and Nutrition Examination Survey, 1988–1994. JAMA. 1998;280:356–62.

37. **Caraballo RS, Giovino GA, Pechacek TF, et al.** Racial and ethnic differences in serum cotinine levels of cigarette smokers: Third National Health and Nutrition Examination Survey, 1988–1991. JAMA. 1998;280:135–139.

38. **Perez-Stable EJ, Herrera B, Jacob P, Berlowitz NL.** Nicotine metabolism and intake in black and white smokers. JAMA. 1998;280:152–6.

39. **Graham H.** Women's smoking and family health. Soc Sci Med. 1987;25:47–56.

40. **Mayer J, Hawkins B, Todd R.** A randomized evaluation of smoking cessation interventions for pregnant women at a WIC clinic. Am J Public Health. 1990;80:76–8.

41. **Fleisher L, Keintz M, Rimer B, et al.** Process evaluation of a minimal-contact smoking cessation program in an urban nutritional assistance (WIC) program. In: Advances in Cancer Control: Screening and Prevention Research. New York: Wiley-Liss; 1990: 95–106.

42a. **Kendrick J, Merritt R.** Women and smoking: an update for the 1990s. Am J Obstet Gynecol. 1996;175:528–35.

42b. **Lantz PM, House IS, Lepkowski JM, et al.** Socioeconomic factors, heath behaviors, and mortality: results from a nationally representative prospective study of U.S. adults. JAMA. 1998;279:1703–8.

43. **Orleans C, Jepson C, Resch N, Rimer B.** Quitting motives and barriers among older smokers: the 1986 Adult Use of Tobacco Survey revisited. Cancer. 1994;74(Suppl 7):2055–61.

44. **Rimer B, Orleans C.** Tailoring smoking cessation for older adults. Cancer. 1994; 74(Suppl 7):2051–4.

45. **Ruzek S.** Towards a more inclusive model of women's health. Am J Public Health. 1993;83:6–8.

46. **American Psychiatric Association.** Diagnostic and Statistical Manual of Mental Disorders. 4th ed. Washington, DC: American Psychiatric Association; 1994.

47. **West R, Hajek P, Belcher M.** Severity of withdrawal symptoms as a predictor of outcome of an attempt to quit smoking. Psychol Med. 1989;19:981–5.

48. **Gritz E, Berman B, Bastani R, Wu M.** A randomized trial of a self-help smoking cessation intervention in a nonvolunteer female population: testing the limits of the public health model. Health Psychol. 1992;11:280–9.

49. **Hughes J, Hatsukami D.** The nicotine withdrawal syndrome: a brief review and update. Int J Smoking Cessation. 1992;1:21–6.

50. **Pomerleau O, Collins A, Shiffman S, Pomerleau C.** Why some people smoke and others do not: new perspectives. J Consult Clin Psychol. 1993;6:723–31.

51. **Bjornson W, Rand C, Connett J, et al.** Gender differences in smoking cessation after 3 years in the Lung Health study. Am J Public Health. 1995;85:223–30.

52. **Jacobson B.** Beating the Ladykillers: Women and Smoking. London: Pluto Press; 1986.

53. **Graham H.** Smoking in pregnancy: the attitudes of expectant mothers. Soc Sci Med. 1976;10:399-405.

54. **Gabe J, Thorogood N.** Prescribed drug use and the management of every day life: the experiences of black and white working class women. Sociol Rev. 1986;34:737–72.

55. **March A, Matheson J.** Smoking attitudes and behavior. London: OPCS, Social Survey Division, HMSO, 1983.

56. **Royce J, Corbett K, Sorensen G, Ockene J.** Gender, social pressure, and smoking cessation: the Community Intervention Trial for Smoking Cessation at Baseline. Soc Sci Med. 1996;44:359–70.

57. **Gritz E, Nielsen I, Brooks L.** Smoking cessation and gender: the influence of physiological, psychological, and behavioral factors. J Am Med Women Assoc. 1996;51: 35–42.

58. **Solomon L, Flynn B.** Women who smoke. In: Orleans C, Slade J (eds). Nicotine Addiction: Principles and Management. New York: Oxford University Press; 1993:339–49.

59. **Sorensen G, Pechacek T.** Attitudes toward smoking cessation among men and women. J Behav Med. 1987;10:129–37.

60. **Shiffman S.** Relapse following smoking cessation: a situational analysis. J Consult Clin Psychol. 1982;50:71–86.

61. **Salive M, Blazer D.** Depression and smoking cessation in older adults: a longitudinal study. J Am Geriatr. 1993;41:1313–6.

62. **Cohen S, Syme S.** Social support and health. Orlando, FL: Academic Press; 1985.

63. **Fisher E, Lowe M, Levenkron J, Newman A.** Reinforcement and structural support of maintained risk reduction. In: Stuart R (ed). Adherence, Compliance, and Generalization in Behavioral Medicine. New York: Brunner/Mazel; 1982:145–68.

64. **Williamson D, Madans J, Anda R, et al.** Smoking cessation and severity of weight gain in a national cohort. N Engl J Med. 1991;324:739–45.

65. **Flegal K, Troiano R, Pamik E, et al.** The influence of smoking cessation on the prevalence of overweight in the United States. N Engl J Med. 1995;333:1165–70.

66. **Hall S, Ginsberg D, Jones R.** Smoking cessation and weight gain. J Consult Clin Psych. 1986;54:342–6.

67. **Pomerleau C, Kurth C.** Willingness of women smokers to tolerate postcessation weight gain. J Subst Abuse Treat. 1996.

68a. **Nides M, Rand C, Dolce J, et al.** Weight gain as a function of smoking cessation and 2-mg nicotine gum use among middle-aged smokers with mild lung impairment in the first 2 years of the Lung Health Study. Health Psychol. 1994;13:354–61.

68b. **Hurt R, Sachs D, Glover E, et al.** A comparison of sustained-released bupropion and placebo for smoking cessation. N Engl J Med. 1997;337:1195–1202.

69. **Ockene I, Ockene J (eds).** Prevention of Coronary Heart Disease. Boston: Little, Brown; 1992.

70. **Ockene J, Kristeller J, Goldberg R, et al.** Smoking cessation and severity of disease: the Coronary Artery Smoking Intervention Study. Health Psychol. 1992;11: 119–26.

71. **DeBusk R, Houston MN, Superko H, et al.** A case-management system for coronary risk factor modification after acute myocardial infarction. Ann Intern Med. 1994;120: 721–9.

72. **Frid D, Ockene I, Ockene J, et al.** Severity of angiographically proven coronary artery disease predicts smoking cessation. Am J Prev Med. 1991;7:131–5.

73. **Rose G, Hamilton P.** A randomized controlled trial of the effect on middle-aged men of advice to stop smoking. J Epidemiol Community Health. 1978;32:275–81.

74. **Becker M.** The Health Belief Model and personal health behavior. Health Educ Monographs. 1974;2:324–473.

75. **Rosenstock I.** The Health Belief Model: explaining health behavior through expectancies. In: Glanz K, Lewis F, Rimer R (eds). Health Behavior and Health Education: Theory, Research, and Practice. San Francisco: Jossey Bass, 1990.

76. **U.S. Department of Health, Education, and Welfare.** Healthy People: the Surgeon General's Report on Health Promotion and Disease Prevention. United States Department of Health and Human Services, Public Health Service; 1979.

77. **Glanz K.** Nutritional intervention: A behavioral and educational perspective. In: Ockene I, Ockene J (eds). Prevention of Coronary Heart Disease. Boston: Little, Brown;1992.

78. **Dunbar J.** Assessment of medication compliance: a review. In: Haynes R, Mattson M, Engebretson T (eds). Patient compliance to prescribed antihypertensive medication regimen. USDHHS, PHS Publication NIH 81-2101; 1988.

79. **Greenfield S, Kaplan S, Ware J, et al.** Patients' participation in medical care: effects on blood sugar control and quality of life in diabetes. J Gen Int Med. 1988;3:448–57.

80. **Waitzkin H.** Information giving in medical care. J Health Soc Behav. 1985;26: 81–101.

81. **Faden R, Becker C, Lewis C, et al.** Disclosure of information to patients in medical care. Med Care. 1981;19:718–33.

82. **U.S. Department of Health and Human Services.** Current Estimates from the National Health Interview Survey. Series 10: Data from the National Health Survey No. 190. Hyattsville, MD: PHS, CDC, NCHS, USDHHS Publication 95-1518; 1994.

83. **Ockene J.** Physician-delivered interventions for smoking cessation: strategies for increasing effectiveness. Prev Med. 1987;16:723–37.

84. **Fiore M, Novotny T, Pierce J, et al.** Methods used to quit smoking in the United States: do cessation programs help? JAMA. 1990;263:2760–5.

85. **Ockene J.** Towards a smoke-free society. Am J Public Health. 1984;74:1198–200.

86. **Owen N, Brown S.** Smokers unlikely to quit. J Behav Med. 1990;14:627–36.

87. **Bertakis K.** The communicating of information from physician to patient: a method for increasing patient retention and satisfaction. J Fam Prac. 1977;5:217–22.

88. **Siegel M.** Mass media anti-smoking campaign: a powerful tool for health promotion. Ann Internal Medicine 1998;129:128–32.

89. **Ockene J.** Smoking intervention: the expanding role of the physician. Am J Public Health. 1987;77:782–3.

90. **Ockene J, Lindsay E, Berger L, Hymowitz N.** Health care providers as key change agents in the Community Intervention Trial for Smoking Cessation (COMMIT). Int Community Health Education. 1991;11:223–37.

91. **Ockene J.** Smoking intervention: a behavioral, educational, and pharmacologic perspective. In: Ockene I, Ockene J (eds). Prevention of Coronary Heart Disease. Boston: Little, Brown; 1992:201–30.

92. **Ockene J, Quirk M, Goldberg R, et al.** A residents training program for the development of smoking intervention skills. Arch Int Med. 1988;148:1039–45.

93. **Division of Preventive and Behavioral Medicine.** Health Care Provider Smoking Intervention Training: Workshop Participant Manual. Worcester, MA: University of Massachusetts Medical School, 1994.

94. **Glynn T, Manley M.** How To Help Your Patients Stop Smoking. Bethesda: NIH, NCI Publication 93-3064; 1993.

95. **Fagerstrom K.** Measuring degree of physical dependency to tobacco smoking with reference to individualization of treatment. Addict Behav. 1978;3:235–41.

96. **Jarvik M, Henningfield J.** Pharmacological treatment of tobacco dependence. Pharmacol Biochem Behav. 1988;30:279–94.

97. **Heatherton T, Kozlowski L, Frecker R, Fagerstrom K.** The Fagerstrom Test for Nicotine Dependence: a revision of the Fagerstrom Tolerance Questionnaire. Brit J Addiction. 1991;86:1119–27.

98. **Foxx R, Brown R.** Nicotine fading and self-monitoring for cigarette abstinence or controlled smoking. J Appl Behav Anal. 1979;12:111–25.

99. **Lam W, Sze P, Sacks H, Chalmers T.** Meta-analysis of randomized controlled trials of nicotine chewing gum. Lancet. 1987;2:27–9.

100a. **Schneider N, Olmstead R, Mody F, et al.** Efficacy of a nicotine nasal spray in smoking cessation: a placebo-controlled, double-blind trial. Addiction. 1995;90: 1671–82.

100b. **Hjalmarson A, Nilsson F, Sjostrom L, Wiklund O.** The nicotine inhaler in smoking cessation. Arch Intern Med. 1997;157:1721–8.

101. **Klesges R, Meyers A, Klesges L, LaVasque M.** Smoking, body weight and their effects on smoking behavior: a comprehensive review of the literature. Psychol Bull. 1989;106:204–30.

102. **Hofstetter A, Schutz Y, Jequier E, Wahren J.** Increased 24-hour energy expenditure in cigarette smokers. N Engl J Med. 1986;314:79–82.

103. **Perkins K.** Metabolic effects of cigarette smoking. J Appl Physiol. 1992;72:401–9.

104. **Grunberg N.** The effects of nicotine and cigarette smoking on food consumption and taste preferences. Addict Behav. 1982;7:317–31.

105. **Wack J, Rodin L.** Smoking and its effects on body weight and the systems of caloric regulation. Am J Clin Nutr. 1982;35:366–80.

106. **Marlatt G, Gordon J.** Determinants of relapse: Implications for the maintenance of behavior change. In: Davidson P, Davidson S (eds). Behavioral Medicine: Changing Health Lifestyles. New York: Brunner/Mazel, 1980:410–52.

107. **Davis J, Glaros A.** Relapse prevention and smoking cessation. Addict Behav. 1986;11: 105–14.

108. **Shiffman S, Read L, Maltese J, et al.** Preventing relapse in ex-smokers: a self-management approach. In: Marlatt A, Gordon J (eds). Relapse Prevention. New York: Guilford Press, 1985.

109. **Robinson M, Laurent S, Little J.** Including smoking status as a new vital sign: it works! J Fam Pract. 1995;40:556–63.

CHAPTER 3

Diabetes and Insulin Resistance

AMI LAWS, MD

Type II diabetes is at one end of a spectrum of disorders caused by insulin resistance. Insulin resistance was first demonstrated by Himsworth and Kerr (1), who administered oral glucose loads and subcutaneous insulin to a number of diabetic patients. Based on the resulting glucose levels, the investigators found they could separate the patients into two groups: those who were sensitive to insulin's effect in lowering glucose and those who were not. The latter group had what is now called type II or non–insulin-dependent diabetes (NIDDM). Persons with type II diabetes comprise about 90% of diabetic patients of all ages and almost all of the diabetic patients over 45 years of age (2).

More sophisticated methods than that used by Himsworth and Kerr have since been developed to measure insulin resistance. With these methods, resistance to insulin-stimulated glucose uptake has been demonstrated in many groups in addition to those with type II diabetes: persons with impaired glucose tolerance (3), persons with normal glucose tolerance with hyperinsulinemia (4), and normoglycemic persons with a family history of type II diabetes (5). Insulin resistance is also present among persons with generalized (6) and upper-body (7) obesity, sedentary (8) persons, and persons with hypertension (9), dyslipidemia (10), and abnormalities of fibrinolysis (11). Insulin resistance is common among ethnic groups that have high prevalences of diabetes—e.g., Mexican Americans (12), African Americans (12), and persons from the Indian subcontinent (13).

Given its widespread prevalence in conditions that are risk factors for type II diabetes and coronary artery disease (CAD), insulin resistance makes a considerable contribution to morbidity and mortality in the United States. This chapter reviews the epidemiology of the spectrum of insulin resistance, behavioral (i.e., preventable) contributors to insulin resistance, and relationships of insulin resistance to CAD risk factors and atherosclerosis. It also discusses treatment of type II diabetes with emphasis on reducing CAD risk.

Insulin Resistance Defined

Insulin-Stimulated Glucose Uptake

In persons with normal carbohydrate metabolism, glucose levels are closely regulated by insulin. Following ingestion of carbohydrate, plasma glucose levels rise, stimulating insulin release from the pancreas. The resulting increased circulating insulin levels promote glucose uptake into muscle and fat tissue and inhibit glucose output from liver. Glucose levels then fall again to their fasting level.

In persons who are insulin resistant, however, this feedback loop is altered because insulin is less effective in stimulating glucose uptake. Higher levels of insulin must be secreted to achieve the same amount of glucose disposal. Some normoglycemic persons have a degree of insulin resistance as high as that seen in persons with type II diabetes (4). If the pancreas of those in the former group can secrete enough insulin, they remain normoglycemic, but at the price of ambient hyperinsulinemia. Unfortunately, as discussed below, hyperinsulinemia is itself a risk factor for CAD.

In the progression from normal glucose tolerance to impaired glucose tolerance (IGT) to type II diabetes, susceptible individuals develop defects in pancreatic secretion of insulin. Impaired insulin secretion that results in levels insufficient to overcome the degree of peripheral insulin resistance causes glucose levels to rise above the normal range. Thus, persons with IGT have hyperglycemia despite high circulating insulin levels. They have been shown to have a degree of insulin resistance equivalent to persons with mild type II diabetes (3).

As pancreatic failure progresses, insulin levels fall further, and glucose levels rise to levels of frank hyperglycemia in persons with type II diabetes. Numerous longitudinal studies have now demonstrated that in the progression from normal glucose tolerance to type II diabetes, individuals pass through three stages in the spectrum of insulin resistance: normal glucose tolerance with hyperinsulinemia, mildly elevated glucose levels with hyperinsulinemia, and hyperglycemia with normal or decreased insulin levels (14-17).

Insulin Suppression of Free Fatty Acid Concentrations

In addition to stimulating glucose uptake, insulin has an equally important function as the major hormone responsible for suppressing plasma free fatty acid (FFA) levels. Insulin does this by suppressing lipolysis of triglycerides in fat cells (18), and possibly by promoting re-esterification of FFAs into triglycerides in fat cells (19).

As with defects in insulin-stimulated glucose uptake, defects in insulin suppression of FFA levels were first demonstrated in persons with type II diabetes (10,20,21). More recently, however, decreases in insulin suppression of FFA concentrations have been demonstrated in persons with IGT (22,23), in men compared with women (23-25), in South Asians compared with persons of European heritage (13), in women (26) and men (27) with upper body obesity, and in sedentary men (25). That is, impaired insulin suppression of FFA is present in many of the same groups demonstrating resistance to insulin-stimulated glucose uptake, and each of these groups is at increased risk for CAD.

Epidemiology of the Spectrum of Insulin Resistance

Survey data in 1993 (2) indicated that there were 7.8 million persons in the United States with diagnosed diabetes. The prevalence of diagnosed diabetes increases with age, from 1.3% of those aged 18 to 44 to greater than 10% of those over 65 years of age. It is estimated that an equal number of persons have undiagnosed diabetes. The percent of persons with diabetes has been steadily increasing over the past 50 years. There are no clear gender differences in prevalence, but there are marked ethnic differences. Mexican Americans, Native Americans, and African Americans have higher rates of diabetes than do Americans of European background (Fig. 3-1).

Paralleling trends in diabetes, IGT prevalence increases with age. It was estimated that 11.2% of the adult population in the United States in 1976-80 had IGT, ranging from 6.4% for the age group 20 to 44 to 22.8% for those aged 65 to 74 (2). As for diabetes, the prevalence of IGT increases with age, and ethnic groups with high rates of diabetes also have high rates of IGT (2). Data from the Second National Health and Nutrition Examination Survey (1976-80) and the Hispanic Health and Nutrition Examination Survey (1982-84) show that the estimated combined prevalence of diagnosed diabetes, undiagnosed diabetes, and IGT is greater than 30% in African Americans and greater than 40% in Mexican Americans aged 45 to 74 years (2). These disorders of insulin resistance, therefore, are highly prevalent in the U.S. population, especially in ethnic minorities.

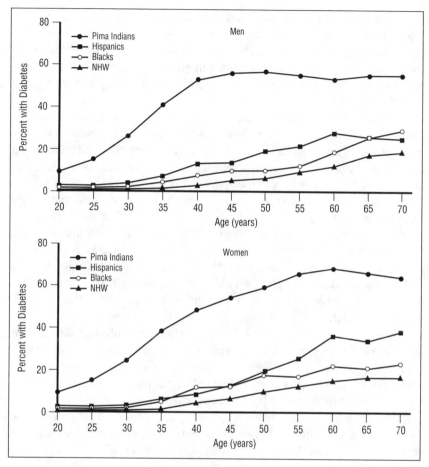

FIGURE 3-1 Prevalence of diabetes in men and women in four ethnic groups in the United States. NHW = non-Hispanic whites. (From Kenny SJ, Aubert RE, Geiss LS. Prevalence and incidence of non-insulin-independent diabetes. In: National Diabetes Data Group. Diabetes in America. 2nd ed. NIH Publication 95-1468; 1995.)

Behavioral (Modifiable) Risk Factors for Insulin Resistance

Overall and Central Obesity

A relationship between obesity and insulin resistance is well-established (6,28). The mechanisms responsible for this are unclear; however, weight loss has been shown to ameliorate the obesity-related defect in insulin-stimulated glucose uptake (6).

It is also established that central or abdominal obesity, as measured by waist-hip ratio or skin-fold thicknesses, is associated with insulin resistance. Kissebah et al (7) and others (29,30) have shown that women with abdominal obesity have decreased insulin-stimulated glucose uptake compared with women with the same degree of overall obesity but with lower body fat distribution.

Given its relation to insulin resistance, it is not surprising that abdominal obesity, independent of overall obesity, is associated with increased risk for development of type II diabetes in women (31) and men (32). The relationship may be more important in women. Haffner et al showed that 8-year incidence of type II diabetes in Mexican Americans was related to the degree of central obesity as measured by the ratio of subscapular to triceps skinfold thicknesses and that the relationship was much stronger for women than men (17).

While abdominal obesity is independently associated with insulin resistance and type II diabetes, it is important to note that overall obesity (e.g., obesity without increased waist-hip ratio) is not metabolically benign (33). In a population study, Young and Gelskey showed that body mass index (BMI), a measure of overall obesity, was as important or more important than abdominal obesity in determining glucose, lipid, and blood pressure levels (33). Furthermore, Landin et al (34) showed that the effects of central fat distribution were far more important in women who were obese compared with those who were lean. More recently, Bonora et al (35), using euglycemic insulin clamps, showed that, among obese women, abdominal but not overall obesity was related to insulin-mediated glucose uptake, whereas for nonobese women the opposite was true. Overall, however, glucose uptake was reduced in the obese women compared with the nonobese women. The important point of these studies is that overall leanness is essential to optimum glucose and insulin metabolism.

Differences in fat distribution between men and women (men tend to have more abdominal obesity) probably play a role in the gender difference in CAD risk, and this is likely mediated by insulin effects on plasma FFA concentrations. This is discussed in more detail below.

Physical Activity

Physical inactivity has been demonstrated to play an important role in the development of insulin resistance and type II diabetes (36,37). Insulin-stimulated glucose uptake has been shown to be directly related to the degree of aerobic fitness in both cross-sectional (38,39) and exercise training studies (8).

Exercise training in nondiabetic persons results in decreased insulin response after oral glucose tolerance load, indicating improved insulin sensitivity (36,39,40). The improvement does not depend on weight loss, since a single 1-hour period of exercise improves muscle insulin sensitivity (41). Furthermore, insulin sensitivity deteriorates in trained athletes who do not exercise for several days despite no change in their body weight or percent body fat (42). In persons with type II diabetes, physical training also improves glucose and insulin responses in oral glucose tests (43).

Several large, prospective studies have shown that regular physical activity reduces type II diabetes incidence (44-47). Manson et al showed that women who engaged in vigorous exercise at least once per week had significantly reduced risk of developing type II diabetes during 8 years of follow-up. The risk reduction was independent of obesity and family history of diabetes (44). In another study, Helmrich et al showed that among male alumni of the University of Pennsylvania leisure-time physical activity, expressed in kilocalories expended per week in walking, stair climbing, and sports, was inversely related to the development of type II diabetes independent of obesity, hypertension, and parental history of diabetes (45). Exercise was the most protective in those at highest risk of developing diabetes. A study of U.S. male physicians showed that the incidence of type II diabetes decreased significantly in men who exercised at least once per week compared with those who exercised less frequently, independent of obesity (46). These investigators found a dose-response relationship, with those exercising five or more times per week at the lowest risk. In the Honolulu Heart Program, age-adjusted 6-year cumulative incidence of diabetes decreased progressively with increasing quintile of physical activity, and the relation was highly statistically significant (47). Taken together, these studies indicate a strong, preventive effect of exercise on the development of type II diabetes. Given the high prevalence of type II diabetes in the population, efforts to increase physical activity to promote public health are therefore warranted.

The mechanisms by which physical activity improves insulin sensitivity have now been worked out (40). During exercise, muscle glycogen stores are reduced, and enhanced glucose uptake following exercise is directed towards repleting these stores. Ebeling et al recently showed that athletes had enhanced muscle blood flow and glucose uptake compared with sedentary controls. On a cellular-molecular level, the muscles of athletes had increased glucose transporter (GLUT-4) units, increased glycogen synthase activity, and increased glucose storage as glycogen (48). Another recent study showed that, compared with lean controls, endurance-trained athletes had higher rates of whole body glucose uptake and nonoxidative glucose disposal (glycogen synthesis) during hyperinsulinemia (49). They also had higher content of glucose transporter (GLUT-4) in muscle cells and higher leg blood flow during insulin stimulation. In a study of persons at increased risk for development of type II diabetes—namely, those with a family history of the disorder—Perseghin et al showed that exercise increased insulin sensitivity by increasing insulin-stimulated glycogen synthesis in muscle (50). The ability of exercise to increase insulin sensitivity in this group has important implications for the prevention of type II diabetes.

In summary, studies of the effects of physical activity on insulin resistance and development of type II diabetes indicate that exercise increases insulin sensitivity and is of primary importance in the prevention and treatment of type II diabetes.

Insulin Resistance, Type II Diabetes, and CAD Risk

Glucose and Insulin Levels in Nondiabetic Persons

Each of the disorders of carbohydrate metabolism caused by insulin resistance has been demonstrated to increase risk for CAD. A number of population-based, prospective studies have shown that high glucose levels in nondiabetic persons predict subsequent development of CAD (51-53a). In the Framingham Offspring Study, glucose intolerance correlated with multiple cardiovascular risk factors including central obesity, hypertension, and low levels of HDL, as well as elevated insulin and triglyceride levels (Fig. 3-2) (53b). Prospective population studies have shown that fasting (52,54) and post-challenge (52) glucose concentrations are related to incident CAD among nondiabetic persons. A recent meta-analysis of 18 studies of over 88,000 nondiabetic subjects, with a mean follow-up of 11.5 years, showed an exponential and continuous relation between blood glucose levels and incident cardiovascular events (55). Compared with those with a fasting glucose level of 75 mg/dL, persons with fasting glucose of 100 mg/dL had a relative risk of incident cardiovascular disease of 2.3. For those with a fasting glucose level of 120 mg/dL, the relative risk increased to 4.7. This study highlights the fact that small increases in fasting glucose level in nondiabetic persons are associated with increasing risk for cardiovascular events. Of note, these levels of fasting glucose are below the current, revised cut point for the diagnosis of type II diabetes—126 mg/dL (56). Also important is that risk increases continuously with increases in glucose level and there is no threshold (i.e., the lower the fasting glucose level, the lower the risk).

Other studies have focused on hyperinsulinemia in normoglycemic persons as a risk factor for CAD, with mixed results (57). The reasons for the conflicting findings have been recently reviewed (58). Three population-based, prospective studies have shown that plasma insulin concentration is a risk factor for CAD in nondiabetic men, independent of other risk factors (59-61). In the Paris Prospective Study of middle-aged men, fasting plasma insulin after oral glucose challenge was related independently to CAD mortality after

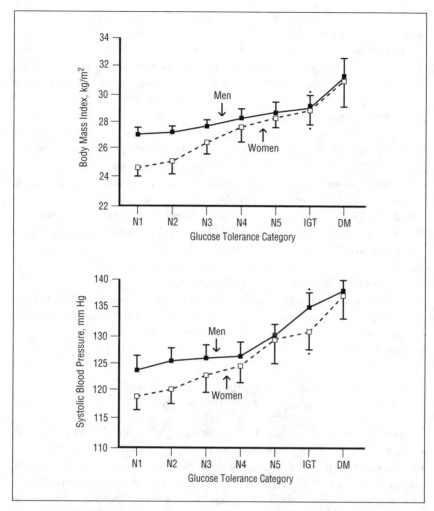

FIGURE 3-2 Distribution of obesity and blood pressure by glucose tolerance category. Mean body mass index (*top*), systolic blood pressure (*bottom*), and 95% confidence intervals (*error bars*) for women and men are given for each glucose tolerance category from the lowest quintile (N1) to the highest quintile (N5) of fasting plasma glucose level among participants with normal glucose tolerance, impaired glucose tolerance (IGT), and previously undiagnosed diabetes mellitus (DM). Means are multivariable adjusted; $p < 0.001$ for trend from the lowest quintile of normal fasting glucose level to impaired glucose tolerance.

approximately 5 years' follow-up (62). A follow-up study showed the relationship persisted up to 10 years (62). In the Busselton Study, 1-hour plasma insulin after oral glucose load predicted CAD mortality at 12 years in men (59).

In the Helsinki Policeman Study, men in the upper quintile of post-oral glucose challenge insulin levels had significantly increased risk of CAD death or nonfatal myocardial infarction (MI) at 7½ years follow-up compared with men in the lower four quartiles, independent of other risk factors including age, blood glucose, plasma cholesterol and triglycerides, blood pressure, body mass index, level of physical activity, and smoking (60). A recent follow-up showed the increased risk persisted for 15 years (63).

Too few studies have examined the relation of baseline hyperinsulinemia to incidence of CAD in women. Two studies have shown no relation of insulin level to CAD in women, but there were far fewer women and a smaller number of events in women than men (59,64). The similar impact of insulin levels on CAD risk factors in men and women (65,66), the greater risk for CAD associated with type II diabetes for women than men, and the fact that insulin is directly atherogenic (67a), all suggest that hyperinsulinemia plays as important a role in CAD in women as in men. A recent meta-analysis that included analysis by race found the relation between insulin and cardiovascular disease greater in white than nonwhite populations (67b).

Degrees of glucose intolerance not in the diabetic range (i.e., IGT) have also consistently been demonstrated to increase the risk of CAD (68). As with type II diabetes, the increase in risk associated with IGT may be greater for women than men (69).

Hyperinsulinemia, Insulin Resistance, and Polycystic Ovary Syndrome

A condition specific to women that is characterized by insulin resistance and hyperinsulinemia is polycystic ovary syndrome (PCO) (70). Women with PCO have elevated levels of circulating androgens; some studies have shown they also have increased triglyceride (71-74) and decreased HDL cholesterol concentrations (72-75) compared with control women. It would be expected, therefore, that women with PCO would have increased CAD risk. One cross-sectional study of women undergoing coronary angiography showed that women with PCO by ultrasound assessment had more extensive coronary artery disease than women with normal ovaries (73). Almost no prospective data on CAD incidence in women with PCO are available; this is an important area for future study.

Insulin Resistance and Atherosclerosis

Recently, studies have shown a relation between insulin resistance, measured directly, and CAD (76-78). Laakso et al showed a significant association of insulin resistance as measured by euglycemic, hyperinsulinemic clamp, and asymptomatic atherosclerosis of the femoral and carotid arteries (76). In a small case-control study of patients with normal glucose tolerance (NGT) and IGT, Shinozaki et al showed that insulin resistance, as measured by the steady-state plasma glucose test, was greater in patients with CAD demonstrated by angiography compared with controls (77). In a large multi-center study, Howard et al showed that decreased insulin sensitivity, as assessed by the frequently sampled glucose tolerance test with minimal model analysis, was associated with intimal-medial thickness of the carotid artery as measured by B-mode ultrasonography (78). This relation was found in Hispanics and in non-Hispanic whites but not in African Americans.

Type II Diabetes

The increased risk for CAD associated with diabetes is well-established (68), and prospective studies have consistently shown that the increased risk for CAD attributable to diabetes is greater for women than for men (Fig. 3-3) (54,69,79-85). This gender difference is accounted for by the fact that nondiabetic women are relatively protected from CAD compared with men, whereas diabetic women have CAD risk similar to that of diabetic men (80,83). The reasons for the relatively greater impact of diabetes on CAD risk in women

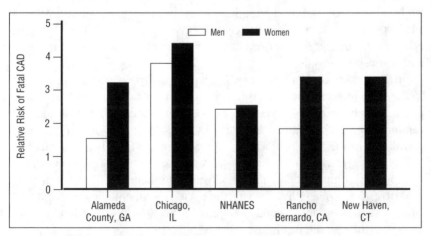

Figure 3-3 Multiple adjusted risk of fatal coronary artery disease in diabetic compared with nondiabetic adults, by sex. Definition of risk: Alameda—relative risk; Chicago, NHANES, Rancho Bernardo—relative hazard; New Haven—odds ratio. (From Davidson MB. Diabetes Mellitus: Diagnosis and Treatment. 4th ed. Philadelphia: WB Saunders; 1998:435; with permission.)

remain undefined but, as discussed below, are likely related to atherogenic lipids and lipoprotein changes associated with insulin resistance (86).

In addition to increasing risk of incident CAD, diabetes confers a higher risk of death following MI (87-95). Several studies have shown that risk of death following MI is higher for diabetic women that for diabetic men (87,89,91,93-95). Some of the increased risk of death following MI among diabetic patients is attributable to cardiac heart failure (CHF) (87-89,92), for which diabetic women appear to be at higher risk than diabetic men (87,89). These studies suggest that aggressive measures for secondary prevention are warranted in diabetic women following MI.

What is the basis for the associations of insulin resistance and type II diabetes to CAD? Insulin resistance is associated with a number of CAD risk factors that are discussed below.

Insulin Resistance and Dyslipidemia

Insulin resistance is related to a number of lipid and lipoprotein abnormalities that are atherogenic; this has recently been reviewed (96). The lipid abnormality most closely associated with insulin resistance and hyperinsulinemia is hypertriglyceridemia (97). Very-low-density lipoprotein (VLDL) triglycerides and total triglycerides are elevated in persons with IGT and type II diabetes (96). In normoglycemic persons, insulin resistance and hyperinsulinemia are associated with increases in VLDL-triglyceride secretion rate and plasma triglyceride concentration (98). Although the exact roles of insulin resistance and hyperinsulinemia in hypertriglyceridemia are disputed, it is clear that persons who are hyperinsulinemic and/or insulin resistant have high triglyceride concentrations (96).

An important consequence of the relation of hyperinsulinemia to high triglyceride levels is that diets high in carbohydrates that result in higher plasma insulin levels also cause hypertriglyceridemia (99). This had been demonstrated in both human and animal studies. In rats fed diets high in carbohydrates in the form of fructose (100) or sucrose (101), hyperinsulinemia and hypertriglyceridemia develop. If these rats are exercise-trained, however, thereby preventing the development of hyperinsulinemia, they do not develop hypertriglyceridemia (102). The effect of these experimental manipulations of diet and exercise on insulin and triglyceride concentrations have implications for treatment that will be discussed below.

As outlined above, in addition to stimulating glucose uptake, insulin has the important role of suppressing FFA release from fat cells. The defect in insulin suppression of FFA concentrations that has been demonstrated in persons with IGT (22,23) and type II diabetes (20) also plays an important role in the development of dyslipidemia (96). Free fatty acids are the major substrate for triglyceride synthesis in liver and, in vitro, they stimulate apolipoprotein B (apo B) release from liver cells (103,104). Elevated FFA levels therefore initiate an atherogenic lipoprotein cascade that results in high triglyceride and VLDL cholesterol levels, and subsequently, through a number of metabolic steps, in low HDL cholesterol and increased small, dense LDL cholesterol (105).

Among normoglycemic persons, resistance to insulin-mediated glucose uptake (13,106-108) and hyperinsulinemia (65,66,109,110) are strongly related to low HDL cholesterol concentrations, independent of obesity, abdominal obesity, and physical fitness level (108). Because low HDL cholesterol level is a strong risk factor for CAD, this is one mechanism through which insulin resistance increases CAD risk. Both HDL cholesterol (111-113) and triglyceride concentrations (114) have been shown to be more important than total or LDL cholesterol in determining CAD risk in women. They also appear to be more important CAD risk factors in women than in men. Thus factors that influence HDL cholesterol and triglyceride levels—namely, insulin resistance and hyperinsulinemia—are important determinants of CAD risk in normoglycemic women.

Among persons with diabetes, prospective epidemiological studies have shown that the dyslipidemia of insulin resistance, specifically high triglycerides (115) and low HDL cholesterol (116), plays a greater role in CAD risk than do total (115,116) or LDL cholesterol (116) concentrations. One recent study suggests the greater risk for CAD associated with type II diabetes in women is due to greater an impact of HDL and VLDL cholesterol on ischemic heart disease risk in diabetic women than diabetic men (117).

Recently, hyperinsulinemia (118), insulin resistance (119), IGT (120), and type II diabetes (120,121) have all been shown to be correlated with small, dense LDL particles (LDL phenotype B) that are highly atherogenic (122).

In summary, insulin resistance is associated with a dyslipidemia characterized by high plasma and VLDL triglyceride concentrations, low HDL cholesterol concentrations and an increase in small, dense LDL cholesterol concentrations. These lipid and lipoprotein abnormalities increase risk for CAD.

Insulin Resistance and Hypertension

Welborn et al first demonstrated that, compared with normotensive persons, hypertensive patients had increased plasma insulin concentrations in response to oral glucose challenge (123). A large number of studies now demonstrate that insulin resistance and hyperinsulinemia are related to the development of hypertension. Studies of different populations have shown that insulin concentration and blood pressure are correlated in normotensive, nondiabetic subjects, independent of obesity (124). Studies that have measured insulin resistance directly have shown it to be increased in persons with hypertension compared with normotensive subjects (125,126).

Interventions that decrease insulin resistance and plasma insulin levels (e.g., weight loss and exercise training) also decrease blood pressure (127,128). This again highlights the importance of optimal body weight and fitness in the prevention and treatment of complications that result from insulin resistance.

Hypertension is more common among persons with diabetes than among nondiabetic persons, and it contributes substantially to CAD risk in diabetes (129,130). In a large cohort of diabetic outpatients in the Schwabing Study, systolic blood pressure was the most consistent predictor of major cardiovascular events at 5-year follow-up in both men and women (129).

Insulin Resistance and Abnormalities of Fibrinolysis

Patients with type II diabetes have defects in fibrinolysis, and the reduction in fibinolytic activity in these patients correlates strongly with levels of plasminogen activator inhibitor of the endothelial cell type 1 (PAI-1) (131,132). PAI-1 inhibits tissue plasminogen activator (t-PA) by irreversibly binding to it to form a t-PA-PAI-1 complex that is rapidly degraded. An increase in PAI-1 level in plasma is a strong risk factor for CAD (133). Relations between insulin resistance, hyperinsulinemia, and PAI-1 have recently been reviewed (11,134). The mechanisms linking insulin levels and insulin resistance to increased PAI-1 levels are currently unclear, but the mediator may be plasma triglyceride concentration (10,111).

Interventions that increase insulin sensitivity and/or decrease insulin concentrations also cause a decrease in PAI-1 levels. Vague et al showed that a 24-hour fast in ten obese women resulted in decreases in insulin, triglyceride, and PAI-1 concentrations (135). Other investigators have shown that low-calorie diets (136,137), physical training (138,139), and metformin (140), all of which lower plasma insulin and triglyceride concentrations, also lower PAI-1 concentrations and improve fibrinolytic activity.

Insulin Resistance and Hyperuricemia

Increased serum uric acid concentration has been shown to be associated with increased risk for CAD (141,142). It has also been shown that persons with hyperuricemia tend to be glucose intolerant and have dyslipidemia and hypertension (142). These findings suggest that hyperuricemia has a relation to insulin resistance, and this has now been demonstrated. A study of normoglycemic subjects showed statistically significant correlations between serum uric acid concentration and both insulin resistance and hyperinsulinemia (143). The relation appeared to be mediated by the effect of insulin resistance on uric acid clearance. Subjects who were insulin resistant had decreased 24-hour uric acid clearance and resulting increases in uric acid levels.

Insulin Resistance Syndrome

From the above discussion, it is clear that insulin resistance and hyperinsulinemia are associated with a number of risk factors for CAD, including IGT and type II diabetes, hypertriglyceridemia, low HDL cholesterol, increased small, dense LDL cholesterol, hyperuricemia, hypertension, and abnormalities of fibrinolysis. This clustering of risk factors has been termed *insulin resistance syndrome* (Box 3-1) (10).

Only recently have investigators demonstrated this clustering of risk factors in various populations (65,118,144-147). One study, by Austin and Selby (118), examined nearly 700 women twins. They found that going from normal to impaired glucose tolerance to type II diabetes, there were increasing proportions of women with atherogenic small, dense LDL cholesterol (subclass phenotype B). They also found that women with LDL subclass phenotype B had, on average, higher body mass indices, higher waist-hip ratios, elevated triglyceride and low HDL-cholesterol concentrations, and higher systolic and diastolic blood pressures. Thus the insulin resistance syndrome was demonstrated in this female sample.

Box 3-1 Characteristics of Insulin Resistance Syndrome

Insulin resistance
Hyperinsulinemia
Non–insulin-dependent diabetes
Hypertriglyceridemia
Low HDL cholesterol concentrations
High VLDL cholesterol concentrations
Small, dense LDL cholesterol
Hyperuricemia
Hypertension
Abnormalities of fibrinolysis

Another important study establishing that CAD risk factors associated with insulin resistance syndrome cluster among individuals in the population was conducted with data from the Atherosclerosis Risk in Communities Study (ARIC) (145). These investigators showed that clustering of dyslipidemia, diabetes, hypertension, and hyperuricemia is present in African American and white men and women. This cluster of CAD risk factors was associated most strongly with high insulin levels, but it was also associated with high body mass index and waist-hip ratio.

Ethnicity and Insulin Resistance Syndrome

Components of the insulin resistance syndrome have been demonstrated in population studies of Mexican Americans (147), African Americans (145), and white Americans (145). Hyperinsulinemia, hypertriglyceridemia, and low HDL cholesterol have also been shown to be associated with insulin resistance in South Asians (13) and to play a major role in CAD risk in this population (146). A recent worksite study of Chinese men and women in Hong Kong showed inter-relationships between glucose intolerance, body mass index, waist-hip ratio, blood pressure, and serum triglyceride and insulin levels (148). Another recent study examined a Japanese community and found that men and women with IGT and type II diabetes had increased triglyceride concentrations and blood pressure levels compared with those with NGT (149). Among men and women with NGT, post-oral glucose load insulin levels were positively correlated with triglyceride concentration and systolic and diastolic blood pressure and negatively correlated with HDL cholesterol (149). Yamada et al (150) also showed relations of hyperinsulinemia to mean blood pressure, plasma triglyceride, and HDL cholesterol concentrations in Japanese subjects. These findings demonstrate that the cluster of CAD risk factors due to insulin resistance exists in most populations and likely contributes significantly to CAD in diverse populations.

One U.S. population at especially increased risk for CAD caused by metabolic abnormalities related to insulin resistance is Native Americans. Data from the Strong Heart Study show that diabetes rates in American Indians are several times higher than those reported in the U.S. population (151). Among American Indians in Arizona, who had the highest age-adjusted rates, 72% of women and 65% of men aged 45 to 74 years had diabetes. In all three centers studied, diabetes was more prevalent in women than men. Diabetes, hypertension, percent body fat, and high plasma insulin and low HDL cholesterol concentrations were the strongest predictors of CAD in this cross-sectional study, suggesting again that components of the insulin resistance syndrome play an important role in development of CAD in this population.

Behavioral Interventions To Improve Insulin Sensitivity in Persons with Type II Diabetes and Nondiabetic Persons

Physical Activity

As discussed above, physical activity is a health behavior with a major impact on insulin sensitivity. Exercise training studies consistently show improvement in glucose and insulin concentrations and in insulin sensitivity after physical training (36,37). In perhaps the most successful study to date, Holloszy et al (43) enrolled patients in a 12-month exercise-training study. Five of the men had type II diabetes, eight had IGT, and eight had high normal plasma glucose values with moderate hyperinsulinemia during OGTT. During the last three months of training, participants averaged 3.7 exercise sessions per week, running 5 to 8 km per session. At the end of the study, three of the diabetic patients had completely normal glucose tolerance, while the other improved to IGT. All eight patients with IGT had completely normalized their glucose tolerance by the end of the study. Finally, all eight patients with high normal glucose levels and hyperinsulinemia had improvement in glucose tolerance and reduction in insulin concentrations on oral glucose tolerance testing. All these changes are compatible with improved insulin sensitivity. Although some of the participants lost weight, improvements in glucose and insulin concentrations were independent of weight loss. This study highlights the powerful effect of aerobic exercise in maintaining and improving insulin sensitivity.

Endurance exercise training has beneficial effects on all of the components of the insulin resistance syndrome. Exercise raises HDL cholesterol concentrations, improves fibrinolysis, and lowers blood pressure (152). For these reasons, physical exercise training would be expected to lower CAD risk in insulin resistant persons, though this had not yet been tested in prospective trials.

Weight Loss and Diet Composition

As discussed above, obesity is a strong risk factor for the development of insulin resistance, and weight loss improves insulin resistance (6). Even modest weight loss can have significant metabolic benefits (153). Unfortunately, despite advances in the behavioral weight control, achieving and maintaining weight loss remains an elusive goal for many patients (154). In cases of morbid obesity, surgical treatment is sometimes indicated and can be successful in alleviating metabolic consequences of obesity (155).

There are special considerations with respect to diet composition among persons with components of the insulin resistance syndrome. These arise from the fact that, in the absence of weight loss, high-carbohydrate diets raise plasma insulin and triglyceride concentrations in normoglycemic persons (156,157) and in persons with type II diabetes (158,159). High-carbohydrate diets also lower HDL cholesterol concentrations in both normoglycemic persons (157) and persons with type II diabetes (159), thereby enhancing metabolic abnormalities that increase risk for CAD. Because equivalent weight loss had been shown to be achievable on either high-fat or low-fat diets with equivalent energy restriction (160,161), and because high-carbohydrate diets have deleterious effects on plasma triglyceride (156-159) and HDL cholesterol (158,159), high-carbohydrate diets should not be recommended for persons with components of the insulin resistance syndrome. Diets high in monounsaturated fats appear to have the most beneficial effect on components of the insulin resistance syndrome, including glucose control, insulin, lipid and lipoprotein levels, and coagulation factors (158,159,162-164).

Management of Type II Diabetes To Reduce CAD Risk

Glycemic Control

Whether glucose levels per se play a role in CAD risk among persons with type II diabetes is currently unclear; this has been the subject of a recent, excellent review (165a). The Swedish DIGAMI (Diabetes Mellitus, Insulin Glucose Infusion in Acute Myocardial Infarction) study recruited 620 patients, of whom 314 served as controls and 306 received intensive insulin treatment (insulin-glucose infusion and then subcutaneous insulin at least four times a day for 3 months.) The treatment group had improved glycemic control with a decrease in all-cause mortality rate (33% vs. 44%; RR = 0.72 [95% CI, 0.55–0.92]; p = 0.011). The mean (range) follow-up was 3.4 (1.6–5.6) years. The greatest benefit was seen in low-risk patients who had not previously received insulin treatment and who were at a low cardiovascular risk (165b). Results of the large, randomized, controlled U.K. clinical trial of the effect of improved glucose control on macrovascular complications are eagerly awaited. In the meantime, because the value of achieving excellent glycemic control to avert microvascular complications is undisputed, it remains an important goal in the management of type II diabetes patients. Fortunately, there are an increased number of agents to aid in pursuit of this goal, including the newer medications metformin and troglitazone. The pharmacologic treatment of hyperglycemia has recently been thoughtfully reviewed (166).

Metformin, which has been used for many years in Europe, was recently introduced in the United States. It improves glucose control without increasing insulin levels (167). It also has been shown in some studies to improve lipid levels (168,169) and blood pressure (169); therefore it would be expected to reduce CAD risk, although this has not yet been demonstrated in prospective studies. Another use for metformin may emerge in the treatment of PCO. Velazquez et al (170) showed that metformin reduced insulin resistance and hyperinsulinemia in women with PCO, resulting in lower androgen levels and resumption of normal menses.

Troglitazone, the newest available agent for treating type II diabetes, lowers glucose levels by improving insulin sensitivity (171). Its effect on related CAD risk factors remains unclear.

Treatment of Hypertension

Control of blood pressure in patients with type II diabetes is essential to preventing both macrovascular and microvascular complications. Optimal treatment of hypertension in type II diabetes has been the subject of several recent reviews (172,173a). Currently angiotensin-converting inhibitors are thought to be the agents of choice because of their important role in reducing microalbuminuria and delaying or preventing diabetic nephropathy. There are increasing data that initiation of angiotensin-converting inhibitor therapy within 24 hours of acute MI especially benefits patients with diabetes (173b). Alpha-1-receptor blockers are also useful because of their beneficial effects on lipid levels (172). Low doses of thiazide diuretics have been shown to reduce cardiovascular events in elderly patients with isolated systolic hypertension (174). Concerns have been expressed about the risk of sudden cardiac death associated with non–potassium-sparing diuretics (175-177); this subject warrants further study.

Treatment of Dyslipidemia

Despite the important role of lipids and lipoproteins in CAD risk in diabetes, no prospective drug treatment trials specifically of patients with type II diabetes have yet been completed. Dyslipidemia is common in black and white type II diabetic adults (Fig. 3-4) (2). However, subgroup analysis of the Scandinavian Simvastatin Survival Study revealed that the incidence of major CAD events was lowered in diabetic persons similarly to nondiabetic persons (178).

Both gemfibrozil (179) and lovastatin (180) have been shown to have beneficial effects on lipid and lipoprotein levels in persons with type II diabetes. A new HMG-CoA reductase inhibitor, atorvastatin, may be particularly useful in hyperlipidemic diabetic patients, because it substantially lowers triglycerides and VLDL cholesterol in addition to lowering LDL cholesterol (181). Prospective trials of effects of various lipid-lowering regiments in reducing CAD risk in persons with type II diabetes are clearly needed.

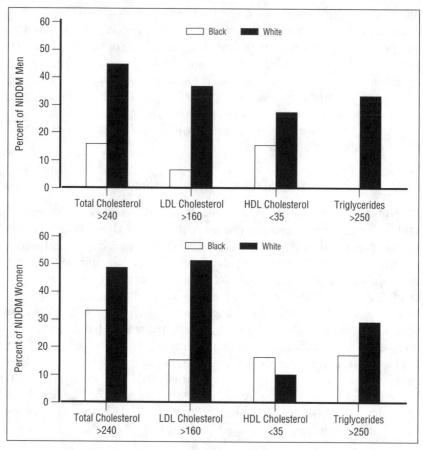

FIGURE 3-4 Dyslipidemia in black and white adults with NIDDM, United States, 1976–80. (From Davidson MB. Diabetes Mellitus: Diagnosis and Treatment. 4th ed. Philadelphia: WB Saunders; 1998:624; with permission.)

Hormone Replacement Therapy

The important question of whether diabetic women benefit from post-menopausal hormone replacement therapy has not yet been answered. One large, cross-sectional study showed that diabetic women appeared to have a blunted response to the HDL-raising effects of estrogen and an exaggerated hypertriglyceridemic response compared with nondiabetic women (182), suggesting limited benefit in reducing CAD risk. However, a double-blind, placebo-controlled, cross-over study of estrogen replacement in diabetic women with hyperandrogenicity showed that androgenicity (as measured by sex hormone-binding globulin and free testosterone) decreased, and blood glucose, glycosylated hemoglobin, and LDL cholesterol decreased, whereas HDL cholesterol increased (183). These changes would be expected to decrease CAD risk. Another double-blind, placebo-controlled trial of oral estradiol-17β in postmenopausal women with type II diabetes showed no change in insulin-stimulated glucose uptake, but decreased glycosylated hemoglobin, LDL cholesterol, and apo B, and increased HDL cholesterol and apo A1 (184). Both of these studies were short-term, however. Prospective clinical trial data of hormone replacement in Type II diabetic women, when they become available, will provide an important contribution to our understanding of CAD risk reduction in this high-risk group.

Summary

Insulin resistance and the resulting metabolic abnormalities known as insulin resistance syndrome are common in diverse populations and increase the risk for CAD. The risk for CAD associated with type II is higher for women than men, and diabetic women are more likely than men to die after MI. Management of disorders associated with insulin resistance, including IGT and type II diabetes, must include multi-factorial CAD risk reduction, including smoking cessation and treatment of hypertension and lipid and lipoprotein abnormalities. Behavioral modification, including weight loss and exercise, is central to the prevention and treatment of disorders of insulin resistance.

REFERENCES

1. **Himsworth HP, Kerr RB.** Insulin-sensitive and insulin-insensitive types of diabetes mellitus. Clin Sci. 1939;4:119-124.
2. **Kenny SJ, Aubert RE, Geiss LS.** Prevalence and incidence of non–insulin-dependent diabetes. In: National Diabetes Data Group. Diabetes in America. 2nd ed. NIH Publication 95-1468; 1995.
3. **Reaven GM, Hollenbeck CB, Chen Y-DI.** Relationship between glucose tolerance, insulin secretion, and insulin action in nonobese individuals with varying degrees of glucose tolerance. Diabetologia. 1989;32:52-5.
4. **Hollenbeck CB, Reaven GM.** Variations in insulin-stimulated glucose uptake in healthy individuals with normal glucose tolerance. J Clin Endocrinol Metab. 1987; 64:1169-73.
5. **Laws A, Stefanick ML, Reaven GM.** Insulin resistance and hypertriglyceridemia in nondiabetic relatives of patients with non–insulin-dependent diabetes mellitus. J Clin Endocrinol Metab. 1989;69:343-7.
6. **Olefsky JM, Reaven GM, Farquhar JW.** Effects of weight reduction on obesity: studies of carbohydrate and lipid metabolism. J Clin Invest. 1974;53:64-76.
7. **Kissebah AH, Vydelingum N, Murray R, et al.** Relation of body fat distribution to metabolic complications of obesity. J Clin Endocrinol Metab. 1982;54:254-60.

8. **DeFronzo RA, Sherwin RS, Kraemer N.** Effect of physical training on insulin action in obesity. Diabetes. 1987;36:689-92.

9. **Ferrannini E, Buzzigoli G, Bonadonna R.** Insulin resistance in essential hypertension. N Engl J Med. 1987;317:350-7.

10. **Reaven GM.** Role of insulin resistance in human disease. Diabetes. 1988;37:1595-1607.

11. **Vague P, Raccah D, Scelles V.** Hypofibrinolysis and the insulin resistance syndrome. Intl J Obesity. 1995;19(suppl 1):S11-5.

12. **Haffner SM, Howard G, Mayer E, et al.** Insulin sensitivity and acute insulin response in African-Americans, non-Hispanic whites, and Hispanics with NIDDM: the Insulin Resistance Atherosclerosis Study. Diabetes. 1997;46:63-9.

13. **Laws A, Jeppesen JL, Maheux PC, et al.** Resistance to insulin-stimulated glucose uptake and dyslipidemia in Asian Americans. Arterioscler Thromb Vasc Biol. 1994;14: 917-22.

14. **Reaven GM, Miller R.** Study of the relationship between glucose and insulin responses to an oral glucose load in man. Diabetes. 1968;17:560-9.

15. **Sicree RA, Zimmet PZ, King HOM, Coventry JS.** Plasma insulin response among Nauruans: prediction of deterioration in glucose tolerance over 6 years. Diabetes. 1987;36:179-86.

16. **Saad MF, Knowler WC, Pettit DJ, et al.** Sequential changes in serum insulin concentration during development of non–insulin-dependent diabetes. Lancet. 1989;1: 1356-9.

17. **Haffner SM, Stern MP, Mitchell BD, et al.** Incidence of type II diabetes in Mexican Americans predicted by fasting insulin and glucose levels, obesity and body-fat distribution. Diabetes. 1990;39:283-8.

18. **Havel RJ.** Some influences on the sympathetic nervous system and insulin on mobilization of fat from adipose tissue: studies on the turnover rates of free fatty acids and glycerol. Ann NY Acad Sci. 1965;131:91-101.

19. **Wolfe RR, Peters EJ.** Lipolytic response to glucose infusion in human subjects. Am J Physiol. 1987;252:E218-23.

20. **Bierman EL, Dole VP, Roberts TN.** An abnormality of nonesterified fatty acid metabolism in diabetes mellitus. Diabetes. 1957;6:475-9.

21. **Swislocki ALM, Chen Y-DI, Golay A, et al.** Insulin suppression of plasma-free fatty acid concentration in normal individuals and patients with Type 2 (non–insulin-dependent) diabetes. Diabetologia. 1987;30:622-6.

22. **Byrne CD, Wareham NJ, Brown DC, et al.** Hypertriglyceridemia in subjects with normal and abnormal glucose tolerance: relative contributions of insulin secretion, insulin resistance and suppression of plasma non-esterified fatty acids. Diabetologia. 1994;37:889-96.

23. **Laws A, Hoen HM, Selby JV, et al, for the Insulin Resistance Atherosclerosis Study (IRAS) Investigators.** Differences in insulin suppression of free fatty acid levels by gender and glucose tolerance status: relation to plasma triglyceride and apolipoprotein B concentrations. Arterioscler Thromb Vasc Biol. 1997;17:64-71.

24. **McKeigue PM, Laws A, Chen Y-DI, et al.** Relation of plasma triglyceride and apolipoprotein B levels to insulin-mediated suppression of non-esterified fatty acids: possible explanation for sex differences in lipoprotein pattern. Arterioscler Thromb Vasc Biol. 1993;13:1187-92.

25. **Byrne CD, Wareham NJ, Day NE, et al.** Decreased non-esterified fatty acid suppression and features of the insulin resistance syndrome occur in a subgroup of individuals with normal glucose tolerance. Diabetologia. 1995;38:1358-66.

26. **Jensen MD, Haymond MW, Rizza RA, et al.** Influence of body fat distribution on free fatty acid metabolism in obesity. J Clin Invest. 1989;83:1168-73.

27. **Coon PJ, Rogus EM, Goldberg AP.** Time course of plasma-free fatty acid concentration in response to insulin: effect of obesity and physical fitness. Metabolism. 1992; 41:711-6.

28. **DeFronzo RA, Soman V, Sherwin RS, et al.** Insulin binding to monocytes and insulin action in human obesity, starvation and refeeding. J Clin Invest. 1978;62: 689-92.

29. **Evans DJ, Hoffmann RG, Kalkhoff RK, Kissebah AH.** Relationship of body fat topography to insulin sensitivity and metabolic profiles in premenopausal women. Metabolism. 1984;33:68-75.

30. **Peiris AN, Struve MF, Mueller RA, et al.** Glucose metabolism in obesity: influence on body fat distribution. J Clin Endocrinol Metab. 1988;67:760-7.

31. **Kaye SA, Folsom AR, Sprafka JM, et al.** Increased incidence of diabetes mellitus in relation to abdominal adiposity in older women. J Clin Epidemiol. 1991;44:329-34.

32. **Ohlson LO, Larsson B, Svardsudd K, et al.** The influence of body fat distribution on the incidence of diabetes mellitus: 13.5 years of follow-up of the participants in the study of men born in 1913. Diabetes. 1985;34:1055-8.

33. **Young TK, Gelskey DE.** Is noncentral obesity metabolically benign? JAMA. 1995; 274:1939-41.

34. **Landin K, Krotkiewski M, Smith U.** Importance of obesity for the metabolic abnormalities associated with an abdominal fat distribution. Metabolism. 1989;38: 572-6.

35. **Bonora E, Del Prato S, Bonadonna RC, et al.** Total body fat content and fat topography are associated differently with in vivo glucose metabolism in nonobese and obese nondiabetic women. Diabetes. 1992;41:1151-9.

36. **Laws A, Reaven GM.** Effect of physical activity on age-related glucose tolerance. Clin Geriatr Med. 1990;6:849-63.

37. **Laws A, Reaven GM.** Physical activity, glucose tolerance, and diabetes in older adults. Ann Behav Med. 1991;13:125-32.

38. **Hollenbeck CB, Haskell W, Rosenthal M, Reaven GM.** Effect of habitual physical activity on regulation of insulin-stimulated glucose disposal in older males. J Am Geriatr Soc. 1985;33:273-7.

39. **Rodnick KJ, Haskell WL, Swislocki ALM, et al.** Improved insulin action in muscle, liver and adipose tissue in physically trained subjects. Am J Physiol. 1987;253:E489-95.

40. **Horton ES.** Exercise and physical training: effects on insulin sensitivity and glucose metabolism. Diabetes Metab Rev. 1996;1:1-17.

41. **Richter EA, Mikines KJ, Galbo H, Kiens B.** Effect of exercise on insulin action in human skeletal muscle. J Appl Physiol. 1989;66:876-85.

42. **King DS, Dalsky GP, Clutter WE, et al.** Effects of exercise and lack of exercise on insulin sensitivity and responsiveness. J Appl Physiol. 1988;64:1942-6.

43. **Holloszy JO, Schultz J, Kusnierkiewicz J, et al.** Effects of exercise on glucose tolerance and insulin resistance: brief review and some preliminary results. Acta Med Scand. 1986;711(suppl):55-65.

44. **Manson JE, Rimm EB, Stampfer MJ, et al.** Physical activity and incidence of non–insulin-dependent diabetes mellitus in women. Lancet. 1991;338:774-8.

45. **Helmrich SP, Ragland DR, Leung RW, Paffenbarger RS.** Physical activity and reduced occurrence of non–insulin-dependent diabetes·mellitus. N Engl J Med. 1991; 325:147-52.

46. **Manson JE, Nathan DM, Krolewski AS, et al.** A prospective study of exercise and incidence of diabetes among U.S. male physicians. JAMA. 1992;268:63-7.

47. **Burchfiel CM, Sharp DS, Curb JD, et al.** Physical activity and incidence of diabetes: the Honolulu Heart Program. Am J Epidemiol. 1995;141:360-8.

48. **Ebeling P, Bourey R, Koranyi L, et al.** Mechanism of enhanced insulin sensitivity in athletes: increased blood flow, muscle glucose transport protein (GLUT-4) concentration, and glycogen synthase activity. J Clin Invest. 1993;92:1623-31.

49. **Hardin DS, Azzarelli B, Edwards J, et al.** Mechanisms of enhanced insulin sensitivity in endurance-trained athletes: effects on blood flow and differential expression of GLUT-4 skeletal muscles. Endocrinol Metab. 1995;80:2437-46.

50. **Perseghin G, Price TB, Petersen KF, et al.** Increased glucose transport, phosphorylation and muscle glycogen synthesis after exercise training in insulin-resistant subjects. N Engl J Med. 1986;335:1357-62.

51. **Fuller JH, Shipley MJ, Rose G, et al.** Coronary heart disease risk and impaired glucose tolerance. Lancet. 1980;1:1373-6.

52. **Barret-Connor E, Wingard DL, Criqui MH, Suarez L.** Is borderline fasting hyperglycemia a risk factor for cardiovascular death? J Chron Dis. 1984;37:773-9.

53a. **Donahue RP, Abbott RD, Reed DM, Yano K.** Postchallenge glucose concentration and coronary heart disease in men of Japanese ancestry: the Honolulu Heart Program. Diabetes. 1987;36:689-92.

53b. **Meigs JB, Nathan DM, Wilson WF, et al.** Metabolic risk factors worsen continuously across the spectrum of nondiabetic glucose tolerance: the Framingham Offspring Study. Ann Intern Med. 1998;128:524-33.

54. **Butler WJ, Ostrander LD, Carman WJ, Lamphiear DE.** Mortality from coronary heart disease in the Tecumseh Study. Am J Epidemiol. 1985;121:541-7.

55. **Coutinho M, Wang Y, Gerstein HC, Yusuf S.** Continuous relationship of glucose with cardiovascular events in nondiabetic subjects: a meta-regression analysis of 18 studies in 88,000 individuals. Circulation. 1996(suppl);94:I-214.

56. **The Expert Committee on the Diagnosis and Classification of Diabetes Mellitus.** Report of the Expert Committee on the Diagnosis and Classification of Diabetes Mellitus. Diabetes Care. 1997;20:1183-97.

57. **Wingard DL, Barrett-Connor EL, Ferrara A.** Is insulin really a heart disease risk factor? Diabetes Care. 1995;18:1299-1304.

58. **McKeigue P, Davey G.** Associations between insulin levels and cardiovascular disease are confounded by comorbidity. Diabetes Care. 1995;9:1294-9.

59. **Welborn TA, Wearne K.** Coronary heart disease incidence and cardiovascular mortality in Busselton with reference to glucose and insulin concentrations. Diabetes Care. 1979;2:154-60.

60. **Pyorala K.** Relationship of glucose tolerance and plasma insulin to the incidence of coronary heart disease: results from two population studies in Finland. Diabetes Care. 1979;2:131-41.

61. **Ducimetiere P, Eschwege E, Papoz L, et al.** Relationship of plasma insulin levels to the incidence of myocardial infarction and coronary heart disease mortality in a middle-aged population. Diabetologia. 1980;19:205-10.

62. **Eschwege E, Richard JL, Thibult N, et al.** Coronary heart disease mortality in relation with diabetes, blood glucose and plasma insulin levels: the Paris Prospective Study, ten years later. Horm Metab Res Suppl. 1985;15:41-5.

63. **Pyorala M, Pyorala K, Laakso M.** Hyperinsulinemia as predictor of coronary heart disease risk: 22-year follow-up results of the Helsinki Policemen Study. Circulation. 1996;94:I-213.

64. **Modan M, Or J, Karaski A, et al.** Hyperinsulinemia, sex, and risk of atherosclerotic cardiovascular disease. Circulation. 1991;84:1165-75.

65. **Laws A, King AC, Haskell WL, Reaven GM.** Relation of fasting plasma insulin concentration to high density lipoprotein cholesterol and triglyceride concentrations in men. Arterioscler Thromb Vasc Biol. 1991;11:1636-42.

66. **Laws A, King AC, Haskell WL, Reaven GM.** Metabolic and behavioral covariates of high-density lipoprotein cholesterol and triglyceride concentrations in postmenopausal women. J Am Geriatr Soc. 1993;41:1289-94.

67a. **Stout RW, Vallance-Owen W.** Insulin and atheroma. Lancet. 1969;1:1078-80.

67b. **Nesto RW, Zarich S.** Acute myocardial infarction in diabetes mellitus: lessons learned form ACE inhibition. Circulation. 1998;97:12-5.

68. **Pyorala K, Laakso M, Uusitupa M.** Diabetes and atherosclerosis: an epidemiologic view. Diabetes Metab Rev. 1987;3:463-524.

69. **Kannel WB, McGee DL.** Diabetes and glucose tolerance as risk factors for cardiovascular disease: the Framingham Study. Diabetes Care. 1979;2:120-6.

70. **Dunaif A, Segal KR, Futterweit W, Dobrjansky A.** Profound peripheral insulin resistance, independent of obesity, in polycystic ovary syndrome. Diabetes. 1989;28: 1165-74.

71. **Mattsson LA, Cullberg G, Hamberger L, et al.** Lipid metabolism in women with polycystic ovary syndrome: possible implications for an increased risk of coronary heart disease. Fertil Steril. 1984;42:579-84.

72. **Wild RA, Painter PC, Coulson PB, et al.** Lipoprotein lipid concentrations and cardiovascular risk in women with polycystic ovary syndrome. J Clin Endocrinol Metab. 1985;61:946-51.

73. **Birdsall MA, Farquhar CM, White HD.** Association between polycystic ovaries and extent of coronary artery disease in women having cardiac catherization. Ann Intern Med. 1997;126:32-5.

74. **Talbott E, Guzick D, Clerici A, et al.** Coronary heart disease risk factors in women with polycystic ovary syndrome. Aterioscler Thromb Vasc Biol. 1995;15:821-6.

75. **Robinson S, Henderson AD, Gelding SV, et al.** Dyslipidaemia is associated with insulin resistance in women with polycystic ovaries. Clin Endocrinol. 1996;44:277-84.

76. **Laakso M, Sarlund H, Salonen R, et al.** Asymptomatic atherosclerosis and insulin resistance. Aterioscler Thromb Vasc Biol. 1991;11:1068-76.

77. **Shinozaki K, Suzuki M, Ikebuchi M, et al.** Demonstration of insulin resistance in coronary artery disease documented with angiography. Diabetes Care. 1996;19:1-6.

78. **Howard G, O'Leary DH, Zaccaro D, et al, for the IRAS Investigators.** Insulin sensitivity and atherosclerosis. Circulation. 1996;93:1809-17.

79. **Heyden S, Heiss G, Bartel AG, Hames CG.** Sex differences in coronary mortality among diabetics in Evans County, Georgia. J Chronic Dis. 1980;33:265-73.

80. **O'Sullivan JB, Mahan CM.** Mortality related to diabetes and blood glucose levels in a community study. Am J Epidemiol. 1982;116:678-84.

81. **Jarrett RJ, McCartney P, Keen H.** The Bedford Study: Ten-year mortality rates in newly diagnosed diabetics, borderline diabetics and normoglycemic controls and risk indices for coronary heart disease in borderline diabetics. Diabetologia. 1982;22: 79-84.

82. **Pan W-H, Cedres LB, Liu K, et al.** Relationship of clinical diabetes and asymptomatic hyperglycemia to risk of coronary heart disease mortality in men and women. Am J Epidemiol. 1986;123:504-16.

83. **Barrett-Connor EL, Cohn BA, Wingard DL, Edelstein SL.** Why is diabetes mellitus a stronger risk factor for fatal ischemic heart disease in women than in men? The Rancho Bernardo Study. JAMA. 1991;265:627-31.

84. **Lee ET, Howard BV, Savage PJ, et al.** Diabetes and impaired glucose tolerance in three American Indian populations aged 45-74: the Strong Heart Study. Diabetes Care. 1995;18:599-610.

85. **Will JC, Casper M.** The contribution of diabetes to early deaths from ischemic heart disease: U.S. gender and racial comparisons. Am J Public Health. 1996;86:576-9.

86. **Walden CE, Knopp RH, Wahl P, et al.** Sex differences in the effect of diabetes mellitus on lipoprotein triglyceride and cholesterol concentrations. N Engl J Med. 1984; 311:953-9.

87. **Abbott RD, Donahue RP, Kannel WB, Wilson PWF.** The impact of diabetes on survival following myocardial infarction in men vs. women: the Framingham Study. JAMA. 1988;260:3456-60.

88. **Lehto S, Pyorala K, Miettinen H, et al.** Myocardial infarct size and mortality in patients with non–insulin-dependent diabetes. J Intern Med. 1994;236:291-7.

89. **Sprafka JM, Burke GL, Folsom AR, et al.** Trends in prevalence of diabetes mellitus in patients with myocardial infarction and effect of diabetes on survival: the Minnesota Heart Survey. Diabetes Care. 1991;14:537-43.

90. **Singer DE, Moulton AW, Nathan DM.** Diabetic myocardial infarction: interaction of diabetes with other preinfarction risk factors. Diabetes. 1989;28:350-7.

91. **Molstad P, Nustad M.** Acute myocardial infarction in diabetic patients. Acta Med Scand. 1987;222:433-7.

92. **Savage MP, Krolewski AS, Kenien GG, et al.** Acute myocardial infarction in diabetes mellitus and significance of congestive heart failure as a prognostic factor. Am J Cardiol. 1988;62:665-9.

93. **Chun BY, Dobson AJ, Heller RF.** The impact of diabetes on survival among patients with first myocardial infarction. Diabetes Care. 1997;20:704-8.

94. **Donahue RP, Goldberg RJ, Chen Z, et al.** The influence of sex and diabetes mellitus on survival following acute myocardial infarction: a community-wide perspective. J Clin Epidemiol. 1993;46:245-52.

95. **Utiger RD.** Insulin and the polycystic ovary syndrome. N Engl J Med. 1996;335: 657-8.

96. **Laws A.** Free fatty acids, insulin resistance and lipoprotein metabolism. Curr Opin Lipidol. 1996;7:172-7.

97. **Olefsky JM, Farquhar JW, Reaven GJ.** Reappraisal of the role of insulin in hyper-triglyceridemia. Am J Med. 1974;57:551-60.

98. **Tobey TA, Greenfield M, Kraemer F, Reaven GM.** Relationship between insulin resis-tance, insulin secretion, very low density lipoprotein kinetics and plasma triglyceride levels in normotriglyceridemic men. Metabolism. 1981;30:165-71.

99. **Farquhar JW, Frank A, Gross RC, Reaven GM.** Glucose, insulin and triglyceride re-sponses to high and low carbohydrate diets in man. J Clin Invest. 1966;45:1648-56.

100. **Wright DW, Hansen RI, Modon CE, Reaven GM.** Sucrose-induced insulin resistance in the rat: modulation by exercise and diet. Am J Clin Nutr. 1983;38:879-83.

101. **Zavaroni I, Chen YD, Reaven GM.** Studies of the mechanism of fructose-induced hy-pertriglyceridemia in the rat. Metabolism. 1982;31:1077-83.

102. **Zavaroni I, Chen YI, Mondon CE, Reaven GM.** Ability of exercise to inhibit carbohy-drate-induced hypertriglyceridemia in rats. Metabolism. 1981;30:417-20.

103. **Pullinger CR, North JD, Teng B-B, et al.** The apolipoprotein B gene is constitutively expressed in HepG2 cells: regulation of secretion by oleic acid, albumin, and insulin, and measurement of the mRNA half-life. J Lipid Res. 1989;30:1065-77.

104. **Byrne CD, Wang TWM, Hales CN.** Control of Hep G2 cell triacylglycerol and apolipoprotein-B synthesis and secretion by polyunsaturated nonesterified fatty acids and insulin. Biochem J. 1992;299:101-7.

105. **Brinton EA, Eisenberg S, Breslow JL.** Human HDL cholesterol levels are deter-mined by ApoA-I fractional catabolic rate, which correlates inversely with estimates of HDL particle size: effects of gender, hepatic and lipoprotein lipases, triglyceride and insulin levels, and body fat distribution. Arterioscler Thromb Vasc Biol. 1994;14: 707-20.

106. **Abbott WG, Lillioja S, Young AA, et al.** Relationships between plasma lipoprotein concentrations and insulin action in an obese hyperinsulinemic population. Dia-betes. 1987;36:897-904.

107. **Laakso M, Sarlund H, Salonen R, et al.** Asymptomatic atherosclerosis and insulin resistance. Arterioscler Thromb Vasc Biol. 1991;11:1068-76.

108. **Laws A, Reaven GM.** Evidence for an independent relationship between insulin re-sistance and fasting plasma HDL-cholesterol, triglyceride and insulin concentra-tions. J Intern Med. 1992;231:25-30.

109. **Stalder M, Pometta D, Wuenram A.** Relationship between plasma insulin levels and high density lipoprotein cholesterol levels in healthy men. Diabetologia. 1981;21: 544-8.

110. **Zavaroni I, Dall'Aglio E, Alpi O, et al.** Evidence for an independent relationship be-tween plasma insulin and concentration of high density lipoprotein cholesterol and triglyceride. Atherosclerosis. 1985;55:259-66.

111. **Crouse JR.** Gender, lipoproteins, diet and cardiovascular risk: sauce for the goose may not be sauce for the gander. Lancet. 1989;1:318-20.

112. **Bush TL, Barrett-Connor E.** Cholesterol, lipoproteins, and coronary heart disease in women. Clin Chem. 1988;34:B60-70.

113. **Jacobs DR, Mebane IL, Bangdiwala SI, et al.** High density lipoprotein cholesterol as a predictor of cardiovascular disease mortality in men and women: the follow-up study of the Lipid Research Clinics Prevalence Study. Am J Epidemiol. 1990;131: 32-47.

114. **Bass KM, Newschaffer CJ, Klag MJ, Bush TL.** Plasma lipoprotein levels as predictors of cardiovascular death in women. Arch Intern Med. 1993;153:2209-16.

115. **Fontbonne A, Eschwege E, Cambien F, et al.** Hypertriglyceridemia as a risk factor of coronary heart disease mortality in subjects with impaired glucose tolerance or diabetes: results from the 11-year follow-up of the Paris Prospective Study. Diabetologia. 1989;32:300-4.

116. **Laws A, Marcus EB, Grove JS, Curb JD.** Lipids and lipoproteins as risk factors for coronary heart disease in men with abnormal glucose tolerance: the Honolulu Heart Program. J Intern Med. 1993;234:471-8.

117. **Goldschmid MG, Barrett-Connor E, Edelstein SL, et al.** Dyslipidemia and ischemic heart disease mortality among men and women with diabetes. Circulation. 1994;89: 991-7.

118. **Austin MA, Selby JV.** LDL subclass phenotypes and the risk factors of the insulin resistance syndrome. Intl J Obesity. 1995;19(suppl 1):S22-6.

119. **Reaven BM, Chen IY-D, Jeppesen J, Krauss RM.** Insulin resistance and hyperinsulinemia in individuals with small, dense, low density lipoprotein particles. J Clin Invest. 1993;92:141-6.

120. **Barakat HA, Carpenter JW, McLendon VD, et al.** Influence of obesity, impaired glucose tolerance and NIDDM on LDL structure and composition: possible link between hyperinsulinemia and atherosclerosis. Diabetes. 1990;39:1527-33.

121. **Haffner SM, Mykkanen L, Stern MP, et al.** Greater effect of diabetes on LDL size in women than in men. Diabetes Care. 1994;17:1164-71.

122. **Austin MA, Breslow JL, Hennekens CH, et al.** Low-density lipoprotein subclass patterns and risk of myocardial infarction. JAMA. 1988;260:1917-21.

123. **Welborn TA, Breckenridge A, Rubenstein AH, et al.** Serum-insulin in essential hypertension and in peripheral vascular disease. Lancet. 1966;1:1336-7.

124. **Donahue RP, Skyler JS, Schneiderman N, Prineas RJ.** Hyperinsulinemia and elevated blood pressure: cause, confounder, or coincidence. Am J Epidemiol. 1990;132:827-36.

125. **Ferrannini E, Buzzigoli G, Bonadonna R.** Insulin resistance in essential hypertension. N Engl J Med. 1987;317:450-7.

126. **Shen DC, Shieh SM, Fuh MM, et al.** Resistance to insulin-stimulated glucose uptake in patients with hypertension. J Clin Endocrinol Metab. 1988;66:580-3.

127. **Reisin E, Abel R, Modan M, et al.** Effect of weight loss without salt restriction in the reduction of blood pressure in overweight hypertensive patients. N Engl J Med. 1978; 298:1-6.

128. **Krotkiewski M, Mandroukas K, Sjostrom L, et al.** Effects of long-term physical training on body fat, metabolism, and blood pressure in obesity. Metabolism. 1979;28:650-8.

129. **Janka HU, Dirschedl P.** Systolic blood pressure as a predictor for cardiovascular disease in diabetes: a 5-year longitudinal study. Hypertension. 1985;7(suppl II):II-90–II-94.

130. **Stamler J, Vaccaro O, Neaton JD, Wentworth D.** Diabetes, other risk factors, and 12-year cardiovascular mortality for men screened in the Multiple Risk Factor Intervention Trial. Diabetes Care. 1993;16:434-4.

131. **Auwerx J, Bouillon R, Cohen D, Geboers J.** Tissue-type plasminogen activator antigen and plasminogen activator inhibitor in diabetes mellitus. Arteriosclerosis. 1988;8:68-72.

132. **Juhan-Vague I, Alessi MC, Vague P.** Increased plasma plasminogen activator inhibitor 1 levels: a possible link between insulin resistance and atherothrombosis. Diabetologia. 1991;34:457-62.

133. **Hamsten A, de Faire U, Walldius G, et al.** Plasminogen activator inhibitor in plasma: risk factor for recurrent myocardial infarction. Lancet. 1987;2:3-9.

134. **Hamsten A, Karpe F, Bavenholm P, Silveira A.** Interactions amongst insulin, lipoproteins and haemostatic function relevant to coronary heart disease. J Intern Med. 1994;236(suppl 736):75-88.

135. **Vague P, Juhan-Vague I, Aillaud MF, et al.** Correlation between blood fibrinolytic activity, plasminogen activator inhibitor level, plasma insulin level and relative body weight in normal and obese subjects. Metabolism. 1986;35:250-3.

136. **Sundell IB, Dahlgren S, Ranby M, et al.** Reduction of elevated plasminogen activator inhibitor levels during modest weight loss. Fibrinolysis. 1989;3:51-3.

137. **Mehrabian M, Peter JB, Barnard RJ, Lusis AJ.** Dietary regulation of fibrinolytic factors. Atherosclerosis. 1990;84:25-32.

138. **Estelles A, Aznar J, Tormo G, et al.** Influence of a rehabilitation sports program on the fibrinolytic activity of patients after myocardial infarction. Thromb Res. 1989;55:203-12.

139. **Gris JC, Schved JF, Aguilar-Martinez P, et al.** Impact of physical training on plasminogen activator inhibitor activity in sedentary men. Fibrinolysis. 1990;4:97-8.

140. **Vague P, Juhan-Bague I, Alessi MC, et al.** Metformin decreases the high plasminogen activatory inhibition capacity, plasma insulin and triglyceride levels in nondiabetic obese subjects. Thromb Haemost. 1987;57:326-8.

141. **Gertler MM, Garn SM, Levine SA.** Serum uric acid in relation to age and physique in health and coronary heart disease. Ann Intern Med. 1951;34:1421-31.

142. **Myers AR, Epstein FH, Dodge JG, Mikkelsen WM.** The relationship of serum uric acid to risk factors in coronary heart disease. Am J Med. 1968;45:520-8.

143. **Facchini F, Chen Y-DI, Hollenbeck CB, Reaven GM.** Relationship between resistance to insulin-mediated glucose uptake, urinary uric acid clearance, and plasma uric acid concentrations. JAMA. 1991;226:3008-11.

144. **Modan M, Halkin H, Lusky A, et al.** Hyperinsulinemia is characterized by jointly disturbed plasma VLDL, LDL, and HDL levels: a population-based study. Arteriosclerosis. 1988;8:227-36.

145. **Schmidt MI, Duncan BB, Watson RL, et al, for the ARIC Study Investigators.** A metabolic syndrome in whites and African-Americans. Diabetes Care. 1996;19:414-8.

146. **McKeigue PM, Shah B, Marmot MG.** Relation of central obesity and insulin resistance with high diabetes prevalence and cardiovascular risk in South Asians. Lancet. 1991;337:382-6.

147. **Haffner SM, Valdez RA, Hazuda HP, et al.** Prospective analysis of the insulin-resistance syndrome (syndrome X). Diabetes. 1992;41:715-22.

148. **Chan JCN, Cheung JCK, Lau EMC, et al.** The metabolic syndrome in Hong Kong Chinese. Diabetes Care. 1996;19:953-9.

149. **Ohmura T, Ueda K, Kiyohara Y, et al.** The association of the insulin resistance syndrome with impaired glucose tolerance and NIDDM in the Japanese general population: the Hisayama Study. Diabetologia. 1994;37:897-904.

150. **Yamada N, Yoshinaga H, Sakurai N, et al.** Increased risk factors for coronary artery disease in Japanese subjects with hyperinsulinemia or glucose intolerance. Diabetes Care. 1994;17:107-14.

151. **Howard BV, Lee ET, Cowan LD, et al.** Coronary heart disease prevalence and its relation to risk factors in American Indians: the Strong Heart Study. Am J Epidemiol. 1995;142:254-68.

152. **Harris SS, Caspersen CJ, DeFriese GH, Estes EH.** Physical activity counseling for healthy adults as a primary preventive intervention in the clinical setting: report for the U.S. Preventive Services Task Force. JAMA. 1989;261:3590-8.

153. **Bosello O, Armellini F, Zamboni M, Fitchet M.** The benefits of modest weight loss in type II diabetes. Intl J Obesity. 1997;21(suppl 1):S10-3.

154. **Wing RR.** Behavioral treatment of obesity: its application to type II diabetes. Diabetes Care. 1993;16:193-9.

155. **Kolanowski J.** Surgical treatment for morbid obesity. British Medical Bulletin. 1997;53:433-44.

156. **Mensink RP, Katan MB.** Effect of monounsaturated fatty acids versus complex carbohydrates on high-density lipoproteins in healthy men and women. Lancet. 1987; 1:122-5.

157. **Borkman M, Campbell LV, Chisholm DJ, Storlein LH.** Comparison of the effects on insulin sensitivity on high carbohydrate and high fat diets in normal subjects. J Clin Endocrinol Metab. 1991;72:432-7.

158. **Garg A, Bonanome A, Grundy SM, et al.** Comparison of a high-carbohydrate diet with a high-monounsaturated fat diet in patients with non–insulin-dependent diabetes mellitus. N Engl J Med. 1988;319:829-34.

159. **Garg A, Grundy SM, Unger RH.** Comparison of effects of high and low carbohydrate diets on plasma lipoproteins and insulin sensitivity in patients with mild NIDDM. Diabetes. 1992;41:1278-85.

160. **Peterson CM, Jovanovic-Peterson L.** Randomized crossover study of 40% vs. 55% carbohydrate weight loss strategies in women with previous gestational diabetes mellitus and nondiabetic women of 130-200% ideal body weight. J Am Coll Nutr. 1995;14:369-75.

161. **Golay A, Allaz A-F, Morel Y, et al.** Similar weight loss with low- or high-carbohydrate diets. Am J Clin Nutr. 1996;64:174-8.

162. **Garg A, Bantle JP, Henry RR, et al.** Effects of varying carbohydrate content of diet in patients with non–insulin-dependent diabetes mellitus. JAMA. 1994;271:1421-8.

163. **Rasmussen OW, Thomsen C, Hansen KW, et al.** Effects on blood pressure, glucose, and lipid levels of a high-monounsaturated fat diet compared with a high-carbohydrate diet in NIDDM subjects. Diabetes Care. 1993;16:1565-71.

164. **Rasmussen O, Thomsen C, Ingerslev J, Hermansen K.** Decrease in von Willebrand factor levels after a high monounsaturated fat diet in non–insulin-dependent diabetic subjects. Metabolism. 1994;43:1406-9.

165a. **Nathan DM, Meigs J, Singer DE.** The epidemiology of cardiovascular disease in type 2 diabetes mellitus: how sweet it is… or is it? Lancet. 1997;350(suppl 1):4-9.

165b. **Malmberg K, for the DIGAMI Study Group.** Prospective randomised study of intensive insulin treatment on long term survival after acute myocardial infarction in patients with diabetes mellitus. BMJ. 1997;314:1512-5.

166. **Bressler R, Johnson DG.** Pharmacological regulation of blood glucose levels in non–insulin-dependent diabetes mellitus. Arch Intern Med. 1997;157:836-48.

167. **DeFronzo RA, Goodman AM, and the Multicenter Metformin Study Group.** Efficacy of metformin in patients with non–insulin-dependent diabetes mellitus. N Engl J Med. 1995;333:541-9.

168. **Jeppesen J, Zhou M-Y, Chen Y-DI, Reaven FM.** Effect of metformin on postprandial lipemia in patients with fairly to poorly controlled NIDDM. Diabetes Care. 1994;17:1093-9.

169. **Fanghanel G, Sanchez-Reyes L, Trujillo C, et al.** Metformin's effects on glucose and lipid metabolism in patients with secondary failure to sulfonylureas. Diabetes Care. 1996;18:1185-9.

170. **Velazquez EM, Mendoza S, Hamer T, et al.** Metformin therapy in polycystic ovary syndrome reduces hyperinsulinemia, insulin resistance, hyperandrogenemia, and systolic blood pressure, while facilitating normal menses and pregnancy. Metabolism. 1994;43:647-54.

171. **Suter SI, Nolan JJ, Wallace P, et al.** Metabolic effects of new oral hypoglycemic agent CS-045 in NIDDM subjects. Diabetes Care. 1992;15:193-203.

172. Consensus statement. Treatment of hypertension in diabetes. Diabetes Care. 1996; 19(suppl 1):S107-13.

173a. **Poulter NR.** Managing the diabetic hypertensive patient. Diabetes Complications. 1996;10:141-3.

173b. **Ruige JB, Assendelft WJJ, Dekker JM, et al.** Insulin and risk of cardiovascular disease: meta-analysis. Circulation. 1998;97:996-1001.

174. **Curb JD, Pressel SL, Cutler JA, et al, for the Systolic Hypertension in the Elderly Program Cooperative Research Group.** Effect of diuretic-based antihypertensive treatment on cardiovascular disease risk in older diabetic patients with isolated systolic hypertension [published erratum appears in JAMA. 1997;277:1356]. JAMA. 1996;276:1886-92.

175. **Warram JH, Laffel LMB, Valsania P, et al.** Excess mortality associated with diuretic therapy in diabetes mellitus. Arch Intern Med. 1991;151:1350-6.

176. **Hoes AW, Grobbee DE, Lubsen J, et al.** Diuretics, beta-blockers, and the risk for sudden cardiac death in hypertensive patients. Ann Intern Med. 1995;123:481-7.

177. **Freis ED.** The efficacy and safety of diuretics in treating hypertension. Ann Intern Med. 1995;122:223-6.

178. **Pyorala K, Pedersen TR, Kjekshus J, et al, for the Scandinavian Simvastatin Survival Study (4S) Group.** Cholesterol lowering with simvastatin improves prognosis of diabetic patients with coronary heart disease: a subgroup analysis of the Scandinavian Simvastatin Survival Study (4S). Diabetes Care. 1997;20:614-20.

179. **Vinik AI, Colwell JA, for the Hyperlipidemia in Diabetes Investigators.** Effects of gemfibrozil on triglyceride levels in patients with NIDDM. Diabetes Care. 1993;16: 37-44.

180. **Garg A, Grundy SM.** Lovastatin for lowering cholesterol levels in non–insulin-dependent diabetes mellitus. N Engl J Med. 1988;318:81-6.

181. **Bakker-Arkema RG, Davidson MH, Goldstein RJ, et al.** Efficacy and safety of a new HMG-CoA reductase inhibitor, atorvastatin, in patients with hypertriglyceridemia. JAMA. 1996;275:128-33.

182. **Robinson JC, Folsom AR, Nabulsi AA, et al, for the Atherosclerosis Risk in Communities Study Investigation.** Can postmenopausal hormone replacement improve plasma lipids in women with diabetes? Diabetes Care. 1996;19:480-5.

183. **Andersson B, Mattsson LA, Hahn L, et al.** Estrogen replacement therapy decreases hyperandrogenicity and improves glucose homeostasis and plasma lipids in postmenopausal women with non–insulin-dependent diabetes mellitus. J Clin Endocrinol Metab. 1997;82:638-43.

184. **Brussaard HE, Bevers Leuven JA, Frolich M, et al.** Short-term estrogen replacement therapy improves insulin resistance, lipids and fibrinolysis in postmenopausal women with NIDDM. Diabetologia. 1997;40:843-9.

CHAPTER 4

Lipids

Natural History and Pharmacologic Management

JUDITH M.E. WALSH, MD, MPH

Hyperlipidemia is a risk factor for the development of coronary artery disease (CAD) in both women and men; however, hyperlipidemia in women and men differs in several important ways. Cholesterol levels change differently with aging in women and men. Low-density lipoprotein (LDL) cholesterol is less predictive of CAD risk in women than in men, whereas high-density lipoprotein (HDL) cholesterol is more predictive. Finally, the role of lipoprotein Lp(a) as a CAD risk factor may differ in women and men (1,2).

Most studies of hyperlipidemia treatment have included predominantly (sometimes entirely) male subjects, and the majority of hyperlipidemia management guidelines are based on the results of these studies. The few studies that have included women contain limited numbers of female subjects. This is especially problematic because at any given age fewer women than men have or are at risk for CAD. In addition, the maximum age for inclusion in most hyperlipidemia treatment studies has been 65 years. Older women, who are at the greatest risk for CAD, largely have been excluded from studies of cholesterol lowering.

The Women's Health Initiative, the largest clinical trial in the history of the nation, will provide critical information on the epidemiology of CAD, CAD risk factors, and cholesterol-lowering interventions in women. Because the results of this trial will not be available until 2006, we must rely on currently available data in the interim. Some observational studies and a limited number of treatment trials have been completed. After we review these trials and consider the potential hazards of pharmacologic therapy, rational guidelines for screening and treatment of hyperlipidemia in women are discussed.

Observational Data About Lipids and Women

Natural History of Cholesterol Levels

Recent data from the National Health and Nutrition Examination Surveys (NHANES) indicate that mean serum cholesterol levels among adults aged 20 to 74 years have been declining consistently from 1960 to 1991. In 1960, the first NHANES survey revealed that the average total cholesterol for a white woman was 223 mg/dL; in 1991, it was 205 mg/dL. During this time period, the proportion of women defined as having high blood cholesterol ($\geq$ 240 mg/dL) has decreased from 28% to 20%. Because HDL and very-low-density lipoprotein (VLDL) fractions have remained relatively constant, the main change is attributed to a decrease in LDL levels. Suggested contributors to this decline include increased public health nutrition education, increased use of cholesterol-lowering diets and drugs, increased use of hormone replacement therapy (HRT), and use of lower-dose oral contraceptives (3).

The natural history of cholesterol levels in women and men is demonstrated in Figure 4-1. Total cholesterol levels in both women and men increase with age. In men, the peak cholesterol level is reached at approximately 50

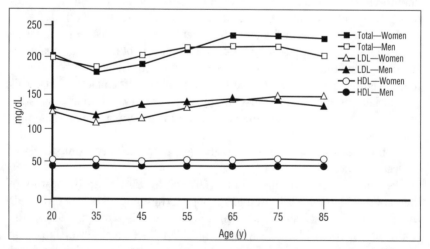

Figure 4-1 Cholesterol levels in men and women by age. LDL = low-density lipoprotein; HDL = high-density lipoprotein.

years of age, with a gradual decline thereafter. Cholesterol levels in women peak later, between the ages of 55 and 64 years, and then decline slightly. Throughout life, women's HDL cholesterol levels are higher than those of men, although HDL levels generally tend to decrease after menopause.

Study of the impact of race and ethnicity on cholesterol levels has been limited. African American women have higher total cholesterol levels than white women, although their HDL cholesterol levels also tend to be higher (4). Interestingly, total cholesterol levels are less likely to change after menopause in black women. Mexican American women have LDL and total cholesterol levels that are similar to those of white women, but their HDL cholesterol levels tend to be lower (5). The lower HDL levels in Mexican American women may be related to body fat distribution or fasting insulin levels (6). Insulin resistance and dyslipidemia, especially low HDL and elevated triglycerides, are reviewed in Chapter 3.

Association of Hyperlipidemia and Coronary Artery Disease Risk in Women

Total Cholesterol

Many observational studies have reported an association between elevated total cholesterol and CAD in women. An NHLBI workshop collected unpublished follow-up data on total, HDL, and LDL cholesterol from 25 populations in 22 U.S. and international cohort studies. Studies that measured serum cholesterol provided follow-up for CAD events and had explicit criteria for CAD end points were eligible for inclusion. Data from these studies, which provided information on approximately 86,000 women, were pooled to assess the association of hyperlipidemia and CAD risk in women. Among women younger than 65 years of age, the pooled relative risk for CAD mortality in women with cholesterol levels equal to or greater than 240 mg/dL compared with those with cholesterol levels less than 200 mg/dL was 2.44 (95% confidence interval [CI]: 2.16, 2.75). In women aged 65 years and over, the relative risk for CAD mortality was 1.12 (95% CI: 1.01, 1.25) (7) (Table 4-1). In the Framingham study, the relationship of total cholesterol to CAD mortality also attenuated with age to the extent that total cholesterol was less important in women and men over 70 years of age (8).

The association between total cholesterol and total mortality was assessed at another NHLBI conference at which data from 11 cohort studies among over 124,000 women were combined. There was no association between total cholesterol and all-cause mortality nor between total cholesterol and total cardiovascular mortality in women. However, in women with cholesterol levels greater than or equal to 240 mg/dL, the relative risk for CAD death was 1.56 compared with women with cholesterol levels of 160 to 199 mg/dL. Total

Table 4-1 Association of Hyperlipidemia and Coronary Artery Disease Risk

	Relative Risks*		
	Total Cholesterol†	LDL Cholesterol‡	HDL Cholesterol§
Women			
< 65 years of age	2.44	3.27	2.13
≥ 65 years of age	1.12	1.13	1.75
Men			
< 65 years of age	1.73	1.92	2.31
≥ 65 years of age	1.32	1.51	1.09

* Includes data from ~86,000 women.
† Comparing women with total cholesterol of ≥ 240 mg/dL to < 200 mg/dL.
‡ Comparing women with LDL-C ≥ 160 mg/dl to < 140 mg/dL.
§ Comparing women with HDL-C < 50 mg/dL to ≥ 60 mg/dL.
HDL = high-density lipoprotein; LDL = low-density lipoprotein.
Adapted from Manolio TM, et al. Cholesterol and heart disease in older persons and women: review of an NHLBI workshop. Ann Epidemiol. 1992; 2:161–76.

cardiovascular mortality was not associated with elevated cholesterol levels, and CAD mortality was increased in women with elevated cholesterol levels; these findings suggest that there was an increase in some other form of cardiovascular mortality in the women with cholesterol levels of 160 to 199 mg/dL. Hemorrhagic stroke was more common in women with low total cholesterol levels, although the small number of hemorrhagic strokes could not fully explain the observed difference. Finally, low cholesterol levels (< 160 mg/dL) were also associated with higher death rates from respiratory and digestive diseases and some cancers (9).

Low- and High-Density Lipoprotein Cholesterol
The roles of LDL and HDL as predictors of CAD mortality may be different in women and men. Although elevated LDL cholesterol is clearly established as a CAD risk factor in men, LDL may be a less important predictor in women. In the NHLBI study among women less than 65 years old, those with LDL cholesterol levels greater than 160 mg/dL had a relative risk for CAD mortality 3.27 times greater than women with LDL cholesterol levels less than 140 mg/dL. For women aged 65 years and over, the relative risk was only 1.13 (7).

HDL cholesterol is a particularly important predictor of CAD risk in women. In a 20-year follow-up of women in the Donolo–Tel Aviv Prospective Coronary Artery Disease Study, women who had a higher percentage of HDL cholesterol had a lower risk of CAD mortality. In addition, a high HDL percentage was protective even in women with elevated total cholesterol levels (10). Other cohort studies have confirmed the role of HDL cholesterol as the strongest predictor of CAD risk in women, with higher levels being protective (11–14).

In the NHLBI study, which pooled data from 86,000 women, the relationship between HDL cholesterol and CAD mortality was assessed. Women less than 65 years of age with an HDL level less than 50 mg/dL had a relative risk for CAD mortality 2.13 times greater than those with an HDL level greater than 60 mg/dL. Among women aged 65 years and over, the comparable relative risk was 1.75 (7) (*see* Table 4-1).

In the NHLBI study, HDL cholesterol was the only significant lipid predictor of CAD mortality in women over the age of 65 years (i.e., those at highest risk for CAD). In a prospective study of 2527 women aged 71 years and over who were followed for 4.4 years, HDL was also found to be important in older women. CAD mortality was inversely related to HDL-cholesterol levels; women with HDL levels 60 mg/dL or greater had a CAD mortality rate half that of those with HDL cholesterol levels of less than 35 mg/dL (15).

Triglycerides

Some cohort studies have shown elevated triglycerides to be an independent risk factor for CAD mortality in women (12,16), but others have not (17,18). Elevated triglycerides are often associated with other CAD risk factors (e.g., obesity, glucose intolerance, low HDL levels), making it more difficult to estimate each factor's independent contribution. In addition, no clinical trial has been performed whose main goal has been lowering triglyceride levels (19,20). In many studies, multivariate analyses that include LDL and HDL cholesterol levels reduce the association between elevated triglycerides and CAD mortality. In one study, however, triglycerides maintained more of their independent effect in women than in men, suggesting that the role of triglycerides in producing atherogenesis may not be the same in the two sexes (21). Finally, the role of diabetes as a major CAD risk factor in women may be partly related to hypertriglyceridemia (22,23).

Lipoprotein Lp(a)

Lp(a) excess has been shown to be an important predictor of CAD in men in several large observational studies (24–29). Two studies of the association between Lp(a) and CAD in women have reached conflicting conclusions (2,30). In the Framingham Offspring Study, the attributable risk associated with Lp(a) excess in women was similar to the risk associated with hypercholesterolemia and low HDL cholesterol levels (2). In the second study of the association between Lp(a) and CAD in women, no association between Lp(a) and CAD was seen, but the study had inadequate statistical power; hence, a true association could have been missed (30).

At least part of the increased risk associated with Lp(a) seems to be associated with concomitant excess of LDL cholesterol (31). Currently, no clinical trial evidence suggests that lowering Lp(a) decreases CAD mortality. Estrogen replacement therapy, however, has been shown to decrease Lp(a) levels by up to 50% (32–37), although the addition of progestin negates some of estrogen's benefit. This lowering of Lp(a) may explain in part the protective effect of estrogen on CAD.

In summary, cohort data from a large number of women suggest an association between lipoprotein levels and CAD, although the risk differs between young and old women. Among young women in whom absolute CAD risk is low, an increased relative risk is associated with elevated total cholesterol, elevated LDL cholesterol, and low HDL cholesterol. However, among women aged 65 years and over who have a higher absolute risk of CAD, only low HDL cholesterol is substantially associated with increased CAD mortality. HDL cholesterol is a strong predictor of CAD risk, whereas LDL cholesterol is a less consistent predictor of risk in women than in men. Guidelines for lipid management that focus on LDL levels may be less useful in women. Hypertriglyceridemia may be particularly important in women with diabetes, and elevated levels of Lp(a) may also be a CAD risk factor in women.

Cohort study data are subject to limitations. The only outcome assessed was mortality; other important CAD-associated morbidities were not included. Information about potential confounding variables (e.g., estrogen use, obesity, and other cardiovascular risk factors) are not available for these women. Finally, although elevated cholesterol levels might be associated with CAD death in women, cohort studies do not provide any information about whether lowering cholesterol levels will change CAD risk. This information is available only from randomized, controlled trials.

Lipid-Lowering Interventions

Primary Prevention

Primary prevention trials in men have shown that cholesterol lowering can reduce mortality from CAD. Muldoon and colleagues (38) pooled data from six randomized primary prevention trials and found a 15% decrease in CAD mortality in men treated for hypercholesterolemia. However, the treated group had a higher mortality from non-CAD causes, total mortality was not decreased, and the decrease in CAD mortality was of borderline statistical significance ($p = 0.06$). In the West of Scotland Coronary Primary Prevention Study, high risk men treated with pravastatin had 31% fewer coronary events than untreated men, and there were no additional deaths from noncardiovascular causes (39).

Only four primary prevention trials with clinical end points have included women: two studies used dietary treatment and two used drug treatment (colestipol or lovastatin). In the Finnish Mental Hospital Study, there were statistically insignificant reductions in CAD death rates (34%) and cardiovascular disease death rates (14%), but all-cause mortality was similar for women in both groups (40). In the Minnesota Coronary Survey, no significant differences in cardiovascular events, CAD or cardiovascular deaths, or total mortality were seen between the groups (41). In the colestipol study, CAD and total mortality rates in women did not differ significantly between treatment groups (42a). In the Air Force/Texas Coronary Atherosclerosis Prevention Study (AFCAPS/TexCAPS) study, which included 997 women (15% of total), there was no significant difference in first major coronary events between treated (lovastatin) and nontreated women (1.4% vs. 2.6%; NS). Coronary artery disease and total mortality rates were not reported separately for women (42b) (Table 4-2).

Because each individual trial had few outcomes, summary estimates of the relative risks were calculated. The summary relative risk based on the two studies that provided confidence intervals was 1.03 (95% CI: 0.62, 1.70) for CAD mortality and 1.15 (95% CI: 0.90, 1.46) for total mortality, neither of which was significant (43).

There are several limitations to the available studies. The participants in both dietary studies were not hypercholesterolemic, and the dietary treatment used in one trial (41) was significantly different from the dietary guidelines currently suggested by the National Cholesterol Education Program (NCEP). Because women were not selected for the presence or absence of CAD, these studies may have enrolled some women with CAD, and hence may not represent true primary prevention. Finally, two of the four studies used

Table 4-2 Primary Prevention Trials in Women

Trial	No. of Women (No. of Patients)	Intervention	CAD Mortality RR in Women (95% CI)	Total Mortality RR in Women (95% CI)
Finnish Mental Hospital Study (40)	6434 (10,612)	Low-saturated-fat diet	0.66 (NA)*	1.06 (NA)*
Minnesota Coronary Survey (41)	4664 (9057)	Low-saturated-fat diet	1.08 (0.59, 1.97)	1.16 (0.89, 1.52)
Colestipol (42a)	1184 (2278)	Colestipol	0.93 (0.38, 2.26)	1.08 (0.59, 1.57)
AFCAPS/TexCAPS (42b)	997 (6605)	Lovastatin	NA	NA

* Cannot calculate CIs from published data.
CAD = coronary artery disease; CI = confindence interval; RR = relative risk.

institutionalized populations that may not be representative of healthy women.

In summary, the data about the effect of cholesterol-lowering in healthy women are limited, and the relatively small numbers of women studied provide inadequate power to detect small differences. When the results from two of the studies were pooled, there were still no significant differences in either CAD or total mortality between treated and nontreated women. Although the available studies have limitations, currently no evidence exists that cholesterol lowering in otherwise healthy women affects subsequent CAD mortality.

Hormone Replacement Therapy

Of the at least 32 observational epidemiologic studies that have assessed the relationship between estrogen replacement therapy and CAD, 16 have been prospective; 15 of the 16 prospective studies have shown a protective effect of estrogen on CAD. Based on all available studies, Stampfer and Colditz calculated a pooled, estimated relative risk of 0.56 (95% CI: 0.50, 0.61) for CAD among estrogen users. Grady and colleagues (44), using slightly different methods, performed a meta-analysis and calculated a pooled relative risk for CAD death among ever users of estrogen compared with nonusers of 0.63 (95% CI: 0.55, 0.72).

Estrogen decreases LDL by 10%–15%, increases HDL by 10%–15%, and decreases Lp(a) by up to 50%. Estrogen also acts as an antioxidant, reduces platelet adhesiveness, and has a direct effect on the coronary vasculature. It has been estimated that only approximately 25%–50% of the effect of estrogen is due to its effects on lipids (45).

Because progestins attenuate the positive effect of estrogen on lipids (i.e., it causes less of an increase in HDL concentrations), there has been concern that the addition of a progestin may negate or diminish the beneficial cardioprotective effects of estrogen. Three prospective cohort studies have assessed the effect of treatment with estrogen plus a progestin on CAD risk in women. In all of these, the risk of CAD among users was lower than among nonusers, and the degree of protection was similar to that seen for estrogen alone (46–48).

Because HRT has other effects on other outcomes in addition to CAD, investigators in the Nurses Health Study recently assessed the relationship between postmenopausal hormone use and total mortality. They found that current hormone users had a relative risk of death that was 0.63 (95% CI: 0.56, 0.70) times that of never users; however, the effect was attenuated with long-term use (RR = 0.80; 95% CI: 0.67, 0.96 after 10 years), because of an increase in breast cancer mortality in long-term users. The relative risk of death for current users of estrogen plus progestin was 0.46 (95% CI: 0.36, 0.58), whereas for current users of estrogen alone it was 0.69 (95% CI: 0.60, 0.80). The largest risk reduction was seen in women at highest risk for cardiac disease, whereas the benefit for women at risk for cardiac disease was significantly lower (RR = 0.51 for high-risk women; RR = 0.89 for low-risk women) (49).

Observational studies of HRT have several problems. Women who choose to take HRT are more likely to be upper middle class, educated, white, and lean; hence, they are at lower risk for CAD (50). Before HRT use, women who elect to take HRT have higher HDL-cholesterol, more leisure time activity, increased alcohol intake, and lower blood pressure, weight, and levels of fasting insulin (51). Observational studies are also prone to physician bias, i.e., physicians may prescribe HRT to healthier women. Finally, although the authors attempt to correct for multiple confounders, there still may be unmeasured confounders. The Hormone Estrogen Replacement Study (HERS), a study of secondary prevention of CAD with hormone therapy, was published in 1998. Women were randomized to either continuous hormone therapy or placebo. There were no significant differences between groups in the primary outcome of nonfatal myocardial infarction (MI) or CAD death (RR = 0.99; 95% CI: 0.80, 1.22). Also, there was a significant time effect, with more events in the hormone group during the first year and fewer in fourth and fifth years (52). Because of these potential biases inherent in observational studies and the surprising results of the secondary prevention study, randomized clinical trials of hormone therapy for primary prevention are needed.

Several ongoing randomized trials with clinical end points are in progress. The largest is the Women's Health Initiative, which has enrolled approximately 63,000 women in the HRT arm but which will not be completed until the year 2006. Meanwhile, several randomized trials using intermediate end points (e.g., lipid levels) are available for review. The earliest of these, a randomized trial of residents of a long-term care facility, was published in 1979 (53). More recent trial participants are healthy and ambulatory.

The Postmenopausal Estrogen Progestin Intervention (PEPI) trial was designed to assess the effects of HRT on multiple heart disease risk factors. Healthy postmenopausal women aged 45 to 64 years were randomized to five groups: 1) placebo, 2) estrogen alone, 3) estrogen plus cyclic medroxyprogesterone, 4) estrogen plus continuous medroxyprogesterone, and 5) estrogen plus cyclic micronized progesterone. The oral preparation of micronized progesterone was developed for this study. The predominantly white subjects were followed over a 3-year period. All active treatments decreased LDL cholesterol levels and increased triglyceride levels. HDL cholesterol levels were increased in all active treatment groups; however, it was increased more in those on estrogen alone and in those on estrogen plus micronized progesterone than in those on estrogen plus either cyclic or continuous medroxyprogesterone. Fibrinogen levels also were decreased in women in the active treatment groups.

The results of the Continuous Hormones as Replacement Therapy (CHART) study were similar to those of PEPI. In the CHART study, 1256 postmenopausal women received various combinations of ethinyl estradiol and norethindrone acetate. LDL cholesterol levels were decreased in all active treatment groups. HDL cholesterol levels were increased in the women on unopposed estrogen, and this effect was attenuated by the addition of norethindrone acetate (54).

Although no trials with clinical end points have compared HRT with lipid-lowering therapy, two trials have compared their effects on lipoproteins. In a randomized crossover trial, 58 postmenopausal women received simvastatin for 8 weeks and HRT (conjugated estrogen plus medroxyprogesterone) for 8 weeks, separated by an 8-week washout period (55). Simvastatin was associated with a greater reduction in total and LDL cholesterol levels than was HRT. HDL cholesterol levels were increased similarly (7%) with either treatment. Lp(a) levels were decreased by 27% with HRT, but were not changed with simvastatin. In a second trial, women were randomized into four groups: 1) conjugated estrogens, 2) pravastatin, 3) conjugated estrogens plus pravastatin, and 4) placebo. HDL cholesterol levels significantly increased in those women taking conjugated estrogens or combined treatment when compared with those taking pravastatin or placebo (56). The differences between the two studies with respect to the effect on HDL cholesterol levels are probably related to the fact that the women in the second study took conjugated estrogens without a progestin.

In summary, estrogen with or without a progestin is associated with an improvement in the lipid profile in healthy women. Increases in HDL cholesterol may be particularly important, given the known cardioprotective effect of HDL in women. In the PEPI trial, micronized progesterone given in a cyclic fashion had a more positive effect on the lipid profile than did medroxyprogesterone, although the effects of continuous micronized progesterone are not known. Estrogen decreases Lp(a) significantly more than statin therapy, which may explain some of its cardioprotective effect. Unanswered questions include whether these changes in cardiovascular risk factors will translate into changes in cardiovascular morbidity and mortality.

Secondary Prevention

Six secondary prevention trials of hyperlipidemia treatment have included women with CAD. All of the subjects had MI, a diagnosis of angina, or obstructed coronary arteries. All trials used drug treatment to lower cholesterol. Four of the studies assessed CAD mortality, one evaluated changes in coronary occlusion using quantitative angiography, and one evaluated both CAD mortality and angiographic changes (Table 4-3).

Table 4-3 Secondary Prevention Trials in Women with Hyperlipidemia

Trial	No. of Women (No. of Patients)	Intervention	CAD Mortality RR in Women (95% CI)	Total Mortality RR in Women (95% CI)
Stockholm Ischaemic Heart Disease Study (57)	103 (555)	Clofibrate and nicotinic acid	Not available*	Not available*
Scottish Society of Physicians (58)	124 (717)	Clofibrate	0.17 (0.02, 1.37)	Not assessed
Newcastle-upon-Tyne (59)	97 (497)	Clofibrate	0.29 (0.19, 1.37)	Not assessed
Scandinavian Simvastatin Survival Study (4S) (60)	827 (4444)	Simvastatin	0.79 (0.37, 1.60)	1.12 (0.65, 1.93)
Program on Surgical Control of the Hyperlipidemias (61,62)	78 (838)	Partial ileal bypass	Not available†	1.7 (0.35, 8.40)
Kane et al (63)	41 (72)	Multidrug treatment	Not available‡	Not available‡

* Women not analyzed separately.
† Unable to calculate because there were no deaths in one group.
‡ Angiographic outcomes only.

The first three treatment trials with CAD death as an end point each used clofibrate. In the Stockholm Ischaemic Heart Disease Study, CAD and total mortality were decreased in the treatment group, but the intervention was not blinded, and outcomes in women were not analyzed separately (57). In the Scottish Society of Physicians' secondary prevention trial, the CAD death rate was not significantly different between women who were treated and women in the control group; total mortality was not assessed (58). Finally, in the Newcastle upon Tyne study, there was no significant difference in CAD death rate between women receiving placebo and those treated with clofibrate, which may be a consequence of the small number of CAD deaths that occurred; again, total mortality was not assessed (59).

More convincing evidence is provided by the Scandinavian Simvastatin Survival Study (4S) in which 827 women (out of a total of 4444 participants) with angina or previous MI were randomized to treatment with simvastatin or placebo. Overall results in the participants revealed that total mortality was decreased in the simvastatin-treated group (RR = 0.70; 95% CI: 0.58, 0.85). CAD mortality was also decreased in the simvastatin-treated group (RR = 0.58; 95% CI: 0.46, 0.73). Among simvastatin-treated women, there was a trend toward decreased CAD mortality. Although there was no significant difference in total mortality, this may be a reflection of the low overall mortality rate in women (60).

Two angiographic studies of subjects with coronary disease included women. In the Program on the Surgical Control of the Hyperlipidemias (POSCH), women in the intervention group underwent partial ileal bypass. In the initial study, angiographic disease progression was significantly lower in treated women, and there were insignificant decreases in overall and CAD mortality in the intervention group. The findings in women paralleled the findings in the overall population (61). Recently, a 5-year post-trial follow-up from POSCH was published. CAD and total mortality were decreased in the treatment group, but the results in women were not analyzed separately (62). In an angiographic study of individuals with heterozygous familial hypercholesterolemia, 41 women were treated with multiple drugs. Mean cross-sectional area of the coronary arteries was reduced in the untreated women but was increased in the treated women, suggesting that treatment with aggressive lipid-lowering therapy in women can cause regression of atherosclerotic plaque. CAD and total mortality were not assessed (63).

A pooled relative risk for lipid lowering in women was calculated based on the three studies that assessed CAD mortality and provided confidence intervals (see Table 4-3). The summary relative risk for CAD mortality was 0.36 (95% CI: 0.25, 0.52). The summary relative risk calculated from the two studies that assessed total mortality was 1.17 (95% CI: 0.70, 1.96) (43).

In each secondary prevention study, the rate of death from cardiac causes in women treated for hypercholesterolemia was lower than in those not treated. When women were analyzed separately, the findings generally paralleled the findings in men. The lack of statistically significant differences may be related in part to the small number of deaths in each study. When pooled, the studies that assessed CAD mortality do suggest a significant reduction in CAD mortality in women treated for hyperlipidemia.

Until recently, the effect of lowering cholesterol in women with documented CAD who have "normal" cholesterol levels was not known. A total of 576 women who had had a recent MI, total cholesterol levels less than 240 mg/dL, and LDL cholesterol levels between 115 and 174 mg/dL were included in the Cholesterol and Recurrent Events (CARE) study. Women were randomized to receive pravastatin 40 mg/d or placebo and were followed for 5 years. Women treated with pravastatin had a 46% lower rate of major coronary events (nonfatal MI and CAD death) than placebo-treated women (64). The corresponding reduction in events in men was only 21%. In addition, a reduction in CAD outcomes with lipid lowering was seen sooner in women than in men, suggesting that cholesterol lowering for secondary prevention may be more efficacious in women (65).

The available data suggest that treatment of hypercholesterolemia in women with documented CAD may decrease subsequent CAD mortality and that therapy may lead to regression of atherosclerotic plaques. Women with CAD who have "normal" cholesterol levels also benefit from cholesterol lowering.

Hormone Replacement Therapy

Several studies have assessed the effects of hormone therapy in women with known CAD. The recent results of the HERS study described previously suggested that hormone therapy was not associated with a reduction in the outcome of nonfatal MI or CAD death in women with known CAD. A significant time effect was seen, however, with more events in the hormone group during the first year and fewer in the fourth and fifth years (52). An earlier prospective observational study had reached different conclusions. Sullivan and colleagues (66) prospectively studied 2268 women referred for angiography. They found that estrogen was associated with increased survival among women who had coronary disease, whereas it had less of an effect on those who did not. Other trials, including those currently in progress, are reviewed in Chapter 10.

Potential Risks of Treatment of Hyperlipidemia

Cholesterol Lowering and Noncardiovascular Mortality

Recent evidence suggests an association between cholesterol lowering for primary prevention in men and elevated deaths due to other causes (e.g., accidents, suicides, violent deaths). There is no evidence that cholesterol lowering for primary or secondary prevention in women is associated with an increase in death rates from noncardiovascular causes (43).

Cholesterol-Lowering Drugs and Cancer

Newman and Hulley (67) tabulated carcinogenicity data from the *Physicians' Desk Reference* for hypolipidemic drugs. They found that the two most commonly used classes of hypolipidemic drugs (statins and fibrates) caused cancer in rodents—some at doses equivalent to those doses used in humans. In contrast, antihypertensives were not carcinogenic.

Are drugs that are carcinogenic in rodents also carcinogenic in humans? Clinical trial results in humans have not shown a consistent relationship between cholesterol lowering and carcinogenesis, but many of the trials have not followed patients long enough for cancer to develop. The statins, for example, are the most popular class of cholesterol-lowering drugs but have been studied for the shortest period of time. Although clinical trial results are promising for reduction of CAD mortality with the statins, no long-term studies of their car-cinogenicity have been done. Short-term statin use was recently evaluated in the CARE study (64). Women who took pravastatin had a higher incidence of breast cancer than women who took placebo (12 cases vs. 1 case). However, the authors suggested that because the incidence of breast cancer in the control group was much lower than would have been expected on the basis of the rate in the general population, this finding may have been an anomaly. Recent results from the AFCAPS/TexCAPS primary prevention study also showed a statistically insignificant increased risk of breast cancer in the women treated with lovastatin (13 cases vs. 9 cases) (42b). Interim results of the ongoing LIPID (Long-Term Intervention with Pravastatin in Ischemic Disease) trial show no increase in breast cancer among women who have been treated with pravastatin for 4 years (68).

Even if there seems to be no short-term risk associated with hypolipidemic agents, an increase in a particular cancer may be delayed for decades after exposure to the drug; thus, any increase in cancer attributable to use of a particular drug may not become evident for many years. Some cholesterol-lowering trials have published extended follow-up data for several years after the conclusion of the trial and have shown no increase in cancer mortality. However, discontinuing a cholesterol lowering drug at the end of a trial is different than continuing the drug throughout the extended follow-up period.

Although the data are limited and problems exist with the extrapolation of rodent data to humans, there are probably some risks in the drug treatment of hyperlipidemia. Given that women tend to develop heart disease at a later age than men and live longer, women may be exposed to cholesterol-lowering drugs for more years. Currently, it is not known whether long-term use of hypolipidemic drugs is associated with increased carcinogenicity in humans. Rather than treating every patient who has a high cholesterol level with a hypolipidemic drug, patients whose risk for CAD outweighs their risk of long-term use of hypolipidemic drugs should be selected for treatment.

Potential Risks of Estrogen Therapy

Women who take estrogen have a lower incidence of CAD; however, the potential risks of taking estrogen, especially breast cancer, must be considered in the decision-making process. (For a detailed discussion of potential risks, see Chapter 11.)

Absolute Risk for Coronary Artery Disease

The dichotomy of primary and secondary prevention is somewhat artificial. Consider the following two women: 1) a female smoker aged 65 years with hypertension and adult onset diabetes mellitus who has a total cholesterol level of 248 mg/dL, an LDL cholesterol level of 157 mg/dL and an HDL cholesterol level of 47 mg/dL; and 2) a healthy woman aged 32 years with no medical problems who has the same cholesterol levels as the older woman. Because neither of these women has clinically evident CAD, treatment of hyperlipidemia in either of them is considered primary prevention. Despite the identical serum cholesterol levels, most clinicians would be more inclined to treat hypercholesterolemia in the first woman than in the second. Rather than dividing women into different groups (i.e., "with CAD" and "without CAD"), it is more useful to consider CAD risk as a continuum and to assess each individual's *absolute risk* of CAD. The first woman's absolute risk of death from CAD is 5.3% per year, whereas the second woman's absolute risk of CAD is 0.0002% per year. Clearly, the first woman has significantly more to gain from hyperlipidemia treatment than the second.

At what level of absolute risk for CAD do the benefits outweigh the risks of hyperlipidemia treatment? Davey-Smith and colleagues (69) pooled trials of cholesterol lowering (both primary and secondary prevention) and found that cholesterol lowering prolonged the lives of those whose risk of CAD was 3% or more per year. The problem with pooling these studies is that the choles-terol-lowering treatments in each were quite different and may have been as-sociated with different risks and benefits. Ideally, such a calculation should be done for each type of therapy.

Furthermore, the meta-analysis did not include any trials of the statins, because the first trial of the effects of the statins on CAD mortality was not published until 1994. In the Scandinavian Simvastatin Survival Study (a sec-ondary prevention study) a survival benefit was seen in a group whose annual risk of CAD death was 1.5% per year. In the first primary prevention study of the statins, the West of Scotland Study, a survival benefit was seen in middle-aged men with an annual risk of CAD death of 0.4% (39). The effectiveness of the statins at lower levels of absolute CAD risk may indicate that the statins have a more favorable risk-benefit profile, but many of the long-term risks of the statins are still not known.

Age is the most important factor in determining CAD risk. Women younger than 54 years of age are unlikely to reach a risk of CAD death of 1.5% per year at any cholesterol level (70). Because CAD risk may be entirely re-versed after 2 years of hyperlipidemia treatment, it may be prudent to wait and screen low-risk women at an older age. Because age is such an important contributor to CAD risk, older women may benefit the most from cholesterol-lowering treatment, although currently no available data from clinical trials exist. Assuming a 15% decrease in CAD mortality with cholesterol lowering, 1000 healthy women aged 60 to 64 years would have to be treated to prevent one CAD death. In contrast, over one million women aged 20 to 24 years would have to be treated to prevent one death from heart disease (43).

Too often the importance of single risk factors is overestimated. Cholesterol is one risk factor that should be viewed in the context of others. An appropriate diagnosis for some patients may be, "Your cholesterol is high, but your CAD risk is not" (70).

National Cholesterol Screening Guidelines

Three sets of National Cholesterol Screening Guidelines have been proposed since 1993. The American College of Physicians (ACP) published its recommendations in the March 1996 issue of the *Annals of Internal Medicine* (71) (Box 4-1). The U.S. Preventive Services Task Force (USPSTF) recommends periodic screening for high blood cholesterol for all men aged 35 to 65 years

---

Box 4-1 American College of Physicians Cholesterol Screening Guidelines

1. Patients in whom screening for lipoprotein abnormalities is appropriate should have their total cholesterol level measured.
2. In patients who are screened for the primary prevention of coronary heart disease, the total cholesterol level should be measured once. Measures should be repeated periodically if the measured value is near a treatment threshold.
3. Screening for total cholesterol levels is not recommended for young men (< 35 years of age) or women (< 45 years of age) unless the history or physical examination suggests a familial lipoprotein disorder or at least two other characteristics increase the risk for coronary heart disease.
4. Screening for total cholesterol in the primary prevention of coronary heart disease is appropriate but not mandatory for men 35–65 years of age or for women 45–65 years of age.
5. Evidence is insufficient to recommend or discourage screening for the primary prevention of coronary heart disease in men and women 65–75 years of age.
6. Screening is not recommended for men or women over 75 years of age.
7. All patients with known coronary heart disease (e.g., history of myocardial infarction, angina pectoris, other evidence of coronary disease) or whose history of other kinds of vascular disease (e.g., stroke or claudication) places them at high risk for coronary heart disease should have lipid analysis, including but not limited to measurement of total cholesterol levels.

Reprinted from American College of Physicians. Guidelines for using serum cholesterol, high-density lipoprotein cholesterol, and triglyceride levels as screening tests for preventing coronary heart disease in adults. Ann Intern Med. 1996;124:515–7.

---

and women aged 45 to 65 years. In addition, USPSTF recommends that all patients receive periodic screening and counseling about other measures to reduce their risk of CAD (72). In contrast, the Adult Treatment Panel II (ATPII) of the NCEP has published guidelines for both screening and treatment of hyperlipidemia (73). NCEP recommends screening all individuals aged 20 years and over for hyperlipidemia at regular intervals. The main difference between the ACP and USPSTF screening guidelines and those of the NCEP is that screening is directed selectively toward those at high risk. Although the NCEP treatment recommendations emphasize degree of CAD risk, the NCEP screening recommendations do not.

When choosing a screening strategy, it is important to consider how the screening test will impact on treatment and management decisions. There are three treatment options for hypercholesterolemia: Step I diet, Step II diet (which includes more stringent dietary management), and drug therapy. As described by the NCEP in the ATPII, the "NCEP's eating pattern recommendation for the general public is similar to the nutrients in the Step I diet" (69). If a low-fat, high-fiber diet with adequate fruit and vegetable intake is recommended to all individuals, will measuring serum cholesterol change that recommendation?

In many low-risk individuals, the results of a cholesterol level check will not change the dietary recommendation. For a healthy premenopausal woman, a low-fat, high-fiber diet will be recommended regardless of whether her cholesterol is 186 or 237 mg/dL. Conversely, if the results of a serum cholesterol measurement will change the treatment (e.g., drug treatment or more stringent diet), then checking the level is appropriate.

Rational Treatment Choices

Rational treatment choices for hyperlipidemia should be based on decreasing total cardiovascular risk, not just decreasing total or LDL cholesterol levels. Cholesterol must be viewed in the context of other risk factors. The level of LDL cholesterol at which treatment is initiated depends on overall risk status. For low-risk women, drug therapy should be initiated at a much higher LDL level than in high-risk women. The NCEP recommends initiation of drug therapy in women with known CAD when the serum LDL cholesterol level is 130 mg/dL or greater, aiming for an LDL target of less than 100 mg/dL. For women with two or more risk factors (HDL cholesterol $\geq$ 60 mg/dL is considered a negative risk factor), the NCEP recommends initiating drug treatment when the LDL cholesterol is 160 mg/dL or greater, aiming for an LDL target of less than 130 mg/dL. For women with less than two risk factors, the NCEP recommends initiating drug treatment when the LDL cholesterol is 190 mg/dL or greater, aiming for an LDL of less than 160 mg/dL. Finally, the NCEP recommends delaying drug therapy in premenopausal women who have an LDL of 190 to 220 mg/dL.

Decisions about the initiation of drug therapy must be individualized and should take into account a woman's total cardiovascular risk, not just her LDL cholesterol. Although drug therapy is probably not indicated in most healthy premenopausal women, it might be considered in a young woman with a family history of premature CAD and familial hyperlipidemia. Conversely, in a healthy postmenopausal woman aged 52 years with an LDL cholesterol level of 168 mg/dL and an HDL cholesterol level of 59 mg/dL, it would be reasonable to continue with nonpharmacologic therapies rather than initiating drug therapy.

Nonpharmacologic Therapies

Nonpharmacologic therapies, including diet, weight loss, and exercise deserve a trial in most women. For low-risk women, nonpharmacologic therapies should be the mainstay of treatment. In higher risk women, even if drug therapy is required, nonpharmacologic therapy should not be abandoned. Finally, modification of other cardiovascular risk factors, including obesity, smoking, inactivity, and diabetes should be part of the overall treatment program. Modification of these other risk factors are associated with an improvement in the lipid profile but, more importantly, will lead to an overall decreased risk of cardiovascular disease.

Diet
Dietary therapy is described in detail in Chapter 5. The Step I diet consists of limiting total fat intake to less than 30% of total calories, with an intake of saturated fat of less than 10% of total calories, and a cholesterol intake of less than 300 mg/d. The Step II diet consists of further reduction of saturated fat intake to less than 7% of total calories, with cholesterol intake of less than 200 mg/d. No primary prevention trials of dietary therapy in women have been associated with a reduction in CAD mortality. Dietary therapy has not been assessed in secondary prevention studies of CAD mortality in women. A low-saturated-fat, low-cholesterol diet is associated with modest decreases in both LDL and HDL cholesterol, although the clinical significance of the decreased HDL is unclear. With dietary therapy, total and LDL cholesterol levels can be lowered by an average of 10%, although responses are variable.

Weight Loss
Obesity is an independent risk factor for CAD, and adiposity is inversely related to HDL cholesterol. Although no data exist to suggest that weight loss

reduces CAD morbidity or mortality, sustained weight loss is associated with an increase in HDL cholesterol, which may be cardioprotective. The low-saturated-fat, low-cholesterol diet recommended for weight loss can reduce HDL cholesterol levels acutely, which theoretically could offset the desired effect of reduced LDL cholesterol. However, when exercise is combined with a low-fat diet, the effects on HDL cholesterol are more favorable (74).

Exercise

The role of exercise in CAD reduction and the impact of exercise on lipids is described further in Chapter 8. Observational data suggest that regular exercise is associated with reduced CAD incidence and mortality. Exercise mediates its positive effects via modification of several CAD risk factors, including its positive effects on LDL and HDL cholesterol.

HDL cholesterol increases with exercise. Although the ideal amount of exercise needed to protect against cardiovascular disease in women is not known currently, there may be a dose-response effect. A recent study of recreational female runners demonstrated that mean HDL cholesterol levels increased with number of miles run per week. Given the known cardioprotective effect of HDL cholesterol in women, more vigorous exercise may lead to lower CAD risk (75).

Exercise can enhance the effect of a low-fat diet on LDL cholesterol. Exercise without diet or weight loss has minimal effects on LDL cholesterol. Overall, the specific effect of exercise on cholesterol levels is less important than its overall impact on reduction of CAD mortality.

Choosing Pharmacologic Therapy

Options for the pharmacologic treatment of hyperlipidemia in women include niacin, statins, bile-acid sequestrants, psyllium, and estrogen replacement. Fibric acids (e.g., gemfibrozil) are not recommended for initial therapy in women due to their minimal effects on LDL cholesterol; their main use is as a treatment of hypertriglyceridemia.

Niacin

Niacin has not been studied in either a primary or secondary prevention study in women. One secondary prevention study in men demonstrated that niacin use was associated with a decrease in CAD mortality (76). Niacin decreases LDL cholesterol levels by 15% to 25% and increases HDL cholesterol levels more than any other hypolipidemic agent. Given that HDL cholesterol seems to be particularly protective in women, niacin may have a unique role in women.

Niacin is very inexpensive but unfortunately has associated side effects that include gastrointestinal distress, glucose intolerance, hyperuricemia, and the well-known flushing reaction. In one study, 40% of patients discontinued niacin due to side effects (77). Hepatic toxicity has been reported with sustained-release preparations. The flushing reaction can be ameliorated by taking low-dose aspirin 30 minutes before the niacin. Compliance can also be improved by starting at a very low dose (e.g.. 100 mg/d) and increasing the dose very slowly and gradually.

HMG Co-A Reductase Inhibitors

HMG Co-A reductase inhibitors (statins) have been associated with decreased CAD mortality in two secondary prevention trials that included women and in a primary prevention trial in high-risk men (39,60,64). Currently, five statins are available: lovastatin, simvastatin, pravastatin, fluvastatin, and atorvastatin. LDL cholesterol levels are decreased an average of 20% to 40% with the statins; the greatest reduction results from the use of atorvastatin. Some data suggest that the statins may have a more favorable risk-benefit profile than other cholesterol-lowering agents. Another advantage to the statin drugs is that they are extremely well tolerated. Gastrointestinal side effects are usually transient; transaminase elevations can occur in a small percentage of those on high doses, but symptomatic hepatitis is uncommon. Myalgias with associated elevations in creatine phosphokinase levels have also been reported with the statins. Ideally, the majority of statins are taken in the evening, because most of the body's cholesterol synthesis occurs at night, but atorvastatin can be taken at any time of the day.

Bile-Acid–Binding Resins

Commonly used bile-acid–binding resins include colestipol and cholestyramine. One primary prevention study in women used colestipol, and no statistically significant difference was seen in CAD mortality between treated and nontreated women. In the Lipid Research Clinics primary prevention study in men, hyperlipidemic men treated with colestipol had a lower rate of CAD events (78). Several secondary prevention studies in women have used colestipol, and meta-analysis suggests a decrease in CAD mortality with treatment. Bile-acid–binding resins lower LDL cholesterol levels by approximately 20%.

Patient acceptance of the bile-acid–binding resins is limited for a variety of reasons. Because they interfere with the absorption of fat-soluble vitamins and other medications, other drugs must be given 2 hours before or 6 hours after the bile-acid–binding resins. Gastrointestinal side effects (e.g., bloating, constipation, heartburn, nausea) are common, although these symptoms tend to abate with time. In one study of elderly men, 37% of patients discontinued the drug because of its side effects (79). Compliance may be enhanced by using smaller doses, by using a fiber supplement to reduce bloating and constipation, or both. In one study that included women, a lower dose of colestipol in conjunction with psyllium was better tolerated and had the same lipid-lowering effects as higher doses of colestipol (80).

Psyllium

Psyllium, which is high in dietary fiber, lowers serum cholesterol levels. No studies in women assess the role of psyllium in the reduction of CAD mortality. Psyllium has been shown in several studies to reduce total cholesterol by 4% to 10% and to reduce LDL cholesterol by 6% to 20% (81–83). Psyllium's effect is independent of weight loss and dietary change (84) and is augmented when used in conjunction with a low-fat diet (85). Finally, psyllium seems to work better when taken with meals rather than between meals (86), which may be due to its bile-acid–binding property. The side effects of psyllium are mainly gastrointestinal, and no serious toxic effects exist at high doses. Given its safety and other potential health benefits (e.g., decreased colon cancer risk, diverticulosis, and irritable bowel syndrome), it is certainly a reasonable adjunct to a low-fat diet, other drug therapy, or both in women with mild to moderate hypercholesterolemia.

Estrogen

Estrogen with or without a progestin has been shown to decrease LDL and increase HDL in postmenopausal women, although it is also associated with an increase in triglycerides (87). Use of estrogen results in a greater increase in HDL cholesterol than use of a statin drug (56), although combined estrogen/progestin therapy does not seem to increase HDL cholesterol more than the statins (55). Estrogen does significantly decrease Lp(a), which may account for some of its cardioprotective effect (33,37,56). In addition, observational studies have shown that women who take estrogen have a significantly lower rate of CAD mortality. However, a recent randomized controlled trial of HRT for secondary prevention concluded that there was no significant difference in nonfatal MI or CAD death among hormone therapy users, although there was a significant time effect, with more events in the hormone therapy group in the first year and fewer in the fourth and fifth years (52). Other known benefits (e.g., osteoporosis prevention) and risks (e.g., breast cancer and deep venous thrombosis) of estrogen must be considered in the decision to treat with estrogen. Estrogen is not currently approved by the FDA for the reduction of CAD risk.

Combination Therapy

When a single drug does not lower cholesterol appropriately, two or three drugs can be used together. Combining statins with gemfibrozil or niacin may be associated with an increased risk of myopathy. Estrogen can be used in conjunction with any other lipid-lowering agent.

Pharmacologic therapy of hyperlipidemia should be used in those women most likely to benefit. Presently, no clinical outcome data exist to direct the choice of hypolipidemic medications in women. Although many experts recommend that statins be the first line of therapy (88), this recommendation does not acknowledge the role of estrogen in women. Although currently, no data compare statins with estrogen replacement for hyperlipidemia and CAD outcomes, the effects on LDL seem to be similar, and the effects on HDL and Lp(a) may be better with estrogen (55,56).

Given its association with decreased CAD mortality in observational studies, estrogen may be a reasonable initial choice for the treatment of hyperlipidemia in women without CAD. When using estrogen for CAD reduction, other considerations should include a woman's risk for osteoporosis and breast cancer as well as her tolerance for potential side effects such as bleeding and breast tenderness.

Statins are also a reasonable choice, given their proven efficacy in secondary prevention in women and in primary prevention for high-risk men as well as their excellent tolerance. The statins, however, have recently been studied only in clinical trials and no long-term follow-up data exist.

Bile-acid–binding resins have been studied for secondary prevention in women and seem to be efficacious in CAD reduction, but their side effects and inconvenience limit their widespread use. Because of its positive effect on HDL, niacin is theoretically an excellent choice in women, although no clinical data on niacin and CAD outcomes in women exist. Both niacin and bile-acid–binding resins seem to be relatively safe for long-term use. Psyllium should be used as an adjunct to dietary therapy in all women who are willing to take it.

Recommendations for Screening and Treatment

Women with Coronary Artery Disease

Limited evidence suggests that treatment of hypercholesterolemia in women with coronary disease may decrease CAD mortality. These women also have a high absolute risk of recurrent CAD events so that the benefits of cholesterol lowering probably outweigh the risks. Because women with peripheral vascular disease or symptomatic carotid artery disease have a risk of CAD equal to that of patients with stable angina (89), they will probably benefit from cholesterol-lowering treatment in the same way as will patients with CAD. Aggressive lowering of LDL cholesterol levels to less than 100 mg/dL is very appropriate in all these high-risk women. Recent data suggest that many women with CAD are not being aggressively treated for hyperlipidemia (90,91). Although no data compare the various pharmacologic therapies, factors that influence the choice of medication include potential effects on HDL cholesterol level, patient tolerance, convenience, cost, side effects, and risk for other diseases such as osteoporosis and breast cancer.

Women at Risk for Coronary Artery Disease

Although there is no evidence about healthy women at high risk of CAD (e.g., those who smoke and have diabetes), these women may also benefit from cholesterol lowering. Efforts at primary prevention should be directed toward those women most likely to benefit from treatment. Because the relative risk for CAD associated with diabetes in women is significantly higher than in men (92,93), diabetics with hyperlipidemia that does not improve with control of their diabetes are candidates for drug therapy. Other women who have failed nonpharmacologic treatment and are at high risk for CAD should be considered for drug therapy.

Hyperlipidemia is a risk factor, not a disease. When treating any risk factor, it is important to consider both the risks and benefits of treatment. Screening should be directed at those women whose management will change as a result, and treatment should be directed at those most likely to benefit from it.

Healthy Women

Cohort study evidence reveals that elevated total and LDL-cholesterol levels are associated with increased CAD risk in women less than 65 years of age but not in older women. Women with elevated HDL cholesterol levels seem relatively protected from CAD independent of LDL cholesterol levels. No evidence from primary prevention suggests that cholesterol lowering affects total mortality or CAD mortality in healthy women, although the available data are very limited. ATPII of NCEP recommends delaying drug treatment for high cholesterol levels in premenopausal women. Interventions should focus on nonpharmacologic attempts at overall CAD reduction rather than specifically on cholesterol levels. Finally, those interventions that increase HDL cholesterol are likely to be most beneficial.

REFERENCES

1. **Stein JH, Rosenson RS.** Lipoprotein Lp(a) excess and coronary heart disease. Arch Intern Med. 1997;157:1170–6.

2. **Bostom AG, Gagnon DR, Cupples LA, et al.** A prospective investigation of elevated lipoprotein(a) detected by electrophoresis and cardiovascular disease in women: the Framingham Heart Study. Circulation. 1994;90:1688–95.

3. **Johnson CL, Rifkind BM, Sempos CT, et al.** Declining serum cholesterol levels among U.S. adults: the National Health and Nutrition Examination surveys. JAMA. 1993;269:3002–8.

4. **Harris-Hooker S, Sanford GL.** Lipids, lipoproteins and coronary heart disease in minority populations. Atherosclerosis. 1994;108(Suppl):S83–104.

5. **Haffner SM, Stern MP, Hazuda MP, et al.** The role of behavior variables and fat patterning in explaining ethnic differences in serum lipids and lipoproteins. Am J Epidemiol. 1986;123:830–9.

6. **Fulton-Kehoe DL, Eckel RH, Shetterly SM, Hamman RF.** Determinations of total HDL lipoprotein cholesterol and high density lipoprotein subfraction levels among Hispanic and non-Hispanic white persons with normal glucose tolerance: the San Luis Valley Diabetes Study. J Clin Epidemiol. 1992;45:1191–200.

7. **Manolio TA, Pearson TA, Wenger NK, et al.** Cholesterol and heart disease in older persons and women: review of an NHLBI workshop. Ann Epidemiol. 1992; 2: 161–76.

8. **Kronmal RA, Cain KC.** Total serum cholesterol levels and mortality risk as a function of age: a report based on the Framingham Data. Arch Intern Med. 1993;153:1065–73.

9. **Jacobs D, Blackburn H, Higgins M, et al.** Report of the conference on low blood cholesterol: mortality associations. Circulation. 1992;86:1046–60.

10. **Brunner D, Weisbort J, Meshulam N, et al.** Relation of serum total cholesterol and high-density cholesterol percentage to the incidence of definite coronary events: twenty-year follow-up of the Donolo-Tel Aviv Prospective Coronary Artery Disease Study. Am J Cardiol. 1987;59:1271–6.

11. **Bass KM, Newschaffer CJ, Koag MJ, Bush TL.** Plasma lipoprotein levels as predictors of cardiovascular death in women. Arch Inter Med. 1993;153:2209–16.

12. **Castelli WP, Garrison RJ, Wilson PWF, et al.** Incidence of coronary heart disease and lipoprotein cholesterol levels: the Framingham study. JAMA. 1986;256:2835–8.

13. **Jacobs DR, Mebane IL, Bangdiwala SI, et al.** High-density lipoprotein cholesterol as a predictor of cardiovascular disease mortality in men and women: the follow-up study of the Lipid Research Clinics Prevalence Study. Am J Epidemiol. 1990;131:32–47.

14. **Kannel WB.** Metabolic risk factors for coronary heart disease in women: perspective from the Framingham study. Am Heart J. 1987;114:413–9.

15. **Corti MC, Guralnik JM, Salive ME, et al.** HDL cholesterol predicts coronary heart disease mortality in older persons. JAMA. 1995;274:539–44.

16. **Bengtsson C.** Ischaemic heart disease in women: a study based on a randomized population sample of women and women with myocardial infarction in Goteborg, Sweden. Acta Med Scand. 1973;549(Suppl):1–128.

17. **Simons LA.** Interrelations of lipids and lipoproteins with coronary artery disease mortality in 19 countries. Am J Cardiol. 1986;57:5–10G.

18. **Criqui MH, Heiss G, Cohn R, et al.** Plasma triglyceride level and mortality from coronary heart disease. N Engl J Med. 1993;328:1220–5.

19. **LaRosa JC.** Triglycerides and coronary risk in women and the elderly. Arch Intern Med. 1997;157:961–8.

20. **NIH Consensus Conference.** Triglyceride, high-density lipoprotein and coronary heart disease. JAMA. 1993;269:505–10.

21. **Stensvold I, Tverdal A, Urdal P, Graff-Iverson S.** Non-fasting serum triglyceride concentration and mortality from coronary heart disease and any cause in middle aged Norwegian women. BMJ. 1993;307:1318–22.

22. **Krolewski AA, Warram JH, Valsania P, et al.** Evolving natural history of coronary artery disease in diabetes mellitus. Am J Med. 1991;90(Suppl):56–61S.

23. **Goldschmid MG, Barrett-Conner E, Edelstein SL, et al.** Dyslipidemia and ischemic heart disease mortality among men and women with diabetes. Circulation. 1994;89:991–7.

24. **Bostom AG, Cupples AG, Jenner JL, et al.** Elevated plasma lipoprotein(a) and coronary heart disease in men aged 55 years and younger: a prospective study. JAMA. 1996;274:544–6.

25. **Schaefer EJ, Lamon-Fava S, Jenner JL, et al.** Lipoprotein(a) levels and risk of coronary heart disease in men. JAMA. 1994;271:999–1003.

26. **Cremer P, Nagel D, Labrot B, et al.** Lp(a) as predictor of myocardial infarction in comparison to fibrinogen, LDL cholesterol and other risk factors: results from the prospective Gottingen Risk Incidence and Prevalence Study (GRIPS). Eur J Clin Invest. 1994;24:444–53.

27. **Wald NJ, Law M, Watt HC, et al.** Apolipoproteins and ischaemic heart disease: implications for screening. Lancet. 1994;343:75–9.

28. **Rosengren A, Wilhelmsen L, Eriksson E, et al.** Lipoprotein(a) and coronary heart disease: a prospective case-control study in a general population sample of middle aged men. BMJ. 1990;301-:1248–51.

29. **Sigurdsson G, Baldursdottir A, Sigvaldason H, et al.** Predictive value of apolipoproteins in a prospective survey of coronary artery disease in men. Am J Cardiol. 1992;69: 1251–4.

30. **Coleman MP, Key TJA, Wang EY, et al.** A prospective study of obesity, lipids, apolipoproteins and ischaemic heart disease in women. Atherosclerosis. 1992;92:177–85.

31. **Armstrong VW, Cremer P, Eberle E, et al.** The association between serum Lp(a) concentrations and angiographically assessed coronary atherosclerosis: dependence on serum LDL levels. Atherosclerosis. 1986;62:249–57.

32. **Soma MR, Osnago-Gadda I, Paoletti R, et al.** The lowering of lipoprotein(a) induced by estrogen plus progesterone replacement therapy in postmenopausal women. Arch Intern Med. 1993;153:1462–8.

33. **Sacks FM, McPherson R, Walsh BW.** Effect of postmenopausal estrogen replacement on plasma Lp(a) lipoprotein concentrations. Arch Intern Med. 1994;154:1106–10.

34. **Kim CJ, Jang HC, Cho DH, Min YK.** Effects of hormone replacement therapy on lipoprotein(a) and lipids in postmenopausal women. Arterioscler Thromb Vasc Biol. 1994;14:275–81.

35. **Kim CJ, Min YK, Ryu WS, et al.** Effect of hormone replacement therapy on lipoprotein(a) and lipid levels in postmenopausal women: influence of various progestogens and duration of therapy. Arch Intern Med. 1996;156:1693–1700.

36. **Shewmon DA, Stock JL, Rosen CJ, et al.** Tamoxifen and estrogen lower circulating lipoprotein(a) concentrations in healthy postmenopausal women. Arterioscler Thromb Vasc Biol. 1994;14:1586–93.

37. **Haines C, Chung T, Chang A, et al.** Effect of oral estradiol on Lp(a) and other lipoproteins in postmenopausal women. Arch Intern Med. 1996;156:866–72.

38. **Muldoon MF, Manuck SB, Matthews KA.** Lowering cholesterol concentrations and mortality: a review of primary prevention trials. BMJ. 1990;301:309–14.

39. **Shepherd J, Cobbe SM, Ford I, et al.** Prevention of coronary heart disease with pravastatin in men with hypercholesterolemia. New Engl J Med. 1995;333:1301–7.

40. **Miettinen M, Turpeinen O, Karvonen MJ, et al.** Effect of cholesterol-lowering diet on mortality from coronary heart disease and other causes:a twelve year clinical trial in men and women. Lancet. 1972;2:835–8.

41. **Frantz ID, Dawson EA, Ashman PL, et al.** Test of effect of lipid lowering by diet on cardiovascular risk: the Minnesota Coronary Survey. 1989;9:129–35.

42a. **Dorr AE, Gunderson K, Schneider JC, et al.** Colestipol hydrochloride in hypercholesterolemic patients: effect on serum cholesterol and mortality. J Chron Dis. 1978;31: 5–14.

42b. **Downs JR, Clearfield M, Weis S, et al.** Primary prevention of acute coronary events with lovastatin in men and women with average cholesterol levels. JAMA, 1998. 279:1615–22.

43. **Walsh J, Grady D.** Treatment of hyperlipidemia in women. JAMA. 1995;274:1152–58.

44. **Grady D, Rubin SM, Petitti DB, et al.** Hormone therapy to prevent disease and prolong life in postmenopausal women. Ann Intern Med. 1992;117:1016–37.

45. **Bush TL, Barrett-Connor E, Cowan L, et al.** Cardiovascular mortality and noncontraceptive use of estrogen in women: results from the Lipid Research Clinics Program Follow-up Study. Circulation. 1987;75:1102–9.

46. **Hunt K, Vessey M, McPherson K.** Mortality in a cohort of long-term users of hormone replacement therapy: an updated analysis. Br J Obstet Gynecol. 1990;97:1080–6.

47. **Falkeborn M, Persson I, Adomami DO, et al.** The risk of acute myocardial infarction after oestrogen and oestrogen and progesteren replacement. Brit J Obstet Gynecol. 1992;99:821–8.

48. **Grodstein F, Stampfer MJ, Manson JE, et al.** Postmenopausal estrogen and progestin use and the risk of cardiovascular disease. New Engl J Med. 1996;335:453–61.

49. **Grodstein R, Stampfer MJ, Colditz GA, et al.** Postmenopausal hormone therapy and mortality. New Engl J Med. 1997;336:1769–75.

50. **Barrett-Connor E, Bush TL.** Estrogen and coronary heart disease in women. JAMA. 1991;265:1861–7.

51. **Matthews KA, Kuller LH, Wing RR, et al.** Prior to use of estrogen replacement therapy: are users healthier than nonusers? Am J Epidemiol. 1996;143:971–8.

52. **Hulley S, Grady D, Bush T, et al.** Randomized trial of estrogen plus progestin for secondary prevention of coronary heart disease in postmenopausal women. JAMA. 1998:280:605–13

53. **Nachtigall LE, Nachtigall RH, Nachtigall RD, et al.** Estrogen replacement therapy II: a prospective study in the relationship to carcinoma and cardiovascular and metabolic problems. Obstet Gynecol. 1979;54:74–9.

54. **Speroff L, Rowan J, Symons J, et al.** The comparative effect on bone density, endometrium, and lipids of continuous hormones as replacement therapy (CHART Study): a randomized controlled trial. JAMA. 1996;276:1397–1403.

55. **Darling GM, Johns JA, McCloud PI, Davis SR.** Estrogen and progestin compared with simvastatin for hypercholesterolemia in postmenopausal women. New Engl J Med. 1997;337:595–601.

56. **Davidson MH, Testolin LM, Maki KC, et al.** A comparison of estrogen replacement, pravastatin, and combined treatment for the management of hypercholesterolemia in postmenopausal women. Arch Intern Med. 1997;157:1186–92.

57. **Carlson LA, Rosenhamer G.** Reduction of mortality in the Stockholm Ischaemic Heart Disease Secondary Prevention Study by combined treatment with clofibrate and nicotinic acid. Acta Med Scand. 1988;223:405–18.

58. **Research Committee of the Scottish Society of Physicians.** Ischemic heart disease: a secondary prevention trial using clofibrate. BMJ. 1971;4:775–84.

59. **Group of Physicians of the Newcastle upon Tyne Region.** Trial of clofibrate in the treatment of ischemic heart disease. BMJ. 1971;4:767–75.

60. **Scandinavian Simvastatin Survival Study Group.** Randomised trial of cholesterol lowering in 4444 patients with coronary heart disease: the Scandinavian Simvastatin Survival Study. Lancet. 1994;344:1383–9.

61. **Buchwald H, Campos C, Matts JP, et al.** Women in the POSCH trial: effects of aggressive cholesterol modification in women with coronary heart disease. Ann Surgery. 1992;216:389–400.

62. **Buchwald H, Campos C, Matts JP, et al.** Effective lipid modification by partial ileal bypass reduced long-term coronary heart disease morality and morbidity: five-year post-trial follow-up report from the POSCH. Arch Intern Med. 1998;158:1253–61.

63. **Kane JP, Malloy MJ, Ports TA, et al.** Regression of coronary atherosclerosis during treatment of familial hypercholesterolemia with combined drug regimens. JAMA. 1990;264:3007–12.

64. **Sacks FM, Pfeffer MA, Moye LA, et al.** The effect of pravastatin on coronary events after myocardial infarction in patients with average cholesterol levels. New Engl J Med. 1996;335:1001–9.

65. **Lewis S, Mitchell J, East C, et al.** Women in CARE have earlier and greater response to pravastatin post myocardial infarction [Abstract]. Circulation. 1996;94:1–12.

66. **Sullivan JM, Vander Zwaag R, Lemp GF, et al.** Postmenopausal estrogen use and coronary atherosclerosis. Ann Intern Med. 1988;108:358–63.

67. **Newman TB, Hulley SB.** Carcinogenicity of lipid-lowering drugs. JAMA. 1996;275: 55–60.

68. **The Lipid Study Group.** Design features and baseline characteristics of the LIPID study: a randomized trial in patients with previous acute myocardial infarction and/or unstable angina pectoris. Am J Cardiol. 1995;76:474–9.

69. **Davey-Smith G, Song F, Sheldon TA.** Cholesterol lowering and mortality: the importance of considering initial level of risk. BMJ. 1993;306:1367–73.

70. **Haq IU, Jackson PR, Yeo WW, Ramsay LE.** Sheffield risk and treatment table for cholesterol lowering for primary prevention of coronary heart disease. Lancet. 1995;346: 1467–71.

71. **American College of Physicians.** Guidelines for using serum cholesterol, high-density lipoprotein cholesterol, and triglyceride levels as screening tests for preventing coronary heart disease in adults. Ann Intern Med. 1996;124:515–7.

72. **U.S. Preventive Services Task Force.** Guide to Clinical Preventive Services. 2nd ed. Alexandria, VA: International Medical Publishing; 1996.

73. **Expert Panel on Detection, Evaluation, and Treatment of High Blood Cholesterol in Adults.** Summary of the Second Report of the National Cholesterol Education Program (NCEP) Expert Panel on Detection, Evaluation, and Treatment of High Blood Cholesterol in Adults (Adult Treatment Panel II). JAMA. 1993;269:3015–23.

74. **Wood PD, Stefanick ML, Williams PT, Haskell W.** The effects on plasma lipoproteins of a prudent weight-reducing diet, with or without exercise, in overweight men and women. New Engl J Med. 1991;325:461–6.

75. **Williams PT.** High-density lipoprotein cholesterol and other risk factors for coronary heart disease in female runners. N Engl J Med. 1996;334:1298–303.

76. **Canner PL, Berge KG, Wenger NK, et al.** Fifteen-year mortality in Coronary Drug Project patients: long-term benefit with niacin. J Amer Coll Cardiol. 1986;8:1245–55.

77. **Gibbons LW, Gonzalez V, Gordon N, Grundy S.** The prevalence of side effects with regular and sustained release nicotinic acid. Am J Med. 1995;99:378–85.

78. **Lipid Research Clinics Program.** The Lipid Research Clinics coronary prevention trial results. JAMA. 1984;251:351–74.

79. **Schectman G, Hiatt J, Hartz A.** Evaluation of the effectiveness of lipid-lowering therapy (bile acid sequestrants, niacin, psyllium and lovastatin) for treating hypercholesterolemia in veterans. Am J Cardiol. 1993;71:759–65.

80. **Spence JD, Huff MW, Heidenheim P, et al.** Combination therapy with colestipol and psyllium mucilloid in patients with hyperlipidemia. Ann Intern Med. 1995;123: 493–99.

81. **Roberts DCK, Truswell AS, Bencke A, et al.** The cholesterol-lowering effect of a breakfast cereal containing psyllium fiber. Med J Aust. 1994;161:660–4.

82. **Wolever TMS, Jenkins DJA, Mueller S, et al.** Psyllium reduces blood lipids in men and women with hyperlipidemia. Am J Med Sci. 1994;307:269–73.

83. **Anderson JW, Ridell-Mason S, Gustafson NJ, et al.** Cholesterol-lowering effects of psyllium-enriched cereal as an adjunct to a prudent diet in the treatment of mild to moderate hypercholesterolemia. Am J Clin Nutr. 1992;56:93–8.

84. **Hunninghake DB, Miller VT, LaRosa JC, et al.** Hypocholesterolemic effects of a dietary fiber supplement. Am J Clin Nutr. 1994;59:1050–4.

85. **Sprecher DL, Harris BV, Goldberg AC, et al.** Efficacy of psyllium in reducing serum cholesterol levels in hypercholesterolemic patients on high- or low-fat diets. Ann Intern Med. 1993;119:545–54.

86. **Wolever TMS, Jenkins DJA, Mueller S, et al.** Method of administration influences the serum cholesterol-lowering effect of psyllium. Am J Clin Nutr. 1994;59:1055–9.

87. **Writing Group for the PEPI Trial.** Effects of estrogen or estrogen/progestin regimens on heart disease risk factors in postmenopausal women: the postmenopausal estrogen/progestin interventions (PEPI) trial. JAMA. 1995;273:199–208.

88. Medical Letter: Choice of lipid-lowering drugs. 1996;38:67–70.

89. **Criqui MH, Langer RD, Fronek A, et al.** Mortality over a period of 10 years in patients with peripheral arterial disease. New Engl J Med. 1992;326:381–6.

90. **Schrott HG, Bittner V, Vittinghoff E, et al.** Adherence to National Cholesterol Education Program treatment goals in postmenopausal women with heart disease: the Heart and Estrogen/Progestin Replacement Study (HERS). JAMA. 1997;277:1281–6.

91. **Lemaitre RN, Furberg CD, Newman AB, et al.** Time trends in the use of cholesterol lowering agents in older adults: the Cardiovascular Health Study. Arch Intern Med. 1998;158:1761–8.

92. **Barrett-Connor E, Wingard DL.** Sex differential in ischemic heart disease mortality in diabetics: a prospective population-based study. Am J Epidemiol. 1983;118:489–96.

93. **Pan WH, Cedres LB, Liu K, et al.** Relationship of clinical diabetes and asymptomatic hyperglycemia to risk of coronary heart disease mortality in men and women. Am J Epidemiol. 1986;123:504–16.

Chapter 5

Nutrition and Lipids

HENRY N. GINSBERG, MD
WAHIDA KARMALLY, MS, RD, CDE

More than 100 years ago, physicians recognized that the atherosclerotic lesion was laden with lipids. For decades, numerous epidemiologic studies of diet, nutrition, and cardiovascular disease have linked human disease to diets high in saturated fat, cholesterol, and calories. During World War II, the incidence of coronary artery disease (CAD) fell dramatically in occupied countries. Subsequently, in the United States, the switch from a farming to an industrial society—together with a change from a high-carbohydrate to a high-fat diet—paralleled the epidemic of CAD in the United States during the 1950s through the 1970s. Simultaneously, the field of lipid and lipoprotein metabolism has rapidly developed from investigations of the human diet to studies of transgenic and "knockout" mouse models. More recent intervention trials in women and men have documented less progression of CAD and fewer coronary events with treatment (1,2).

The roles of both genetic and environmental factors in the occurrence of CAD have been explored in numerous long-term prospective studies, including Framingham, the Honolulu Heart Study, and the Chicago Gas and Electric Company Study (3). Hypercholesterolemia, hypertension, tobacco exposure, and diabetes are the major risk factors for CAD and stroke. Although total plasma cholesterol has been known as a risk factor for a long time, a low level of high-density lipoprotein (HDL) cholesterol is now recognized as an important risk factor as well.

The prevalence of individual risk factors may differ by age, race, or gender, but the major risk factors are usually of similar importance across racial and gender lines. Premenopausal women have lower total and low-density lipoprotein (LDL) cholesterol levels and higher HDL cholesterol concentrations than postmenopausal women. Hormone replacement therapy usually lowers total and LDL cholesterol and raises HDL cholesterol. The National

---

Box 5-1 Risk Status Based on Presence of Coronary Artery Disease Risk Factors Other Than Low-Density Lipoprotein Cholesterol*

Positive risk factors

Age

Men ≥ 45 years of age

Women ≥ 55 years of age (or premature menopause without ERT)

Family history of premature CAD

Definite MI or sudden death < 55 years of age in father or other male first-degree relative or < 65 years of age in mother or other female first-degree relative

Current cigarette smoking

Hypertension

≥ 140/90 mm Hg[†] or on antihypertensive medication

Low HDL cholesterol levels (≤ 35 mg/dL)[†]

Diabetes mellitus

Negative risk factor[‡]

High HDL cholesterol levels (≥ 60 mg/dL)

CAD = coronary artery disease; ERT = estrogen replacement therapy; HDL = high-density lipoprotein; MI = myocardial infarction.

* High risk (defined as two or more CAD risk factors) leads to more vigorous intervention. Age (defined differently for women and men) is treated as a risk factor because CAD rates are higher in the elderly than in the young and higher in men than in women of the same age. Obesity is not listed as a risk factor because it operates through other risk factors that are included (e.g., hypertension, hyperlipidemia, decreased HDL cholesterol levels, diabetes mellitus), but it should be considered a target for intervention. Physical inactivity is also not listed as a risk factor, but it too should be considered a target for intervention, and it is recommended as desirable for everyone.

[†] Confirmed by measurements on several occasions.

[‡] If the HDL cholesterol level is ≥ 60 mg/dL, subtract one risk factor (because high HDL cholesterol levels decrease CAD risk).

Adapted from National Cholesterol Education Program Adult Treatment Panel II. Summary of the second report of the NCEP expert panel on detection, evaluation, and treatment of high blood cholesterol in adults. JAMA. 1993;269:3015–23.

Cholesterol Education Program (NCEP) guidelines provide a list of the major risk factors (Box 5-1).

In this chapter, the effects of specific dietary components on lipid and lipoprotein metabolism are reviewed; the evidence that these interactions impact directly on the risk of CAD is also discussed. The link between dietary components and lipid and lipoprotein levels in blood are presented in detail, followed by a discussion of dietary carbohydrates, fiber, protein, total calories, alcohol, vitamins, and minerals.

Nutrition and Lipoproteins

Dietary fatty acids are divided into three major classes: saturated, monounsaturated, and polyunsaturated fatty acids. The foods that contribute to saturated fatty-acid intake include 1) red meats (e.g., beef, pork, lamb, veal, processed meat products, poultry with skin), 2) milk and other dairy products (e.g., butter, cheese, ice cream, puddings, yogurt), and 3) tropical fats (e.g., coconut, palm, palm kernel oils). The saturated fatty-acid content of beef and veal is 48%, and the saturated fatty-acid content of coconut oil is 87%. Fats that have a high percentage of saturated fatty acids are solid at room temperature. As a group, the different saturated fatty acids (which range in length from 8–18 carbon atoms) raise plasma LDL cholesterol levels; however, each acid may vary in its hypercholesterolemic effect.

Polyunsaturated fatty acids are divided into two major categories: the omega-6 and omega-3 fatty acids. The main omega-6 fatty acid in commonly consumed foods is linoleic acid, which is an essential fatty acid. Dietary sources of linoleic acid are safflower, sunflower, corn, and soybean oils. The omega-3 fatty acids are α-linolenic acid (found in canola oil and purslane), and eicosapentaenoic acid, and docosahexaenoic acid (found in salmon, bluefish, mackerel, and tuna).

Monounsaturated fatty acids are mainly present as oleic acid in olive oil, canola oil, avocado, hazelnuts, peanuts, pecans, almonds, and macadamia nuts. The oleic acid found in the typical U.S. diet is usually derived from animal fats, which are also high in saturated fatty acids. The *trans* form of oleic acid is elaidic acid and can be found in hydrogenated products (e.g., margarine, shortenings).

Dietary Fat and Fatty Acids

This section focuses on the effects of the three major classes of dietary fatty acids (i.e., saturated, monounsaturated, and polyunsaturated) on plasma lipids and lipoproteins. When appropriate, more details on individual fatty acids are presented. Many well-controlled diet studies have shown the effects of different fats, fat classes, and fatty acids on plasma lipids and lipoproteins. These studies have been used to generate blood-cholesterol-predictive equations (Box 5-2) to assess the effects of fat quality on plasma total cholesterol and lipoprotein cholesterol levels. The blood-cholesterol-predictive equations consistently show that saturated fatty acids raise blood cholesterol levels approximately twice as much as polyunsaturated fatty acids lower them. Monounsaturated fatty acids are either neutral or mildly hypocholesterolemic. Stearic acid has a neutral blood-cholesterol response.

Effects of Saturated Fatty Acids on Plasma Concentrations of Total and Low-Density Lipoprotein Cholesterol

The classic studies of Keys and colleagues (4) and Hegsted and colleagues (5) clearly demonstrated that increases in the percent of calories from saturated fat predicted increases in total plasma cholesterol levels. Although numerous studies (6–8) have been carried out since, the regression coefficients proposed in those original investigations generally have stood the test of time. The response in total cholesterol is mirrored by changes in LDL cholesterol and

---

Box 5-2 Predictive Equations for Estimating Changes in Plasma and Lipoprotein Cholesterol Levels in Response to Dietary Fatty Acids and Cholesterol*

Keys equation (4)
$$\Delta TC = 1.35(2\Delta S - \Delta P) + 1.52\Delta Z$$
Hegsted equation (5)
$$\Delta TC = 2.16\Delta S - 1.65\Delta P + 0.067\Delta C - 0.53$$
Mensink and Katan equation (7)
$$\Delta TC = 1.51\Delta S - 0.12\Delta M - 0.60\Delta P$$
$$\Delta LDL\text{-}C = 1.28\Delta S - 0.24\Delta M - 0.55\Delta P$$
$$\Delta HDL\text{-}C = 0.47\Delta S + 0.34\Delta M + 0.28\Delta P$$
Yu equation (8)
$$\Delta TC = 2.02\Delta 12{:}0\text{-}16{:}0 - 0.30\Delta 18{:}0 - 0.48\Delta M - 0.96\Delta P$$
$$\Delta LDL\text{-}C = 1.46\Delta 12{:}0\text{-}16{:}0 + 0.07\Delta 18{:}0 - 0.69\Delta M - 0.96\Delta P$$
$$\Delta HDL\text{-}C = 0.62\Delta 12{:}0\text{-}16{:}0 - 0.06\Delta 18{:}0 + 0.39\Delta M + 0.24\Delta P$$

* Where ΔTC = changes in plasma total cholesterol levels in mg/dL; $\Delta LDL\text{-}C$ = changes in plasma low-density lipoprotein cholesterol levels in mg/dL; $\Delta HDL\text{-}C$ = changes in plasma high-density lipoprotein cholesterol levels in mg/dL; ΔS = change in percentage of daily energy from saturated fatty acids; ΔM = change in percentage of daily energy from monounsaturated fats; ΔP = change in percentage of daily energy from polyunsaturated fats; ΔZ = change in the square root of dietary cholesterol levels in mg/1000 kcal; and ΔC = change in dietary cholesterol levels in mg/dL (Hegsted) mg/1000 kcal (Keys).

apoB levels and is similar in women and men, older and younger individuals, pre- and post-menopausal women, and whites and blacks (9). Children also respond to reductions in dietary saturated fat intake, with expected reductions in total and LDL cholesterol levels.

The mechanisms by which saturated fatty acids raise LDL cholesterol levels have been investigated intensely (10,11). In a variety of animal models, down-regulation of the LDL receptors, coupled with increased production of cholesterol carrying lipoproteins from the liver, accounts for the rise in plasma LDL levels. In primary hepatocytes from rats fed saturated fat, levels of LDL-receptor mRNA are depressed; similar effects have been observed in other rodents and in nonhuman primates. Less is known about the mechanisms that control increased formation and production of lipoprotein cholesterol; data are conflicting on the effects of intracellular cholesterol on apoB secretion. Several studies of the effects of saturated fats on human lipoprotein metabolism have been conducted. In a study of normal and hypercholesterolemic men, Turner and colleagues (12) found that high-fat diets with very low P:S ratios were associated with increased rates of production and slightly reduced rates of clearance of LDL apoB compared with diets with very high P:S ratios. Shepherd and colleagues (13) found that similar diets altered clearance rates in normal subjects. Cortese and colleagues (14) fed high-fat diets with varying P:S ratios and a low-fat diet to hyperlipidemic men. The investigators found that saturated fats increased 1) the number of very-low-density lipoprotein (VLDL) secreted by the liver, and 2) the conversion of VLDL to LDL.

In the same series of studies from which both Keys and Hegsted generated regression coefficients for saturated fats as a class, coefficients were estimated for each of the individual saturated fatty acids from C12 through C18. In the succeeding years, interest in the individual saturated fatty acids increased intermittently; recently, interest has peaked once again, in part because of technological advances that allow production of specific fatty acid blends that may be useful in food production. What follows is a brief review of the present database of individual saturated fatty acids; obviously, more studies are needed.

In the original studies by both Keys and Hegsted, contrasting effects of lauric acid (C12:0) were observed. Keys had assigned lauric acid a coefficient equal to that of palmitic acid and myristic acid, whereas Hegsted found it to have only a mild cholesterol-raising effect. In a more recent study, the effect of lauric acid was compared with palmitic acid and oleic acid using liquid formula diets fed to individuals for 3 weeks, each in random order. The results of the study indicated that relative to oleic acid, lauric acid raised LDL cholesterol only two thirds as much as that seen on the high palmitic acid diet. On the other hand, another study suggested that a diet rich in lauric acid raised LDL cholesterol concentrations more than a high palmitic acid diet.

Data from both the Keys and Hegsted trials suggested that myristic acid (C14:0) may be four to six times more cholesterolemic than palmitic acid. In a recent trial (15), the effect of myristic acid was tested on a large group of volunteers. Compared with both palmitic and oleic acids, myristic acid significantly raised both total and LDL cholesterol levels. Myristic acid raised cholesterol levels approximately 1.5 times as much as palmitic acid. In contrast, another study reported no increase in total and LDL cholesterol when myristic acid was substituted for palmitic acid. Thus, relative to the other major saturated fatty acids, the cholesterol-raising effects of myristic acid remains in question.

In addition to the aforementioned studies, several other investigations have revealed that palmitic acid (C16:0) is less hypercholesterolemic than a combination of lauric acid and myristic acid when substituted for lauric plus myristic acid over a range of energy intake of 5% to 18%.

Finally, both the earlier studies of Keys and Hegsted assigned a neutral role to stearic acid (C18:0), a role confirmed by more recent studies (16). It must be noted, however, that relative to unsaturated fats like linoleic acid, stearic acid raises total cholesterol and LDL cholesterol. Recently, Yu and colleagues (8) developed a new regression equation based on 18 studies that reported data on stearic and other fatty acids. In this equation, stearic was found to be neutral. The lack of a cholesterol-raising effect of stearic acid is due in part to its desaturation to oleic acid shortly after absorption as well as its higher incorporation into phosphatidylcholine (versus triglyceride and cholesteryl esters) compared with palmitic acid. Saturated fatty acids, with the exception of stearic acid (C18:0), suppress clearance of receptor-dependent LDL cholesterol from the circulation.

Food choices made by individuals can impact intake of the different saturated fatty acids. Selecting leaner cuts of meat (e.g., sirloin and round steak, which are high in palmitic acid) and limiting the amount of lean meat, skinless chicken, or fish to less than 6 oz/d would help in lowering saturated fat intake. Milk and other dairy products are high in myristic acid content. Substituting skim milk and nonfat dairy products for whole milk products will result in a reduction of saturated fat and myristic acid intake. Because food fats are a mixture of different fatty acids in varying amounts, multiple strategies have to be included to lower intakes of the saturated fatty acids that raise serum cholesterol levels.

Effects of Polyunsaturated Fatty Acids on Plasma Concentrations of Total and Low-Density Lipoprotein Cholesterol

Results of human feeding studies conducted during the early 1950s suggested that polyunsaturated fats had unique properties that reduced plasma cholesterol concentrations. Both the Keys and Hegsted studies estimated negative regression coefficients for this class of fatty acids. When individuals were fed diets high in polyunsaturated fats, their total cholesterol levels were reduced, and although these reductions were confounded in many studies by concomitant reductions in HDL cholesterol levels (7), LDL cholesterol levels fell as well. Indeed, the reductions in LDL levels seem to be not only a response to replacement of saturates by polyunsaturated fats in many studies but also a direct result of some activity of polyunsaturated fatty acids. Thus, after many years, several meta-analyses of well-controlled diet studies have confirmed a direct LDL-lowering effect of polyunsaturated fatty acids in humans, although this effect is not as potent as when saturated fats are reduced (7,8). This effect may be difficult to observe in single studies in which modest increases in polyunsaturated fats are achieved. Additionally, polyunsaturated fats may be potent only when they are added to diets lacking or extremely low in this class of fats. Hayes (17) has suggested that a level of 5% of calories from polyunsaturated fatty acids is at the top of the dose-response curve for the LDL cholesterol-lowering effect.

The mechanisms for lowering LDL levels during consumption of diets high in polyunsaturated fats are the opposite of those demonstrated for saturates: increased LDL-receptor function and reduced lipoprotein-cholesterol secretion from the liver. The human studies cited in the discussion of saturated fatty acids all used polyunsaturated fats as the comparison fatty acid class.

Effects of Monounsaturated Fatty Acids on Plasma Concentrations of Total and Low-Density Lipoprotein Cholesterol

Recently, the effects of monounsaturated fatty acids has generated much interest because of the low rates of CAD and all atherosclerotic cardiovascular disease in the Mediterranean area where diets are high in fats that come mainly from olive oil. In both the Keys and Hegsted studies, monounsaturated fats (specifically *cis*-oleic acid, which is found in olive oil) were found to have negligible independent cholesterol-lowering effects. This was an accepted fact until the mid-1980s, when other investigators demonstrated that monounsaturated fats could lower total and LDL cholesterol levels. Those studies, however, used diets in which monounsaturated fatty acids replaced saturated fatty acids. In a study in young, healthy men by Ginsberg and colleagues (18), the replacement of 7% of calories from carbohydrates with *cis*-oleic acid in an otherwise Step 1 diet (defined by the American Heart Association [AHA] later in this chapter) did not cause a further lowering of total or LDL cholesterol levels. This finding is in accord with the predictive regression coefficient based on a meta-analysis of the effects of fatty acids published by Mensink and Katan (7), although Yu and colleagues (8) recently developed a predictive equation in which monounsaturated fats minimally lowered cholesterol levels. Overall, the addition of moderate amounts of *cis*-oleic acid to the diet (in the range of 5%–10% of total calories) is unlikely to have a discernible effect on total and LDL cholesterol. Other monounsaturated fats (e.g., palmitoleic acid) are found in very low amounts in the typical U.S. diet; palmitoleic acid levels are higher in individuals whose diets include many types of nuts.

A unique but commercially important monounsaturated fatty acid is elaidic acid, the *trans*-isomer of *cis*-oleic acid (Fig. 5-1). Individuals receive some *trans*-fatty acids from dairy foods and ruminant meats, but most people obtain them from products containing commercially hydrogenated vegetable oils (e.g., margarine, shortening, baked goods). Early work by Mattson and colleagues (19) in the 1960s led to the belief that elaidic acid acted like *cis*-oleic acid; it had no effect on plasma cholesterol concentrations. Work published a few years later, however, suggested a slight cholesterol-raising effect of *trans*-fatty acids. Finally, in 1990, Mensink and colleagues (6) published the first of a series of papers indicating that *trans*-fatty acids might behave more like saturated fatty acids. LDL levels increased in a dose-response manner to the replacement of dietary oleic acid by moderate to large amounts of elaidic acid. Interestingly, HDL levels fell and lipoprotein(a) (Lp[a]) levels increased on the diet high in elaidic acid. The findings for LDL have been confirmed in other studies (20,21), whereas the fall in HDL was observed in some (21,22) but not all studies (20). Additionally, an increase in Lp(a) was not seen in the

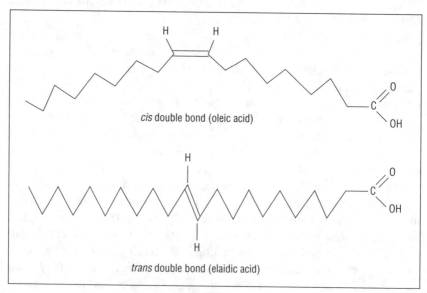

FIGURE 5-1 Structure of *cis*- and *trans*-fatty acids.

study by Lichtenstein and colleagues (22), although it was observed by Nestel and colleagues (20). The average intake of *trans*-fatty acids is estimated at 5% to 6% of calories (23), which is appreciably lower than the 12% intake of saturated fatty acids (NHANES III).

The Joint Task Force of the American Society for Clinical Nutrition and the American Institute of Nutrition concluded that 1) the effects of *trans*-unsaturated fats are less adverse than those of saturated fats, and 2) *trans*-fats are reasonable substitutes for saturated fats but not for polyunsaturated fats (24). Subsequent studies have raised further questions about the safety of consuming *trans*-fatty acids. Table 5-1 lists the *trans*-fatty acid content of foods in the U.S. diet.

Some epidemiologic data indicate a negative effect of *trans*-fatty acid intake on morbidity and mortality. The Framingham study found that after the first decade of follow-up, the relative risk of coronary heart disease was 1.1 for each additional teaspoon of margarine eaten each day (25). In a prospective study in 80,802 women who were 34 to 59 years of age and had no coronary disease, Hu and colleagues (26) suggested that replacing saturated fats with unhydrogenated monounsaturated and polyunsaturated fats is more effective in preventing CAD in women than reducing overall fat intake. Reports of this

Table 5-1 Estimated Average Daily Intake of Total Fat and *Trans*-Fat from Primary Food Sources of *Trans*-Fatty Acids

Food Source	Total Fat (g/d)*	*Trans*-Fat (g/d)[†]
Vegetable		
Breads (commercial)	4.0	0.3
Fried foods[‡]	3.9	0.8
Cakes, related baked goods	2.9	0.3
Savory snacks	2.3	0.3
Margarine (sticks)[§]	1.7	0.5
Margarine (soft, spreads)[§]	1.2	0.2
Cookies	1.2	0.2
Crackers	0.5	0.1
Household shortening[§]	0.4	0.1
Animal		
Milk	5.5	0.2
Ground beef	3.4	0.1
Butter	1.3	0.1

* Total fat values are 3-day averages from the U.S. Department of Agriculture Continuing Surveys of Food Intakes by Individuals, 1989–90 and 1990–91. Total fat intake is 69 g/d; total energy intake is 7.355 MJ/d (1758 kcal/d).

[†] *Trans*-fat composition data adapted from Nutrient Data Bank Bulletin Board (USDA/Agriculture Research Service, Riverdale, MD).

[‡] Home and restaurants combined.

[§] Intake of these foods does not include use as ingredients in foods already listed in table.

study were interpreted as "Butter is better than margarine" by the news media. Reducing the levels of *trans*-fatty acids in foods and avoiding the mistake of replacing *trans*-fatty acids with saturated fats in cooking and baking could have meaningful effects on the public's health (27). This can be achieved by decreasing intake of total at or substituting with unhydrogenated unsaturated oils (28a).

Effects of Fatty Acids on Plasma Concentrations of High-Density Lipoprotein Cholesterol

In their early studies, both Keys and Hegsted examined only total plasma cholesterol levels on different diets. Indeed, it wasn't until the late 1970s—after the rediscovery of the importance of HDL cholesterol as a protective factor for CAD—that studies of the effects of dietary fatty acids on HDL cholesterol began to appear. In many of the early studies, large quantities of polyunsaturated fatty acids were used, making up as much as 20% to 30% of total calories. Those studies demonstrated reductions in HDL cholesterol concentrations (along with lowering of LDL cholesterol levels). In the studies by Mattson and Grundy (28b) in which monounsaturated fats were compared with polyunsaturated fatty acids as replacements for saturated fats, the "high-poly" diets were associated with much lower HDL cholesterol levels compared with the "high-mono" diets. LDL cholesterol concentrations were similar in the two diets. In several recent studies in which smaller quantities of polyunsaturated fatty acids were added to an AHA Step 1 diet, smaller HDL lowering was observed (29).

A more systematic look at the effects of each class of fatty acids on HDL cholesterol levels can be achieved using the meta-analysis approach. In reports by Mensink and Katan (7), and more recently by Yu and colleagues (8), saturated, polyunsaturated, and monounsaturated fatty acids were all found to actually have raised HDL cholesterol levels; however, the relative potency of these classes was saturated > monounsaturated >> polyunsaturated. Thus, if monounsaturated fats were used as a replacement for saturated fats, the fall in HDL levels was very slight (monounsaturated fats raise HDL levels slightly less than saturates) but was statistically insignificant in most of the small diet studies. If polyunsaturated fats replaced saturated fats, the fall in HDL cholesterol levels was greater (polyunsaturated fats raise HDL only ~40% as much as saturated fats) and was statistically significant in most previous studies. This scheme makes it clear why replacement of total fat (with any fatty-acid distribution) with carbohydrates (which are neutral in regards to HDL cholesterol) results in significant reductions in HDL levels: all fats raise HDL.

Three human studies focused on the mechanisms by which HDL levels fall during consumption of diets with different total fat content. Blum and colleagues (30) first studied HDL apoAI metabolism in subjects consuming a diet very high in carbohydrates (80% of total calories) and low in fats (5% of total calories) compared with diets high in fats (40% of total calories) with a typical carbohydrate content (40% of total calories). The investigators demonstrated that the fall in HDL cholesterol and apoAI levels was associated with increased fractional clearance of apoAI. Brinton and colleagues (31) performed a similar experiment several years later in which they fed subjects diets containing either 40% or 10% fat. They found that the fall in HDL cholesterol levels on the low-fat diet was associated mainly with reduced apoAI production. Fractional clearance of apoAI increased as well. Shepherd and colleagues (32) compared diets that were very high and very low in polyunsaturated fat; they found that the lower HDL levels observed in subjects on the high-polyunsaturated-fat diet had significantly reduced rates of apoAI appearance in plasma. In summarizing these studies, the consistent theme is that fatty acids somehow increase secretion of apoAI from the liver, intestine, or both. Furthermore, saturated fats stimulate apoAI secretion more than polyunsaturated fats; it is assumed that monounsaturated fats are close to saturated fats in this regard. Replacing fatty acids with carbohydrates also may result in increased fractional clearance of apoAI and lower plasma levels of this protein. Under most conditions, altered levels of apoAI will result in altered plasma concentrations of HDL cholesterol.

Effects of Fatty Acids on Plasma Concentrations of Triglycerides

In general, saturated fatty acids increase plasma triglyceride levels moderately, whereas polyunsaturated fatty acids reduce them to a similar degree. An exception to the moderate effects of fatty acids on plasma triglycerides are those observed when large amounts of omega-3 fatty acids (4–8 g/d) are consumed (33). This class of fatty acids, which includes α-linolenic acid, eicosapentaenoic acid, and docosahexaenoic acid, is found mainly in the fat tissue of cold-water fish (Box 5-3). Consumption of large quantities of salmon oil was shown to reduce significantly the secretion of VLDL from livers in normal and hypertriglyceridemic humans. Omega-3 fatty acids also reduce postprandial triglyceride levels. Both eicosapentaenoic and docosahexaenoic acids can increase the intracellular degradation of nascent apoB in cultured liver cells. Capsules of concentrated omega-3 fatty acids have been used to treat patients with severe hypertriglyceridemia.

Effects of Fatty Acids on Lipoprotein(a) Levels

Lipoprotein(a) is a subclass of LDL that contains apo(a) in addition to apoB. Some epidemiologic studies have indicated increased risk for CAD as Lp(a) increases. Although some studies have suggested that greater than 90% of the variability in Lp(a) levels seem to be genetically determined, recent studies have found that increases in plasma Lp(a) levels occur in normal and dyslipi-

---

Box 5-3 Major Dietary Fatty Acids by Class

Saturated fatty acids
  Lauric acid (12:0)
  Myristic acid (14:0)
  Palmitic acid (16:0)
  Stearic acid (18:0)
Monounsaturated fatty acids
  Oleic acid (18:1n-9)
Polyunsaturated fatty acids
  Omega-6
    Linoleic acid (18:2n-6)
  Omega-3
    Alpha-linoleic acid (18:3n-3)
    Eicosapentaenoic acid (20:5n-3)
    Docosahexaenoic acid (22:6n-3)

---

demic individuals when saturated fatty acids are removed from the diet (9,34). In several previous studies, Lp(a) concentrations were not altered by changes in dietary saturated fats or cholesterol (35). In contrast, Lp(a) levels did rise in the majority of studies in which *trans*-fatty acids were increased (7,20,22). Further studies will be needed to confirm and investigate the mechanisms underlying these effects of fatty acids on Lp(a) concentrations in plasma.

Dietary Cholesterol

The role of dietary cholesterol in both development of hypercholesterolemia and atherosclerosis has been the focus of many investigators over the past century. The studies by Ignatovski (36) and later by Anitschkow and Chalatow (37) indicated the importance of dietary cholesterol. Their work in rabbits has been supported by many studies in other animal models and in human diet and epidemiologic investigations (38a). However, other investigators have come to opposite conclusions after reviewing numerous human feeding studies (although many continue to support the view that dietary cholesterol is the major atherogenic nutrient in the diet). This controversy has been evident in the changing prominence of dietary cholesterol in the AHA Diet Statements published every several years.

One reason for this controversy is that the animal models may not be appropriate to humans; clearly, humans do not respond to dietary cholesterol with the marked increases in plasma cholesterol observed in rabbits. Even ro-

dent species, which are resistant to atherosclerosis, respond to dietary cholesterol and fat with larger increases in lipid levels than do humans. Another
problem is that the amounts of cholesterol fed to animals in most early studies were much beyond the highest intakes reported in humans. More recently,
however, diets with modest increases in cholesterol content have been shown
to increase plasma cholesterol significantly in nonhuman primates, with concomitant development of atherosclerosis.

Many studies of the effects of dietary cholesterol on plasma cholesterol levels in humans have been published during the past several decades. Many
were of poor quality, however, with little control over nutrient intake other
than cholesterol. Several excellent studies deserve review. First, as always, the
classic studies of Keys and Hegsted both provided regression coefficients for
the effects of dietary cholesterol on total plasma cholesterol levels. These coefficients suggested that for each 100 mg of dietary cholesterol added per day,
plasma cholesterol would rise between 3 and 6 mg/dL. In a later review of
more experiments, Hegsted (38b) lowered his previous estimate of the effect of
dietary cholesterol to be in line with that of the original Keys study. Ginsberg
and colleagues (39,40) carried out two well-controlled studies in healthy
young men (39) and women (40). Dietary cholesterol ranged from approximately 125 to 750 mg/d and was part of the NCEP Step 1 diet. Four (39) or
three (40) levels of cholesterol were fed to individuals, allowing for estimation
of the results by regression analysis. For each addition of one egg (~200 mg of
cholesterol), LDL cholesterol levels increased approximately 3 to 4 mg/dL
(Fig. 5-2). This change was statistically significant, but obviously modest, particularly in the setting of baseline LDL cholesterol levels of approximately 100
mg/dL. The changes observed amounted to approximately 60% of the original
estimate of response proposed by Keys and colleagues (4). HDL cholesterol
levels tended to increase in the men and significantly increased in the women
(1 mg/dL for each egg added to the diet).

Human metabolic studies of the effects of dietary cholesterol on lipoprotein production and degradation have added to our knowledge of the mechanism underlying effects on plasma levels. Within the range of typical intakes,
dietary cholesterol does not seem to affect VLDL production by the liver, although increased entry of intermediate-density lipoprotein (IDL) into the circulation has been observed in a small group of subjects fed very high levels of
cholesterol. Several studies of HMG CoA reductase inhibitors, which reduce
endogenous cholesterol synthesis, have demonstrated reduced secretion of
VLDL in vivo. Thus, the effects of dietary cholesterol on VLDL (and IDL) as-
sembly and secretion remains incompletely characterized.

A number of studies have focused on the effects of dietary cholesterol on
LDL metabolism. Ginsberg and colleagues (41) determined LDL apoB turnover
in five healthy men on diets containing either 300 or 1200 mg/d of cholesterol.

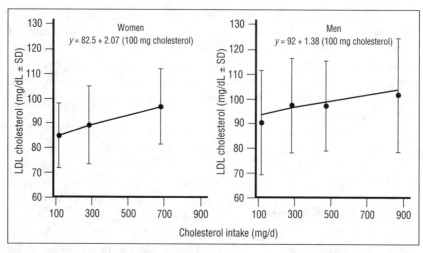

Figure 5-2 Low-density lipoprotein (LDL) cholesterol levels in women and men. (Adapted from Ginsberg HN, Karmally W, Siddiqui M, et al. A dose-response study of the effects of dietary cholesterol on fasting and postprandial lipid and lipoprotein metabolism in healthy young men. Arterioscler Thromb Vasc Biol. 1994;14:576–86; and Ginsberg HN, Karmally W, Siddiqui M, et al. Increases in dietary cholesterol are associated with modest increases in both low-density and high-density lipoprotein cholesterol in healthy young women. Arterioscler Thromb Vasc Biol. 1995;15:169–78.)

Both diets contained 40% of calories as fat, with a P:S ratio of 0.4. The fourfold increase in dietary cholesterol had no effect on LDL production or fractional clearance, and LDL cholesterol levels did not change. In a similar study by Packard and colleagues (42), an eightfold increase in dietary cholesterol (40% of calories from fat; P:S of 0.2) increased plasma cholesterol levels and was associated with both increased LDL production and decreased LDL fractional removal. The differing results in these two studies may be related to the greater absolute cholesterol load in the study by Packard and Shepherd (1800 mg/d) or to the lower P:S ratio in their study.

Dietary Carbohydrates

Dietary recommendations to lower total fat intake include increasing dietary carbohydrate intake, because favorable plasma lipid and lipoprotein levels have been reported for populations and individuals whose habitual diet is high in carbohydrates. There is, however, concern over reports of high carbohydrate consumption being associated with a decrease in HDL cholesterol levels and an elevation of plasma triglyceride levels. Individuals who eat a high-carbohydrate diet have low plasma HDL cholesterol levels and low CAD rates. Plasma triglyceride levels are not significantly elevated in these individuals, possibly because obesity is rare. Another issue being studied currently is whether it is advisable to recommend high-carbohydrate diets to individuals with insulin resistance and diabetes who may have high plasma triglyceride and low HDL cholesterol levels (43). The concern is that high-carbohydrate diets may exacerbate the risk for heart disease. In a well-controlled multicenter study, small differences were found in plasma HDL cholesterol and triglyceride levels in women and men who were fed diets higher in carbohydrates or higher in monounsaturated fatty acids. The diet higher in monounsaturated fatty acids was associated with slightly higher HDL cholesterol levels and slightly lower triglyceride levels (unpublished data).

A study on postmenopausal women revealed that hypertriglyceridemia caused by an eucaloric high-carbohydrate intake is not associated with a decrease in LDL particle size (44). The authors allow for the possibility that carbohydrate-induced hypertriglyceridemia may affect LDL particle size differently in premenopausal women or in men. In postmenopausal women, however, carbohydrate-induced hypertriglyceridemia may not have the same atherogenic implications as genetic disorders such as combined hyperlipidemia or hypertriglyceridemia.

Dietary Fiber

Studies have shown that only water-soluble fiber plays a role in lipoprotein metabolism in humans. The soluble fiber content of oats, barley, guar gum, beans, and psyllium seeds is related to CAD. A meta-analysis of 20 studies found that intake of oat products reduces serum cholesterol levels (45). The lipid-lowering effect is dose related and is most significant in individuals with the highest cholesterol levels. A daily intake of approximately 3 g of soluble fiber from oats has been reported to reduce serum cholesterol levels by 5.6 mg/dL. The hypocholesterolemic effects of oats depend on the bran, which contains beta-glucan, a water-soluble fiber. Controlled trials with psyllium have shown that a daily intake of 5.1 to 10.4 g of psyllium can lower total cholesterol levels by 4.8% to 14.8% and LDL cholesterol levels by 5.7% to 20.2% within 6 to 16 weeks; this amount of psyllium is also well tolerated.

The mechanism by which dietary fiber affects plasma lipid levels has not been established. Insoluble fibers in wheat and vegetables do not seem to reduce serum cholesterol, but they do have other beneficial effects.

Dietary Protein

Forty years ago, population studies indicated that people who ate large amounts of soy protein had lower rates of atherosclerosis. Soy protein has been shown to lower serum cholesterol levels in animals and in hypercholesterolemic individuals when compared with casein (a dairy protein) and beef proteins. A meta-analysis of 38 studies included data from 730 subjects (46). Twenty-one of the studies used isolated soy protein, 14 studies used textured soy protein, and three studies used a combination of the two types of protein. Four of the studies were in children and 34 were in adults. In these 38 studies, there was a 12.9% reduction in LDL cholesterol levels, a 2.4% rise in HDL levels, and a 10.5% reduction in triglyceride levels when the average intake of soy protein was 47 g/d. The mechanism underlying these changes is not clear. It has been stated that soy protein may affect cholesterol absorption, bile-acid absorption, the insulin–glucagon ratio, serum thyroxin levels, and hepatic LDL-receptor activity. It is also believed that the soy isoflavone, genistein (a molecule that resembles estradiol), may play a role in cholesterol metabolism.

Proteins may differ in amino acid composition, and this may affect cardiovascular risk. Chronic dietary supplement of L-arginine in animals has been shown to decrease platelet aggregation and the adhesiveness of aortic endothelium for monocytes, to prevent the intimal thickening of coronary arteries, and to reverse endothelial dysfunction. These effects seem to be due to the metabolism of L-arginine to nitric oxide, whose many biologic roles have been reviewed recently (47). L-arginine has also been shown to improve endothelial dysfunction of both coronary microvasculature and epicardial coronary arteries in cardiac transplant recipients. Platelet aggregation in hypercholesterolemic individuals is also reduced by L-arginine supplements. These findings are intriguing because L-arginine availability should not be rate limiting for nitric oxide synthesis under most dietary conditions. Arginine (levels of which are generally higher in plant proteins) seems to have a hypocholesterolemic effect, whereas lysine and methionine (amino acids found generally in animal proteins) seem to raise plasma cholesterol concentrations.

Calories

The states of being overweight (body mass index [BMI] > 25 kg/m^2) or obese (BMI > 30 kg/m^2) are the result of calorie intake in excess of energy expenditure. A well-established association exists between obesity and an increased risk for cardiovascular disease in both women and men (48,49). For a given level of BMI, abdominal obesity is a significant and independent predictor of CAD and is associated with insulin resistance, hypertension, and hyperlipidemia. Even levels of body fat that are not labeled as overweight and are average for the U.S. population can increase the risk of plasma lipid level elevation, glucose intolerance, and high blood pressure. The leanest individuals have a lower risk than those with average degrees of adiposity, suggesting that weight reduction may also benefit individuals who are not overtly overweight. A meta-analysis of 70 studies indicated that weight reduction was associated with increases in HDL cholesterol levels and significant decreases in total, LDL, and VLDL cholesterol and triglyceride levels (50).

In a cohort of middle-aged female nurses studied by Manson and colleagues (51), body weight was an important determinant of mortality. BMI was more strongly associated with deaths from CAD and other cardiovascular diseases than with deaths from other causes. (A more extensive discussion can be found in Chapter 7.)

Alcohol

Epidemiologic studies have shown a reverse trend between low to moderate alcohol consumption and CAD in both women and men (52). This protective effect had been associated with an increased concentration of plasma HDL cholesterol as well as some HDL apoproteins (i.e., A-I, A-II, and A-IV). Among the major subclasses of HDL, HDL-2 and HDL-3 are both increased by alcohol consumption. Reduced platelet aggregation and blood coagulation and increased fibrinolytic activity are all associated with alcohol consumption; these may be viewed as possible additional underlying mechanisms for the cardioprotective effect of alcohol. These findings have led physicians to recommend daily consumption of moderate amounts of alcohol (i.e., one 5-ounce glass of wine, 12 ounces of beer, or 1.5 ounces of distilled spirits per day for women and no more than twice that for men). These recommendations continue to be controversial; the data on alcohol are difficult to assess because of the lack of enough controlled human studies and the lack of clarity in the description of "moderate" and "heavy" drinking in relation to the pathophysiology of atherosclerosis. Excessive ethanol consumption can result in alcoholic cardiomyopathy. In addition, regular alcohol consumption raises blood pressure and contributes significantly to the prevalence of hypertension in drinking populations (53). Finally, although moderate drinking (< 40 g/d pure ethanol for men; < 30 g/d for women) seems to have benefits (e.g., inverse correlation with CAD risk), any possible benefits must be balanced against the risks, which include stroke, motor vehicle accidents, cancer, birth defects, and dangerous interactions with drugs. In addition, when people do not adhere to moderate recommendations, social and health problems increase.

A potential metabolic risk arises from the observation that alcohol given in moderate amounts increases hepatic synthesis of VLDL. Similar responses were not seen with isocaloric amounts of either carbohydrates or fats. Plasma triglyceride levels can be increased in fasting individuals after alcohol ingestion for several hours to several days (54). As noted above, HDL cholesterol levels are increased modestly by alcohol, so the alcohol-induced hypertriglyceridemia is the exception to the rule that higher triglycerides are associated with lower HDL cholesterol levels. Low or subnormal levels of LDL cholesterol have been found consistently in chronic alcoholics. One possible explanation is that VLDL is converted less readily to LDL in alcoholics. Alternatively, excessive alcohol intake usually is associated with malnutrition and weight loss, and these may result in lower LDL levels.

Chromium

Trials in humans show that chromium elevated serum HDL levels and lowered total serum cholesterol levels (55,56a). Serum HDL levels increased by 5.8 mg/dL in men who received β-blockers (commonly used antihypertensive drugs that tend to lower HDL cholesterol levels) with three daily doses of 200 μg of chromium for 8 weeks. In a randomized, double-blind, placebo-controlled study, no significant changes were seen in LDL or triglyceride levels. In a study of 28 moderately obese non–insulin-dependent diabetic patients, 2 months of chromium picolinate supplements lowered plasma triglyceride levels by 17.4% (56b). A range of chromium intakes between 50 and 200 μg/d is recommended tentatively for adults by the National Academy of Science. In the U.S. population, chromium intake from self-selected meals can be as low as 25 μg/d.

Diet and Atherosclerosis

Dietary Lipids

The twentieth century has seen the continuous growth of a base of information supporting a significant role for diet in the atherogenic process. Following the groundbreaking studies in rabbits by Ignatowski (36) and Anitschkow and Chalatow (37), scientists were able to observe and record the "natural" experiment associated with World War II, in which the incidence of CAD fell in occupied countries (57). The similar patterns of association between increases in dietary fat intake and CAD seen in Japanese men who migrated to Hawaii and the mainland United States (58) and in all Americans between 1950 and 1970 provided strong evidence for the link between diet and heart disease. At the same time, Keys and colleagues (59), using epidemiologic approaches to support his clinical diet studies, reported the Seven Countries Study, which showed remarkable relationships between heart disease mortality and dietary intake of saturated fatty acids.

Cohort studies such as the Ireland-Boston Heart Study and the Western Electric Study have added further support for hypotheses linking CAD to dietary saturated fatty acids, cholesterol, or both. A detailed review of these data is provided in the Diet and Health report of the National Research Council (3) and the Surgeon General's Report (60). Probably the most convincing data derive from the clinical trials that have been carried out using only dietary interventions. In the early study by Dayton and colleagues (61), increasing polyunsaturated fats in the diet was associated with lower CAD events in an elderly population. The Finnish Mental Hospital Study (Miettinen et al, 1983) demonstrated reduced CAD in women and men who received lower dietary saturated fat and cholesterol. More recently, the Oslo Heart Study (62) found that men given diets high in polyunsaturated and low in saturated fatty acids had fewer fatal and nonfatal CAD events. Both the Lifestyle Heart Trial (1) and the St. Thomas Atherosclerosis Regression Study (STARS) trial (2) showed less progression and regression of coronary atherosclerosis in men treated with lower fat and cholesterol diets. STARS also demonstrated fewer CAD events in the treated group compared with controls.

Overall, the link between dietary saturated fatty acids and CAD is clear and convincing; similar, but less convincing data are available for dietary cholesterol. The association between these dietary factors and atherosclerosis is almost certainly based on their effects on plasma lipid and lipoproteins, although separate effects on thrombogenic factors must be considered as well (63).

Antioxidants

The concept that oxidatively modified LDL is pro-atherogenic and exists in vivo is supported by a growing body of data. In animal models, antioxidant supplementation inhibited the progression of atherosclerosis. The nutrients studied in these experiments were ascorbic acid, alpha-tocopherol (vitamin E), and beta-carotene. At present, there is insufficient clinical trial data to make recommendations about the use of antioxidant supplements to the diet (64).

A significant inverse relationship was found between plasma vitamin C and CAD in epidemiologic studies (65). Ascorbate concentrations were also found to be lower in the aortas of people with atherosclerosis, diabetes, and CAD and in smokers and nonsmokers when compared with unaffected controls. It has been hypothesized that low concentrations of ascorbate in the arterial wall may predispose LDL to oxidation, which could promote atherogenesis. In the NHANES study, which included 11,349 U.S. women and men, there was an inverse association between cardiovascular mortality and ascorbic acid intake (66).

Alpha-tocopherol is the predominant lipophilic antioxidant in plasma membranes and tissue and is the most abundant antioxidant in LDL. On average, there are six molecules of alpha-tocopherol per LDL particle; they can function as antioxidants by trapping free radicals. Low plasma levels of alpha-tocopherol were inversely correlated with CAD in a cross-sectional study and with angina pectoris in a case control study. In prospective studies, alpha-tocopherol supplementation seemed to reduce the risk of coronary events in both women and men (67,68). In the female Nurses Health Study, there was an inverse association between CAD events and alpha-tocopherol intake (67). In a randomized, placebo-controlled study in men, the LDL oxidation kinetics in a group supplemented with 800 IU was similar to the kinetics in the group that received combined supplementation with 1.0 g ascorbate, 30 mg beta-carotene, and 800 IU alpha-tocopherol. There was a 40% decrease in the oxidation rate after 3 months of supplementation (68). Miwa and colleagues found plasma vitamin E levels were significantly lower in patients (both women and men) with active variant angina than in patients without coronary spasm (69). In a cohort of 34,486 postmenopausal women, dietary vitamin E was found to be protective in women in the highest quintile of dietary vitamin E intake (70).

Randomized clinical trials investigating the effect of antioxidant intake on CAD have shown mixed results. In the Alpha-Tocopherol, Beta-Carotene (ATBC) Cancer Prevention Study (71), no benefit with respect to CAD for alpha-tocopherol or beta-carotene was seen. However, the dosage of alpha-tocopherol (50 mg/d) was below the protective range suggested by the Nurses Health Study. In the Cambridge Heart Antioxidant Study (CHAOS) in which 2002 British women and men with angiographically proved CAD were included, a 77% reduction was seen in nonfatal myocardial infarction in subjects taking vitamin E as compared with those on placebo (72); however, an increase in cardiovascular and overall mortality was also seen.

Beta-carotene has been shown to inhibit oxidation of LDL and Lp(a) (73). Smokers have lower LDL beta-carotene levels relative to nonsmokers. The Physicians Health Study, however, did not demonstrate benefit from beta-carotene supplementation (74). The Beta-Carotene and Retinol Efficacy Trial (CARET) was stopped 21 months early because the beta-carotene group had 285 more lung cancer cases and 17% more deaths than the control group (75). Cardiovascular mortality was also increased in the beta-carotene group.

Primary and secondary prevention trials with vitamin E and C supplementation are ongoing. These studies are including women and patients with diabetes mellitus and coronary and peripheral vascular disease. Although vitamin E seems promising, the evidence currently available does not support any public health policy recommendations for antioxidant supplementation. In the meantime, the U.S. population should be encouraged to increase consumption of fruits and vegetables because of their unique antioxidant content as well as being low in fat and high in fiber. (For a more extensive discussion, see Chapter 9).

Nutrient Intake Deficiency Associated with Homocysteinemia

Elevated levels of homocysteine in the blood have been associated with an increased risk of cardiovascular disease (76). Recent clinical studies have linked moderate hyperhomocysteinemia to peripheral vascular, cerebrovascular, and coronary heart disease. A prospective study of male physicians indicated that plasma homocysteine concentrations of 17 μmol/L (or 12% above the upper limit of normal) were associated with a three- to four-fold increase in the risk of acute myocardial infarction (77). A high plasma homocysteine concentration and low levels of folate and vitamin B_6, through their role in homocysteine metabolism, were also associated with an increased risk of extracranial carotid artery stenosis. The effect of homocysteine is independent of the established risk factors (e.g., hyperlipidemia and hypertension). Elevated homocysteine level may reflect inadequate availability of folate or vitamins B_6 or B_{12}. The female Nurses Health Study (78) demonstrated a significant inverse relationship between dietary intake of folate and vitamin B_6 and cerebrovascular disease mortality and morbidity. Supplementation with these vitamins, particularly folic acid, may normalize plasma homocysteine levels. (See Chapter 9 for a detailed discussion.)

Iron

Iron overload on the myocardium as a potential risk for CAD was indicated in animal experiments in which iron overload increased myocardial damage caused by anoxia and reperfusion. A role for iron in promoting oxidation of LDL cholesterol and atherosclerosis has been proposed, but convincing data are lacking. A prospective study in Finland reported a twofold increase in acute myocardial infarction among men with serum ferritin levels above 200 μg/L (79). A study of U.S. physicians (80) and a cohort study of Icelandic women and men (81) showed no association between serum levels of ferritin or iron and the risk of myocardial infarction. In the same study, serum total iron-binding capacity was inversely correlated with the risk of myocardial infarction. Increased risk for myocardial infarction also has been directly correlated with high serum iron concentrations but not with serum transferrin saturation levels. In summary, the data presently available for a link between iron and CAD are inconsistent and do not justify changes in food fortification policy or dietary recommendations.

Selenium

Selenium is an integral part of the antioxidant enzyme glutathione peroxidase and has been studied in relation to CAD. A reduced plasma selenium level has been associated with an increased risk of cardiovascular disease and death in some studies (82); however, other studies did not show this association (83). Whereas high intake levels of selenium may not be protective, low intake of selenium could be a risk factor; however, in a cross-sectional study of random population samples of apparently healthy middle-aged men in four European countries, selenium levels did not correlate with the reported rates of CAD (84).

Dietary Treatment of Hypercholesterolemia

Efforts to optimize plasma lipid and lipoprotein levels and reduce the risk for CAD should start with diet modification:

1. Reducing the intake of saturated fatty acids
2. Reducing caloric intake in excess of energy requirements
3. Reducing the intake of dietary cholesterol

The most important nutritional intervention for hypercholesterolemia is lowering the intake of saturated fatty acids and cholesterol. For most people with elevated plasma cholesterol levels, dietary changes aimed at lowering saturated fat and cholesterol intake will be the only intervention required to lower serum cholesterol levels, thereby lowering the risk for CAD (71). The degree to which an individual's blood cholesterol level drops after initiation of diet therapy depends on their eating patterns before diet modification is initiated and their inherent degree of responsiveness. Individuals exhibit great biologic variability. Usually, patients with high cholesterol levels experience the greatest reduction in total and LDL cholesterol.

The NCEP has recommended a two-step approach to lower plasma total cholesterol concentrations by progressively reducing intakes of saturated fatty acids and cholesterol and to promote weight loss in overweight patients by reducing total caloric intake. The Step 1 diet, which is similar to the diet recommended by the American Heart Association, is a population-based ap-

Table 5-2 Two-Step Approach to Treating Hypercholesterolemia

Nutrient	Recommended Intake	
	Step 1 Diet	Step 2 Diet
Total fat	< 30% of total calories	< 30% of total calories
Saturated fatty acids	< 10% of total calories	< 7% of total calories
Polyunsaturated fatty acids	≥ 10% of total calories	≥ 10% of total calories
Monounsaturated fatty acids	10%–15% of total calories	10%–15% of total calories
Carbohydrates	50%–60% of total calories	50%–60% of total calories
Protein	10%–20% of total calories	10%–20% of total calories
Cholesterol	< 300 mg/d	< 200 mg/d
Total calories	To achieve and maintain desirable weight	To achieve and maintain desirable weight

proach for lowering blood cholesterol. The recommendations (Table 5-2) include a total fat intake of 30% or less of total calories, an intake of saturated fat between 8% and 10% of total calories, an intake of polyunsaturated fat up to 10% of total calories, and an intake of monounsaturated fat between 10% and 15% of total calories. Cholesterol intake should be less than 300 mg/d. Dietary treatment should be aimed to achieve and maintain a healthy body weight and eating patterns, with a permanent change in eating behavior. The Step 1 diet should be followed for a minimum of 3 months to maximize the time for the desired response expected with good adherence. If the response is not achieved, the NCEP recommendation is to progress to the Step 2 diet. The Step 1 diet should reduce plasma cholesterol levels approximately 10% from baseline, depending on previous diet pattern and inherent characteristics of responsiveness. Advancement to the Step 2 diet may achieve a further 5% drop in plasma total cholesterol. The individual variability in responsiveness is significant, however, and the range of reduction in plasma cholesterol is from 0% to 25%.

The Step 2 diet (*see* Table 5-2) is recommended if the response to the Step 1 diet is not optimum. It calls for reducing further the intake of saturated fatty acids to less than 7% of calories and for reducing cholesterol intake to less than 200 mg/d. Both the Step 1 and Step 2 diets recommend that patients achieve and maintain ideal body weight. Implementation of the Step 2 diet may require intensive nutrition counseling by a registered dietitian to lower the saturated fat and cholesterol content of the diet even further, without jeopardizing food palatability and acceptability. The total fat intake, however, can be maintained at 30% of calories. This allows the individual to use sources of monounsaturated fatty acids (e.g., olive and canola oils) or polyunsaturated fatty acids (e.g., corn and safflower oils) as a replacement for the additional removal of saturated fats, thereby providing satiety attributable to the fat content of the meal.

The major contributors to the intake of saturated fatty acids are the higher fat red meats (especially hamburger, veal, lamb, pork, and processed meat products), poultry with skin, and whole milk and dairy products. Fats that have a high percentage of saturated fat are solid at room temperature and are used in commercial baking of cakes, pastries, cereals, and granola. The "nondairy" creamers and dairy substitutes for whipped cream and sour cream, which may be labeled as containing no cholesterol because they are derived from plants, are usually made with highly saturated coconut or palm oil or hydrogenated vegetable oil. These vegetable fats are frequently used commercially because they are inexpensive and resist oxidation (which extends their shelf life).

The polyunsaturated fatty acids are composed of two major categories: the omega-6 and omega-3 fatty acids. The main omega-6 fat is linoleic acid, which is an essential fatty acid present in large amounts in safflower, sunflower, soybean, and corn oils. The oils in most cold-water fish are major sources of omega-3 fatty acids (e.g., eicosapentaenoic and docosahexaenoic acids). As noted earlier, these fatty acids are effective in lowering triglyceride levels when fed in large amounts. They have not been shown to be helpful in lowering LDL cholesterol levels and, therefore, are not recommended for the treatment of hypercholesterolemia. However, both high-fat fish (e.g., salmon, mackerel, bluefish) that are rich in omega-3 fatty acids and low-fat fish (e.g., sole, flounder, cod, halibut) should be included in the diet plan because they are a good source of protein and can be a useful substitute for meat that is high in saturated fatty acids.

Monounsaturated fatty acids are present mainly as oleic acid in olive oil and canola oil. Monounsaturated fats should make up 10% to 15% of calories. The current U.S. diet supplies as much oleic acid as is recommended, but the oleic acid is usually derived from animal fats that are also high in saturates. When the intake of animal fat is decreased, vegetable oils and nuts can be included in the meal plan to increase monounsaturated fat intake.

There is no universal agreement about the value of the NCEP dietary guidelines for all U.S. citizens. The effect of carbohydrates on lowering HDL cholesterol levels and raising triglyceride levels is a cause for concern. The alternative to the Step 1 and Step 2 diets is the approach to replace saturated fat with monounsaturated fat.

Cholesterol from food sources is supplied only by animal foods. The organ meats (e.g., brain, liver, kidney, sweetbread) are very rich sources of cholesterol. Meat (both muscle and fat) contains cholesterol. There is no significant difference in the cholesterol content of beef, lamb, pork, chicken, or turkey. Fish (except some shellfish such as shrimp) are slightly lower in cholesterol than meat or poultry.

The intake of protein that is recommended by the U.S. Department of Agriculture is approximately 15% of total caloric intake. This level of intake still meets the recommended dietary allowance (RDA) for a woman consuming 1200 kcal/d. The sources of protein should be from a variety of low-fat animal foods and plant foods such as legumes and grains. The amount of lean animal foods recommended could be a maximum of 5 or 6 oz/d. High-protein foods are usually associated with a high fat content. The exceptions are egg whites and isolated soy protein and casein supplements. High-protein diets used in weight-reducing, fad diet programs can have significant adverse effects on serum cholesterol levels because of the simultaneous increase in saturated fat and cholesterol intake.

The carbohydrate content of the therapeutic diet should be approximately 55% of the total calories. Dietary carbohydrates include simple sugars (the monosaccharides and mainly the disaccharide sucrose used in the preparation of food) and the complex carbohydrates (both the digestible starch and the indigestible fibers). The recommendation is to eat more of the nutrient-rich complex carbohydrates and less of the nutritionally devoid simple carbohydrates that provide only "empty" calories.

Indigestible carbohydrates are also known as dietary fiber and can be separated by whether they are soluble or insoluble in the gastrointestinal tract. Insoluble fiber provides bulk and aids in the movement of food and water through the intestine. It is found in food sources such as whole wheat, whole-grain cereals (*caution:* granolas made with animal fats, vegetable shortenings, or both are high in saturated fatty acids), corn, and vegetables. Insoluble fiber may protect and help in the prevention and treatment of diseases of the intestinal tract (e.g., constipation, diverticulosis, hemorrhoids, cancer of the colon and rectum).

Rich sources of soluble fiber include oatmeal, oat bran, psyllium seeds, legumes containing gums (e.g., dried peas and beans, which contain β-glucan), and some fruits containing pectin (e.g., grapefruit, apples). Soluble fiber has shown to lower LDL cholesterol, help diabetes control by slowing absorption of glucose, and aid in appetite control by creating satiety. Some studies have suggested that large amounts of oat bran (providing 15–25 g of soluble fiber) eaten daily can lower plasma cholesterol by 3% to 15%. Saturated fat intake was reduced concomitantly in the studies that showed the larger effects on plasma cholesterol concentrations. Adding foods containing soluble fiber to the diet could be a valuable adjunct to a low-saturated-fat, low-cholesterol diet. Because eating large quantities of fiber can cause gastrointestinal side effects, it is important to add fiber-rich foods slowly to the diet to help the body adjust and improve tolerance. It is also important to optimize the fluid intake when high-fiber diets are consumed.

Fat Replacers

In the effort to lower fat intake, the development of fat substitutes has generated great interest. Currently available fat replacers include carbohydrate-based gums, protein-based microparticulated proteins, and the sucrose polyester marketed as olestra (Olean). Olestra is made from two common ingredients: sucrose and vegetable oil. Its structure is analogous to a triglyceride molecule, with a sucrose core instead of glycerol and from six to eight fatty-acid side chains attached to the sucrose core. Because of the large size of the olestra molecule, it is not absorbed or digested and serves as a noncaloric fat replacer. The physical properties and heat stability of olestra are similar to those of conventional fats and oils.

In 1996, the Food and Drug Administration (FDA) approved the use of olestra to replace 100% of the vegetable oil used in the preparation of savory snacks. FDA approval of olestra is confined to its use in "savory snack foods," such as potato chips, tortilla chips, and crackers. These snacks must contain vitamins A, D, E, and K to compensate for the malabsorption of fat-soluble vitamins. In addition, the package must bear a label stating, "This product contains olestra. Olestra may cause abdominal cramping and loose stools. Olestra inhibits the absorption of some vitamins and other nutrients. Vitamins A, D, E, and K have been added." The FDA also requires studies that monitor consumption and long-term effects of olestra. So far, virtually all the data are from studies carried out by the manufacturer of olestra, Procter and Gamble (85). The FDA has passed on to the public the responsibility of testing its long-term safety by asking people to report complaints about the product. In its position on fat replacers, the American Dietetic Association (86) stated that "individuals who choose such foods should do so within the content of a diet consistent with the dietary guidelines for Americans."

Summary

The practical approach to dietary treatment is to apply cholesterol-lowering recommendations to individual food patterns of patients. This means translating the nutritional principles described above into food choices relevant to the individual so that drastic changes do not have to be made to follow a heart-healthy eating plan. Several minor changes in the right direction can have a significant cumulative effect on the attainment of the treatment goals. Physicians will be more effective in helping people make healthy food choices by using positive messages such as "choose more of," "for a change you should try," or "experiment with" instead of issuing a series of "don'ts." The diet that is described as percentages of energy derived from fats, carbohydrates, and proteins to maintain the concept of balance is meaningless to an individual who buys food and not nutrients in a supermarket. Moreover, the concept of a balance of nutrients may not be achieved in restaurants, where meals may have a higher fat content than foods prepared at home. Here, again, the individual should be taught to monitor his daily fat and cholesterol intake so that the higher fat meals can be balanced with meals that are lower in fat, particularly saturated fat and cholesterol.

Encouraging the patient to involve family and friends in healthy eating could remove some of the roadblocks to adherence. Traditionally, women have had the primary responsibility for food purchasing and preparation; educational efforts for healthy eating target the women in the typical U.S. household. This focusing was recently confirmed as reflecting current realities (87).

The physician plays an important role either as a primary counselor or as a supporter of the patient's efforts to make changes in his or her eating styles. If the physician emphasizes the importance of the low-saturated-fat, low-cholesterol diet as the primary strategy in treating hypercholesterolemia, the patient will believe that diet modification is an essential and necessary therapeutic measure. The majority of individuals would much rather modify their diet than take medication. It is the role of the physician and his or her staff and the registered dietitian to assist the patient in reaching this goal.

REFERENCES

1. **Ornish D, Brown SE, Scherwitz LW, et al.** Can lifestyle changes reverse coronary heart disease? The Lifestyle Heart Trial. Lancet. 1990;336:129–33.

2. **Watts GF, Lewis B, Brunt JN, et al.** Effects on coronary artery disease of lipid-lowering diet, or diet plus cholestyramine, in the St. Thomas Atherosclerosis Regression Study (STARS). Lancet. 1992;339:1241–2.

3. Diet and Health: Implications for Reducing Chronic Disease Risk. Washington, DC: National Academy Press; 1989.

4. **Keys A, Anderson JT, Grande F.** Serum cholesterol response to changes in the diet, part IV: particular saturated fatty acids in the diet. Metabolism. 1965;14:776–87.

5. **Hegsted DM, McGandy RB, Myers ML, Stare FJ.** Quantitative effects of dietary fat on serum cholesterol in man. Am J Clin Nutr. 1965;17:281–95.

6. **Mensink RP, Katan MB.** Effect of dietary *trans*-fatty acids on high-density and low-density lipoprotein cholesterol levels in healthy subjects. N Engl J Med. 1990;323:439–45.

7. **Mensink RP, Katan MB.** Effect of dietary fatty acids on serum lipids and lipoproteins. Arterioscler Thromb Vasc Biol. 1992;12:911–9.

8. **Yu S, Derr J, Etherton TD, Kris-Etherton PM.** Plasma cholesterol-predictive equations demonstrate that stearic acid is neutral and monounsaturated fatty acids are hypocholesterolemic. Am J Clin Nutr. 1995;61:1129–39.

9. **Ginsberg HN, Kris-Etherton P, Dennis B, et al.** Effects of reducing dietary saturated fatty acids on plasma lipids and lipoproteins in healthy subjects: the Delta Study, Protocol 1. Arterioscler Thromb Vasc Biol. 1998; 18:441–49.

10. **Woollett LA, Spady DK, Dietschy JM.** Saturated and unsaturated fatty acids independently regulate low-density lipoprotein receptor activity and production rate. J Lipid Res. 1992;33:77–88.

11. **Woollett LA, Spady DK, Dietschy JM.** Regulatory effects of the saturated fatty acids 6:0 through 18:0 on hepatic low density lipoprotein receptor activity in the hamster. J Clin Invest. 1992;89:1133–41.

12. **Turner JD, Le NA, Brown WV.** Effect of changing dietary fat saturation on low density lipoprotein metabolism in man. Am J Physiol. 1981;241:E57–63.

13. **Shepherd J, Packard CJ, Grundy SM, et al.** Effects of saturated and polyunsaturated fat diets on the chemical composition and metabolism of low-density lipoproteins in man. J Lipid Res. 1980;21:91–8.

14. **Cortese C, Levy Y, Janus ED, et al.** Modes of action of lipid-lowering diets in man: studies of apolipoprotein B kinetics in relation to fat consumption and dietary fatty acid composition. Eur J Clin Invest. 1983;13:79–85.

15. **Welty TK, Lee ET, Yeh J, et al.** Cardiovascular disease risk factors among American Indians: the Strong Heart Study. Am J Epidemiol. 1995;142:269–87.

16. **Bonanome A, Grundy SM.** Effect of dietary stearic acid on plasma cholesterol and lipoprotein levels. N Engl J Med. 1988;318:1244–8.

17. **Hayes KC.** Dietary fatty acid thresholds and cholesterolemia. FASEB J. 1992;6:2600–7.

18. **Ginsberg HN, Barr SL, Karmally W, et al.** Reduction of plasma cholesterol levels in normal men on an American Heart Association Step 1 diet or a Step 1 diet with added monounsaturated fat. New Engl J Med. 1990;322:574–79.

19. **Mattson FH, Hollenbach EJ, Kligman AM.** Effect of hydrogenated fat on the plasma cholesterol and triglyceride levels of man. Am J Clin Nutr 1975;28:726–731.

20. **Nestel P, Noakes M, Belling B, et al.** Plasma lipoprotein lipid and Lp(a) changes with substitution of elaidic acid for oleic acid in the diet. J Lipid Res. 1992;33:1029–36.

21. **Judd JT, Clevidence BA, Muesing RA, et al.** Dietary *trans*-fatty acids: effects on plasma lipids and lipoproteins of healthy men and women. Am J Clin Nutr. 1994;59: 861-868.

22. **Lichtenstein AH, Ausman LM, Carrasco W, et al.** Hydrogenation impairs the hypolipidemic effect of corn oil in humans: hydrogenation, *trans*-fatty acids, and plasma lipids. Arterioscler Thromb Vasc Biol. 1993;13:154–61.

23. **NIH Consensus Conference.** Triglyceride, high-density lipoprotein, and coronary heart disease. JAMA. 1995;269:505–10.

24. **ASCN/AIN Task Force on *Trans*-Fatty Acids.** Position paper on *trans*-fatty acids. Am J Clin Nutr 1996;63:663–70.

25. **Gillman MW, Cuppica LA, Yagnon D, et al.** Margarine intake and subsequent coronary heart disease in men. Epidemiology. 1997;8:144–9.

26. **Hu FB, Stampfer MJ, Manson JE, et al.** Dietary fat intake and the risk of coronary heart disease in women. N Engl J Med. 1997;337:1491.

27. **Byers T.** Hardened fats, hardened arteries. N Engl J Med. 1997;337:1544–5.

28a. **Lichtenstein AH.** *Trans*-fatty acids, plasma lipid levels, and risk of developing cardiovascular disease: a statement for health care professionals from the Amercian Heart Association. Circulation. 1997;95:2588–90.

28b. **Mattson FH, Grundy SM.** Comparison of effects of dietary saturated, monounsaturated, and polyunsaturated fatty acids on plasma lipids and lipoproteins in man. J Lipid Res. 1985;26:194–202.

29. **Ginsberg HN, Karmally W, Barr SL, et al.** Effects of increasing dietary polyunsaturated fatty acids within the guidelines of the AHA Step 1 diet on plasma lipid and lipoprotein levels in normal males. Arterioscler Thromb Vasc Biol. 1994;14:892–901.

30. **Blum CB, Levy R, Eisenberg S, et al.** High-density lipoprotein metabolism in man. J Clin Invest. 1997;60:795–807.

31. **Brinton EA, Eisenberg S, Breslow JL.** A low-fat diet decreases high density lipoprotein (HDL) cholesterol levels by decreasing HDL apolipoprotein transport rates. J Clin Invest. 1990;85:144–51.

32. **Shepherd J, Packard CJ, Patsch JR, et al.** Effects of dietary polyunsaturated and saturated fat on the properties of high-density lipoproteins and the metabolism of apolipoprotein A-I. J Clin Invest. 1978;62:1582–92.

33. **Harris WS, Connor WE, Illingworth DR, et al.** Effects of fish oil on VLDL triglyceride kinetics in humans. J Lipid Res. 1990;31:1549–58.

34. **Lefevre M, Ginsberg HN, Kris-Etherton P, et al.** ApoE genotype does not predict lipid response to changes in dietary saturated fatty acids in a heterogeneous normolipidemic population. Arterioscler Thromb Vasc Biol. 1997;17:2914–23.

35. **Berglund L.** Diet and drug therapy for lipoprotein(a). Curr Opin Lipidol. 1995;6:48–56.

36. **Ignatowski AI.** Influence of animal food on the organism of rabbits. Izv Imp Voyenno-Med Akad Peter. 1908;16:154–76.

37. **Anitschkow N, Chalatow S.** Ueber experimentelle cholesterinsteatose und ihre bedeutung fur die entstehung einiger pathologischer prozesse. Zentralbl Allg Pathol Anat. 1913;24:1–9.

38a. **Stamler J, Shekelle R.** Dietary cholesterol and human coronary heart disease. Arch Pathol Lab Med. 1988;112:1032–40.

38b. **Hegsted DM.** Serum cholesterol response to dietary cholesterol: a re-evaluation. Am J Clin Nutr. 1986;44:299–305.

39. **Ginsberg HN, Karmally W, Siddiqui M, et al.** A dose-response study of the effects of dietary cholesterol on fasting and postprandial lipid and lipoprotein metabolism in healthy young men. Arterioscler Thromb Vasc Biol. 1994;14:576–86.

40. **Ginsberg HN, Karmally W, Siddiqui M, et al.** Increases in dietary cholesterol are associated with modest increases in both low-density and high-density lipoprotein cholesterol in healthy young women. Arterioscler Thromb Vasc Biol. 1995;15:169–78.

41. **Ginsberg H, Le N, Mays C, et al.** Lipoprotein metabolism in non-responders to increased dietary cholesterol. Arteriosclerosis. 1981;1:463–70.

42. **Packard CJ, McKinney L, Carr K, Shepherd J.** Cholesterol feeding increases low-density lipoprotein synthesis. J Clin Invest. 1983;72:45–51.

43. **Garg A, Bantle JP, Henry RR, et al.** Effects of varying carbohydrate content of diet in patients with non–insulin-dependent diabetes mellitus. JAMA. 1994;271:1421–8.

44. **Kasim-Karakas SE, Lane E, Almario R, et al.** Effects of dietary fat restriction on particle size of plasma lipoproteins in postmenopausal women. Metabolism. 1997;46:431–6.

45. **Ripsin CM, Keenan JM, Jacobs DR Jr, et al.** Oat products and lipid lowering: a meta-analysis. JAMA. 1992;267:3317–25.

46. **Anderson JW, Johnstone BM, Cook-Newell ME.** Meta-analysis of the effects of soy protein intake on serum lipids. New Engl J Med. 1995;333:276–82.

47. **Loscalzo J.** Nitric oxide and vascular disease. N Engl J Med. 1995;333:251–3.

48. **Manson JE, Colditz GA, Stampfer MJ.** A prospective study of obesity and risk of coronary heart disease in women. N Engl J Med. 1990;322:882–9.

49. **Donahue RP, Abbott RD, Bloom E.** Central obesity and coronary heart disease in men. Lancet. 1987;1:821–4.

50. **Dattilo AM, Kris-Etherton PM.** Effects of weight reduction on blood lipids and lipoproteins: a meta-analysis. Am J Clin Nutr. 1992;56:320–8.

51. **Manson JE, Willitt WC, Stampfer MJ, et al.** Body weight and mortality among women. N Engl J Med. 1995;333:677–85.

52. **Kannel WB.** Alcohol and cardiovascular disease. ProcNutr Soc. 1998;47:99–110.

53. **Beilin LJ, Puddey IB.** Alcohol, hypertension, and cardiovascular disease: implications for management [Review]. Clin Exper Hypertens. 1993;15:1157–70.

54. **Ginsberg H, Olefsky J, Farquhar J, Reaven G.** Moderate ethanol ingestion and plasma triglyceride levels. Ann Intern Med. 1974;80:143–9.

55. Chromium status and serum lipids. Nutr Rev. 1993;41:307–10.

56a. **Roeback JR, Hia KM, Chambless LE, Fletcher RH.** Effects of chromium supplementation on serum high-density lipoprotein cholesterol levels in men taking beta-blockers: a randomized controlled trial. Ann Intern Med. 1991;115:917–24.

56b. **Lee NA, Reasner CA.** Beneficial effect of chromium supplementation on serum triglyceride levels in NIDDM. Diabetes Care. 1994;17:1449–52.

57. **Malmros H.** Diet, lipids, and atherosclerosis. Acta Med Scan. 1980;207:207–14.

58. **Kato H, Tillotson J, Nichaman MZ.** Epidemiologic studies of coronary heart disease and stroke in Japanese men living in Japan, Hawaii and California. Am J Epidemiol. 1973;97:373–85.

59. **Keys A, Menotti A, Karvonen MJ, et al.** The diet and 15-year death rate in the Seven Countries Study. Am J Epidemiol. 1986;124:903–15.

60. **U.S. Department of Health and Human Services.** The Surgeon General's Report on Nutrition and Health. Washington, DC: USDHHS; 1988.

61. **Dayton S, Pearce ML, Goldman H, et al.** Controlled trial of a diet high in unsaturated fat for prevention of atherosclerotic complications. Lancet. 1986;2:1060–2.

62. **Hjermann I, Holme I, Leren P.** Oslo study diet and antismoking trial: results after 102 months. Am J Med. 1986;80:7–11.

63. **Miller GJ.** Lipoproteins and thrombosis: effects of lipid lowering. Curr Opin Lipidol. 1995;6:38–42.

64. **Jha P, Flather M, Lonn E, et al.** The antioxidant vitamins and cardiovascular disease: a critical review of epidemiologic and clinical trial data. Ann Intern Med. 1995;123: 860–72.

65. **Gey KF, Brubacher GB, Stahelin HB.** Plasma levels of antioxidant vitamins in relation to ischemic heart disease and cancer. Am J Clin Nutr. 1987;45:1368–77.

66. **Enstrom JE, Karim LE, Klein MA.** Vitamin C intake and mortality among a sample of the United States population. Epidemiology. 1992;3:194–202.

67. **Stampfer MJ, Hennekens CH, Manson JE, et al.** Vitamin E consumption and the risk of coronary heart disease in women. N Engl J Med. 1993;328:1450–6.

68. **Rimm EB, Stampfer MJ, Ascherio A, et al.** Vitamin E consumption and the risk of coronary heart disease in men. N Engl J Med. 1993;328:1450–6.

69. **Miwa K, Miyagi Y, Igawa A, et al.** Vitamin E deficiency in variant angina. Circulation. 1996;94:14–8.

70. **Kushi LH, Folsom AR, Prineas RJ, et al.** Dietary antioxidant vitamins and death from coronary heart disease in postmenopausal women. N Engl J Med. 1996;334:1156–62.

71. **National Cholesterol Education Program Adult Treatment Panel II.** Summary of the Second Report of the NCEP Expert Panel on Detection, Evaluation, and Treatment of High Blood Cholesterol in Adults. JAMA. 1993;269:3015–23.

72. **Stephens NG, Parsons A, Schofield PM, et al.** Randomized controlled trial of vitamin E in patients with coronary disease: Cambridge Heart Antioxidant Study (CHAOS). Lancet. 1996;347:781–6.

73. **Jialal I, Norkus E, Cristol I, Grundy SM.** Beta-carotene inhibits the oxidative modifications of low-density lipoprotein. Biochem Biophys Acta. 1991;1086:134–8.

74. **Hennekens CH, Buning JE, Manson JE.** Lack of effect of long-term supplementation with beta carotene on the incidence of malignant neoplasms and cardiovascular disease. N Engl J Med. 1996;334:1145–9.

75. **Omenn GS, Goodman GE, Thornquist MD, et al.** Effects of a combination of beta-carotene and vitamin A on lung cancer and cardiovascular disease. N Engl J Med. 1996;334:1150–5.

76. **van Poppel G, Kardinaal A, Princen H, Kok FJ.** Antioxidants and coronary heart disease. Ann Med. 1994;26:429–34.

77. **Stampfer MJ, Malinow MR, Willett WC.** A prospective study of plasma homocyst(e)ine and risk of myocardial infarction in U.S. physicians. JAMA. 1992;268:877–81.

78. **Rimin EB, Willett WC, Hu FB.** Folate and vitamin B6 from diet and supplement in relation to risk of coronary heart disease among women. JAMA. 1998;279:359–64.

79. **Salonen JT, Nyyssonen K, Korpela H, et al.** High stored iron levels are associated with excess risk of myocardial infarction in eastern Finnish men. Circulation. 1992;86:1036–7.

80. **Stampfer MJ, et al.** A prospective study of plasma ferritin and risk of myocardial infarction in U.S. physicians. Circulation. 1993;87:688.

81. **Jonsson JJ, Johannesson GM, Sigfusson N, et al.** Prevalence of iron deficiency and iron overload in the adult Icelandic population. J Clin Epidemiol. 1991;44:1289–97.

82. **Salonen JT, Alfthan G, Huttunen JK.** Association between cardiovascular death and myocardial infarction and serum selenium in a matched-pair longitudinal study. Lancet. 1982;2:175–9.

83. **Salonen JT.** Selenium in ischaemic heart disease. Int J Epidemiol. 1987;16:323–8.

84. **Riemersma RA, Oliver M, Elton RA, et al.** Plasma antioxidants and coronary heart disease: vitamins C, E, and selenium. Eur J Clin Nutr. 1990;44:143–50.

85. **Blackburn H.** Olestra and the FDA. N Engl J Med. 1996;3341:984–6.

86. **American Dietetic Association.** Position paper on fat replacers. J Am Diet Assoc. 1998;98:463–8.

87. **Harnack L, Story M, Martinson B, et al.** Guess who's cooking? The role of men in meal planning, shopping, and preparation in U.S. families. J Am Diet Assoc. 1998;98:995–1000.

CHAPTER 6

Hypertension

ELLEN COHEN, MD
DEBORAH M. SWIDERSKI, MD
MARY E. WHEAT, MD
PAMELA CHARNEY, MD

Hypertension as a risk factor for coronary artery disease (CAD) and its treatment have been studied extensively in recent decades. Increasingly, an examination of the role of gender has been incorporated into this research.

The current definition of hypertension emphasizes that cardiovascular risk increases with an increasing level of blood pressure. In the United States the threshold for defining hypertension has gradually been lowered during the past 30 years. In the Framingham study, hypertension was defined as greater than 160/95, with a borderline category encompassing those with blood pressures between 140/90 and 160/95. Since 1984, however, the Joint National Committee (JNC) on Detection, Evaluation, and Treatment of High Blood Pressure has defined hypertension as beginning at 140/90. In the sixth JNC report (JNC VI; published in 1997), normal blood pressure was defined as <135 systolic and <85 diastolic, whereas optimal blood pressure was defined as <120 systolic and <80 diastolic (1).

This chapter examines the relationship between hypertension and CAD in women, starting with a review of the epidemiology of hypertension with attention to gender, race, and age. Evidence of the importance of hypertension as a cardiovascular risk factor is considered next. Finally, the pharmacologic management and nonpharmacologic management of hypertension are discussed.

Epidemiology: A Gender Perspective

When examining gender and hypertension as cardiovascular risk factors, it is critical to be aware of differences between studies both in terms of blood pressure assessment techniques (e.g., number of measurements) and variations in the definition of hypertension. In addition, most older clinical studies of hypertension focused on diastolic and combined systolic/diastolic hypertension, whereas in the last 15 to 20 years more attention has been paid to isolated systolic hypertension as a cardiovascular risk factor, especially in patients over 60 years of age.

National surveys based on probability samples of the entire population have examined the epidemiology of hypertension in the United States according to gender and race, particularly amongst blacks and whites. Some information is available on hypertension in Latinos, but no population-based data have been reported for Asian-Americans. The National Health and Nutrition Examination Survey II (NHANES II) reported the prevalence of several different categories of hypertension in persons aged 18 to 74 years (Table 6-1) (2). When one looks at all hypertensive persons (defined by SBP > 160 or DBP > 95 or as taking antihypertensive medications), blacks, both women and men, clearly have much higher prevalence rates than whites in all age groups. Among blacks and whites, hypertensive women have a much greater likelihood than men of having their blood pressure effectively controlled at the time of screening. This observation is supported by data from other studies, such as the large, population-based, multicenter Hypertension Detection and Follow-up Program (HDFP) (3). These studies also indicate that women are more likely than men to know that they have high blood pressure and to be taking antihypertensive medications at the time of screening. It is interesting that most studies show a higher prevalence of labile, or "white coat," hypertension in women than in men (4).

Table 6-1 Race-Sex and Hypertension Prevalence in NHANES II

Race and Sex	% Hypertensive with Uncontrolled Blood Pressure (±SE)	% Hypertensive with Controlled Blood Pressure (±SE)
Black women	39.8 (±1.96)	38.3 (±4.35)
Black men	28.3 (±1.86)	16.1 (±3.72)
White women	20.0 (±0.66)	40.3 (±2.99)
White men	21.2 (±1.04)	20.9 (±2.01)

Data from National Center for Health Statistics, Rowland M, Roberts J. Blood pressure levels and hypertension in persons ages 6-74 years: United States, 1976-1980. In: Advance Data from Vital and Health Statistics of the National Center for Health Statistics of the National Center for Health Sciences. No. 84. 84th ed. Rockville, Maryland: Public Health Service; 1982:1-12.

The only survey that has examined the prevalence of hypertension in different Latino subgroups in this country is the Hispanic Health and Nutrition Examination Survey (HHANES) (5). The population prevalence found in HHANES is lower than that noted previously in blacks or whites and lower than most other surveys including either Mexican-Americans or Puerto Ricans. Several methodologic problems have been identified that may make this an unreliable estimate of hypertension in Latin women (6a). Nonetheless, among older age groups, the prevalence of hypertension in Mexican-American women and men equalled that in whites, but the prevalence in Cuban-Americans and Puerto Ricans continued to be lower. As in whites, the prevalence of hypertension in Mexican-American and Cuban-American women exceeded that in men after age 65. In older subjects, there were lower levels of controlled hypertension among Mexican-Americans than among white and black populations. However, as in black and white populations, women were more likely to have controlled hypertension than men (6b).

Another way to look at gender differences in hypertension is to examine incidence rates. Data for black and white women and men are provided by the NHANES I Epidemiologic Follow-up Study (NHEFS), which looked at the development of newly detected hypertension a mean of 9.5 years after initial screening for NHANES I (7). In NHEFS women and men, hypertension developed at similar rates in all age groups, with steadily increasing incidence rates at each 10-year age interval. At all ages, black women and men consistently had incidence rates at least twice those of their white counterparts. As the population ages, women and men develop hypertension at similarly increasing rates, yet men die at younger ages than women. Thus, by age 65, hypertensive women actually outnumber hypertensive men in the overall population (Fig. 6-1).

Hypertension as a Cardiovascular Disease Risk Factor

The major potential sequelae of hypertension include myocardial infarction (MI), congestive heart failure, stroke, and renal insufficiency. Treatment of hypertension is justified by documenting a reduction of such end points when blood pressure is reduced, ultimately translating into a reduction of overall mortality. Because cardiovascular disease is the major cause of morbidity and mortality in U.S. women and men over 60 years old, the most clinically relevant way to look at the relative risk of hypertension in women and men is in terms of its contribution to cardiovascular events. Men (whether hypertensive or not) have a higher incidence of cardiovascular end points than do women at all ages, as demonstrated by follow-up data from the Framingham study (8).

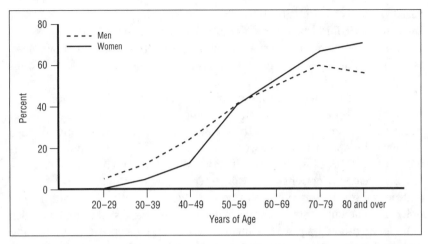

Figure 6-1 Prevalence of hypertension among persons 20 years of age and over by sex and age—United States, 1988-91. A *person with hypertension* is defined as either having elevated blood pressure (systolic pressure of at least 140 mm Hg or diastolic pressure of at least 90 mm Hg) or taking antihypertensive medicine. Percents are based on an average of six measurements of blood pressure. (Reprinted from Centers for Disease Control and Prevention, National Center for Health Statistics, National Health and Nutrition Examination Survey III (Phase I). Health—United States, 1995. Hyattsville, Maryland: Public Health Service; 1996:34.)

Overall, cardiovascular disease is the leading cause of death in both women and men. As W.B. Kannel states, "Coronary disease is the most common and most lethal sequela of hypertension, equaling in incidence all the other cardiovascular outcomes combined" (9). Examining the association of hypertension and coronary disease end points in women reveals an association at least as strong as that observed in men.

Looking at more specific data, a 30-year follow-up of the original Framingham cohort demonstrated that SBP (which closely paralleled DBP) correlated very strongly with risk of CAD events, especially for women aged 35 to 64 years and men over age 65 years at enrollment (10). The Walnut Creek Contraceptive Drug Study, an observational study of more than 10,000 premenopausal or early postmenopausal women, found that high blood pressure (>140 mm Hg SBP or >90 mm Hg DBP) was second only to diabetes mellitus as an independent predictor of cardiovascular mortality (11). Data on risk factors for CAD in blacks compared with whites have been elucidated by longitudinal cohort studies such as the Charleston Heart Study, which published 30-year follow-up data showing that SBP was the most consistent predictor of CAD risk in black and white women and men (12). Hypertension carried the greatest population-attributable risk for development of congestive heart failure (CHF) in multivariate analysis of results from the Framingham study, accounting for 59% of the cases of CHF in women and 39% of the cases in men (13). These observational data confirm that hypertension is common in women, that many women are treated for hypertension, and that such treatment, if effective in reducing adverse outcomes, may have major public health implications.

Another way to look at cardiovascular risk associated with hypertension is to consider its presence and course in women with established heart disease. Studies of gender differences in the incidence and survival rates after MI have provided the opportunity to assess the presence of hypertension in women with known CAD. Most, but not all, studies have shown an increased prevalence of treated hypertension in women compared with men at presentation with initial MI. It is important to note that women with an initial MI were older than men in all studies that provided data on age distribution by gender (14). As mentioned above, the incidence of hypertension increases steadily with age. However, in age-adjusted studies (15a), hypertension still occurs significantly more frequently in women. Higher pre-MI blood pressure may predict an increased risk of death with MI for both women and men (15b). Mortality from MI varies by gender even when adjusted for age and premorbid risk factors. Several studies demonstrate increased early mortality in women compared with men (15c), but women's survival at 1 year is at least as favorable as men's (see Chapter 16). What contribution, if any, hypertension and its treatment makes to these differences in mortality is unknown.

Preventing damage to target organs is an important goal of reducing elevated blood pressure. As discussed above, men have a higher incidence rate of total cardiovascular end points than women at all ages. However, when one considers a specific outcome such as stroke, which is most associated with hypertension as a risk factor, hypertensive women and men both have an increased risk ratio for stroke over time (2.6 for women versus 3.8 for men at 36 years' follow-up in the Framingham study) (9). Similarly, for coronary disease, which is more common than stroke, hypertensive women and men have almost identical risk ratios (2.2 for women versus 2.0 for men at 36 years' follow-up in the Framingham study) (9).

The significance of left ventricular hypertrophy (LVH) as a sequela of hypertension has also been elucidated by the Framingham study. Echocardiographically proven LVH was independently associated with increased risk of all measured end points (16). For all cardiovascular disease end points, women and men with LVH had a similarly increased relative risk (women, 1.49; men, 1.57). For cardiovascular death and death from all causes, women with LVH had a greater increase in relative risk than men (women: 2.12 and 2.01; men: 1.73 and 1.49).

Because evidence of LVH confers increased CAD risk, it is important to recognize what forms of elevated blood pressure are associated with the presence of LVH. Several studies have demonstrated that both isolated systolic and combined diastolic/systolic hypertension are associated with increased risk of LVH (17). Gender-specific analysis of echocardiographic data from the Framingham study demonstrated that women with isolated systolic hypertension had more than twice the odds of having LVH as did their male counterparts (odds ratio: 5.94 in women [95% CI, 3.06 to 11.53]; 2.58 in men [95% CI, 0.97 to 6.86]). It was also noted that women had both increased LV mass and increased wall thickness, whereas men had increased LV mass and LV dilatation without a significant change in wall thickness (18a). In several studies completed on participants in the Hypertension Optimal Treatment (HOT) Study, the relationship between hypertension and LVH was further explored (18b-d). Concentric hypertrophy was more common in women than men (53% versus 40%, $p < 0.05$). Women with uncontrolled hypertension at time of enrollment had greater LV mass than women who had controlled hypertension, whereas LV mass was similar in men regardless of blood pressure control (18b). Women at least aged 65, compared with women after age 50, were more likely to have smaller LV systolic dimensions and thicker LV walls, whereas in men there was no change with increasing age at enrollment (18c).

Although their significance is not clear, these observations may reflect gender differences in cardiac performance and adaptation to stress. In this regard, it is intriguing to note recent data from two studies that compared echocardiographic findings in a group of normotensive, true hypertensive, and "white-coat hypertensive" patients (based on a comparison of office and ambulatory blood pressure recordings). These studies found patients with "white-coat" hypertension to have LV wall mass and LV diastolic function between those for normotensive and true hypertensive patients (18e,19).

To date, there are no adequate data documenting the effect of antihypertensive therapy on the course of LVH in women (20,21). It is interesting that in the Framingham data ECG evidence of LVH was associated with a threefold increase in the risk of a CAD event during more than 30 years of follow-up in both women and men. The regression of ECG voltage changes on serial follow-up was associated with lower cardiovascular risk for both women and men when compared with those who had no serial change (22). However, better data are clearly still needed to address the issue of whether antihypertensive therapy leads to LVH regression in women and whether LVH regression in fact leads to lower CAD risk in both women and men.

Overall, it appears that women and men suffer similar cardiovascular consequences of hypertension, at fairly comparable rates. As with men, hypertensive women should be monitored for the development of cardiovascular symptoms as well as for cerebrovascular disease and renal insufficiency. Whether hypertensive women or men should routinely be evaluated echocardiographically for the presence of LVH remains controversial.

Management of Hypertension

Evaluation for Secondary Causes

Of the multiple secondary causes of elevated blood pressure that occur in women (Box 6-1), the most common, which may be overlooked by clinicians, are noncompliance with medications, increased weight or alcohol use (see section on Nonpharmacological Therapy), and oral contraceptives (OCP).

Oral contraceptives are cited as the most frequent reversible cause of secondary hypertension. Cohort studies of women taking higher-dose OCP have reported an average 5 to 7 mm Hg increase in SBP, with a smaller 1 to 2 mm Hg rise in DBP. The most recent, and largest, data set in this area comes from the Nurses Health Study and involves only self-reported blood pressure (23). This study of more than 68,000 nurses free of hypertension, diabetes mellitus, CAD, and cerebrovascular accident at baseline showed an age-adjusted relative risk of developing hypertension of 1.5 to 1.8 for current OCP users, without a significant effect of age or ethnicity. However, this amounted to only 41.5 cases per 10,000 person-years of observation. Some data suggest that these changes differ among races (24-26). Increases in blood pressure seem to be attributable to both estrogenic and progestogenic content. Few data are available on the risks of hypertension associated with progesterone-only methods (e.g., Norplant, minipill). Women using OCP need periodic monitoring of their blood pressure. If overt hypertension occurs, the medication should be stopped; in most cases blood pressure normalizes within 3 months. For women whose blood pressure increases in the high-normal range and who have high cardiovascular risk profiles, other contraceptive options should be explored, and the risks of an unwanted pregnancy weighed against the risks of an increase in blood pressure.

Regarding estrogen replacement therapy in postmenopausal women, the relative doses of estrogen and progesterone are substantially lower. It is only recently that the relationship between hormonal status, the renin-angiotensin system, and blood pressure has been studied. In a population-based sample in Germany (27), women using estrogen replacement therapy were

---

Box 6-1 Evaluation for Secondary Causes of Hypertension

Noncompliance with treatment regimen	Oral contraceptives
Increased weight	Renovascular disease
High salt use in salt-sensitive individuals	Pheochromocytoma
Alcohol or cocaine abuse	

less likely to report the use of antihypertensive medication and had lower renin and higher angiotensin levels than other women, regardless of their blood pressure. Other studies have demonstrated that oral estrogen, with or without progesterone, does not affect blood pressure (28).

Renovascular disease, the cause of elevated blood pressure in about 0.5% of all hypertensives, is important to diagnose because its treatment may enable the cessation of antihypertensive therapy. Atherosclerosis is responsible for about two thirds of all renovascular hypertension and occurs twice as frequently in younger men than women, with the gender distribution equalizing in the elderly. Fibromuscular dysplasia, on the other hand, is the most common cause of renovascular hypertension under age 40 and occurs predominantly in women (29,30). Findings suggestive of renovascular hypertension include abdominal bruits and lack of response to intensive pharmacotherapy.

Pheochromocytoma is an exceedingly rare cause of hypertension (0.1%) but should be considered in women because it may first appear during pregnancy and, if not identified, be associated with adverse outcomes. Orthostatic hypotension, sweating, pallor, and tachycardia should alert the clinician to the possibility of pheochromocytoma (31). Thyroid disease occurs ten times more frequently in women than men; however, its role as a cause of hypertension remains unclear (32).

Treating Hypertension To Prevent Cardiovascular Disease

Because it is clear from the above discussion that elevated blood pressure, both systolic and diastolic, confers increased risk of adverse coronary events in both women and men, it is of obvious importance to examine the data on prevention of CAD by blood pressure–lowering therapy. Many of the early hypertension treatment trials included primarily young and middle-aged patients, which meant there were few atherosclerotic events observed, particularly in the female subjects.

The first large hypertension treatment trial to include women was the Hypertension and Detection Follow-Up Program (HDFP), which was composed of more than 10,000 participants, 46% of whom were women, aged 30 to 51 at entry, with a DBP greater than 90 mm Hg (33). This study involved randomization of the experimental group to treatment in special centers, using a stepped-care regimen beginning with diuretics. The control group participants were only advised to obtain treatment for an elevated blood pressure from their usual source of care. Gender-specific data analysis was only performed post hoc. This study showed reductions in stroke rates with active treatment in all race-gender groups; however, for other cardiovascular events, black women were found to benefit from treatment, whereas the treatment benefit for white women was questionable (34). Although HDFP terminated at 5 years, a subsequent analysis of the cohort that had been followed for 8.3 years revealed reductions in all-cause mortality with stepped care, in all four race-gender groups, including white women (35). In addition, a subsequent meta-analysis of the impact of pharmacologic treatment in white women confirmed the benefit of treatment (36). Post hoc analysis of the 5-year incidence of coronary artery disease revealed a 15.2% decrease in patients treated with stepped care in special centers.

Because the incidence of CAD increases with age in both women and men, studies of older patients have had greater power to demonstrate reductions in atherosclerotic event rates with the treatment of hypertension. Recent trials have focused on the treatment of systolic and diastolic hypertension in older populations. The Swedish Trial in Old Patients with Hypertension (STOP) enrolled patients 70 to 84 years of age, 63% of whom were women (37,38), with either diastolic or combined hypertension. Patients were treated with metoprolol CR, atenolol, pindolol, or hydrochlorothiazide, with each treatment center choosing any of the four drugs to use versus placebo throughout the study. STOP was prematurely terminated at 25 months of follow-up because of the dramatic decrease in end points in the actively treated group. Specifically, the risk of stroke decreased by 42% and the risk of MI and sudden death decreased by 21%. Gender analysis revealed that "women seemed to benefit more from treatment then men, even though the differences for neither MI nor stroke were statistically significant" (38).

The Systolic Hypertension in the Elderly Program (SHEP) focused on the treatment of isolated systolic hypertension after age 59 (39). The study enrolled almost 5000 subjects, 57% of whom were women and 14% black, with SBP 160 to 219 mm Hg and DBP less than 90. Subjects were randomized to receive either low-dose chlorthalidone or placebo, with subsequent addition of atenolol or placebo if goal blood pressure was not achieved (SBP ≤ 180, or 20 mm Hg decline for baseline SBP of 160 to 179). By the end of the trial, almost half of the subjects had their blood pressure controlled with chlorthalidone alone. SHEP showed that participants who received active treatment had substantial relative risk reduction in stroke (37%) and MI (33%) in this largely female, elderly population. In addition, the SHEP trial has published results demonstrating a 49% reduction in the risk of congestive heart failure in the actively treated group (40).

The Skaraborg HTN Project was an observational cohort study designed to assess the impact of blood pressure reduction with beta-blockers and thiazides on the incidence of MI (41a). The study population of 2574 individuals 40 to 69 years of age, 56% of whom were women, was followed for 7.4 years. Blood pressure control improved with treatment (women: –5 mm Hg SBP and –2 mm Hg DBP). Although the risk of MI at 7.4 years follow-up was not significantly related to DBP or SBP in women, LVH was the strongest predictor of MI for both women and men (relative risk = 2.87 in women and 2.48 in men with LVH).

A recent meta-analysis of gender differences in outcome after pharmacologic treatment for hypertension has been completed, including data from most of the major randomized controlled hypertensive treatment trials (36). Gender differences in cardiovascular risk factors were significant for higher SBP in women (170.9 ± 20.9 mm Hg compared with 162.6 ± 19.9 mm Hg in men) as well as higher total cholesterol and less tobacco use. Women and men treated with thiazides or beta-blockers as first-line agents had comparable absolute risk reductions for all major categories of cardiovascular events given equivalent untreated cardiovascular risk. Although women did not have a statistically significant reduction in all-cause or cardiovascular mortality, or in major coronary events, this may be because of the fact that the underlying rate of these events was lower in women than in men (i.e., the analyses of data in women had less statistical power). This observation is not surprising given that by far the largest number of subjects in this meta-analysis were from HDFP and the Medical Research Council trial of treatment of mild hypertension, with a mean age of 51 and 52 years respectively, and concomitantly low CAD event rates in women subjects. Table 6-2 provides the number needed to treat (NNT) to prevent one coronary artery and one cardiovascular event in women and men from trials (HDFP, STOP, SHEP) discussed earlier.

The goal for treatment of hypertension has been to achieve SBP < 140 and DBP < 90 mm Hg (1). Because of concern about a possible J-point phenomenon (that lower blood pressures might be dangerous), the Hypertension Optimal Treatment (HOT) randomized clinical trial was developed to define the most advantageous blood pressure goal (41b). The impact on cardiovascular

Table 6-2 Number Needed To Treat To Prevent Coronary Artery Disease Event and All Cardiovascular Events in Women and Men from Three Trials

Treatment Studies	NNT* To Prevent CAD Event		NNT* To Prevent Any Cardiovascular Event†	
	Women	Men	Women	Men
HDFP‡	143	59	55	42
STOP§	83	77	21	27
SHEP‖	50	111	223	31

*NNT = Number needed to treat for prevention of an event over 25 months (STOP) or 5 years (HDFP and SHEP).
†All myocardial infarction and stroke and sudden death.
‡HDFP = Hypertension Detection and Follow-up Program.
§STOP = Swedish Trial in Older Patients with Hypertension.
‖SHEP = Systolic Hypertension in the Elderly Program.

outcomes of achieving diastolic targets of <90, <85, or <80 mm Hg was explored in this multicenter trial of 18,790 subjects aged 50 to 80 years old who had an initial DBP of 100 to 115 mm Hg. Initial therapy was felodipine, a calcium channel blocker, followed by either a beta-blocker or angiotensin-converting enzyme (ACE) inhibitor, or then a diuretic. Additionally, half the participants were randomized to receive 75 mg aspirin daily. Women were 47% of trial participants, but gender-specific data analysis is not yet available. Because of a low cardiovascular event rate, follow-up was increased from 2.5 years to 3.8 years. Most participants had a substantial decrease in both DBP and SBP. Overall, cardiovascular event differences between groups were small, with the exception of subjects with diabetes at baseline. For those diabetics, the rate of major cardiovascular events (all MIs and strokes and other cardiovascular deaths) was 50% lower with a DBP ≤ 80 mm Hg compared to those with a DBP ≤ 90 mm Hg [p < 0.005]). Otherwise, the impact of the achievement of a specific DBP on cardiovascular events was less dramatic. The lowest risk of major cardiovascular events was noted at a DBP of 82.6 and a SBP of 138.5 mm Hg. Once DBP was less than 90 mm Hg, the additional benefit was slight although complications were not more frequent. In comparison, aspirin decreased major cardiovascular events by 15% (p = 0.03) without an increase in number of strokes. All MIs (including silent only found on EKG) were 36% less common in those randomized to aspirin (p = 0.002).

In summary, hypertension is more common overall in women than men. Because both systolic hypertension and CAD are more common with increasing age, it is to be expected that hypertension might be particularly important in the prevention of CAD in older women. And, in fact, the importance of treatment of systolic hypertension to prevent CAD is perhaps greater for women than men (34,36,42). Hypertensive patients benefit from the addition of low-dose aspirin to their treatment regimen.

Pharmacologic Therapy

The goal of antihypertensive therapy is the reduction of cardiovascular morbidity and mortality, with a concomitant decrease in total morbidity and mortality (Table 6-3). Many trials (including HDFP, STOP, and SHEP) employed thiazide diuretics and beta-blockers as their first-line antihypertensive agents. As noted above, although women have a much lower rate of cardiovascular end points in all studies in which they are included, women receiving active treatment obtain comparable risk reductions to men for all major categories of end points, after adjusting for baseline cardiovascular risk. Based on these findings, the JNC VI advised generally beginning treatment with thiazides and beta-blockers in all patients without contraindications to their use (1).

Table 6-3 Individualizing Antihypertensive Therapy

Drug Class	Comorbid Conditions	Contraindications or Special Monitoring Required
Initial Therapy		
Thiazide diuretics	Osteoporosis	Pre-eclampsia, IHSS[t]
	CHF*	Hypercholesteremia, gout, glucose intolerance
Loop diuretics	Renal insufficiency	Diabetes, gout
Potassium-sparing diuretics	. . .	Renal insufficiency, ACE[‡]-inhibitor use
β-Blockers	Angina, IHSS, post-MI	Bronchospasm, bradycardia, heart block
	Migraine headache	Peripheral artery disease, CHF
ACE inhibitors	CHF, diabetes	Pregnancy or pregnancy planning, IHSS
	Renal insufficiency	Renal artery stenosis, cough side effect more common in women
Calcium-antagonists block	Angina, diabetes, migraine headache	CHF, bradycardia, IHSS (diltiazem, verapamil)
α-Antagonists	Hypercholesteremia	IHSS
Supplemental Therapy		
α₂-Agonists	Pregnancy or pregnancy planning§, depression	Liver disease§
Direct vasodilators	Pregnancy or pregnancy planning‖	Post-MI, angina, IHSS
Reserpine	. . .	Depression, peptic ulcer disease

*CHF = congestive heart failure.
[t]IHSS = idiopathic hypertrophic subaortic stenosis.
[‡]ACE = angiotensin-converting enzyme.
§Alpha-methyl dopa.
‖Hydralazine.

Concern has been raised about the potential side effects of the thiazide diuretics, perhaps most importantly the alteration of serum lipids. Because lipid physiology differs for women and men, including changes with menopausal status, these effects are potentially important in predicting cardiovascular risk for women. Few studies of antihypertensive therapy have included a gender analysis of effects on lipids (43). Although the Medical Research Council (MRC) Trial did show an increase in total cholesterol in both women and men treated with bendrofluazide, propranolol, or methyldopa, neither specific lipoproteins nor menopausal status was reported. Boehringer et al found that chlorthalidone treatment was associated with an increase in both low-density lipoproteins and total cholesterol in postmenopausal but not premenopausal women, although menopausal status was defined by age alone (44). The Trial Antihypertensive Interventions and Management (TAIM) study compared various pharmacologic and nonpharmacologic interventions and found that chlorthalidone raised total cholesterol whereas nutritional therapy lowered it. A multiple regression analysis of factors related to change in total cholesterol showed that gender was not a significant predictor (45a). All of these findings may be put into a different perspective by more recent work (SHEP), which indicates that the use of lower doses of thiazide diuretics does not seem to cause changes in lipoprotein levels (45b).

From a beneficial point of view, there is evidence to suggest that thiazide diuretics may decrease the risk of hip fracture by reducing urinary excretion of calcium, thereby enhancing bone density (46,47). Meta-analysis of several observational cohort studies (48) suggested that current use of thiazide diuretics, especially with long-term use, may decrease the risk of hip fracture by as much as 20%. Although this suggestion awaits confirmation by a randomized study involving adequate numbers of patients, it provides additional impetus to use this medication in hypertensive women.

There are no studies that demonstrate a gender differential in the effects of beta-blockers. As discussed above, they are demonstrated to be effective as first-line therapy in hypertension. They have also been studied in secondary prevention after MI and found to be effective in decreasing the risk of a second MI in both women and men (49a). There is also increasing data suggesting the benefit of beta-blockers in patients with congestive heart failure.

Evidence for gender-specific efficacy of either calcium antagonists or ACE inhibitors is quite limited, and prevention of cardiovascular end points through their use as antihypertensive agents has not been adequately documented (49b). Several small studies have focused on their efficacy in lowering blood pressure, with some conflicting results. Applegate et al studied 240 women over the age of 65, comparing atenolol, enalapril, and diltiazem over a 16-week period (50). Again, all three drugs were effective in lowering blood pressure, although diltiazem was significantly more effective in lowering diastolic pressure. Total rates of adverse events were equal for all three drugs. Three other trials included women and men and analyzed blood pressure effects by gender. In the Amlodipine Cardiovascular Community Trial (ACCT), slightly more than 1000 patients (about 33% women, 20% black) received amlodipine as a sole agent for 18 weeks (51). This study demonstrated that women reached goal blood pressure significantly more often than men (91% versus 83%, $p < 0.001$) and that women on treatment had a significantly greater decrease in SBP and DBP than men ($p < 0.0001$), even after adjustment for baseline blood pressure, age, weight and dose. This decrease was not affected by the presence or absence of hormone replacement therapy. The Hydrochlorothiazide, Atenolol, Nitrendipine, Enalapril Study (HANE) trial compared the efficacy of hydrochlorothiazide, atenolol, nitrendipine, and enalapril in a double-blind, multicenter, 48-week trial (52). Slightly less than 50% of the 868 patients were women. In the total study group there was a significantly higher response rate with atenolol than any of the other three drugs. This difference persisted to 48 weeks for all drugs except enalapril and held true for women when subgroup analysis by gender was performed. In addition, gender analysis showed that enalapril was significantly more effective in women than in men (59% response rate compared with 42%, $p < 0.015$). In both women and men, the highest dropout rate occurred among those taking nitrendipine. Finally, in the Verapamil-Diuretic (VERDI) Trial, 364 patients (about equal numbers of women and men, ages 21 to 71) were treated with either hydrochlorothiazide or verapamil over 48 weeks (53). Verapamil was significantly more effective as a single agent in mild-to-moderate hypertension, with similar rates of withdrawal because of side effects for both drugs. Although no analysis by gender was presented, it is mentioned that results were similar in women and men.

ACE inhibitor agents have been prescribed more frequently for diabetic and nondiabetic patients since being shown to improve survival after congestive heart failure and MI as well as to retard progression of renal failure in diabetics (see Chapter 21). For hypertensive women, many of whom are in their reproductive years, the implications of possible teratogenic effects should be considered. Limited data suggest that the greatest risk of fetal abnormalities and death occur after the first trimester (54). Ideally, women considering pregnancy should not use ACE inhibitors and, if pregnancy occurs, the drug should be rapidly changed to avoid fetal complications. The most common side effect of ACE inhibitor use is a dry cough, which occurs more frequently in women than men (55).

In summary, it seems reasonable to continue to use thiazides and beta-blockers as first-line antihypertensive agents in most women and to choose newer agents when concomitant clinical circumstances warrant it (e.g., ACE inhibitors in diabetics; calcium channel blockers in women with angina). Only thiazides and beta-blockers have been found to decrease MI, sudden death, and congestive heart failure in women as well as men. Limited clinical data are available now on the blood pressure lowering effects of specific classes of medication in women compared with men.

Nonpharmacologic Therapy

JNC VI emphasizes lifestyle modification as definitive or adjunctive therapy for the prevention and treatment of high blood pressure (1). Moderate sodium restriction, potassium supplementation, weight reduction, increased physical activity, relaxation training, and restriction of alcohol have all been shown to have some antihypertensive efficacy, although the consistency of effect and quality of evidence are variable. Nonpharmacologic therapy may carry particular benefit for treating hypertension as a coronary risk factor, because several lifestyle maneuvers (e.g., physical activity and weight management) favorably affect the coronary risk factors (e.g., glucose intolerance, obesity, and dyslipidemia) that often cluster with hypertension and act synergistically with it to increase cardiac risk (56,57).

Evidence consistently supports the importance of weight as a risk factor for hypertension. In a prospective population-based study from Belgium, body mass index explained 27.6% of the SBP variance in women compared with 9.9% in men (58). Data from the Framingham Offspring Study (59) confirm the importance of weight as a predictor of hypertension, even among those who are normotensive at baseline. Obese women between 30 and 39 years old were seven times more likely to develop hypertension than lean women of the same age. Weight reduction is also an effective treatment for hypertension. Randomized controlled trials have demonstrated that weight loss reduces blood pressure in both normotensive and hypertensive women (45,60-63) and is effective as both sole and adjunctive therapy.

Weight loss may be more difficult to achieve in women, however (64-66). A gender-specific analysis of Treatment of Mild Hypertension Study (TOMHS) participants indicated that women randomized to lifestyle intervention alone were less likely to lose weight, to increase their physical activity, and to successfully have their blood pressure controlled than their male counterparts. Hence, although compelling evidence supports the efficacy of even modest weight loss in reducing blood pressure, achievement of this goal may be particularly problematic for women.

Physical activity is an important component of any weight reduction program; however, its independent effect on blood pressure has been much less studied in women than men (67,68). Sedentary lifestyle has been well documented as a CAD risk factor in men. The effect of exercise on CAD appears to be similar in women and men (see Chapter 8). Firm epidemiologic evidence to confirm the independent utility of exercise for the primary prevention of CAD in women is not yet available (69). However, because of its documented benefit in weight management, diabetes, and lipid profiles (69-71), as well as reduced overall mortality and osteoporosis (69,72), its inclusion as a potentially useful antihypertensive modality is justified.

An extensive body of literature also supports the efficacy of sodium restriction in reducing blood pressure, both in normotensive (primary prevention) and hypertensive individuals (73). Many of these trials have included women, but gender analyses have rarely been performed. Investigators have noted a heterogeneity of response to sodium manipulation and the interaction of sodium sensitivity with potassium and calcium intake (74). One recent small study of patients aged 55 to 75 with untreated mild-to-moderate hypertension demonstrated a reduction of SBP/DBP of 7.6/3.3 mm Hg after replacement of sodium salt with a low-sodium, high-potassium, high-magnesium mineral salt, without weight reduction or other dietary changes. Results in this study were comparable for women and men (75).

Weinberger's group noted that plasma renin activity was significantly lower in individuals sensitive to sodium than in those who were sodium resistant, although renin profiles alone were not accurate in predicting sodium sensitivity (76). Data from the Trial of Antihypertensive Interventions and Management (TAIM) indicated an interaction between plasma renin levels and DBP response to a multicomponent, nonpharmacologic intervention (weight reduction, low sodium/high potassium) (77). Alderman (78) indicated an increased risk of MI associated with low urinary sodium with a high renin-sodium profile among treated hypertensive men. There was no apparent association between low urinary sodium excretion and MI in women; however, the small number of events ($n = 9$) precludes definitive analysis. Hypertensive women have been observed to have lower renin levels than hypertensive men (79); furthermore, estrogen replacement therapy may lower plasma renin levels despite an increase in angiotensin (27). Thus, gender analyses of response to sodium manipulation, including menopausal and hormonal status, should be undertaken in future research. Data examining other dietary maneuvers, such as potassium, calcium, or magnesium supplementation have yielded mixed results (80,81). A recent meta-analysis of 33 randomized, controlled trials examining oral potassium supplementation indicated a 3 mm/2 mm Hg reduction in SBP/DBP (82). Women were present in 21 of these trials and represented one third or more of the participants in 14 of them. Effect size was comparable in women and men; it was greater in black participants and in those with greater sodium intake. Regardless of the effect of potassium on blood pressure, however, data from the Rancho Bernardo study demonstrate a relative risk of 4.8 for stroke-associated mortality among women in the lowest tertile of potassium intake (compared with 2.6 for men) (83).

Heterogeneity has also been noted in epidemiologic associations between calcium and magnesium intake and blood pressure levels as well as in the blood pressure response to calcium or magnesium supplementation (84,85). The potential interaction of these ions with dietary sodium has already been mentioned. Similarly, serum-ionized calcium and magnesium levels vary with plasma renin activity, although in opposite directions (86). Because of the possibility of a gender interaction with plasma renin activity, gender may be an important consideration in delineating groups likely to benefit from particular dietary advice and therefore deserves specific investigation. Obviously, comorbid conditions (e.g., osteoporosis and renal calculi) should be included in the consideration of such supplementation.

Certain complex dietary patterns, such as vegan or religious vegetarian diets, have also been associated with reduced blood pressure in population studies (87,88). It is unclear whether this effect is owing to a specific nutrient (e.g., saturated fat or animal protein [89,90]) or represents a complex interaction not only of nutrients but of lifestyle factors associated with eating, such as physical activity, psychosocial functioning, age, and body mass index (91,92).

An association between alcohol intake and increased blood pressure has been observed in several large cross-sectional and cohort studies that included large numbers of women and gender analyses (93-97). The risk of increased blood pressure rises significantly at intakes greater than 2 or 3 drinks per day. It is lowest in women reporting 1 to 7 drinks per week, thus following a J-shaped curve similar to that noted in men and similar to the association of alcohol with coronary disease risk (98). The Hypertension Control Project, which enrolled participants from the HDFP trial, combined alcohol reduction with other nutritional changes (weight loss and sodium restriction) to improve blood pressure effectively (99a), although a post hoc regression analysis did not report alcohol as a significant factor in the study effect. Forty percent of trial participants were women, but no gender analysis was performed. The Prevention and Treatment of Hypertension Study (PATHS) enrolled predominantly male veterans in a clinical trial with the goal of reducing alcohol consumption to 50% of baseline use or less than 14 drinks weekly (99b). By 6 and 24 months, alcohol use had decreased by 1.3 drinks daily without significant changes in blood pressure. JNC VI has noted that because women absorb more ethanol than men, and people who weigh less are more susceptible to the effects of alcohol, these individuals should be advised to drink no more than 0.5 oz of ethanol per day (1).

Relaxation techniques have been shown to reduce blood pressure in some studies (100) but not in others (60,101,102). Women have been participants in these studies, but no gender analyses have been performed. A recent small, randomized trial in older blacks compared twice-daily transcendental meditation with progressive muscle relaxation and education about JNC V–defined lifestyle changes. These researchers demonstrated a respective reduction in SBP and DBP of 10.4/6.6 mm Hg in women compared with 12.7/8.1 mm Hg in men. Because data suggest that blood pressure reactivity is greater among women than men (103,104), as well as a possible association between hormonal status and blood pressure changes during mental stress (105), future studies should continue to explore the efficacy of relaxation training and/or biofeedback in reducing blood pressure and blood pressure reactivity in women. Interestingly, Framingham data suggest that although anxiety is more common among middle-aged women than men, it is a risk factor for the development of hypertension only in men (106).

Evidence increasingly suggests comparable efficacy of antihypertensive therapy in women and men. All pharmacologic therapy carries financial cost as well as potential side effects, even when efficacious. Gender analyses of women's response to nonpharmacologic therapy remain necessary. Responses to manipulation of sodium, calcium and other ions, blood pressure reactivity, and effective approaches to weight management and exercise deserve particular priority.

Summary

Hypertension is common in women as they age and confers considerable risk upon them for the development of CAD. When a woman has been diagnosed with mild-to-moderate hypertension (SBP: 140–179 mm Hg; DBP: 90–99 mm Hg), a vigorous 3- to 6-month trial of indicated nonpharmacologic therapy should generally be pursued. The presence of established CAD, other cardiac risk factors, or target-organ damage should dictate earlier institution of pharmacologic therapy. The goals of aggressive pharmacologic treatment of hypertension should include achieving DBP of at least less than 90 mm Hg and SBP of less than 140 mm Hg (1), daily aspirin use (41b), and management of other risk factors (such as hyperlipidemia) in addition to nonpharmacologic interventions.

The most compelling evidence supporting pharmacologic therapy of hypertension in women to prevent coronary events derives from the recent meta-analysis of major treatment trials, which were composed largely of young and middle-aged subjects. This may explain why statistical significance was not achieved for prevention of all categories of cardiovascular events. There was, however, a consistent trend towards prevention of coronary outcomes by active drug treatment in women. These data, combined with the consistent reduction in stroke rates with active treatment of hypertension in women in all treatment trials, strongly support pharmacologic intervention when blood pressure is not effectively lowered by nonpharmacologic therapy. Because all the major long-term hypertension treatment trials to date have used thiazide diuretics and beta-blockers, these drugs should be employed as first-line therapy in patients who do not have contraindications to their use or specific reasons for using other agents. The utility of thiazides is particularly compelling for women in light of their lower renin profiles and should be strongly favored in women at risk for osteoporosis. The role of newer antihypertensive agents in preventing coronary events remains to be further elucidated by future studies.

REFERENCES

1. **Joint National Committee on Prevention, Detection, Evaluation and Treatment of High Blood Pressure.** The Sixth Report of the Joint National Committee on Preven-

tion, Detection, Evaluation, and Treatment of High Blood Pressure. Arch Intern Med. 1997;157:2413-46.

2. **National Center for Health Statistics, Rowland M, Roberts J.** Blood pressure levels and hypertension in persons ages 6-74 years: United States, 1976-1980. In: Advance Data from Vital and Health Statistics of the National Center for Health Statistics of the National Center for Health Sciences. Publication No. 84. 84th ed. Rockville, Maryland: Public Health Service; 1982:1-12.

3. **Hypertension Detection and Follow-up Program Cooperative Group.** Blood pressure studies in 14 communities: a two-stage screen for hypertension. JAMA. 1977;237:2385-91.

4. **Pickering TG.** White coat hypertension. In: Laragh JH, Brenner BM, eds. Hypertension: Pathophysiology, Diagnosis, and Management. 2nd ed. New York: Raven Press; 1995:1913-25.

5. **Pappas G, Gergen PJ, Carroll M.** Hypertension prevalence and the status of awareness, treatment, and control in the Hispanic Health and Nutrition Examination Survey (HHANES), 1982-84. Am J Public Health. 1990;80:1431-6.

6a. **Geronimus AT, Neidert LJ, Bound J.** A note on the measurement of hypertension in HHANES. Am J Public Health. 1990;80:1437-42.

6b. **Satish S, Stroup-Benham CA, Espino DV, et al.** Undertreatment of hypertension in older Mexican-Americans. J Am Geriatr Soc. 1998;46:405-10.

7. **Cornoni-Huntley J, LaCroix AZ, Havlik RJ.** Race and sex differentials in the impact of hypertension in the United States: the National Health and Nutrition Examination Survey: I—Epidemiologic follow-up study. Arch Intern Med. 1989;149:780-8.

8. **Lerner DJ, Kannel WB.** Patterns of coronary heart disease morbidity and mortality in the sexes: a 26-year follow-up of the Framingham population. Am Heart J. 1986; 111:383-90.

9. **Kannel WB.** Blood pressure as a cardiovascular risk factor: prevention and treatment. JAMA. 1996;275:1571-6.

10. **Stokes J, Kannel WB, Wolf PA, et al.** Blood pressure as a risk factor for cardiovascular disease: the Framingham Study—30 years of follow-up. Hypertension. 1989;13(suppl I):I-13-8.

11. **Perlman JA, Wolf PH, Ray R, Lieberknecht G.** Cardiovascular risk factors, premature heart disease, and all-cause mortality in a cohort of Northern California women. Am J Obstet Gynecol. 1988;158:1568-74.

12. **Keil JE, Sutherland SE, Knapp RG, et al.** Mortality rates and risk factors for coronary disease in black as compared with white men and women. N Engl J Med. 1993;329:73-8.

13. **Levy D, Larson M, Vasan RS, et al.** The progression from hypertension to congestive heart failure. JAMA. 1996;275:1557-62.

14. **Vaccarino V, Krumholz HM, Berkman LF, Horwitz RI.** Sex differences in mortality after myocardial infarction: is there evidence for an increased risk for women? Circulation. 1995;91:1861-71.

15a. **Johansson S, Bergstrand R, Ulvenstam G, et al.** Sex differences in preinfarction characteristics and longterm survival among patients with myocardial infarction. Am J Epidemiol. 1984;119:610-23.

15b. **Njolstad I, Arnesen E.** Preinfarction blood pressure and smoking are determinants for a fatal outcome of myocardial infarction: a prospective analysis from the Finmark Study. Arch Intern Med. 1998;158:1326-32.

15c. **Chandra NC, Ziegelstein RC, Rogers WJ, Tiefenbrunn AJ.** Observations of the treatment of women in the United States with myocardial infarction: a report from the National Registry of Myocardial Infarction—I. Arch Intern Med. 1998;158:981-8.

16. **Levy D, Garrison RJ, Savage DD, et al.** Prognostic implications of echocardiographically determined left ventricular mass in the Framingham Heart Study. N Engl J Med. 1990;322:1561-6.

17. **Psaty BM, Furberg CD, Kuller LH, et al.** Isolated systolic hypertension and subclinical cardiovascular disease in the elderly: initial findings from the Cardiovascular Health Study. JAMA. 1992;268:1287-91.

18a. **Krumholz HM, Larson M, Levy D.** Sex differences in cardiac adaptation to isolated systolic hypertension. Am J Cardiol. 1993;72:310-3.

18b. **Zabalgoitia M, Noor Ur Rahman S, Haley WE, et al.** Comparison of left ventricular mass and geometric remodeling in treated and untreated men and women >50 years of age with systemic hypertension. Am J Cardiol. 1997;80:648-51.

18c. **Zabalgoitia M, Noor Ur Rahman S, Haley WE, et al.** Comparison in systemic hypertension of left ventricular mass and geometry with systolic and diastolic function in patients < 65 to ≥ 65 years of age. Am J Cardiol. 1998;82:604-8.

18d. **Zabalgoitia M, Noor Ur Rahman S, Haley WE, et al.** Impact of ethnicity on left ventricular mass and relative wall thickness in essential hypertension. Am J Cardiol. 1998;81:412-7.

18e. **Palatini P, Mormino P, Santonastaso M, et al.** Target-organ damage in Stage 1 hypertensive subjects with white coat hypertension and sustained hypertension: results from the HARVEST study. Hypertension. 1998;31(part 1):57-63.

19. **Kuwajima I, Suzuki Y, Fujisawa A, Kuramoto K.** Is white coat hypertension innocent? Structure and function of the heart in the elderly. Hypertension. 1993;22:826-31.

20. **Schulman SP, Weiss JL, Becker LC, et al.** The effects of antihypertensive therapy on left ventricular mass in elderly patients. N Engl J Med. 1990;322:1350-5.

21. **McFate Smith W.** Epidemiology of congestive heart failure. Am J Cardiol. 1985;55:3A-8A.

22. **Levy D, Salomon M, D'Agostino RB, et al.** Prognostic implications of baseline electrocardiographic features and their serial changes in subjects with left ventricular hypertrophy. Circulation. 1994;90:1786-93.

23. **Chasan-Taber L, Willett WC, Manson JE, et al.** Prospective study of oral contraceptives and hypertension among women in the United States. Circulation. 1996;94:483-9.

24. **Khaw K, Peart WS.** Blood pressure and contraceptive use. BMJ. 1982;285:402-7.

25. **Layde PM, Beral V, Kay CR.** Further analyses of mortality in oral contraceptive users: Royal College of General Practioners Oral Contraception Study. Lancet. 1981;1:541-6.

26. **Blumenstein BA, Douglas MB, Hall WD.** Blood pressure changes and oral contraceptive use: a study of 2676 black women in the Southeastern United States. Am J Epidemiol. 1980;112:539-52.

27. **Schunkert H, Jan Danser AH, Hense HW, et al.** Effects of estrogen replacement therapy on the renin-angiotensin system in postmenopausal women. Circulation. 1997;95:39-45.

28. **Writing Goup for the PEPI Trial.** Effects of estrogen or estrogen/progestin regimens on heart disease risk factors in postmenopausal women: the Postmenopausal Estrogen/Progestin Interventions (PEPI) Trial. JAMA. 1995;273:199-208.

29. **Mann SJ, Pickering TC.** Detection of renovascular hypertension: state of the art. Ann Intern Med. 1992;117:945-53.

30. **Ram C, Venkata S.** Renovascular hypertension. Cardiol Clin. 1988;6:483-508.

31. **Manger WM, Gifford RW.** Pheochromocytoma. In: Laragh JH, Brenner BM, eds. Hypertension: Pathophysiology, Diagnosis and Management. New York: Raven Press; 1990:1639-57.

32. **Klein I.** Thyroid hormone and blood pressure regulation. In: Laragh JH, Brenner BM, eds. Hypertension: Pathophysiology, Diagnosis, and Managment. New York: Raven Press; 1990;1661-72.

33. **Hypertension Detection and Follow-up Program Cooperative Group.** Effect of stepped care treatment on the incidence of myocardial infarction and angina pectoris: 5-year findings of the Hypertension Detection and Follow-up Program. Hypertension. 1984;6 (suppl I):I-198-206.

34. **Anastos K, Charney P, Charon RA, et al.** Hypertension in women: what is really known? Ann Intern Med. 1991;115:287-93.

35. **Hypertension Detection and Follow-up Program Cooperative Group.** Persistence of reduction in blood pressure and mortality in the hypertension detection and follow-up program. JAMA. 1988;259:2113-22.

36. **Gueyffier F, Boutitie F, Boissel JP, et al.** Effects of antihypertensive drug treatment on cardiovascular outcomes in women and men: a meta-analysis of individual patient data from randomized, controlled trials. Ann Intern Med. 1997;126:761-7.

37. **Dahlof B, Hansson L, Lindholm LH, et al.** Swedish Trial in Older Patients with Hypertension (STOP-Hypertension) analyses performed up to 1992. Clin Exper Hypertens. 1993;15:925-39.

38. **Dahlof B, Lindholm LH, Hansson L, et al.** Morbidity and mortality in the Swedish Trial in Older Patients with Hypertension (STOP-Hypertension). Lancet. 1991;338:1281-5.

39. **SHEP Cooperative Research Group.** Prevention of stroke by antihypertensive drug treatment in older persons with isolated systolic hypertension: final results of the Systolic Hypertension in the Elderly Program (SHEP). JAMA. 1991;265:3255-64.

40. **Kostis JB, Davis BR, Cutler JA, et al.** Prevention of heart failure by antihypertensive drug treatment in older persons with isolated systolic hypertension. JAMA. 1997;278:212-6.

41a. **Lindblad U, Rastam L, Ryden L, et al.** Control of blood pressure and risk of first myocardial infarction: the Skaraborg hypertension project. BMJ. 1994;308:681-6.

41b. **Hansson L, Zanchetti A, Carruthers SG, et al.** Effects of intensive blood-pressure lowering and low-dose aspirin in patients with hypertension: principal results of the Hypertension Optimal Treatment (HOT) randomised trial. Lancet. 1998;351:1755-62.

42. **Kitler ME.** Differences in men and women in coronary artery disease, systemic hypertension and their treatment. Am J Cardiol. 1992;70:1077-80.

43. **Lardinois CK, Neuman SL.** The effects of antihypertensive agents on serum lipids and lipoproteins. Arch Intern Med. 1988;148:1280-9.

44. **Boehringer K, Weidmann P, Mordasini R, et al.** Menopause-dependent plasma lipoprotein alterations in diuretic-treated women. Ann Intern Med. 1982;97:206-9.

45a. **Oberman A, Wassertheil-Smoller S, Langford HG, et al.** Pharmacologic and nutritional treatment of mild hypertension: changes in cardiovascular risk status. Ann Intern Med. 1990;112:89-95.

45b. **Systolic Hypertension in the Elderly Program.** Influence of long-term, low-dose, diuretic-based antihypertensive therapy on glucose, lipid, uric acid, and potassium levels in older men and women with isolated systolic hypertension. Arch Intern Med. 1998;158:741-51.

46. **LaCroix AZ, Wienpahl J, White LR, et al.** Thiazide diuretic agents and the incidence of hip fracture. N Engl J Med. 1990;322:286-90.

47. **Cauley JA, Cummings SR, Seeley DG.** Effect of thiazide diuretic therapy on bone mass, fracture and falls. Ann Intern Med. 1993;118:666-73.

48. **Jones G, Nguyen T, Sambrook PN, Eismann JA.** Thiazide diuretics and fractures: can meta-analysis help? J Bone Mineral Res. 1995;10:106-11.

49a. **Beta-blocker Heart Attack Trial Research Group.** A randomized trial of propranolol in patients with acute myocardial infarction: mortality results. JAMA. 1982;247:1707-14.

49b. **Michels KB, Rosner BA, Manson JE, et al.** Prospective study of calcium channel blocker use, cardiovascular disease, and total mortality among hypertensive women: the Nurses' Health Study. Circulation. 1998;97:1540-8.

50. **Applegate WB, Phillips HL, Schnaper J, et al.** A randomized controlled trial of the effects of three antihypertensive agents on blood pressure control and quality of life in older women. Arch Intern Med. 1991;151:1817-23.

51. **Kloner R, Sowers J, DiBona G, et al.** Sex- and age-related antihypertensive effects of amlodipine. Am J Cardiol. 1996;77:713-22.

52. **Philipp T, Anlauf M, Distler A, et al.** Randomized, double blind, multicentre comparison of hydrochlorothiazide, atenolol, nitrendipine, and enalapril in antihypertensive treatment: results of the HANE study. BMJ. 1997;315:154-9.

53. **Holzgreve H, Distler A, Michaelis J, et al.** Verapamil versus hydrochlorothiazide in the treatment of hypertension: results of a long-term, double-blind comparative trial. BMJ. 1989;299:881-6.

54. **Feldkamp M, Jones KL, Ornoy A, et al.** Postmarketing surveillance for angiotensin-coverting enzyme inhibitor use during the first trimester of pregnancy—United States, Canada, and Israel, 1987-1995. MMWR Morb Mortal Wkly Rep. 1997;46:240-2.

55. **Os I, Bratland B, Dahlof B, et al.** Female preponderance for lisinopril-induced cough in hypertension. Am J Hypertens. 1997;7:1012-5.

56. **Reaven GM.** Insulin resistance and compensatory hyperinsulinemia: role in hypertension, dyslipidemia and coronary heart disease. Am Heart J. 1991;121:1283-8.

57. **Grimm RH, Jr., Flack JM, Grandits GA, et al.** Long-term effects on plasma lipids of diet and drugs to treat hypertension. JAMA. 1996;275:1549-56.

58. **Staessen JA, Roels H, Fagard R.** Lead exposure and conventional and ambulatory blood pressure. JAMA. 1996;275:1563-70.

59. **Garrison RJ, Kannel WB, Stokes J, Castelli WP.** Incidence and precursors of hypertension in young adults: the Framingham offspring study. Prev Med. 1987;16:235-51.

60. **The Trials of Hypertension Prevention Collaborative Reserach Group.** The effects of nonpharmacologic interventions on blood pressure of persons with high normal levels: results of the Trials of Hypertension Prevention—Phase I. JAMA. 1992;267:1213-20.

61. **Stamler R, Stamler J, Gosch FC, et al.** Primary prevention of hypertension by nutritional-hygenic means: final report of a randomized, controlled trial. JAMA. 1989;262:1801-7.

62. **Langford HG, Blaufox MD, Oberman A, et al.** Dietary therapy slows the return of hypertension after stopping prolonged medication. JAMA. 1985;253:657-64.

63. **Hypetension Prevention Trial Research Group.** The Hypertension Prevention Trial: three-year effects of dietary changes on blood pressure. Arch Intern Med. 1990;150:153-62.

64. **Lewis CE, Grandits GA, Flack JM, et al, for the TOMHS Research Group.** Efficacy and tolerance of antihypertensive treatment in men and women with stage I diastolic hypertension: results of Treatment of Mild Hypertension Study. Arch Intern Med. 1996;156:377-85.

65. **Kramer FM, Jeffrey RW, Forster JL, Snell MK.** Long-term follow-up of behavioral treatment of obesity: patterns of weight regain among men and women. Int J Obes Relat Metab Disord. 1989;13:123-36.

66. **Stevens VJ, Corrigan SA, Obarzanek E, et al.** Weight loss intervention in Phase I of the Trials of Hypertension Prevention. Arch Intern Med. 1993;153:849-58.

67. **Arroll B, Beaglehole R.** Does physical activity lower blood pressure? A critical review of the clinical trials. J Clin Epidemiol. 1992;45:439-47.

68. **Kokkinos PF, Narayan P, Colleran JA, et al.** Effects of regular exercise on blood pressure and left ventricular hypertrophy in African-American men with severe hypertension. N Engl J Med. 1995;333:1462-7.

69. **Blair SN, Kohl HW, Paffenberger RS, et al.** Physical fitness and all-cause mortality: a prospective study of men and women. JAMA. 1989;262:2395-401.

70. **Blair SN.** Evidence for success of exercise in weight loss and control. Ann Intern Med. 1993;119(7 pt.2):702-6.

71. **Helmrich SP, Ragland SR, Leung RW, Paffenberger RS.** Physical activity and reduced occurrence of non–insulin-dependent diabetes mellitus. N Engl J Med. 1991; 325:147-52.

72. **Chow R, Harrison JE, Notarius C.** Effect of two randomized exercise programs on bone mass of healthy postmenopausal women. BMJ. 1987;295:1441-4.

73. **Culter JA, Follman D, Elliott P, Suh I.** An overview of randomized trials of sodium reduction and blood pressure. Hypertension. 1991;17:I-27-33.

74. **Weinberger MH.** Clinical studies of the role of dietary sodium in blood pressure. In: Laragh JH, Brenner BM, eds. Hypertension: Pathophysiology, Diagnosis, and Management. New York: Raven Press; 1990:1999-2007.

75. **Geleijnse JM, Witteman JCM, den Breeijen JH, Grobbee DE.** Reduction in blood pressure with a low sodium, high potassium, high magnesium salt in older subjects with mild to moderate hypertension. BMJ. 1994;309:436-40.

76. **Weinberger MH, Miller JZ, Luft FC, et al.** Definitions and characteristics of sodium sensitivity and blood pressure resistance. Hypertension. 1986;8:II-127-34.

77. **Blaufox MD, Lee HB, Davis B, et al.** The effects of nonpharmacologic interventions on blood pressure of persons with high normal levels. JAMA. 1992;267:1221-5.

78. **Alderman MH, Madhavan S, Ooi WL, et al.** Association of the renin-sodium profile with the risk of myocardial infarction in patients with hypertension. N Engl J Med. 1991;324:1098-103.

79. **Meade TW, Imeson JD, Gordon D, Peart WS.** The epidemiology of plasma renin. Clin Science. 1983;64:273-80.

80. **Kaplan NM.** Long-term effectiveness of nonpharmacological treatment of hypertension. Hypertension. 1991;18:I-153-60.

81. **Canadian Consensus Conference on Non-Pharmacological Approaches to the Management of High Blood Pressure.** Recommendations of the Canadian Consensus Conference on non-pharmacological approaches to the management of high blood pressure. Can Med Assoc J. 1990;142:1397-409.

82. **Whelton PK, He J, Cutler JA, et al.** Effects of oral potassium on blood pressure: meta-analysis of randomized controlled clinical trials. JAMA. 1997;277:1624-32.

83. **Khaw K, Barrett-Connor E.** Dietary potassium and stroke-associated mortality. N Engl J Med. 1987;316:235-9.

84. **Cutler JA, Brittain E.** Calcium and blood pressure: an epidemiologic perspective. Am J Hypertens. 1990;3:137S-46S.

85. **Whelton PK, Klag MJ.** Magnesium and blood pressure: review of the epidemiologic and clinical trial experience. Am J Cardiol. 1989;63:26G-30G.

86. **Resnick LM, Laragh JH, Sealey JE, Alderman MA.** Divalent cations in essential hypertension: relations between serium ionized calcium, magnesium, and plasma renin activity. N Engl J Med. 1983;309:888-91.

87. **Sacks FM, Rosner B, Kass EH.** Blood pressure in vegetarians. Am J Epidemiol. 1974;100:390-8.

88. **Armstrong B, VanMerwyk AJ, Coates H.** Blood pressure in Seventh Day Adventist vegetarians. Am J Epidemiol. 1977;105:444-9.

89. **Obarzanek E, Velletri PA, Cutler JA.** Dietary protein and blood pressure. JAMA. 1996;275:1598-603.

90. **Sacks FM.** Dietary fats and blood pressure: a critical review of the evidence. Nutr Rev. 1989;47:291-300.

91. **Beilin LJ.** Vegetarian and other complex diets, fats, fiber, and hypertension. Am J Clin Nutr. 1994;59(suppl):1130-5S.

92. **Appel LJ, Moore TJ, Obarzanek E, et al.** A clinical trial of the effects of dietary patterns on blood pressure. N Engl J Med. 1997;336:1117-24.

93. **Ueshima H, Ozawa H, Baba S, et al.** Alcohol drinking and high blood pressure: data from a 1980 national cardiovascular survey of Japan. J Clin Epidemiol. 1992;45:667-73.

94. **Witteman JCM, Willette WC, Stampfer MJ, et al.** Relation of moderate alcohol consumption and risk of systemic hypertension in women. Am J Cardiol. 1990;65:633-7.

95. **Moore RD, Levine DM, Southard J, et al.** Alcohol consumption and blood pressure in the 1982 Maryland Hypertension Survey. Am J Hypertens. 1990;3:1-7.

96. **Gruchow HW, Sobocinski KA, Barboriak JJ.** Alcohol, nutrient intake, and hypertension in U.S. adults. JAMA. 1985;253:1567-70.

97. **Klatsky A, Friedman G, Armstrong M.** The relationship between alcoholic beverage use and other traits to blood pressure: a new Kaiser Permanente study. Circulation. 1986;73:628-36.

98. **Stampfer MJ, Colditz GA, Willet WC, et al.** A prospective study of moderate alcohol consumption and the risk of coronary artery disease in women. N Engl J Med. 1988; 319:267-73.

99a. **Stamler R, Stamler J, Grimm R, et al.** Nutritional therapy for high blood pressure: final report of a four-year randomized controlled trial—The Hypertension Control Program. JAMA. 1987;257:1484-91.

99b. **Cushman WC, Cutler JA, Hanna E, et al.** Prevention and Treatment of Hypertension Study (PATHS): effect of an alcohol treatment program on blood pressure. Arch Intern Med. 1998;158:1197-2107.

100. **Patel C, Marmot MG, Terry DJ, et al.** Trial of relaxation in reducing coronary risk: four-year follow-up. BMJ. 1985;290:1103-6.

101. **van Montfrans GA, Karemaker JM, Wieling W, Dunning AJ.** Relaxation therapy and continuous ambulatory blood pressure in mild hypertension: a controlled study. BMJ. 1990;300:1368-72.

102. **Johnston DW, Gold A, Kentish J, et al.** Effects of stress management on blood pressure in mild primary hypertension. BMJ. 1993;306:963-6.

103. **Pickering TG, James GD, Boddie C, et al.** How common is white coat hypertension? JAMA. 1988;259:225-8.

104. **Perloff D, Sokolow M, Cowman R.** The prognostic value of ambulatory blood pressures. JAMA. 1983;249:2792-8.

105. **Owens JF, Stoney CM, Matthews KA.** Menopausal status influences ambulatory blood pressure levels and blood pressure changes during mental stress. Circulation. 1993;88:2794-802.

106. **Markovitz JH, Matthews KA, Kannel WB, et al.** Psychological predictors of hypertension in the Framingham study: is there tension in hypertension? JAMA. 1993; 270:2493-43.

CHAPTER 7

Obesity and Other Cardiovascular Risk Factors in Young Women

GERALD SANDERS BERENSON, MD

PAMELA CHARNEY, MD

SATHANUR RAMACHANDARAN SRINIVASAN, PHD

WENDY ANN WATTIGNEY, MS

WEIHANG BAO, PHD

KURT JOSEPH GREENLUND, PHD

THERESA ANN NICKLAS, DRPH

Obesity has become increasingly common among Americans of all ages (1,2a,2b). It is often associated with abnormal carbohydrate and/or insulin metabolism, hypertension, and dyslipidemia, all of which have additive or multiplicative adverse effects on cardiac outcomes (3).

Adult obesity is increasingly defined by body mass index (BMI) [weight (kilograms)/height (meters)^2] rather than by weight alone, because BMI better defines total body-fat mass (4a). Although obesity or being overweight may be defined by selected BMI cut points, for most outcomes there is a continuous relationship with the degree of obesity when subjects of different weights are compared. Women with a BMI above 25 are considered overweight (4b), and marked obesity is often defined as a BMI above 30 (e.g., a woman 180 cm tall who weighs more than 75 kg is markedly obese) (4a). In the United States and most Western countries, the prevalence of obesity has been steadily rising.

Obesity is increasingly common as women and men age. Although energy requirements decrease with aging, most individuals are sedentary and tend to increase, not decrease, their caloric intake. Even small changes in either input or output gradually translate into considerable changes in weight (1,4).

The prevalence of obesity and other cardiovascular risk factors in the young has been well documented in several studies (5-8) (Fig. 7-1). Although the incidence of coronary artery disease (CAD) tends to be decreasing, especially in men, it appears to be increasing among young women with high tobacco use and a high prevalence of obesity. The Bogalusa Heart Study has elucidated cardiovascular risk from early life through young adulthood by a long-term epidemiologic study of cardiovascular disease risk factors in a biracial (black-white) semi-rural community (9,10). The subclinical stages of atherosclerosis begin in youth and progress dramatically in young adulthood (11,12). Furthermore, tobacco use and increasing obesity in younger populations has accelerated the incidence of atherosclerosis.

Historically internists have primarily focused on the increasing prevalence of obesity in mid-life; yet internists also have an important role to play in the care of younger adults, where efforts may be more successful. Concern for patient offspring is encouraged, because parental obesity substantially increases an offspring's risk of obesity (13). The impact of obesity on the personal health of family members needs to be addressed.

In this chapter the prevalence and increasing frequency of obesity in women are discussed with special attention to age and race. The evidence of

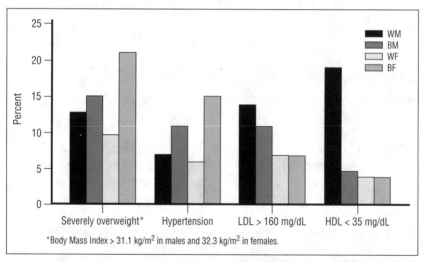

FIGURE 7-1 Prevalence of adverse risk factors in 19- to 32-year-olds by sex and race. Note the large percentage of young adults that are beginning to show clinical evidence of abnormal risk factors, especially the high prevalence of obesity and hypertension in black females. LDL = low-density lipoproteins; HDL = high-density lipoproteins. Data from the Bogalusa Heart Study. (From Wattigney WA, Webber LS, Srinivasan SR, Berenson GS. The emergence of clinically abnormal levels of cardiovascular disease risk factor variables among young adults: the Bogalusa Heart Study. Prev Med. 1995;24:617-26; with permission.)

the relationship between obesity and cardiovascular risk factors such as hypertension, serum lipids and lipoproteins, carbohydrate metabolism, and diabetes is reviewed. Finally, treatment modalities for the prevention and management of obesity are discussed.

Obesity: An Increasing Problem

Most Americans are overweight by recent definitions. The National Health and Nutrition Examination Survey III in 1988-91 defined overweight subjects as having a BMI ≥ 27.3 (2a). In 1998 The Expert Panel on the Identification, Evaluation, and Treatment of Overweight and Obesity in Adults defined normal BMI as less than 25 (2b). In the Bogalusa Heart Study, young black females tended to be 10 to 12 kg heavier than whites at the 90th percentile, with a BMI 5 to 6 units greater at the 90th percentile (14), which is consistent with the high prevalence of obesity in black women (15). Poverty increases the prevalence of obesity (Fig. 7-2).

Observations of secular increases of obesity have now been documented both in adults and children across the U.S. population (8,16,17). Comparison of national surveys of women aged 20 to 74 in 1976-80 and 1988-91 reveal the age-adjusted prevalence of BMI ≥ 27.3 increased from 27% to 34% of women. The increase was similar in black, Hispanic, and white women. Higher rates of obesity have especially occurred in women less than 60 years of age (2).

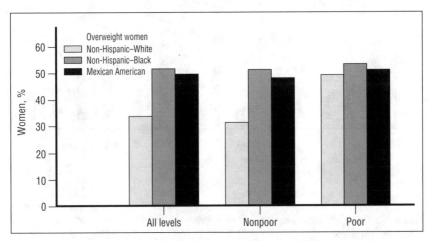

FIGURE 7-2 Prevalence of overweight among women 20 years of age and over by race, Hispanic origin, and poverty status: United States, 1988-91. (Adapted from Health, United States–1995. Chart Book. US Department of Health and Human Services. Public Health Service. DHHS Pub. No. 96-12232-1; Fig. 23.)

Repeated observations in the Bogalusa Heart Study since 1973 have demonstrated secular trends of increasing obesity beginning in childhood (8,17). During the 1970s body weight increased 2.5 kg without an increase in height; during the 1980s the increase was 5 kg (Fig. 7-3). This trend is more prominent in black females and may be explained by greater inactivity and television watching with a decreasing emphasis on physical education for school children (18,19). Furthermore, ease of transportation and easy access to fast-food have contributed to this problem. Depression, lower levels of achievement, and personal adjustment problems also contribute to the development of obesity in women (20).

Generally, weight is inversely related to family income and education. Rural and southern black women are more overweight than their urban or northern and western counterparts (21). The Bogalusa community is poor and representative of many small communities in the Southeast. The prevalence of obesity in women living in such rural settings represents a major health problem, because obesity relates strongly to other cardiovascular risk factors and underlies the occurrence of multiple risk factors in an individual.

Distribution of Body Fat: The Importance of Central Obesity

Although the importance of obesity as an independent risk factor for CAD remains controversial, its influence on other risk factors is quite evident (22).

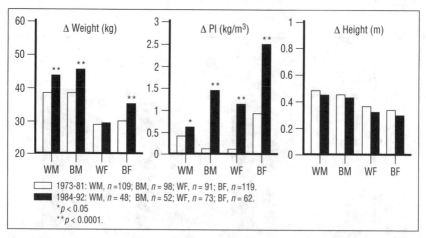

FIGURE 7-3 Change in anthropometric measurements of 7- to 9-year-old children by sex and race over two 8-year periods, cohort 1 (1973-81) and cohort 2 (1984-92). A trend of increasing obesity has occurred over the past two decades of observation. Data from the Bogalusa Heart Study. (From Gidding SS, Bao W, Srinivasan SR, Berenson GS. Effects of secular trends in obesity on coronary risk factors in children: the Bogalusa Heart Study. J Pediatr. 1995;127:868-74; with permission.)

Obesity or weight gain aggravates most cardiovascular risk factors. However, the pattern of fat distribution may be especially important prognostically (23). In women, abdominal or central obesity, frequently determined by an increased waist/hip ratio, appears to be a stronger risk factor for CAD than BMI (24). An independent relationship has been documented between waist/hip ratio and many cardiovascular risk factors often associated with obesity (insulin resistance, diabetes, hypertension, low high-density lipoprotein [HDL], and high triglycerides) (4,23). An elevated waist/hip ratio is much more common in men than women. Mechanisms to explain the etiology of this obesity pattern have not yet been fully elucidated, although cortisol metabolism by omental fat cells has been implicated (25).

As illustrated in the Manitoba Heart Health survey, this does not imply that noncentral obesity is prognostically benign (26). In our studies of children and adolescents, waist measurements alone or waist adjusted for height may be equally or even more reflective of the impact of obesity on risk factors. Similar results in adults were found by Lean et al (27). Subscapular skinfolds, like waist measurements, also indicate a central fat distribution and associates strongly with other risk factors.

Obesity and central fat distribution may be the driving force of this metabolic cluster of risk factors, Syndrome X (28) or the Deadly Quartet (29), which includes insulin resistance/hyperinsulinemia, dyslipidemia, and hypertension. Overweight children tend to become overweight adults, having higher ratios of serum total cholesterol to HDL cholesterol and higher levels of plasma insulin and systolic blood pressure, conditions all related to Syndrome X (Table 7-1) (30).

Ethnicity Differences in Obesity

There are substantial ethnic variations in the prevalence of obesity. Overweight black women exceed overweight white women by a ratio of approximately 2:1 (15). Hispanic children tend to have smaller stature but are fatter than blacks and whites in childhood (31). Striking black-white differences of obesity occur in young women (Table 7-2). In childhood, black females tend to be 2.4 kg heavier than the age-matched white females. The excess obesity in black girls versus white girls appears to begin at about 9 years of age, and this difference becomes more pronounced at 21 years of age. Forty percent of young black women are obese (7).

The patterns of skinfold thickness of females also differ (14). Triceps skinfold thickness for white females are greater than levels for black females until 22 years of age; thereafter levels for black women increase dramatically. This is particularly pronounced at the 90th percentile, with black women showing

Table 7-1 Relation of Adolescent-Onset Adult Overweight Status to the Clustering of Cardiovascular Risk Factors: the Bogalusa Heart Study

	Coexisting Conditions (>75th Percentile)*		
Serum total cholesterol/HDL cholesterol ratio	+	−	+
Insulin	+	+	+
Systolic blood pressure[†]	−	+	+
Overweight cohort (n = 110)[‡]			
Frequency (%)	36	34	19
Risk ratio[‖]	5.8[¶]	5.4[¶]	3.0[¶]
Lean cohort (n = 81)[§]			
Frequency (%)	9	3	3
Risk ratio[‖]	1.4	0.5	0.5

* Young adults.
† Includes patients on medication for hypertension.
‡ BMI ≥ 75th percentile.
‖ Observed frequency/expected frequency.
§ BMI = 25th to 50th percentile.
¶ $p < 0.0001$.
From Srinivasan SR, Bao W, Wattigney WA, Berenson GS. Adolescent overweight is associated with adult overweight and related multiple cardiovascular risk factors: the Bogalusa Heart Study. Metabolism. 1996;45:235-40; with permission.

triceps skinfold thickness as much as 12 mm greater than white women. At the subscapular site, beginning in adolescence, black females show increased skinfold thickness and at the uppermost decile the values for black females exceed those of white females by 10 mm. Thus, obese black girls develop into markedly obese young women.

Not only are black women most likely to be obese and hypertensive (see Fig. 7-1) but the mortality rate from acute myocardial infarction is highest for black women (32). Poor survival in black women has been postulated as caused by a delay in seeking medical care and a lack of access to same, but the high prevalence of obesity, diabetes mellitus, and severe hypertension is likely contributory. As will be discussed later in this chapter, the prevalence of co-morbid conditions also increases with increasing obesity.

Obesity in Older Age Groups

In the most recent National Health and Nutrition Examination Survey III (conducted in 1988-91), 27% of younger women (aged 20 to 39) were overweight, whereas about 40% of women aged 40 to 74 were overweight (2).

Table 7-2 Prevalence of Overweight and Severely Overweight Status Among Young Women: the Bogalusa Heart Study*

Age	White (n = 702)		Black (n = 339)	
	Overweight (%)	Severely Overweight (%)	Overweight (%)	Severely Overweight (%)
19–22	18.8	6.3	33.0	19.8
23–25	23.9	10.9	29.7	15.4
26–27	27.1	9.5	45.8	23.6
28–32	18.0	8.2	45.9	22.4

* Overweight: body mass index ≥ 27.3; severely overweight: body mass index ≥ 32.3.

Menopause did not have an impact on weight for participants in the Health and Women Study, initially aged 42 to 50, although participants gained an average of 2.25 kg (SD = 4.2 kg) over a 3-year follow up, with 20% of the women gaining more than 4.5 kg (33). Weight changes, especially in the elderly, may be related to the development of other medical conditions.

Obesity and the Risk of Coronary Events

The Nurses Health Study (34) has provided important data on the relationship of obesity and changes in weight with the risk of coronary events (coronary death, myocardial infarction, angina with stress test with at least 1 mm of ST segment depression or 70% obstruction on angiography, angioplasty, or bypass surgery). With 605 events over 8 years of observation, the risk of each type of coronary event increased with greater BMI. After adjusting for tobacco use and age, the rate of nonfatal myocardial infarction and coronary death was 32/100,000 person-years in the lowest BMI group compared with 106/100,000 person years in the highest BMI group. Obesity explained 70% of these events in the largest BMI group. In addition, although estimated BMI at age 18 was less predictive than current weight, weight gain over the previous 4 years was also a predictor of coronary events. In a retrospective cohort study from the Group Health Cooperative of Puget Sound, BMI has also been associated with the reinfarction rate of myocardial infarction (35).

Subsequent evaluation by the Nurses Health Study of women in "normal" weight ranges revealed a graded increase in the risk of myocardial infarction or coronary death with higher weight and BMI over 14 years of follow-up (36). Although only 20% of women had a BMI > 23.3 at age 18, nearly half reached this BMI by 1976. Even women with a BMI > 21 have a substantial increased risk of coronary events compared with women with a lower BMI. Both increasing BMI and weight gain equal to or greater than 5 kg after age 18 were significant predictors of coronary events, especially in nonsmoking women.

There is limited literature on the relationship between obesity and coronary events in the elderly. The incidence of cardiac events was defined in white participants aged 70 to 86 years without a history of previous coronary events in the National Health and Nutrition Examination Survey (NHANES) of 1982 to 1984 who were initially part of NHANES I (1971-75). Greater BMI at the first examination and weight loss between examinations were associated with more coronary events but not weight gain. Older subjects experiencing weight loss were more likely to report a history of diabetes, stroke, fair or poor health, and decreased ability to walk. Weight loss was not only common (23% of the women had lost 10% or more of body weight between examinations) but associated with an increased risk of coronary events (37).

Cardiovascular Risk Factors Related to Obesity

Several cardiovascular risk factors frequently occur together and are often associated with obesity: hypertension, serum lipids and lipoproteins, carbohydrate metabolism, adult-onset diabetes, tobacco use, sedentary lifestyles, low sociocultural environment, and dietary patterns. These are individually reviewed in the following sections. The prevalence of each of these risk factors increases with age, and it is often the combination of these risk factors that is particularly lethal. The presence of these risk factors can also identify women at especially high risk for cardiovascular events at an early age.

Hypertension

Hypertension is a major risk factor for coronary artery disease. A 10 mm Hg increase in systolic blood pressure correlates with a 20% to 30% increased risk of coronary artery disease or stroke in an older woman (38). The relationship between weight and blood pressure has been studied throughout the life span. Higher blood pressure levels occur in black girls than in white girls, even without obesity (39). Although not yet recognized as abnormal by clinical standards, higher blood pressure often presages rampant hypertensive disease and ultimately cardiovascular events.

The relationship between obesity, ethnicity, and blood pressure is complex and not fully elucidated. Black and white populations have been the most extensively studied (40-43). Hispanic populations of Mexican American descent have been studied more than other Hispanic groups (44). Mexican American women and men have a similar or slightly lower prevalence and incidence of hypertension than whites. This is consistent with data that Hispanic girls have a lower systolic blood pressure than other ethnic groups (43). There are limited data about most other ethnic groups.

It is well known that blacks have higher blood pressure levels as children (39) and often develop hypertension at an earlier age than white populations with subsequent greater morbidity and mortality. The increasing obesity that is seen in young adult black women certainly has the potential to accelerate the complications of hypertension as well as diabetes. Some 15% of young black women aged 19 to 32 years already have hypertension compared with about 5% of their white counterparts (see Fig. 7-1) (7). Although obesity is known to have an adverse impact on blood pressure levels, this association seems to be more evident in white females than in black females at an early age (14).

A marked black-white difference is seen early in life for a number of related variables. Black children have lower heart rates, lower renin and dopamine beta-hydroxylase levels, less urinary excretion of potassium, and higher insulin-glucose ratios compared with white children (45,46). The observation of lower urinary excretion of potassium is of particular interest in black children, because exposure to a high sodium intake coupled with low calcium, magnesium, and potassium intake may exacerbate the intrinsic susceptibility to hypertension in blacks (47,48). In addition, hyperinsulinemia caused by reduced hepatic clearance of insulin and high prevalence of obesity likely contributes to their excessive hypertension (49,50).

Left ventricular hypertrophy, a common complication of hypertension, is associated with an increased risk of myocardial infarction, congestive heart failure, and stroke (51,52). Early studies diagnosed left ventricular hypertrophy by electrocardiography (large QRS voltage associated with ST segment depression and T wave inversion) and found that both hypertension and obesity were frequent precursors to the development of left ventricular hypertrophy (51). Subsequently, echocardiography has been used to explore the relationship between left ventricular hypertrophy and obesity. A Framingham follow-up of 1822 nonhypertensive women with no previous history of cardiac events assessed the relationship of BMI to left ventricular hypertrophy by echocardiography. In normotensive subjects, both left ventricular mass and left ventricular wall thickness increased with greater BMI. This relationship was obvious throughout the BMI range; there was a 41% increase in left ventricular mass (normalized for height) when women with a BMI of 30 were compared with women with BMI < 23 (52). In a smaller study comparing normotensive and hypertensive adults, BMI was also predictive of left ventricular hypertrophy in both normotensive and hypertensive adults (53). Similarly, in the younger population (aged 23 to 35) of Coronary Artery Risk Development in Young Adults (CARDIA), left ventricular mass was also related to weight and systolic blood pressure (54). Similar observations have been published in the

Bogalusa Heart Study where children and adolescents showed a relation between high blood pressure and obesity and the development of left ventricular
hypertrophy (55).

Serum Lipids and Lipoproteins

Although HDL cholesterol levels are inversely related to CAD in both women
and men, data from the Framingham Study suggest that HDL cholesterol levels profoundly affect the risk of CAD in women (Fig. 7-4) (56). In women, as
in men, serum total and low-density lipoprotein (LDL) cholesterol levels are
directly related to the incidence of CAD events, although LDL cholesterol levels appear not to be as powerful a predictor of CAD in premenopausal women
as in men (57). Similarly, elevated triglyceride levels are more strongly associated with risk of CAD in women than men (58). Epidemiologic studies of the
interaction of sex, age, race, obesity, and lipoprotein levels follow.

Considerable changes in serum lipid and lipoprotein levels that influence
the development of CAD occur during sexual maturation and after menopause
(59,60). Mean serum total cholesterol levels in childhood approach those seen
in young adults. During the first decade of life, black and white girls tend to
have higher LDL cholesterol, triglycerides, and very low-density lipoprotein
(VLDL) cholesterol and lower HDL cholesterol levels than boys. Serum total
cholesterol levels decline during puberty in females but not as greatly as in

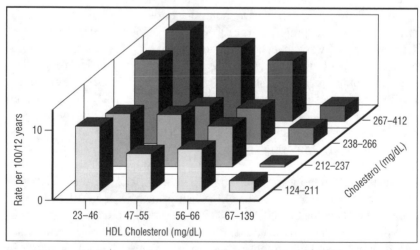

FIGURE 7-4 Twelve-year incidence of myocardial infarction in women. Data from the Framingham Cohort-Women. (From Abbott RD, Wilson PW, Kannel WB, Castelli WP. High-density
lipoprotein cholesterol, total cholesterol screening, and myocardial infarction. Arteriosclerosis. 1988;8:207-11; with permission.)

males. Further, HDL cholesterol levels decrease dramatically only in white males. After sexual maturation, LDL cholesterol levels along with triglycerides and VLDL cholesterol levels tend to increase in females. However, these increases are relatively modest compared with those in males, especially white males. Clearly, the lipoprotein patterns of decreased levels of triglycerides, VLDL and LDL cholesterol, and elevated levels of HDL cholesterol in white women compared with white men is established during transition from adolescence to young adulthood. Blacks, on the other hand, show no such consistent gender-related differences.

Data from the Bogalusa Heart Study and the CARDIA Study suggest that the lipoprotein profiles of women versus men, both black and white, entering into young adulthood generally are beneficial in terms of cardiovascular risk (61,62). However, adverse levels are found in a considerable number of young women (7). The overall favorable lipoprotein profiles and lower blood pressure levels may account for the slower progression in women than men of atherosclerotic fibrous plaque raised lesions found in the aorta and coronary vessels (Fig. 7-5). These observations imply an overall hormonal protection before menopause; however, although these data show an average difference and slower development of coronary atherosclerosis in general, individual variations do occur. Some young adult women demonstrate a severity of atherosclerosis equal to that of young adult males.

In premenopausal women, including adolescents, increased adiposity adversely affects the lipoprotein profile (8,63). The magnitude of this adverse re-

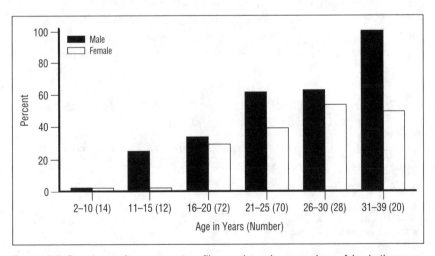

Figure 7-5 Prevalence of coronary artery fibrous plaque by sex and age. A lag in the severity of lesions occurs in females across the age span of 2 to 39 years. Data from the Bogalusa Heart Study.

lationship increases with age, although the association is somewhat weaker in black females. In addition, the use of oral contraceptives and cigarette smoking, especially in combination, results in an unfavorable lipoprotein profile, particularly in whites (64). (Serum lipids and lipoproteins in middle age and older women are discussed in Chapter 4.)

Carbohydrate Metabolism

The influence of obesity on cardiovascular risk is suggested to be mediated through hyperinsulinemia/insulin resistance, a key factor in carbohydrate and lipid metabolism. Obesity is strongly related to parameters of insulin metabolism, even in adolescents (Table 7-3) (65). Insulin and glucose levels are higher in more obese individuals and progressively increase as BMI increases in longitudinal follow-up (65,66).

A comparison of insulin metabolic parameters in obese (BMI > 90th percentile) versus nonobese (BMI < 90th percentile) adolescents shows obese individuals with higher values of plasma insulin, C-peptide, and insulin-to-glucose ratio, as well as lower C-peptide-to-insulin ratio, than nonobese individuals (see Table 7-3). Black females have consistently higher insulin levels than other race-sex groups during adolescence and young adulthood (49,66,67). Furthermore, insulin response to a glucose load is also highest in black females even at the earliest stage of sexual maturation (67). Lower C-peptide values and C-peptide-to-insulin ratios in blacks suggest reduced hepatic insulin clearance (49,65). Persistently high insulin levels could further lead to impaired insulin sensitivity as reflected in the fact that the lowest glucose-to-insulin ratio occurs in black females. These observations are consistent with reports showing that black women display among the highest incidence of non-insulin-dependent diabetes mellitus (68-70). An

Table 7-3 Comparison of Insulin Metabolism Parameters in Adolescents by Obesity Status: the Bogalusa Heart Study

Variables	Nonobese* (*n* = 1047)	Obese† (*n* = 110)
C-peptide (ng/mL)	1.74 ± 0.75	2.66 ± 0.93‡
Insulin (μU/mL)	11.7 ± 6.9	23.7 ± 12.3‡
C-peptide/insulin ratio	0.16 ± 0.06	0.13 ± 0.04‡
Insulin/glucose ratio	0.16 ± 0.08	0.29 ± 0.15‡

* BMI ≤ 90th percentile.
† BMI > 90th percentile.
‡ $p < 0.001$ (adjusted for age).
From Jiang X, Srinivasan SR, Berenson GS. Relation of obesity to insulin secretion and clearance in adolescents: the Bogalusa Heart Study. Int J Obes. 1996;20:951-6; with permission.

equally high incidence of diabetes occurs in Hispanic women and Native Americans (68,69).

Adult-Onset Diabetes Mellitus

As noted in the previous section, populations with higher rates of obesity are more likely to develop type II diabetes. Weight gain after age 18 and duration of weight gain are important predictors of the development of diabetes (70). Additionally, central fat distribution increases the subsequent risk of developing diabetes.

Diabetes is a major risk factor for heart attacks and coronary atherosclerosis in women (see Chapter 3). Data from the National Health Interview Survey in 1986 revealed that women aged 45 to 64 who die from CAD are substantially more likely to have diabetes. The CAD mortality rate for diabetic women compared with nondiabetic women was almost seven times greater for black women and nine times greater for white women (71,72). Because this study determined the presence of diabetes by questioning a relative or close friend and undiagnosed diabetes and glucose intolerance are common, these rates are probably a substantial underestimation of the impact of diabetes on coronary disease mortality. In those diagnosed with non-insulin-requiring diabetes, heart disease is the cause of about half of all deaths, with CAD the predominant etiology (3).

Women with diabetes are also at much greater risk for early CAD (3,71) and death after acute myocardial infarction (73). In the Nurses' Health Study, the attributed risk for cardiovascular disease from diabetes was three-fold greater in the presence of hypertension, smoking, and obesity (74). Thus, it is apparent that a combination of risk factors in women, especially involving alterations in insulin-carbohydrate metabolism, is important (3). Weight loss in diabetic women has been documented to improve glycemic control, insulin resistance, hypertension, and dyslipidemia (70).

Tobacco Use

Cigarette smoking is a major risk factor for CAD in women (75-77). Women who smoke have twice the risk of myocardial infarction as nonsmoking women and have their first myocardial infarction 19 years earlier. Although the total number of adult women who smoke has decreased since 1960, the number of teen-age girls or young women who smoke has actually increased (78). Secular trends in the Bogalusa Heart Study in recent years show a decrease of cigarette smoking in all the race-sex groups except in white girls (Fig. 7-6) (79). (For a more detailed discussion, see Chapter 2.)

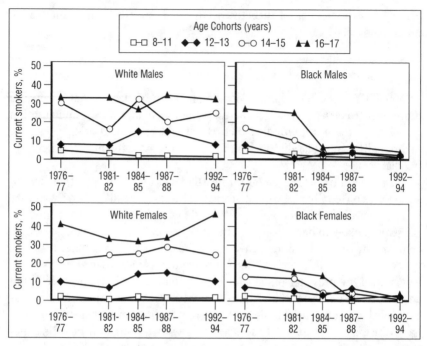

FIGURE 7-6 Trends in prevalence of current smoking status (at least 1 cigarette/week) in children aged 8 to 17 years, 1976-94. Note the continued high incidence of smoking in white females. Data from the Bogalusa Heart Study. (From Greenlund KJ, Johnson CC, Wattigney WA, et al. Trends in cigarette smoking among children in a Southern community, 1976-94: the Bogalusa Heart Study. Ann Epidemiol. 1996;6:467-82; with permission.)

Sedentary Lifestyles

Sedentary lifestyles are a common risk factor for CAD and contribute to the development and maintenance of obesity. Population studies have documented an inverse relationship between physical activity levels and obesity (80). Children aged 8 to 16 studied within the National Health and Nutrition Examination Survey III who watched more than 4 hours of television daily had a greater BMI than those who watched less than 2 hours a day. Although 80% of children overall reported three or more episodes of vigorous exercise weekly, this was more than reported by black (69%) and Mexican American (73%) girls (19).

A sedentary lifestyle was defined in National Health and Nutrition Survey III interviews (1988-91) as no leisure-time physical activity within the past month. (81). Although, overall, after age 19, 27% of women and 17% of men had sedentary lifestyles, there was substantial ethnic diversity. No leisure time activity was reported by 46% of Mexican American women, 40% of black women, and 23% of white women. Vigorous leisure-time activity at least three times a week was reported by only 3% of women, regardless of ethnicity, compared with 9% to 10% of men (depending on ethnicity). The 1990 National Health Interview Survey reviewed rates of regular exercise over the past 2 weeks and found women reported less leisure exercise than men in all age groups, although regular exercise was more often reported (82). In the 2 weeks before the interview, 37.8% of women aged 18 to 44 reported one or more activities at least three times a week compared with 31.8% of women aged 45 to 65 and 23% of women over age 65 (80). In both surveys, walking, gardening, and yard work were the most common forms of leisure-time exercise (80,82).

Socioeconomic Factors

Lower socioeconomic status is associated with a 25% higher risk of death from CAD than in the overall population (83). As described earlier, poor women are more likely to be obese. Lower social class at birth in Britain predicted higher rates of obesity as well as lower educational and employment achievement (84). Because in the United States lower socio-economic status results in less access to care and lower completion rates of health maintenance activities (83), prevention may be more difficult to implement.

Dietary Patterns

Dietary intake is a major determinant of cardiovascular risk. Observations from the Bogalusa Heart Study have shown that dietary intakes of young adult females aged 19 to 28 years do not vary according to race (85). Overall, women consumed 1945 kcal; with 14% of total energy from protein, 36% from fat (12% from saturated fat), and 50% from carbohydrates. A high percentage of young adult females exceeded the current dietary recommendations for total fat (73%), saturated fat (66%), and dietary cholesterol (53%).

Although dietary intakes between races are similar, specific foods contributing to nutrient intake vary by ethnicity (86). The major food contributors of total fat, saturated fat, dietary cholesterol, and sodium vary between races. In black women's diets a higher percentage of these nutrients came from pork, eggs, and snacks; in white women's diets from beef, fats and oils, and cheese.

Many American women, of all ages and body weights, attempt to lose weight by dietary restriction (87). The range of dietary patterns includes both subclinical and clinical eating disorders. There are obese women with bulimia or binge-purge patterns. Other women perceive themselves as being more overweight than they are, an essential element for the diagnosis of anorexia nervosa. Any discussion of dietary restriction with individual women should include screening for clinical eating disorders because dietary restriction is more complicated in this setting. Asking "Are you satisfied with your eating pattern?" and "Do you ever eat in secret?" has been found to be effective in screening for bulimia (88). Screening should include asking women their personal perception of their weight and open-ended exploration about what methods of weight loss have been attempted, including the use of exercise, emetics, and laxatives.

Implications and Management of Cardiovascular Risk in Early Life

Although it is easy to identify cardiovascular risk factors in childhood and to follow risk factor progression into young adulthood, screening for risk factors at any age is controversial (89) and not generally applied. Our observations do not agree with that approach. Prevention must begin early to achieve its maximum benefit. One approach is through education to deal with health values, improve dietary practices, and increase exercise activity directed to the prevention of obesity in young women. Further, ethnic differences related to cardiovascular disease have not yet generally been addressed in prevention programs.

We have, however, made an effort to begin prevention in early life with a public health approach. A comprehensive health education model, Health Ahead/Heart Smart, has been developed to address the large childhood population already at risk (90,91). This model shows the need for more medical professional involvement. Health promotion is introduced at a young age and designed to encourage healthier lifestyles throughout the entire school environment. Health Ahead/Health Smart begins in kindergarten and has been developed for elementary school. The program consists of a comprehensive health education curriculum and protocols for improving school nutrition and exercise activities. It involves parents and teachers and encourages them to improve their own lifestyles. The program addresses social problems faced by schools (e.g., drugs, alcohol abuse, dropouts, teenage pregnancy, violent behavior) by encouraging self-esteem beginning in kindergarten. It also encourages family and the community to become involved in the health education process. The potential for such a program is enormous.

An extension of our health education efforts has involved the development of a nutrition program for high school students (92). Although the program is not comprehensive in all health education aspects, it is an initial attempt to promote healthier eating habits in a nutritionally vulnerable, hard-to-reach population. Additional programs focusing on preventing weight gain, avoiding cigarette smoking, and increasing physical activity are needed for young women. These programs must be culturally sensitive, targeting specific foods that are major contributors of total fat, saturated fat, dietary cholesterol, and sodium in women's diets.

Implications and Management of Obesity in Middle-Aged and Older Adults

Throughout most of the life span, weight and BMI increase. The risk of coronary events and the development of diabetes, hypertension, and hyperlipidemia are related to BMI and the degree of excessive weight gain. Although most individuals gain weight incrementally over time, with increasing age it is substantially more difficult to lose significant amounts and maintain a lower weight. Fortunately, even modest weight loss has beneficial effects on blood pressure, glucose, and lipid profiles (4, 93). Weight loss without dieting, especially in the elderly, may indicate a serious medical problem (e.g., cancer, hyperthyroidism, cardiac or pulmonary cachexia). In patients over age 70 within NHANES follow-up, weight loss was often associated with constitutional illness (37). Frequently used modalities for weight loss include diet, exercise, behavioral therapy, and, less often, medications or surgical procedures such as a vertical-banded gastroplasty.

Dietary recommendations for weight loss utilize caloric reduction. The number of calories should be adjusted for the woman's level of physical activity. Effective weight loss can be achieved with either a high- or low-carbohydrate (high protein) diet (94). The high-carbohydrate diet is generally consistent with a healthy heart diet (see Chapter 5). The importance of small regular meals has been stressed (95). There are, however, negative behavioral and psychological implications in those who were previously normal eaters, greater irritability than those not experiencing food restriction, and an increased tendency to eat for reasons other than hunger (96). Diet and exercise are more effective than either modality alone (4).

Regular exercise, especially in conjunction with a proper diet, may help control obesity and improve the control of hypertension, diabetes, and improve insulin, glucose and lipoprotein levels (4, 97). Daily low-intensity exercise (walking) is usually better tolerated and more successfully adopted than high-intensity exercise, even if the daily caloric output is less (4). Long-term home exercise programs may be more effective than group exercise programs (98). Visceral fat reduction may be facilitated by exercise, especially aerobic exercise (99). (See Chapter 8 for a more extensive discussion of exercise recommendations and their implementation.)

Behavioral therapies for the management of obesity include individual and group counseling sessions that use techniques such as keeping a food diary, looking for and managing triggers for overeating, and changing the environment where one eats (for example, not engaging in other activities such as watching television while eating). Behavioral therapies without medications after 21 weeks resulted in an average 8.5 kg weight loss, although at a mean of 53 weeks follow-up an average weight loss of only 5.6 kg had been maintained (100). As with other modalities, the success of behavioral modalities with less intensive programs may be even smaller (70).

Other modalities for weight loss include pharmacological agents and vertical banding gastroplasty. Most trials of pharmacological agents for the treatment of obesity have been less than 6 months' duration, when the rate of weight loss tends to plateau. When combined with behavioral and exercise interventions, pharmacological agents may improve weight loss at 1 year, although information about long-term safety and side effects is limited (100). Surgical gastric procedures for those with BMI > 40 resulted in 30 to 40 kg weight loss. Most experts would only consider stapling in patients with BMI > 35 who have associated medical problems not responding to other modalities (4).

Even after successful short-term weight loss, weight maintenance is difficult to achieve (101,102). Adolescents have been found to be more effective in weight maintenance than middle aged adults (103), which is yet another reason for internists to focus on this group. One randomized intensive year-long trial of adults found that weight maintenance was more effective with a long-term, ad lib, low-fat, and high-carbohydrate diet than with fixed energy intake (104). Exercise may not only improve weight maintenance (99) but with or without weight loss be of cardiovascular benefit (72,97).

When weight maintenance is not achieved, weight cycling (recurrent weight loss followed by weight gain) occurs. Review of the published literature on weight cycling, from 1966 through 1994, revealed many methodologic limitations, especially in exploring the relationship between weight cycling, morbidity, and mortality. However, evidence that repeated weight loss efforts are metabolically different is lacking, although dietary compliance may be more difficult (105). In summary, the benefits of weight loss in obese women are greater than current theoretical concerns about weight cycling.

Summary

Of the 60 million children in the United States, half being girls, essentially 50% will ultimately die of cardiovascular disease but will have begun to show clinical evidence of heart disease at ages 30 to 40 years. The recognition of cardiovascular risk already associated with silent vascular lesions in adolescence and young adulthood emphasizes the importance of beginning preventive efforts in early life. This has been the message of the Bogalusa Heart

Study implicating the marked influence of obesity on cardiovascular risk beginning in childhood. It clearly shows that clinical cardiovascular risk factors can be identified in childhood and that these relate to underlying atherosclerotic and hypertensive disease. Health education models for children, like Health Ahead/Heart Smart and other programs (90,91,106) encouraging primary health promotion are needed to prevent obesity in the general population at a young age.

Successful programs for younger populations are critical because interventions in adult populations have been of limited success. In recent years, the U.S. population has become more overweight and obese, and the relationships between excess weight in women and the development of CAD events and multiple risk factors are now clearly evident. The prevention of obesity in women should begin in childhood.

Acknowledgments

The Bogalusa Heart Study represents the collaborative efforts of many people whose cooperation is gratefully acknowledged.

This work was supported by Grants HL38844 and HL 32194 from the National Heart, Lung, and Blood Institute of the U.S. Public Health Service.

REFERENCES

1. **Rosenbaum M, Leibel RL, Hirsch J. Obesity.** N Engl J Med.1997;337:396-407.
2a. **US Department of Health and Human Services.** Health, United States—1995. Chart Book. DHHS Pub. No. 96-12232-1.
2b. Executive summary of the clinical guidelines in the identification, evaluation and treatment of overweight and obesity in adults. Arch Intern Med. 1998;158:1855-67.
3. **Kannel WB.** Lipids, diabetes and coronary heart disease: insights from the Framingham Study. Am Heart J. 1985;110:1100-6.
4a. **Bjorntorp P.** Obesity. Lancet. 1997;350:423-6.
4b. **Eckel RH, Krauss RM, for the AHA Nutrition Committee.** American Heart Association Call to Action: obesity as a major risk factor for coronary heart disease. Circulation. 1998; 97:2099-2100.
5. **Johnston FE.** Health implications of childhood obesity. Ann Intern Med. 1985;103: 1068-72.
6. **Must A, Jacques PF, Dallal GE, et al.** Long term morbidity and mortality of overweight adolescents: a follow-up of the Harvard Growth Study of 1892 to 1935. N Engl J Med. 1992;327:1350-5.
7. **Wattigney WA, Webber LS, Srinivasan SR, Berenson GS.** The emergence of clinically abnormal levels of cardiovascular disease risk factor variables among young adults: the Bogalusa Heart Study. Prev Med. 1995;24:617-26.
8. **Gidding SS, Bao W, Srinivasan SR, Berenson GS.** Effects of secular trends in obesity on coronary risk factors in children: the Bogalusa Heart Study. J Pediatr. 1995;127: 868-74.

9. **Berenson GS, McMahan CA, Voors AW, et al.** Cardiovascular Risk Factors in Children: The Early Natural History of Atherosclerosis and Essential Hypertension. New York: Oxford Univ Pr; 1980.

10. **Berenson GS, ed.** Causation of Cardiovascular Risk Factors in Children: Perspectives on Cardiovascular Risk in Early Life. New York: Raven Pr; 1986.

11. Relationship of atherosclerosis in young men to serum lipoprotein cholesterol concentrations and smoking: a preliminary report from the Pathobiological Determinants of Atherosclerosis in Youth (PDAY) Research Group. JAMA. 1990;264:3018-29.

12. **Berenson GS, Srinivasan SR, Bao W, et al.** Association between multiple cardiovascular risk factors and atherosclerosis in children and young adults. N Engl J Med. 1998;338:1650-6.

13. **Whitaker RC, Wright JA, Pepe MS, et al.** Predicting obesity in young adulthood from childhood and parental obesity. N Engl J Med. 1997;337:869-73.

14. **Webber LS, Wattigney WA, Srinivasan SR, Berenson GS.** Obesity studies in Bogalusa. Am J Med Sci. 1995;310(Suppl 1):S53-S61.

15. **Kumanyika S.** Obesity in black women. Epidemiol Rev. 1987;9:31-50.

16. **Williamson DF, Kahn HS, Remington PL, Anda RF.** The ten-year incidence of overweight and major weight gain among United States adults. Arch Intern Med. 1990; 150:665-72.

17. **Freedman DS, Srinivasan SR, Valdez RA, et al.** Secular increases in relative weight and adiposity among children over two decades: the Bogalusa Heart Study. Pediatrics. 1997;99:420-6.

18. **Dietz WH, Gortmaker SL.** Do we fatten our children at the television set? Obesity and television viewing in children and adolescents. Pediatrics. 1985;75:807-12.

19. **Andersen RE, Crespo CJ, Bartlett SJ, et al.** Relationship of physical activity and television watching with body weight and level of fatness among children: results from the Third NHANES. JAMA. 1998;279:938-42.

20. **Friedman MA, Brownell KD.** Psychological correlates of obesity: moving to the next research generation. Psychol Bull. 1995;117:3-20.

21. **Gillum RF.** Overweight and obesity in black women: a review of published data from the National Center for Health Statistics. J Natl Med Assoc. 1987;79:865-71.

22. **Barrett-Connor EL.** Obesity, atherosclerosis, and coronary artery disease. Ann Intern Med. 1985;103:1010-8.

23. **Despres JP, Moorjani S, Lupien PJ, et al.** Regional distribution of body fat, plasma lipoproteins, and cardiovascular disease. Arteriosclerosis. 1990;10:497-511.

24. **Folsom AR, Kaye SA, Sellers TA, et al.** Body fat distribution and 5-year risk of death in older women. JAMA. 1993;269:483-7.

25. **Barrett-Connor E.** Sex differences in coronary heart disease: why are women so superior? The 1995 Ancel Keys lecture. Circulation. 1997;95:252-64.

26. **Young TK, Gelskey DE.** Is non-central obesity metabolically benign? Implications for prevention from a population survey. JAMA. 1995;274:1939-41.

27. **Lean MEJ, Han TX, Seidell JC.** Impairment of health and quality of life in people with large waist circumference. Lancet. 1998;351:853-6.

28. **Reaven GM.** Role of insulin resistance in human disease: Banting Lecture 1988. Diabetes. 1988;37:1595-1607.

29. **Kaplan NM.** The deadly quartet: upper-body adiposity, glucose intolerance, hypertriglyceridemia and hypertension. Arch Intern Med. 1989; 149:1514-20.

30. **Srinivasan SR, Bao W, Wattigney WA, Berenson GS.** Adolescent overweight is associated with adult overweight and related multiple cardiovascular risk factors: the Bogalusa Heart Study. Metabolism. 1996;45:235-40.

31. **Webber LS, Harsha DW, Phillips GT, et al.** Cardiovascular risk factors in Hispanic, white, and black children: the Brooks County and Bogalusa Heart Studies. Am J Epidemiol. 1991;133:704-14.

32. **Cooper RS, Simmons B, Castaner A, et al.** Survival rates and prehospital delay during myocardial infarction among black persons. Am J Cardiol. 1986;57:208-11.

33. **Wing RR, Matthews KA, Kuller LH, et al.** Weight gain at the time of menopause. Arch Intern Med. 1981;151:97-102.

34. **Manson JE, Colditz GA, Stampfer MJ, et al.** Prospective study of obesity and risk of coronary heart disease in women. N Engl J Med. 1990;322:882-9.

35. **Newton KM, LaCroix AZ.** Association of body mass index with reinfarction and survival after first myocardial infarction in women. J Womens Health. 1996;5:433-44.

36. **Willett WC, Manson JE, Stampfer MJ, et al.** Weight, weight change, and coronary heart disease in women: risk within the normal weight range. JAMA. 1995;273:461-5.

37. **Harris TB, Launer LJ, Feldman JJ.** Cohort study of effect of being overweight and change in weight on risk of coronary heart disease in old age. BMJ. 1997;314:1791-4.

38. **Bush TL.** The epidemiology of cardiovascular disease in postmenopausal women. Ann NY Acad Sci. 1990;592:263-71.

39. **Berenson GS, Wattigney WA, Webber LS.** Blood pressure in children and factors predisposing to hypertensive disease in adults. In: Pediatric Cardiology. Vol 4. (Godman MJ, ed). Edinburgh: Churchill Livingstone; 1981:591-600.

40. **Voors AW, Webber LS, Berenson GS.** Epidemiology of essential hypertension in youth: implications for clinical practice. Pediatr Clin North Am. 1978;25:15-27.

41. **Falkner B, Kushner H, Onesti B, Angelakos ET.** Cardiovascular characteristics in adolescents who develop essential hypertension. Hypertension. 1981;3:521-7.

42. **Murphy JK, Alpert BS, Moss DM, Sands GW.** Race and cardiovascular reactivity: a neglected relationship. Hypertension. 1986;8:1075-83.

43. **Berenson GS, Wattigney WA, Webber LS.** Epidemiology of hypertension from childhood to young adulthood in black, white and Hispanic population samples. Public Health Rep. 1996;111:3-6.

44. **Haffner SM.** Hypertension in the San Antonio Heart Study and the Mexico City Diabetes Study: clinical and metabolic correlates. Public Health Rep. 1996;111:11-14.

45. **Voors AW, Berenson GS, Dalferes ER Jr., et al.** Racial differences in blood pressure control. Science. 1979;204:1091-4.

46. **Berenson GS, Voors AW, Webber LS, et al.** Racial differences of parameters associated with blood pressure levels in children: the Bogalusa Heart Study. Metabolism. 1979;28:1218-28.

47. **Voors AW, Berenson GS, Shuler SE, Webber LS.** Blood pressure electrolyte clearance, and plasma renin activity in children sampled from an entire community. J Appl Biochem. 1980;2:87-99.

48. **Voors AW, Dalferes ER Jr, Frank GC, et al.** Relation between ingested potassium and sodium balance in young blacks and whites. Am J Clin Nutr. 1983;37:583-94.

49. **Jiang X, Srinivasan SR, Radhakrishnamurthy B, et al.** Racial (black-white) differences in insulin secretion and clearance in adolescents: the Bogalusa Heart Study. Pediatrics. 1996;97:357-60.

50. **Jiang X, Srinivasan SR, Bao W, Berenson GS.** Association of fasting insulin with blood pressure in young individuals: the Bogalusa Heart Study. Arch Intern Med. 1993;153:323-8.

51. **Kannel WB, Abbott RD.** A prognostic comparison of asymptomatic left ventricular hypertrophy and unrecognized myocardial infarction: the Framingham study. Am Heart J. 1986;111:391-7.

52. **Lauer MS, Anderson KM, Kannel WB, Levy D.** The impact of obesity on left ventricular mass and geometry: Framingham Heart Study. JAMA. 1991;266:231-6.

53. **de Simone G, Devereux RB, Roman MJ, et al.** Relation of obesity and gender to left ventricular hypertrophy in normotensive and hypertensive adults. Hypertension. 1994;23:600-6.

54. **Gardin JM, Wagenknecht LY, Anton-Culver H, et al.** Relationship of cardiovascular risk factors to echocardiographic left ventricular mass in healthy black and white adult men and women: the CARDIA study. Circulation 1995;92:380-7.

55. **Urbina EM, Gidding SS, Boa W, et al.** Effect of body size ponderosity and blood pressure in left ventricular growth children and young adults: the Bogalusa Heart Study. Circulation. 1995;91:2400-6.

56. **Gordon T, Castelli WP, Hjortland MC, et al.** High-density lipoprotein as a protective factor against coronary heart disease: the Framingham Study. Am J Med. 1977;62:707-14.

57. **Elveback LR, Connolly DC, Melton LJ.** Coronary heart disease in residents of Rochester, Minnesota. VII. Incidence—1950-1982. Mayo Clinic Proc. 1986;61:896-900.

58. **Castelli WP.** The triglyceride issue: a view from Framingham. Am Heart J. 1986;112:432-7.

59. **Berenson GS, Srinivasan SR, Cresanta JL, et al.** Dynamic changes in serum lipoproteins in children during adolescence and sexual maturation. Am J Epidemiol. 1981;113:157-70.

60. The Lipid Research Clinics Population Studies Databook. Vol 1. The Prevalence Study. Washington, DC: US Department of Health and Human Services, 1980; NIH Publication No. 80-1527.

61. **Donahue RP, Jacobs DR, Sidney S, et al.** Distribution of lipoproteins and apolipoproteins in young adults: the CARDIA Study. Arteriosclerosis. 1989;9:656-64.

62. **Srinivasan SR, Wattigney W, Webber LS, Berenson GS.** Race and gender differences in serum lipoproteins of children, adolescents, and young adults: emergence of an adverse lipoprotein pattern in white males: the Bogalusa Heart Study. Prev Med. 1991;20:671-84.

63. **Bao W, Srinivasan SR, Wattigney WA, Berenson GS.** Persistence of multiple cardiovascular risk clustering related to syndrome X from childhood to young adulthood: the Bogalusa Heart Study. Arch Intern Med. 1994;154:1842-7.

64. **Voors AW, Srinivasan SR, Hunter SM, et al.** Smoking, oral contraceptives, and serum lipid and lipoprotein levels in children of a total biracial community. Prev Med. 1982;11:1-12.

65. **Jiang X, Srinivasan SR, Berenson GS.** Relation of obesity to insulin secretion and clearance in adolescents: the Bogalusa Heart Study. Int J Obes. 1996;20:951-6.

66. **Folsom AR, Jacobs DR, Wagenknecht LE, et al.** Increase in fasting insulin and glucose over seven years with increasing weight and inactivity of young adults: the CARDIA Study. Am J Epidemiol. 1996;144:235-46.

67. **Svec F, Natasi K, Hilton C, et al.** Black-white contrasts in insulin levels during pubertal development: the Bogalusa Heart Study. Diabetes. 1992;41:313-7.

68. **Carter JS, Pugh JA, Monterossa A.** Non–insulin-dependent diabetes in minorities in the United States. Ann Int Med. 1996;125:221-32.

69. **Harris MI, Hadden WC, Knowler WC, Bennett PH.** Prevalence of diabetes and impaired glucose tolerance and plasma glucose levels in US population ages 20-74 yr. Diabetes. 1987;36:523-4.

70. **Maggio CA, Pi-Sunyer EX.** The prevention and treatment of obesity: application to type 2 diabetes. Diabetes Care. 1997;20:1744-65.

71. **Will JC, Casper M.** The contribution of diabetes to early death from ischemic heart disease: US gender and race comparisons. Am J Pub Health. 1996;86:576-9.

72. **Mosca R, Manson JE, Sutherland SE, et al.** Cardiovascular health in women: a statement for health care professionals from the American Heart Association. Circulation. 1997;96:2468-82.

73. **Behar S, Boyko V, Reicher-Reiss, Goldbourt U.** Ten-year survival after acute myocardial infarction: comparison of patients with and without diabetes. Am Heart J. 1997; 133:290-6.

74. **Manson JE, Colditz GA, Stampfer MJ, et al.** A prospective study of obesity and risk of coronary heart disease in women. N Engl J Med. 1990;322:882-9.

75. **Rigotti, N.** Cigarette smoking and body weight [Editorial]. N Engl J Med. 1989;320: 931-3.

76. **Hansen EF, Andersen LT, Von Eyben FE, et al.** Cigarette smoking and age at first onset of myocardial infarction, and influence of gender and extent of smoking. Am J Cardiol. 1993;71:1439-42.

77. **Johnson A.** Sex differentials in coronary heart disease: the explanatory role of primary risk factors. J Health Soc Behav. 1977;18:46-54.

78. Tobacco use among high school students-United States, 1997. MMWR Morb Mortal Wkly Rpt. 1998;47:224-33.

79. **Greenlund KJ, Johnson CC, Wattigney WA, et al.** Trends in cigarette smoking among children in a Southern community, 1976-1994: the Bogalusa Heart Study. Ann Epidemiol. 1996;6:476-82.

80. **NIH Consensus Development Panel on Physical Activity and Cardiovascular Health.** Physical activity and cardiovascular health. JAMA. 1996;276:241-6.

81. **Crespo, CJ, Keteyian SJ, Heath GW. Sempos CT.** Leisure-time physical activity among US adults: results from the Third National Health and Nutrition Examination Survey. Arch Intern Med. 1996;156:93-8.

82. **Yusuf HR, Croft JB, Giles WH, et al.** Leisure-time physical activity among older adults: United States, 1990. Arch Intern Med. 1996;156:1321-6.

83. **Kahn HS, Williamson DF.** Is race associated with weight change in US adults after adjustment for income, education and marital factors? Am J Clin Nutr. 1991;15:66S-70S.

84. **Power C, Matthews S.** Origins of health inequalities in a national population sample. Lancet. 1997;350:1584-9.

85. **Nicklas TA, Johnson CC, Myers L, et al.** Eating patterns nutrient intakes and alcohol consumption patterns of young adults. Medicine, Exercise, Nutrition, and Health (MENH). 1995;4:316-24.

86. **O'Neil CE, Nicklas TA, Myers L, et al.** Racial differences in dietary intakes of young adult females: the Bogalusa Heart Study. J Am Diet Assoc. 1996;96(Suppl):A57.

87. **Manore MA.** Chronic dieting in active women: what are the health consequences? Womens Health Issues. 1996;6:332-41.

88. **Freund KM, Graham SM, Lesky LG, Moskowitz MA.** Detection of bulimia in a primary care setting. J Gen Intern Med. 1993;8:236-42.

89. **Garber AM, Browner WS, Hulley SB.** Cholesterol screening in asymptomatic adults revisited. Ann Int Med. 1996;124:518-31.

90. **Downey AM, Butcher AH, Frank GC, et al.** Development and implementation of a school health promotion program for the reduction of cardiovascular risk factors in children and prevention of adult coronary heart disease: "Heart Smart." In: Berenson GS, ed. Cardiovascular Risk Factors in Childhood: Epidemiology and Prevention Hetzel. Amsterdam: Elsevier Science Publishers; 1987;103-21.

91. **Downey AM, Cresanta JL, Berenson GS.** Cardiovascular health promotion: "Heart Smart" and the changing role of the physician. Am J Prev Med. 1989;5:279-95.

92. **Nicklas TA, Johnson CC, Farris R, et al.** Development of a school-based nutrition intervention for high school students: Gimme 5. Am J Health Promotion (in press).

93. **Wilding J.** Science, medicine and the future: obesity treatment. BMJ. 1997;315:997-1000.

94. **Golay A, Eigenheer C, Morel Y, et al.** Weight-loss with low or high carbohydrate diet? Int J Obes. 1996;20:1067-72.

95. **Monteleone GP, Browning DG.** Nutrition in women: assessment and counseling. Prim Care. 1997;24:37-51.

96. **Polivy J.** Psychological consequences of food restriction. J Am Diet Assoc. 1996;96:589-92.

97. **Blair SN.** Evidence for success of exercise in weight loss and control. Ann Intern Med. 1993;119:702-6.

98. **Perri MG, Martin AD, Leemakers EA, et al.** Effects of group- versus home-based exercise in the treatment of obesity. J Consult Clin Psychol. 1997;65:278-85.

99. **Garber CE.** The benefits of physical activity on coronary heart disease and coronary heart disease risk factors in women. Womens Health Issues. 1997;7:17-23.

100. **National Task Force on the Prevention and Treatment of Obesity.** Long-term pharmacotherapy in the management of obesity. JAMA. 1996;276:1907-15.

101. **Robison JI, Hoerr SL, Standmark J, Mavis B.** Obesity, weight loss and health. J Am Diet Assoc. 1993;93:444-9.

102. **Grodstein F, Levine R, Spencer T, et al.** Three-year follow-up of participants in a commercial weight loss program: can you keep it off? Arch Intern Med. 1966; 156:1302-6.

103. **Epstein LH, Valoski AM, Kalarchian MA, McCurley J.** Do children lose and maintain weight easier than adults?: a comparison of child and parent weight changes from six months to ten years. Obes Res. 1995;3:411-7.

104. **Toubro S, Astrup A.** Randomized comparison of diets for maintaining obese subjects weight after major weight loss: add lib, low fat, high carbohydrate diet vs. fixed energy intake. BMJ. 1997;314:29-34.

105. **National Task Force on the Prevention and Treatment of Obesity.** Weight cycling. JAMA. 1994;272:1196-1202.

106. **National Institutes of Health.** National Heart, Lung and Blood Institute Cardiovascular Health Promotion Project. Heart Memo, Special Edition. NHLBI Information Center: Bethesda, MD; 1996:10.

CHAPTER 8

Exercise as Primary and Secondary Prevention

JOAN M. FAIR, RN, NP, PHD
KATHLEEN BERRA, MSN, ANP
ABBY C. KING, PHD

Hippocrates advised taking exercise for health. Today, the admonition might well be "Run (or at least walk) for your life."

Increasing evidence suggests that regular, moderate physical activity promotes health and longevity for both women and men (1,2). In spite of the health benefits attributed to exercise, current estimates find that 40% to 55% of American adults report little or no leisure-time physical activity (LTPA) (2,3). Further, approximately 10% of men and only 3% of women report participating in vigorous LTPAs at least three times per week (3). Among adult women, survey data reveal that only 27% report participating in moderate activities five or more days per week, with lower rates of participation among Hispanic women (24.7%) and black non-Hispanic women (17.5%) (4). Thus, more than 70% of women are underactive and are not deriving the health benefits associated with moderate or more vigorous regular physical activity. In the Third National Health and Nutrition Examination Survey, lower socioeconomic class was associated with greater physical inactivity (5). This chapter focuses on the health benefits of physical activity, particularly as they apply to women. The relationship between physical activity and coronary artery disease is discussed. Finally, recommendations and strategies for enhancing the exercise health benefits among women are given.

Physical Activity and Health

A sedentary lifestyle has been associated with increased risk of premature death for all leading causes of death (6). Physical inactivity has been linked to the development of coronary artery disease (CAD) (1,7), stroke (8), cancers of the colon and breast (9,10), non–insulin-dependent diabetes (11,12), obesity (13,14), osteoporosis (15), and decrements in psychologic health and well-being (16,17). It is estimated that 12% of all deaths in the United States are related to physical inactivity (18).

Coronary artery disease is the leading cause of death and disability for adult women and men. Although mortality rates from CAD have declined over the last decade in the U.S. population, current trends suggest that CAD mortality rates are increasing for women (18). In 1992, 51.9% of CAD deaths occurred in women. This trend, coupled with a low prevalence of physical activity among women, warrants an examination of the evidence linking CAD and sedentary lifestyles.

Physical Activity and Coronary Artery Disease

Over 40 published studies have examined the relationship between physical activity and mortality. These studies have used various measures to determine physical activity levels ranging from occupational codes, to self-report ratings, to objective measures of physical fitness. Meta-analysis of these studies concluded that studies using sound methods consistently found an inverse relationship between the level of physical activity and the incidence of CAD death (19,20). When the highest level of physical activity was compared with the lowest level, the strength of the association was estimated as a relative risk for CAD death of 1.6 to 1.8 (20). As shown in Table 8-1, comparisons of CAD risk factors reveal that the strength of the association between physical activity and CAD is similar to that of well-recognized CAD risk factors such as smoking and hyperlipidemia.

Many of the studies included in the above meta-analyses were controlled for confounding factors, such as age and the presence of other CAD risk factors; however, as with other CAD risk factor studies, few have included women in sufficient numbers to permit gender-specific analysis. In those studies that did include specific analyses of women, the association of physical activity and cardiovascular mortality was inconsistent.

One of the first studies to report such gender analysis was a Finnish study of 3688 women and 3978 men aged 30 to 59 years and followed for 7 years (27). After adjustment for other cardiovascular risk factors, a low level of occupational activity was associated with an increased risk of acute myocardial

Table 8-1 Comparisons of Estimated Reductions in Coronary Artery Disease with Risk Factor Modification

Risk Factor	Estimated Reduction in CAD Risk
Cessation of cigarette smoking	50%–70% (21)
Decrease in blood cholesterol levels	1 mg/dL decrease in cholesterol is associated with 2%–3% decrease in CAD risk (22)
	Dietary modification lowers cholesterol ~5%–15% (23)
	Drug therapies lower cholesterol ~15%–35% (24)
Increase in HDL cholesterol levels	1 mg/dL increase in HDL is associated with 3%–5% decrease in CAD risk (25)
Treatment of hypertension	1 mm Hg reduction associated with 2%–3% in CAD
	Average reductions in clinical trials are ~5–6 mm Hg (21)
Physically active lifestyle	25%–55% reduction in CAD risk as compared with sedentary lifestyle (21, 26)

CAD = coronary artery disease; HDL = high-density lipoprotein.

infarction (MI) for both women (relative risk [RR]: 2.4; 90% confidence interval [CI]: 1.5–3.7) and men (RR: 1.5; 90% CI: 1.2–2.0). When LTPA was used as the activity measure and other coronary risk factors were similarly controlled, relative risks for acute MI did not reach statistically significant levels for either women or men.

In the Framingham study of 1404 women aged 50 to 74 years that were followed for 16 years, those with the highest levels of self-reported physical activity had approximately 30% lower overall mortality rates as compared with sedentary women (28). There was, however, no significant association between physical activity level and the incidence of cardiovascular disease or cardiovascular death, suggesting that increased survival among physically active women is due to factors other than cardiovascular disease. To clarify this issue, Blair and colleagues (29) measured both physical fitness (assessed by a maximal exercise test) and self-reported LTPAs or recreational activities in more than 3,000 women and 10,000 men. After an average follow-up of 8 years, low physical fitness was associated significantly with increased all-cause mortality in both women and men; however, low levels of self-reported physical activity were associated with increased mortality only in men. This study raised the possibility that traditional self-reported measures of physical activity do not capture sources of physical activity among women. In a subsequent study, Blair and colleagues (30) demonstrated that low physical fitness was associated with increased risks for both all-cause (RR: 1.52; 95% CI: 1.3–1.8) as well as cardiovascular (RR: 1.70; 95% CI: 1.3–2.3) mortality in men. Among the smaller sample of women being followed, low physical fitness was significantly associated with all-cause (RR: 2.10; 95% CI: 1.4–3.3) but not cardiovascular (RR: 2.42; 95% CI: 0.99–5.92) mortality.

In contrast to these results, LaCroix and colleagues (31) found that walking more than 4 hours per week was associated with a significantly reduced risk for cardiovascular hospitalizations and deaths for women (RR: 0.63; 95% CI: 0.44–0.90). Among men, a similar magnitude of reduced risk of events was observed; however, statistical significance was not achieved due to the small number of events in this subset (RR: 0.67; 95% CI: 0.44–0.1.02). This study included 1030 women and 615 men aged 65 years and older, without a history of CAD at baseline. The older ages in this sample, the larger sample of women compared with men, and a focus on the most commonly reported exercise activity for women likely contributed to the associations reported in this study. Recently reported data from the Nurses Health Study confirmed that longer walking time each week is associated with a lower risk of CAD and stroke (32).

The preceding studies, although they report some inconsistent results, demonstrate overall that the magnitude of risks associated with low levels of physical activity and physical fitness are similar for women and men; in fact, the relative risk may be higher for women (33). The strength of the association when fitness rather than physical activity is assessed is at least as strong as that for men. The lack of a consistent association between physical activity and CAD in women has been attributed to both the small numbers of women included in studies and to difficulties in measuring physical activity. Most studies have focused on occupational or leisure-time sports activity and have failed to estimate energy expenditure for household tasks and walking, two activities that are likely more representative of female activities (34). The achievement of statistical significance among the female subgroups in these studies has also been limited by restricting the sample age to less than 65 years, thereby reducing the number of CAD end points among women. In a 7-year follow-up of a large cohort of over 40,000 postmenopausal women, a graded inverse relationship between physical activity and all-cause as well as cardiovascular mortality was observed (35). This study suggests that the beneficial effects of physical activity extend to older as well as younger women and that the benefits are at least equal to those observed in men.

Physical Activity and Secondary Prevention

The evidence supporting the role of physical activity in the secondary prevention of CAD primarily comes from meta-analysis of randomized clinical trials that examined the protective effect of exercise and recurrent coronary events (16,36,37). The exercise interventions in the studies included in these meta-analysis consisted of exercise alone or exercise in combination with multifactorial risk reduction. These analyses found that patients randomized to exercise interventions following MI had an approximate 25% reduction in total and cardiovascular mortality after 3 years of follow-up as compared with control patients. Exercise interventions have resulted in mortality reductions similar to that of beta-blocker use after MI (37). It should be noted that these studies included few women (3% of the overall meta-analysis sample), which limited the ability to generalize these benefits to women (38).

Recent evidence from the angiographic regression trials provided further evidence to support the notion that exercise may slow the progression of atherosclerosis and stabilize coronary lesions. Three of the angiographic regression studies included an exercise component as a part of the multifactorial study interventions (39–41). The exercise programs consisted of moderate-intensity aerobic programs. In these studies, there was significantly less progression of coronary disease in the intervention groups than in the control groups. Regression of disease, likewise, favored the intervention groups. Generally, the use of multifactorial interventions has not permitted determination of the unique contributions of physical activity. However, using multivariate regression, the Heidelberg study found that low-density lipoprotein (LDL) level at 1 year, the 1-year change in the ratio of cholesterol to high-density lipoprotein (HDL), and LTPA were significant independent predictors of change in coronary diameters (41). In the Stanford Coronary Risk Intervention Project (SCRIP), the best two-variable model included change in treadmill exercise performance and the change in the Framingham risk score (a composite score based on blood pressure, total and HDL cholesterol, and cigarette smoking) (39). An increase in treadmill exercise performance was predictive of a slower rate of atherosclerotic progression.

As with many other cardiovascular intervention studies, few women were included in the angiographic regression trials. In the SCRIP study (39), angiographic rates of progression in the treatment group were slightly less for women (–0.016 mm/y) as compared with men (–0.026 mm/y). The rate of change among the control group was similar for women and men (–0.046 mm/y and –0.045 mm/y, respectively). Although the magnitude of the difference in angiographic progression was greater for women, this difference did not achieve statistical significance due to the small number of women ($n = 30$). These studies, however, provide further evidence that exercise is an important component of secondary prevention of CAD and that the benefit likely extends to women as well as men. Given this evidence, recent guidelines mandate the inclusion of regular physical activity as an important component for the overall treatment and management of the coronary patient (42,43).

Exercise-based cardiac rehabilitation programs have the potential to play a significant role in secondary prevention. Despite continuing evidence of the efficacy of exercise in secondary prevention, survey data show that less than 20% of patients with CAD participate in such programs (44,45). In 1990, a survey of cardiac rehabilitation programs in the United States estimated that

6.9% of women and 13.3% of men participated in cardiac rehabilitation programs after MI (45). One of the reasons suggested for this disparity is that women experience heart disease at an older age and older patients are less likely to participate in exercise programs; however, in a study of coronary patients over 62 years of age, participation was greater for men than women (25% and 15%, respectively) (46). This suggests that age may not account entirely for the disparity. These studies have found that physician endorsement and referral is one of the strongest predictors of participation for older patients (46) and for women (47). Other studies suggest that women and men have different experiences and preferences with respect to exercise. Women, for example, report more pain and fatigue with exercise than men (48). In addition, women have lower exercise tolerance and are more anxious about exercise (49). Women generally have more comorbidities, such as arthritis, hypertension, and diabetes (48), and have less favorable coronary risk factor profiles (50). These differing experiences likely influence entry into exercise-based programs; however, women do gain substantial benefits from participation in such programs. Following 12 weeks of program participation, both women and men have improvements in exercise capacity. Cannistra and colleagues (50) found that although women had lower baseline functional capacity than men (4.5 METs and 5.5 METs, respectively), post-training exercise capacity increased by 20% for women and 15% for men, suggesting that the magnitude of improvement in exercise capacity is similar for both (50). Modest improvements in other coronary risk factors (e.g., lipid levels) have been observed following participation in cardiac rehabilitation programs, and the magnitude of change is again similar for both sexes (50,51). Thus, for both women and men, secondary prevention can be achieved by participation in cardiac rehabilitation programs.

Physical Activity: Mechanisms

Effect on Risk Factors for Coronary Artery Disease

Although there is considerable evidence that physical activity exerts an independent effect on CAD risk, physical activity also influences other known coronary risk factors, including plasma lipids and lipoproteins, glucose metabolism, hypertension, and obesity. The effects of exercise training on lipids has been studied extensively. Most cross-sectional comparisons of exercisers compared with sedentary controls suggest that long-term exercise training results in increased HDL levels (52,53). However, when sedentary subjects are randomized to training regimes, the confounding effects of exercise-induced weight loss often obscure the relationship. Studies comparing weight loss by diet with weight loss by exercise training show that diet-induced effects that lower HDL levels are counteracted by the addition of exercise training in both women and men (52). Similarly, exercise training alone appears to have little effect on LDL levels (54). Some evidence, however, suggests that the exercisers have less of the small, dense, atherogenic LDL subfraction compared with sedentary controls (52). Exercise has been shown to enhance consistently lipoprotein lipase activity and the clearance of circulating triglycerides, which results in lower levels of triglycerides and very-low-density lipoprotein (VLDL) (52). This effect is observed in both women and men and results in an improved ratio of total cholesterol to HDL in response to exercise training (55).

The majority of exercise training studies have used vigorous forms of exercise (e.g., jogging). However, recent evidence suggests that more moderate-intensity forms of regular physical activity (e.g., walking) can have a positive impact on the HDL cholesterol levels of both premenopausal (56) and postmenopausal women (57) that is independent of noticeable changes in body weight. Furthermore, it appears that exercise-related changes in HDL-C levels may take a longer period of time (i.e., up to 2 years) to become evident in older women (57).

Glucose intolerance and the presence of diabetes are considered risk factors for CAD and pose a significantly greater CAD risk for women compared with men (30). For both women and men, regular physical activity is associated with a reduced incidence of non–insulin-dependent diabetes (58,59). Exercise has direct metabolic effects on glucose metabolism, reducing glucose intolerance and improving insulin sensitivity. Exercise increases blood flow and glucose transport to skeletal muscle, increasing glucose uptake and resulting in lowered plasma glucose and insulin levels (12). Importantly for women, moderate-intensity exercises such as walking are equally as effective as higher intensity exercises in provoking these changes (11). In addition, it appears that the acute effects of exercise, rather than the training effect, are most responsible for these benefits (60). This underscores the importance of regular exercise.

An inverse relationship between blood pressure and physical activity level has been demonstrated for both women and men (61). Reaven and colleagues (62) found that both systolic and diastolic blood pressures were significantly lower among women in all categories of physical activity intensity (light, moderate, or heavy) compared with sedentary women. These relationships persisted after adjustment for age, body weight, and insulin levels. Blood pressure is controlled by a variety of mechanisms, many of which are altered by exercise training. For example, exercise increases peripheral vascular vasodilation and reduces catecholamine activity and plasma insulin levels. It is likely that all of these mechanisms play a role in lowering blood pressure among the physically active.

Obesity, particularly abdominal obesity (truncal obesity), has been linked to hypertension, glucose intolerance, hyperinsulinemia, and lipid disorders; these factors in combination seem to enhance CAD risk in particular (63). Physical activity has been suggested as an important treatment strategy for obesity. Reviews of the role of exercise in weight regulation suggest that exercise enhances both initial and long-term maintenance of weight loss (14); however, exercise appears to be a less effective weight-loss modality for women than for men (64). When patterns of fat distribution are considered, women with abdominal or male-pattern obesity respond to exercise with greater loss of fat mass compared with women with gluteal–femoral obesity (13).

Epidemiologic studies have suggested that fibrinogen levels are related to the development of CAD for both women (65) and men (66). Several factors, including exercise training, have been linked to fibrinogen levels in men (67); however, this relationship has not been fully supported in studies including women. In a study of 874 postmenopausal women, LTPA was significantly inversely associated with fibrinogen level (68). In multivariate analysis, however, physical activity level was no longer predictive of fibrinogen level once factors such as age, body mass index, smoking status, alcohol intake, and hormone use were taken into account. Clearly, more research is needed to determine the effects of hemostatic factors on CAD development and to clarify the role of exercise in modifying these factors.

Effects on the Cardiovascular System

In addition to the influence of physical activity on risk factors known to contribute to the development of CAD, physical activity has direct physiologic effects on the cardiovascular system. Exercise increases heart rate, stroke volume, and blood flow to skeletal muscles, resulting in decreased peripheral vascular resistance and enhanced cardiac output (69,70). Adaptation to exercise training results in increased cross-sectional muscle fiber area, increased numbers of capillaries, improved extraction and use of energy substrates, and greater perfusion pressures and vasodilatory responses of coronary arteries (69). Exercise training also results in lower resting and submaximal exercise heart rates, increases in plasma volume, and improved exercise tolerance.

Some differences in cardiac functioning are apparent between women and men. Because women have smaller heart and artery sizes compared with men (71), cardiac output is increased primarily by increasing heart rate, with smaller contributions resulting from increased stroke volume. As a result, women have lower maximum oxygen uptake and a lower work capacity than men. In addition, women in general have lower hemoglobin levels than men, further reducing their oxygen-carrying capacity (71). When exercise training effects are compared, women have a percentage increase in exercise capacity that is similar to men. In fact, some researchers suggest that women may have a greater benefit from exercise training because a lower threshold of intensity is required to obtain a similar magnitude of change in exercise capacity as compared with men (72).

Psychological Benefits Associated with Exercise

The recent scientific literature suggests that psychosocial factors, such as a predisposition to anger arousal or anxiety, and a disengagement cluster that includes depression may be determinants of diseases such as CAD (73,74). The presence of these factors may also alter responses to treatment and result in poorer health outcomes. In the cardiovascular literature, depression and anxiety have been linked in several prospective longitudinal studies to an increased risk of CAD (75) as well as poor health outcomes following MI (76). Negative emotional states have also been associated with physical inactivity. For example, it has been reported that depressive symptoms are twice as common among the physically inactive (77). Similarly, physical activity and physical fitness are associated with reduced anxiety levels (78). Several studies have examined the effect of physical activity on measures of negative mood states and on perceptions of well-being, self-esteem enhancement, and quality of life (79). Exercise training appears to decrease ratings of stress and anxiety and to enhance perceptions of physical functioning and well-being (15,80–84). Exercise effects on depression are mixed. Exercise is more effective in reducing depression among those with manifestations of clinical depression; however, excessive exercise training has been associated with an increase in depressive symptoms among nondepressed athletes (85). In the few studies that have included women, it has been shown that more moderate-intensity exercises, such as walking, confer the exercise and psychosocial benefits described above (80,84).

In summary, it is clear that regular physical activity of moderate or more vigorous intensity can provide women of all ages with a variety of benefits, ranging from prevention and control of cardiovascular disease and other chronic conditions to the promotion of improved physical and psychological functioning and quality of life. The challenge remains how to adequately inform and motivate women to increase their physical activity levels. It is here, as discussed in the next section, that the physician and other health care professionals can play an important role.

Guidelines for Physical Activity

As noted previously, physical activity is critical to health and quality of life throughout the life span. Many factors influence physical activity levels, including social, behavioral, cultural, genetic, and biological determinants. Factors such as age, health status, psychological variables, and sociodemographics all play a role. Earlier in this chapter, the epidemiology and health effects of physical activity were discussed. This section describes guidelines for physical activity, including specifics of exercise prescription, health education to promote physical activity participation, sign and symptom monitoring, and adherence counseling. Safety is discussed also, because it remains a major consideration in the process of evaluation and counseling. Our goal is to familiarize the reader with practical approaches to the development of physical activity recommendations for women without evidence of CAD and for those at high risk for or with established CAD.

Recommendations for Physical Activity

Physicians and other health care providers are important in influencing the adoption and maintenance of positive exercise habits. *Healthy People 2000* identifies physician counseling for physical activity as an important objective (86). This objective is also supported by the U.S. Preventive Services Task Force, which recommends physician counseling for all sedentary patients (87). Williford and colleagues (88) reported that in one sample of physicians, 91% encouraged their sedentary patients to exercise regularly. Another study, however, reported only 39% of private practice physicians counseled their inactive patients (89). Freidman and colleagues (90) surveyed patients and found only 15% of sedentary patients reporting physician advice to become more active. Clearly, it is difficult from the available data to determine accurate estimates of physician advice about physical activity in sedentary patients. The effect of physician counseling in the adoption of physical activity has been evaluated in only a few studies. Two of the studies indicated that physician advice was effective in increasing activity levels (91,92), whereas one study reported less convincing results (93). It remains important, however, for physicians to be involved in the counseling and advice efforts to increase physical activity levels.

The recent Report of the Surgeon General on Physical Activity and Health summarizes the current national physical activity recommendations (Box 8-1), providing guidelines that are credible and easily understood (77). The physician's role is to urge strongly that patients participate in a safe exercise program. Safety relates to cardiovascular, musculoskeletal, and psychologic health. The "art" of recommending physical activity encompasses the physician's ability to assess current activity patterns and to identify barriers to regular participation and potential safety issues. Assessment of physical activity can be as simple as asking, "At least once a week, do you engage in any regular physical activity, such as brisk walking, jogging, or bicycling, long enough to work up a sweat? If so, how many days per week?" The validity of these questions in evaluating physical activity levels, including their use in women,

---

Box 8-1 Summary of Recent Physical Activity Recommendations

- All people over the age of 2 years should accumulate at least 30 minutes of endurance-type physical activity of at least moderate intensity on most (preferably all) days of the week.
- Additional health and functional benefits of physical activity can be achieved by spending more time in moderate-intensity activity or by substituting more vigorous activity.
- People with symptomatic cardiovascular disease, diabetes, or other chronic health problems who would like to increase their physical activity should be evaluated by a physician and provided with an exercise program appropriate for their clinical status.
- Inactive men over 40 years of age, women over 50 years of age, and people at high risk for cardiovascular disease should consult a physician before embarking on a program of vigorous physical activity to which they are unaccustomed.
- Strength-developing activities (e.g., resistance training) should be performed at least twice per week. At least 8–10 strength-developing exercises that use major muscle groups of the legs, trunk, arms, and shoulders should be performed at each session, with one or two sets of 8–12 repetitions of each exercise.

Reprinted from U.S. Department of Health and Human Services. Physical Activity and Health: A Report of the Surgeon General. Atlanta, GA: U.S. Department of Health and Human Services, Centers for Disease Control and Prevention, National Center for Chronic Disease Prevention and Health Promotion; 1996.

---

has been described extensively (94,95). Questions of this type are particularly useful in clinical practice to assess activity levels, with the caveat that one might risk underestimating lower intensity physical activity habits in older women.

The American College of Sports Medicine (ACSM) has developed recommendations to aid physicians and other health professionals in determining the need for a medical examination or clinical exercise evaluation before participation in a regular exercise program (96). These recommendations are based on the presence of coronary risk factors, age, and known cardiac, pulmonary, or metabolic disease. ACSM recommendations for medical examination and exercise testing before participation and physician supervision of exercise tests are described in Table 8-2. Women at low risk for a clinical cardiac event can be advised to safely participate in home-based exercise or in formal exercise programs. Home-based programs include walking, hiking, biking, swimming, and many recreational sports. More formal programs vary

Table 8-2   American College of Sports Medicine Recommendations for Medical Examination and Exercise Testing Before Participation in Physical Activity and Physician Supervision of Exercise Testing

Examination and Exercise Testing Recommended Before	Apparently Healthy		Increased Risk*		Known Disease†
	Younger‡	Older	Asymptomatic	Symptomatic	
Moderate exercise§	No¶	No	No	Yes	Yes
Vigorous exercise**	No	Yes††	Yes	Yes	Yes
Physician Supervision Recommended During					
Submaximal exercise testing	No¶	No	No	Yes	Yes
Maximal exercise testing	No	Yes††	Yes	Yes	Yes

* Individuals with two or more coronary risk factors or one or more signs or symptoms of CAD.
† Individuals with known cardiac, pulmonary, or metabolic disease.
‡ Men ≤ 40 years of age and women ≤ 50 years of age.
§ Intensity of 40%–60% Vo_2 max or well within the individual's current capacity, i.e., activity that 1) can be sustained for a long period (~60 min), 2) has gradual initiation and progression, and 3) is generally non-competitive.
¶ A "No" response indicates that the recommendation is not necessary, not that it should not be done.
** Intensity > 60% Vo_2 max or an intense enough exercise to represent a substantial cardiorespiratory challenge or to elicit fatigue within 20 minutes.
†† A "Yes" response indicates that the recommendation is necessary; a "Yes" response under "Physician Supervision" indicates that a physician should be in close proximity and available in case of an emergency.

widely from dance aerobics to personal training. The American Heart Association (AHA) has stratified adults according to cardiovascular risk factor status as well as the presence and severity of CAD to determine the need for supervision during exercise (97). These guidelines assist physicians and other health professionals in stratifying their patients and making referrals to cardiac programs when applicable. Cardiac rehabilitation program models will be discussed later in this chapter.

Exercise Prescription

Specific physical activity guidelines should include recommendations as to the type, intensity, frequency, and duration of the exercise routine. A woman's current physical activity patterns as well as preferences should be considered before recommending physical activity prescriptions. Ideally, effective cardiovascular programs should include warm-up, cardiovascular conditioning, stretching, muscle strengthening, and cool-down exercises. Women and men are more likely to participate regularly in physical activity programs if they perceive an overall benefit, feel competent and safe performing the activity, and find it enjoyable, easily accessible, and convenient with respect to their daily routine. Also important are the low cost, a minimum of perceived negative consequences (e.g., injury or boredom), and the ability to balance time pressures (77).

Type and Intensity

The recent report of the Behavioral Risk Factor Surveillance System reviewed self-reported physical activity levels in adults over the age of 18 years (98). In this report, 55,506 women were included and reported on the frequency, intensity, and duration of their LTPAs. Twenty-seven percent of all women respondents reported activity levels in accordance with recent recommendations (i.e., > 30 minutes of moderate activities > 5 times/wk). This was in contrast to the 30.2% who reported no LTPA. Women participating in no LTPA increased with increasing age from 25.6% (18–35 y) to 42.1% (> 65 y). In addition, LTPA was inversely related to income and associated with ethnicity. Black non-Hispanic women were less likely to be physically active (43.6% were inactive) compared with Hispanic women (40.2% were inactive), and both groups were less active than Caucasian women (27.6% were inactive) (99). These results are supported by other research evaluating physical activity levels in American women (94,100,101). These data indicate the importance of insuring that older and minority women receive clear messages from physicians and other health professionals about the need for regular physical activity for improved health and day-to-day functioning.

Hawkes and Holm (102) reported that predictors of participation in LTPA for women include health self-determination (the tendency to practice preventive health behaviors) and social influences. Negative attitudes toward exercise also influenced participation, especially among those with a poor perception of their health status (102). Sallis and colleagues (103) studied predictors of physical activity levels in women and men and found that preferences for exercise intensity differed for women and men. Women participated in more moderate levels of activity, whereas men participated in more vigorous activity levels. These results have been confirmed by others (18,95). College-aged women tend to seek physical activity programs that will enhance weight management and appearance as opposed to similar-aged men who prefer competitive programs (104). Eaton and colleagues (95) evaluated the results of a survey that assessed physical activity change in a New England community between 1987 and 1991. The physicians determined that women were more likely to adopt or maintain regular exercise patterns if they had experienced previous success with weight loss and exercise or were encouraged to exercise by their school-aged children. Also, the women were less likely to adopt or maintain exercise if they worked outside the home.

These data suggest that reasons for exercising and the intensity of the recommended physical activity prescription may influence participation. Such information is helpful to health care providers in determining counseling strategies for adoption and maintenance of regular physical activity. Knowing that intense physical activity programs are preferred less by women and are likely to result in poor compliance, recommendations for activities that can be undertaken in a more moderate fashion (e.g., brisk walking, bicycling, and swimming) remain important exercise choices for women. Studies assessing intensity of physical activity in women have confirmed this preference (80,81). This becomes more important as women age or develop signs of clinical CAD or osteoporosis.

Frequency and Duration

Frequency (numbers of exercise sessions per week) and duration (length of time per exercise session) recommendations for physical activity will likely influence adherence and personal enjoyment. The dose-response concept is one that treats physical activity much like a medication. The "dose" (i.e., intensity, frequency, and duration) of the exercise will likely determine some of the benefits as well as some of the risks. Very-low-intensity exercise will likely not confer adequate health-related benefits, whereas vigorous exercise may result in cardiovascular or musculoskeletal harm in some at-risk populations. Current research, however, indicates that the greatest health benefit from regular physical activity is seen in those who move from being physically inactive to more moderately active (33,77). This important finding supports the need for physicians and other health professionals to evaluate, discuss, and encourage increased physical activity levels in all patients, but particularly in those who are the most sedentary. Frequency and duration should be considered as a continuum, with longer, more frequent bouts of exercise balancing the need for increased intensity.

Safety of Exercise

The safety of moderate regular physical activity programs is well established. Although there is a risk associated with any physical activity, the incidence of serious and life-threatening cardiac events is very low. The exercise risk data suggest an acute cardiac event rate of 1 in 187,500 person-hours of vigorous exercise (105). Thompson and colleagues (106) showed a death rate in male joggers of 1 in 396,000 person-hours of jogging. Unfortunately, similar data are not readily available for women. It is important to know that the risk of an acute event appears to be associated with *strenuous* exercise. Because women generally perform less strenuous physical activities compared with men, they may be at somewhat less risk during exercise.

Of concern to most physicians is the issue of safety in their patients who are at high risk for a clinical cardiac event. Van Camp and Peterson (107) examined the safety of exercise in cardiac rehabilitation programs and found the risk of AMI was

1 in 300,000 patient-exercise hours, with a death occurring at a rate of 1 in 790,000 patient-exercise hours. Formal exercise-based cardiac rehabilitation (CR) programs have been an important service for people with CAD in the United States since the 1960s. The Van Camp and Peterson survey indicates that medically prescribed and supervised exercise programs are safe for people with CAD. CR programs in the 1990s offer medically prescribed and supervised exercise along with risk-factor education and modification. The goals of CR are to return patients to optimal physiologic, psychologic, social, vocational, and emotional status (108). CR programs stratify patients by risk based on standard classifications defined by the American Heart Association (AHA) and provide levels of medical supervision based on this evaluation (97). The AHA standards for risk stratification take into account the presence and severity of CAD, including ischemic symptoms, arrhythmias, and clinical congestive heart failure. The patient's ability to self-monitor is also a consideration when defining the need for medical supervision during exercise (97). Additionally, patients in CR programs receive comprehensive risk factor interventions designed to reduce the risk of future coronary events by 1) normalizing blood pressure, lipoproteins, blood sugar, and body weight; 2) reducing saturated fat and cholesterol intake; 3) promoting cigarette smoking cessation; and 4) encouraging stress management practices (108). These services are offered in tandem with exercise therapy sessions. Many people with CAD derive great benefits from participation in formal programs.

The Agency for Health Care Policy and Research has recently published a clinical practice guideline for CR services (109). This document critically analyzed over 900 scientific studies related to CR services. The strength of the evidence ratings were based on study design and methods as well as the reproducibility of the results. Well-designed, randomized, controlled trials were given the highest ratings, with the least weight applied to observational data. In summary, the Guidelines Panel found that participation in CR programs resulted in improvements in exercise tolerance, clinical cardiac symptoms, psychologic well-being, and blood lipid levels. In addition, reductions in cigarette smoking, stress levels, and overall mortality were reported. In meta-analyses of cardiac rehabilitation program outcomes, Oldridge and colleagues (17) and O'Connor and colleagues (37) found a reproducible decrease in mortality of approximately 25% without significant changes in morbidity. Furthermore, adherence to risk reduction strategies may be enhanced by participation in CR programs, although few studies have evaluated this directly. What we do know is that smoking cessation, lipid management, and hypertension control require multifaceted lifestyle interventions and, often, pharmacologic therapies. CR programs can offer systematic support and evaluation of these interventions for referring physicians. As a result, physicians may find CR program staff their best ally in attempts to institute and support lifestyle change in patients with CAD. The limited cost-effectiveness data available also suggest an economic benefit to participation in CR programs

(109). More research is needed to determine the most medically beneficial and cost-effective CR program models.

Self-Monitoring Skills

All cardiac patients participating in exercise programs must be provided with self-monitoring skills designed to provide greater safety and self-confidence. These self-monitoring skills include regular tracking of exercise frequency and duration, evaluation of intensity of effort, presence of ischemic symptoms, presence and severity of arrhythmias, and evaluation of musculoskeletal symptoms. Such self-monitoring practices have also been found to be a beneficial aid for promoting adherence in healthy women and men (110,111). In addition to regular self-monitoring, provision of regular support and feedback about progress are also instrumental factors in promoting regular physical activity participation (110,111).

Intensity of Effort

The rating of perceived exertion (RPE) is frequently assessed during exercise testing as well as during exercise programs and can be an extremely useful measure of exercise intensity. Measurement of RPE was developed by Borg and Linderholm (112) and is commonly referred to as the "Borg Scale." This scale was originally a 15-point scale ranging from 6 to 20, with verbal descriptions of levels of effort at every odd number. Today, a revised scale is generally used with a range from 0 to 10 as a measure of perceived exertion (Table 8-3). Borg and Linderholm showed a linear relationship between heart rate, RPE, and work intensity with a variety of exercises. When heart rate is expressed relative to the percentage of maximum oxygen uptake, RPE values are similar for all age groups (and for obese as well as lean people) and can account for the differing effects of drug therapy on heart rate (e.g., propanolol). The scale provides subjective information about levels of fatigue. RPE is also used in the assessment of exercise tolerance during cardiac rehabilitation exercise sessions (108). For example, RPE can indicate that a patient is exercising within a relatively safe heart rate zone. In addition, RPE can be used as an indicator of exercise intensity.

Ischemic Symptoms

Ischemic symptoms need to be well understood by the cardiac patient before engaging in any unsupervised exercise. Patients should be able to describe their usual symptoms (including triggers, frequency, and duration) and their successful methods of symptom relief (e.g., rest, use of nitrates). For women, it is particularly important to include all symptoms of ischemia, such as shortness of breath and fatigue. Shortness of breath could be related to left ventricular dysfunction during exercise and, as a result, is important to observe, measure, and evaluate. Rating of anginal symptoms during exercise is important in the

Table 8-3 Revised Perceived Exertion Scale (Borg Scale)

Rating	Perceived Exertion
0	Nothing at all
0.5	Very, very weak
1	Very weak
2	Weak
3	Moderately weak
4	Somewhat strong
5	Strong
6	
7	Very Strong
8	
9	Very, very strong
10	Maximal

evaluation of the presence and severity of ischemic symptoms. For most patients, this can be accomplished by using a symptom severity rating scale of 1 to 4 (113). It is also valuable to monitor the length of time that ischemic symptoms take to resolve after onset during exercise. Similarly, cardiac patients can also be taught to record and evaluate the presence of arrhythmias during exercise. A scale that measures the presence of irregular heartbeats, including triggers and number of irregular beats occurring per minute, can be very useful in educating and reassuring patients as well measuring the actual presence of irregularities. If patients take more control of monitoring their symptoms, it is likely that they may have less anxiety and more self-confidence to exercise regularly. Tables 8-4 and 8-5 show symptom ratings scales for angina and arrhythmia, respectively.

Adherence Counseling

Effective strategies for exercise adherence counseling need to consider the person's gender, age, education, prior exercise history, available physical and economic resources, time, and health status among other factors (110,111). A single working mother with preschool-age children will have very different concerns and barriers to regular physical activity compared with an older woman with diabetes and CAD who lives alone. Assessing barriers to regular physical activity can be an effective means of beginning to encourage the adoption of exercise. Barriers include negative beliefs or attitudes, lack of social support, and exercise program complexities (111). Acknowledging these issues, discussing options, and promoting problem-solving skills may improve the patient's exercise adherence regardless of her health status. Effective ways of increasing the use of brief exercise counseling by primary care

Table 8-4 Example of Angina Log

Daily Log for Angina								
No. of Episodes								
Triggered								
Spontaneous								
Grade (1–4)*								
Duration								
Management								
Rest								
Nitroglycerin								
Other								

* Grade 1 is the onset of angina. Grade 2 is worse in location or intensity. Grade 3 is fairly severe and you would definitely stop what you are doing and rest. Grade 4 is the worst.
Reprinted from Fry G, Berra K. YMCArdiac Therapy. National Council of YMCAs. San Francisco: Caroline Bean Assoc.; 1981; with permission.

Table 8-5 Example of Arrhythmia Log

Daily Log for Arrhythmia								
No. of Episodes								
Triggered (e.g., by coffee, alcohol, stress)								
Associated with lightheadedness, fainting?								
Number of irregular beats per minute while exercising								
Occurring at rest?								
Resolve upon stopping exercise?								

Reprinted from Fry G, Berra K. YMCArdiac Therapy. National Council of YMCAs. San Francisco: Caroline Bean Assoc.; 1981; with permission.

physicians have been reported recently as having resulted in significant positive effects on both patient activity levels and on patient ratings of readiness to adopt physical activity (91). Women may also find motivation and support for exercise from printed materials and community resources. A brief list of useful printed materials can be found after the References section.

It is interesting that attrition in CR programs seems to be as high as is seen in the healthy population (82,114). This is surprising because one might imagine that there would be a greater motivation to exercise in people with known CAD. Both in the healthy population and in people with known CAD, attrition seems to be highest during the first 3 to 6 months of participation (72,115). Ongoing supervision by means of telephone or written follow-up seem to be helpful strategies for improving long-term exercise maintenance in both healthy and cardiac populations (110,116). Methods to achieve such ongoing supervision can be provided by clinic-based health educators or nurses, if available, or by referral to the many exercise experts and programs already available in many communities throughout the United States.

Summary

Almost 50 years of epidemiologic, clinical, and laboratory research have provided a prodigious amount of evidence in support of the important role that regular physical activity plays in the prevention and control of cardiovascular and other chronic diseases and conditions. Although, as noted throughout this chapter, the majority of the data collected to date have focused primarily on men, a growing number of studies provide evidence that the benefits achieved in men apply similarly to women.

The challenge remains to develop strategies to promote the regular amounts of moderate intensity or more vigorous physical activity that are crucial for achieving many of these health and psychological benefits. The physician, along with other health providers, continues to play a potentially powerful role in helping to achieve the national goals in this important health area (86). Although time, knowledge, and cost issues currently serve as barriers that prevent many physicians from providing physical activity counseling to their patients, a number of simple strategies can be put into place by physicians that will provide the impetus for many patients to become more active. Such strategies include the following:

1. Give clear, unambiguous messages to the patient about the importance of regular physical activity to the patient's health, both now and in the future.

2. Increase the salience of the physical activity message for the patient by identifying specific health problems or conditions experienced by the patient that can be improved or controlled through regular physical activity.

3. Provide readily available materials from organizations, such as the

American Heart Association, that discuss (often in simple terms) useful strategies for becoming more active.

4. Whenever possible, refer the patient to specific, generally available community programs that provide physical activity.

By asking the patient how active she currently is, by explaining the usefulness of routine forms of moderately intense activity (e.g., walking, stair-climbing) in helping to improve health and functioning, by referring the patient to suitable programs in the community, and by briefly following up with the patient at subsequent clinic visits, the physician and other health professionals can set the stage for increased physical activity interest and participation. It is likely that public health objectives in the physical activity area will be reached only through the efforts described above in combination with other efforts occurring at multiple levels of impact across the nation (e.g., personal, organizational, environmental, policy level).

REFERENCES

1. **Paffenbarger RS Jr, Hyde RT, Wing AL, et al.** Some interrelations of physical activity, physiological fitness, health, and longevity. In: Bouchard C, Shephard RJ, Stephens T, eds. Physical Activity, Fitness and Health: International Proceedings and Consensus Statement. Champagne, IL: Human Kinetics Publishers; 1994:119–35.

2. **Davis MA, Neuhaus JM, Moritz DJ, et al.** Health behaviors and survival among middle-aged men and women in the NHANES I Epidemiologic Follow-up Study. Prev Med. 1994;23:369–76.

3. **Crespo CJ, Keteyian SJ, Heath GW, Sempos CT.** Leisure-time physical activity among U.S. adults. Arch Intern Med. 1996;156:93–8.

4. CDC Report. Prevalence of recommended levels of physical activity among women: Behavioral Risk Factor Surveillance System, 1992. JAMA. 1995;273:986–7.

5. **Winkleby MA, Kraemer HC, Ahn DK, Vardy AN.** Ethnic and socioeconomic differences in cardiovascular disease risk factor: findings for women from the Third National Health and Nutrition Examination Survey, 1986– 1994. JAMA 1998;280:356–2.

6. **McGinnis JM, Foege WH.** Actual causes of death in the United States. JAMA. 1993;270:2207–12.

7. **Kannel WB, Belanger A, D'Agostino R, Israel I.** Physical activity and physical demand on the job and risk of cardiovascular disease and death: the Framingham study. Am Heart J. 1986;112:820–5

8. **Kannel WB, Sorlie P.** Some health benefits of physical activity: the Framingham study. Arch Int Med 1979;139:857–61.

9. **Sternfeld B.** Cancer and the protective effect of physical activity: the epidemiology evidence. Med Sci Sports Exerc. 1992;24:1195–209.

10. **Bernstein L, Henderson BE, Hanish R, et al.** Physical exercise and reduced risk of breast cancer in young women. J Natl Cancer Inst. 1994; 86:1403–8.

11. **Braun B, Zimmermann MB, Kretchmer N.** Effects of exercise intensity on insulin sensitivity in women with non–insulin-dependent diabetes mellitus. J Appl Physiol. 1995;78:300–6.

12. **Rosenthal MW, Haskell WL, Solomon R, et al.** Demonstration of a relationship between level of physical training and insulin-stimulated glucose utilization in normal humans. Diabetes. 1983;VOLUME:408–11.

13. **Krotkiewski M, Bjorntrop P.** Muscle tissue in obesity with different distribution of adipose tissue: effects of physical training. Int J Obes. 1986;10:331–41.

14. **King AC, Tribble DL.** The role of exercise in weight regulation in nonathletes. Sports Med. 1991;11:331–49.

15. **Kohrt WM, Snead DB, Slatopolsky E, Birge SJ.** Additive effects of weight-bearing exercise and estrogen on bone mineral density in older women. J Bone Miner Res. 1995;10:1303–11.

16. **King AC, Taylor CB, Haskell WL, DeBusk RF.** Influence of regular aerobic exercise on psychological health: a randomized, controlled trial of healthy middle-aged adults. Health Psychol. 1989;8:305–24.

17. **Oldridge NB, Guyatt GH, Fischer ME, Rimm AA.** Cardiac rehabilitation after myocardial infarction: combined experience of randomized trials. JAMA. 1988;260:945–50.

18. **American Heart Association.** Heart and Stroke Facts: 1996. Statistical Supplement.

19. **Powell KE, Thompson PD, Caspersen CJ, Kendrick JS.** Physical activity and the incidence of coronary heart disease. Annu Rev Public Health. 1987;8:253–87.

20. **Berlin JA, Colditz GA.** A meta-analysis of physical activity in the prevention of coronary heat disease. Am J Epidemiol. 1990;132:612–28.

21. **Manson JE, Tosteson H, Ridker PM, et al.** The primary prevention of myocardial infarction. N Engl J Med. 1992;1406–16.

22. **Lipid Research Clinics Program.** The Lipid Research Clinics Coronary Primary Prevention Trials results. Part II: The relationship or reduction in incidence of coronary heart disease to cholesterol lowering. JAMA. 1984;251:365–74.

23. **Schaefer EJ, Lichtenstein AH, Lamon-Fava S, et al.** Body weight and low-density lipoprotein cholesterol changes after consumption of a low-fat ad libitum diet. JAMA. 1995;274:1450–5.

24. **Gould KL.** Reversal of coronary atherosclerosis: clinical promise as the basis for noninvasive management of coronary artery disease. Circulation. 1994;90:1558–71.

25. **Gordon DJ, Knoke J, Probsfield JL, et al.** High-density lipoprotein cholesterol and coronary heart disease in hypercholesterolemic men: the Lipid Research Clinics Primary Prevention Trial. Circulation. 1986;74:1217–25.

26. **Haskell WL, Leon AS, Caspersen CJ, et al.** Cardiovascular benefits and assessment of physical activity and physical fitness in adults. Med Sci Sports Exerc. 1992;24(Suppl): S201–20.

27. **Salonen JT, Puska P, Tuomilehto J.** Physical activity and risk of myocardial infarction, cerebral stroke, and death. Am J Epidemiol. 1982;115:526–37.

28. **Sherman SE, D'Agostino RB, Cobb JL, Kannel WB.** Physical activity and mortality in women in the Framingham Heart Study. Am Heart J. 1994;128:879–84.

29. **Blair SN, Kohl HW, Barlow CE.** Physical activity, physical fitness, and all-cause mortality in women: do women need to be active? J Am Coll Nutr. 1993;12:368–71.

30. **Blair SN, Kampert JB, Kohl HW, et al.** Influences of cardiorespiratory fitness and other precursors on cardiovascular disease and all-cause mortality in men and women. JAMA. 1996;276:205–10.

31. **LaCroix AZ, Leveille SG, Hecht JA, et al.** Does walking decrease the risk of cardiovascular disease hospitalizations and death in older adults? J Am Geriatr Soc. 1996;44:113–20.

32. **Manson JE, Rich-Edwards JW, Colditz JA, et al.** The role of walking in the prevention of cardiovascular disease in women. Circulation. 1996;94(Suppl):S339.

33. **Blair SN, Kohl HW III, Paffenbarger RS Jr., et al.** Physical fitness and all cause mortality: a prospective study of health of men and women. JAMA. 1989;262:2395–401.

34. **Masse LC, Ainsworth BE, Tortolero S, et al.** Measuring physical activity in midlife older and minority women: issues from an expert panel. J Womens Health. 1998;7: 57–67.

35. **Kushi LH, Fee RM, Folsom AR, et al.** Physical activity and mortality in postmenopausal women. JAMA. 1997;277:1287–92.

36. **May GS, Eberlein KA, Furberg CD, et al.** Secondary prevention after myocardial infarction: a review of the long-term trials. Prog Cardiovasc Dis. 1982;24:331–62.

37. **O'Connor GT, Buring GE, Yusaf S, et al.** An overview of randomized trials of rehabilitation with exercise after myocardial infarction. Circulation. 1989;80:234–44.

38. **Douglas PS, Clarkson TB, Flowers NC, et al.** Exercise and atherosclerotic heart disease. Med Sci Sports Exerc. 1992;24(Suppl):S266–76.

39. **Haskell WL, Alderman EL, Fair JM, et al.** Effects of intensive multiple risk factor reduction on coronary atherosclerosis and clinical cardiac events in men and women with coronary artery disease. Circulation. 1994;89,975–90.

40. **Ornish DM, Scherwitz LW, Brown SE, et al.** Can lifestyle changes reverse atherosclerosis? Lancet. 1990;336,129–33.

41. **Schuler G, Hambrecht R, Schlierf G, et al.** Regular physical exercise and low-fat diet: effects on progression of coronary artery disease. Circulation. 1992;86:1–11.

42. **Smith SC, Blair SN, Criqui MH, et al.** Preventing heart attack and death in patients with coronary disease. Circulation. 1995;92:2–4.

43. **Fuster V, Pearson TA.** 27th Bethesda Conference: matching the intensity of risk factor management with the hazard for coronary disease events. J Am Coll Cardiol. 1996;27: 957–1047.

44. **Franklin BA, Hall L, Timmis GC.** Contemporary rehabilitation services. Am J Cardiol. 1997:79:1075–7.

45. **Thomas RJ, Houston Miller N, Lamendola C, et al.** National survey on gender differences in cardiac rehabilitation programs. J Cardiopul Rehabil. 1996;16:402–12.

46. **Ades PA, Waldmann ML, McCann WJ, Weaver MS.** Predictors of cardiac rehabilitation participation in older coronary patients. Arch Int Med. 1992;152:1033–35.

47. **Moore SM.** Women's views of cardiac rehabilitation programs. J Cardiopul Rehabil. 1996;16:123–9.

48. **Moore SM.** Women's and men's preference for cardiac rehabilitation program features. J Cardiopul Rehabil. 1996;16:163–8.

49. **Schuster PM, Waldron J.** Gender differences in cardiac rehabilitation patients. Rehabilitation Nursing. 1991;16:248–53.

50. **Cannistra LB, Balady GJ, O'Malley CJ, et al.** Comparison of the clinical profile and outcome of women and men in cardiac rehabilitation. Am J Cardiol. 1992;69:1274–9.

51. **Lavie CJ, Milani RV.** Factors predicting improvements in lipid values following cardiac rehabilitation and exercise training. Arch Intern Med. 1993;153:982–8.

52. **Stefanick ML, Wood PD.** Physical activity, lipid and lipoprotein metabolism, and lipid transport. In: Bouchard C, Shephard RJ, Stephens T, eds. Physical Activity, Fitness, and Health: International Proceedings and Consensus Statement. Champagne IL: Human Kinetics Publishers; 1994:417–31.

53. **Thune I, Njolstad I, Lochen M, Forde OH.** Physical activity improves the metabolic risk profiles in men and women. Arch Intern Med. 1998;158:1633–40.

54. **Stefanick ML, Mackey S, Sheehan M, et al.** Effects of diet and exercise in men and women and postmenopausal women with low levels of HDL cholesterol and high levels of LDL cholesterol. New Engl J Med. 1998;339:12–20.

55. **Lokey EA, Tran ZV.** Effects of exercise training on serum lipid and lipoprotein concentrations in women: a meta-analysis. Int J Sports Med. 1989;10:424–9.

56. **Duncan JJ, Gordon NF, Scott CB.** Women walking for health and fitness: how much is enough? JAMA. 1991;266:3295–329.

57. **King AC, Haskell WL, Young DR, et al.** Long-term effects of varying intensities and formats of physical activity on participation rates, fitness, and lipoproteins in men and women aged 50 to 65 years. Circulation. 1995;91:2596–604.

58. **Manson JE, Rimm EB, Stampfer MJ, et al.** Physical activity and incidence of non–insulin-dependent diabetes mellitus in women. Lancet. 1991;338:774–8.

59. **Helmrick SP, Ragland DR, Leung RW, Paffenbarger RS.** Physical activity and reduced occurrence of non–insulin-dependent diabetes. N Engl J Med. 1991;325:147–52.

60. **Laws A, Reaven GM.** Physical activity, glucose tolerance, and diabetes in older adults. Ann Behav Med. 1991, 13:125–31.

61. **Blair SN, Goodyear NN, Gibbons LW, Cooper KH.** Physical fitness and incidence of hypertension in health normotensive men and women. JAMA. 1984;252:487–90.

62. **Reaven PD, Barrett-Connor A, Edelstein S.** Relation between leisure-time physical activity and blood pressure in older women. Circulation. 1991;83:559–65.

63. **Kaplan NM.** The deadly quartet: upper-body obesity, glucose intolerance, hypertriglyceridemia, and hypertension. Arch Int Med. 1989;149:1514–20.

64. **Gleim GW.** Exercise is not an effective weight loss modality in women. J Am Coll Nutr. 1993;12:363–7.

65. **Kannel WB, Wolf PA, Castelli WP, D'Agnostino RB.** Fibrinogen and risk of cardiovascular disease: the Framingham Heart Study. JAMA. 1987;258:1183–6.

66. **Yarnell JWG, Baker IA, Sweetnam PM, et al.** Fibrinogen, viscosity and white blood cell count are major risk factors for ischemic heart disease: the Caerphilly and Speedwell Collaborative Heart Disease studies. Circulation. 1991;83:836–44.

67. **Ernst E.** Regular exercise reduces fibrinogen levels: a review of longitudinal studies. Br J Sports Med. 1993;27:175–6.

68. **Stefanick ML, Legault C, Tracy RP, et al.** Distribution and correlates of plasma fibrinogen in middle-aged women: initial findings of the Postmenopausal Estrogen/Progesterone Interventions (PEPI) study. Arterioscler Thromb Vasc Biol. 1995;15:2085–93.

69. **McLaughlin MH, McAllister RM, Delp MD.** Physical activity and the microcirculation in cardiac and skeletal muscle. In: Bouchard C, Shephard RJ, Stephens T, eds. Physical Activity, Fitness, and Health: International Proceedings and Consensus Statement. Champagne, IL: Human Kinetics Publishers; 1994:PAGES.

70. **Oka RK.** Cardiovascular response to exercise. Cardiovasc Nurs. 1990;26:31–5.

71. **Cowley AW, Dzau V, Buttrick P, et al.** Working group on noncoronary cardiovascular disease and exercise in women. Med Sci Sports Med. 1992; 24(Suppl):S277–87.

72. **Ades PA, Waldmann ML, Polk DM, Coflesky JR.** Referral patterns and exercise response in the rehabilitation of female coronary patients aged greater than or equal to 62 years. Am J Cardiol. 1992;69:1422–5.

73. **Sobel DS.** Rethinking medicine: improving health outcomes with cost-effective psychosocial interventions. Psychosom Med. 1995;57:234–44.

74. **Scheier MF, Bridges MW.** Person variables and health: personality predispositions and acute psychological states as shared determinants for disease. Psychosom Med. 1995;57:255–68.

75. **Jenkins CD.** Psychosocial and behavioral factors. In: Kaplan NM, Stamler J, eds. Prevention of Coronary Heart Disease: Practical Management of the Risk Factors. Philadelphia: WB Saunders; 1983:98–112.

76. **Frasure-Smith, N, Lesperance F, Talajic M.** The impact of negative emotions on prognosis following myocardial infarction: is it more than depression? Health Psychol. 1995;14:388–98.

77. **US Department of Health and Human Services.** Physical Activity and Health: A Report of the Surgeon General. Atlanta, GA: U.S. Department of Health and Human Services, Centers for Disease Control and Prevention, National Center for Chronic Disease Prevention and Health Promotion; 1996.

78. **Landers DM, Petruzzello SJ.** Physical activity, fitness, and anxiety. In: Bouchard C, Shephard RJ, Stephens T, eds. Physical Activity, Fitness, and Health: International Proceedings and Consensus Statement. Champagne IL: Human Kinetics Publishers. 1994:868–82.

79. **McAuley E.** Physical activity and psychosocial outcomes. In: Bouchard C, Shephard RJ, Stephens T, eds. Physical Activity, Fitness, and Health: International Proceedings and Consensus Statement. Champagne, IL: Human Kinetics Publishers. 1994:551–68.

80. **King AC, Taylor CB, Haskell WL.** The effects of differing intensities and formats of twelve months of exercise training on psychological outcomes. Health Psychol. 1993;12:292–302.

81. **Pereira MA, Kriska AM, Day RD, et al.** A randomized walking trial in postmenopausal women: effects on physical activity and health 10 years later. Arch Inter Med. 1998; 158:1695–1701.

82. **Oldridge N, Guyatt GH, Jones N, et al.** Effects on quality of life with comprehensive rehabilitation after acute myocardial infarction. Am J Card. 1991;67:1084–9.

83. **Denollet J.** Emotional distress and fatigue in coronary heart disease: the Global Mood Scale (GMS). Psychol Med. 1993;23:111–21.

84. **Brown DR, Wang Y, Ward A, et al.** Chronic psychological effects of exercise and exercise plus cognitive strategies. Med Sci Sports Exerc. 1995:27:765–75.

85. **Morgan WP, Costill DL, Flynn MG, et al.** Mood disturbance following increased training in swimmers. Med Sci Sports Med. 1988;20:408–14.

86. **US Department of Health and Human Services.** Healthy People 2000: National Health Promotion and Disease Prevention Objectives. Washington, DC: U.S. Department of Health and Human Services; 1990. [DHHS Publication No. (PHS) 91-50212.]

87. **Harris SS, Casperson CJ, DeFriese, Estes EH.** Physical activity counseling for healthy adults as a primary intervention in the clinical setting: report for the U.S. Preventive Services Task Force. JAMA. 1989;261:3590–8.

88. **Williford HN, Barfield BR, Lazenby RB, Olson MS.** A survey of physicians' attitudes and practices related to exercise promotion. Prev Med. 1992;21:630–6.

89. **Orleans CT, George LK, Houpt JL, Brodie KH.** Health promotion in primary care: a survey of U.S. family practitioners. Prev Med. 1985;14:636–47.

90. **Friedman C, Brownson RC, Peterson DE, Wilkerson JC.** Physician advice to reduce chronic disease risk factors. Am J Prev Med. 1994;106:367–71.

91. **Calfas KJ, Long BJ, Sallis JF, et al.** A controlled trial of physician advice to promote the adoption of physical activity. Prev Med. 1996;25:225–33.

92. **Lewis BS, Lynch WD.** The effect of physician advice on exercise behavior. Prev Med. 1993;22:110–21.

93. **Graham-Clarke P, Oldenberg B.** The effectiveness of a general-practice-based physical activity intervention on patient physical activity status. Behav Change. 1994,11:132–44.

94. **Paffenbarger RS Jr, Hyde RT, Wing AK, Hsieh CC.** Physical activity, all-cause mortality and longevity of college alumni. N Engl J Med. 1986;314: 605–13.

95. **Eaton CB, Reynes J, Assaf AR, et al.** Predicting physical activity change in men and women in two New England communities. Am J Prev Med. 1993;9:209–19.

96. **American College of Sports Medicine.** Guidelines for Exercise Testing and Prescription. 5th ed. Williams & Wilkins: Baltimore, MD; 1995.

97. **Fletcher GF, Ballady G, Froelicher VF, et al.** Exercise standards: a statement for health professionals from the American Heart Association. Circulation. 1995;91: 580–615.

98. Prevalence of recommended physical activity levels among women: Behavioral Risk Factor Surveillance System, 1992. MMWR Morbidity Mortality Weekly Report. 1995; 44:105–8.

99. **Wells CL.** Physical activity and women's health. In: Physical Activity and Fitness Research Digest. Series 2. No 5. Washington, DC: President's Council on Physical Fitness and Sports; 1996.

100. **Casperson CJ, Christenson GM, Pollard RA.** Status of the 1990 physical fitness and exercise objectives: evidence from NHIS. Public Health Rep. 1995;101:587–92.

101. **Ford ES, Merritt RK, Health GW, et al.** Physical activity behaviors in lower and higher socioeconomic status populations. Am J Epidemiol. 1991;133:1246–56.

102. **Hawkes JM, Holm K.** Gender differences in exercise determinants. Nurs Res. 1993; 42:166–172.

103. **Sallis JF, Haskell WL, Fortmann SP, et al.** Predictors of adoption and maintenance of physical activity in a community sample. Prev Med. 1986;15:331–41.

104. **Finkenberg ME, DiNucci JM, McCune SL, McCune ED.** Analysis of course type, gender, and personal incentives to exercise. Percept Mot Skills. 1994;78:155–95.

105. **Gibbons LW, Blair SN, Kohl HW, Cooper KH.** The safety of maximal exercise testing. Circulation. 1989;80:846–52.

106. **Thompson PD, Funk EJ, Carleton RA, Sturner WQ.** The incidence of death during jogging in Rhode Island from 1975 to 1980. JAMA. 1982;247:2535–8.

107. **Van Camp SP, Peterson RA.** Cardiovascular complications of outpatient cardiac rehabilitation programs. JAMA 1986;256:1160–3.

108. **American Association of Cardiovascular and Pulmonary Rehabilitation.** Guidelines for Cardiac Rehabilitation Programs. 2nd ed. Champaign, IL: Human Kinetics; 1995.

109. **Wenger NK, Froelicher ES, Smith LK, et al.** Cardiac Rehabilitation: Clinical Practice Guideline No 17. Washington, DC: US Department of Health and Human Services; 1995. [AHCPR Publication No. 96-0672.]

110. **King AC, Martin JE.** Adherence to exercise. In: Resource Manual for Guidelines for Exercise Testing and Prescription. Malvern, PA: Lea & Febiger; 1988:335–44.

111. **King AC, Blair SN, Bild DE, et al.** Determinants of physical activity and interventions in adults. Med Sci Sports Exerc. 1992;24(Suppl):S221–36.

112. **Borg G, Linderholm H.** Perceived exertion and pulse rate during graded exercise in various age groups. Acta Med Scand. 1967;472(Suppl):S194–206.

113. **Fry G, Berra K.** YMCArdiac Therapy. San Francisco: Caroline Bean Associates: 1981.

114. **Dishman RK.** Exercise Adherence. Champaign, IL: Human Kinetics; 1988.

115. **Carmody TP, Senner JW, Manilow MR, Matarazzo JD.** Physical exercise rehabilitation: long-term drop out rate in cardiac patients. J Behav Med. 1980;3:163–8.

116. **Houston MN.** Home exercise training for coronary patients. In: Resource Manual for Guidelines for Exercise Testing and Prescription. Malvern, PA: Lea & Febiger; 1993: 350–5.

PATIENT EDUCATION MATERIALS

BOOKS

Fresh Start: Stanford Medical School Health and Fitness Program. Stanford, CA: Stanford Medical School; 1997.

Nash J. The New Maximize Your Body Potential. 2nd ed. Patlo Alto, CA: Bull Publishing; 1997.

Nelson ME, Wernick S. Strong Women Stay Young. New York: Bantam Books; 1997.

Paffenberger RS Jr. Lifefit: An Effective Program for Optimal Health and a Longer Life. Champagne, IL: Human Kinetics Publishing; 1996.

OTHER RESOURCES

Women's Health Resource
Mayo Clinic
Rochester, Minnesota

University of California at Berkeley Wellness Letter
School of Public Health
University of California–Berkeley
Berkeley, California

HealthNews
New England Journal of Medicine
Massachusetts Medical Society
Waltham, Massachusetts

Women's Health Advocate Newsletter
Palm Coast, Florida

Women's Health Watch
Harvard Medical School
Boston, Massachusetts

CHAPTER 9

Aspirin, Antioxidants, and Alcohol

CHRISTINE M. ALBERT, MD, MPH

JOANN E. MANSON, MD, DRPH

Cardiovascular diseases, especially coronary artery disease (CAD) and cerebrovascular disease, are the leading cause of morbidity and mortality in women and are responsible for approximately 480,000 deaths annually, or 46% percent of all fatalities in the United States (1). Although the rates of mortality from CAD have been falling since the 1960s, the rate of decline has been slower among women than men since 1979, and CAD remains the leading cause of death among women 60 years of age and older (2). Despite the magnitude of the problem, we have insufficient information about preventive strategies, responses to medical and surgical therapies, and other aspects of CAD in women. Prevention is critical in women because 40% of all coronary events are fatal and 67% of all sudden deaths occur in those without a history of CAD (3). Of the women who do not initially die, it is estimated that 36% of women aged 55 to 64 and 55% of those 75 years or older will be disabled from CAD (4).

Preventive efforts aimed at the modification of risk factors for CAD are equally important in women. Most of the risk factors for CAD in men are also risk factors in women (1), but the magnitude of their effects may be different. In addition to risk factor modification, pharmacologic strategies for the prevention of CAD may reduce CAD incidence in women with or without established risk factors for CAD. In this chapter, we review the rationales and the existing epidemiologic data in women on three of these pharmacologic agents: aspirin, antioxidant vitamins, and alcohol. We also review randomized

236

trials in men (which have reached completion) and those currently ongoing in women.

For the most part, the only direct data available in women for these agents (with the exception of aspirin in secondary prevention of CAD) are observational. Although informative and hypothesis-generating, observational studies are limited in their ability to prove causation. Unmeasured and residual confounding by other dietary and lifestyle factors remains an alternative explanation for the findings of these studies. For example, lifestyle and dietary patterns differ substantially between people with high antioxidant intake (dietary and supplemental) compared with those with low intake. Women with high intake of antioxidant vitamins are less likely to smoke and more likely to be lean and physically active, to use postmenopausal estrogen supplements, and to practice other healthy lifestyle behaviors. Randomized trials can eliminate the potentially confounding effects of these variables and assess the true effect of the intervention. (This will be illustrated further when we discuss the results of randomized trials of beta-carotene.) Thus, randomized clinical trials of sufficient size and duration are necessary to either substantiate or refute apparent benefits suggested by epidemiologic studies before firm conclusions on the efficacy of these pharmacologic interventions can be made.

Aspirin

Aspirin irreversibly acetylates platelet cyclooxygenase, resulting in the inhibition of the synthesis of thromboxane A_2, a potent promoter of platelet aggregation (5,6). This inhibition of platelet function has been hypothesized to be one of the mechanisms for aspirin's benefit on CAD by reducing the risk of acute thrombosis associated with plaque rupture and by inhibiting the chronic effects of platelet activation on atherosclerotic plaque formation. Pharmacologic studies have indicated that the dose of aspirin necessary to inhibit platelet aggregation may be lower than 80 mg (7). At higher doses, aspirin's inhibition of vascular prostacyclin, which is synthesized by endothelial cells and causes vasodilation and inhibition of platelets, becomes more pronounced. Unlike platelet inhibition, which persists for at least 72 hours after a single dose of aspirin, endothelial cell inhibition lasts only 6 hours due to the endothelial cell's capacity to resynthesize the cyclooxygenase enzyme (8). These data provide a theoretical basis for a protective effect of lower doses of aspirin at longer dosage intervals. In addition, recent data have implicated inflammation in the pathogenesis of atherosclerosis, raising the possibility that part of the benefit of aspirin may be due to its anti-inflammatory effects (9). Conflicting evidence exists about the presence or absence of a sex difference in responsiveness to the antithrombotic effect of aspirin. Overall, little evidence supports a sex differential in vivo because the pharmacokinetics of aspirin and its cyclooxygenase inhibition are similar in both sexes (10). Even without a sex difference in action, the risk-to-benefit ratio may still differ between women and men due to established sex-related differences in the relative frequency of outcomes that aspirin may prevent (e.g., myocardial infarction [MI]) (11) or precipitate (e.g., hemorrhagic stroke) (12).

Secondary Prevention

Randomized trials have demonstrated conclusively the efficacy of aspirin in the secondary prevention of cardiovascular events among both women and men who have survived a previous cardiovascular end point. The results of most of these trials suggest a benefit, but the individual sample sizes were too small to provide reliable results. In 1988, an overview was conducted of 25 randomized trials of antiplatelet therapy (including aspirin and/or dipyridamole or sulfinpyrazone) that studied 29,000 patients with previous MI, stroke, transient ischemic attacks (TIAs), or unstable angina. The overview revealed a 32% reduction in subsequent nonfatal MI, a 27% reduction in nonfatal stroke, a 15% reduction in cardiovascular mortality, and a 25% reduction in total important vascular events among patients assigned to antiplatelet therapy (13). The benefit of aspirin in acute evolving MI was demonstrated among 17,187 men and women in the Second International Study of Infarct Survival (ISIS-2). Patients who were assigned to daily aspirin therapy (162.5 mg) within 24 hours of onset of symptoms for 1 month had a 23% reduction in vascular death, 49% reduction in nonfatal reinfarction, and 46% reduction in nonfatal stroke after 5 weeks (14). Despite the limited number of women (< 23% of trial participants), a statistically significant reduction in vascular death was apparent among women when they were analyzed separately.

The findings from the original overview and ISIS-2 were strengthened and extended in a 1994 updated overview that included an additional 40,000 patients with previous cardiovascular disease from 118 trials. This overview included new patient populations, including approximately 20,000 patients with chronic stable angina, coronary revascularization, peripheral vascular disease, atrial fibrillation, and valve surgery and also approximately 20,000 patients with acute MI (primarily from ISIS-2) (15). Among the entire group of 69,000 high-risk patients, there was a 35% reduction in the risk of subsequent nonfatal MI, a 31% reduction in the risk of nonfatal stroke, and an 18% reduction in the risk of vascular death in patients assigned to antiplatelet therapy as compared with controls ($p < 0.00001$). These benefits translated into a 27% reduction in total important vascular events and a 17% reduction in total mortality. When the four major subdivisions of high-risk patients (those who had previous MI, acute MI, previous stroke or TIAs, etc.) were analyzed separately, similar reductions in each end point were demonstrated in each subgroup (Table 9-1). Separate data were available for approximately 10,000 women and 40,000 men from 29 of the trials. Similar benefits in reducing vascular events were found among the women when analyzed separately, with reductions of 33 events for women ($p < 0.0001$) and 37 events for men ($p < 0.00001$) per 1000 patients treated. There was no evidence that higher doses of aspirin or any other antiplatelet regimen was any more effective than low- to medium-dose aspirin (75–325 mg) in reducing the risk of occlusive vascular events. When analyzed separately, the approximately 5000 patients who were randomized in trials testing 75 mg of aspirin per day were found to have a statistically significant 29% reduction in vascular events even at this low dose ($p < 0.0001$).

In summary, the extensive randomized trial data support the use of low to medium doses of aspirin (75–325 mg) among women and men who have a history of previous MI, stroke, TIAs, unstable angina, or other significant cardiovascular disease and who are at high risk for occlusive vascular events. The risk-to-benefit ratio seems to be similar in women when overt cardiovascular disease is present. Women also benefit from aspirin therapy if initiated during the first 24 hours of acute evolving MI. In this and other acute settings (e.g., unstable angina) at least 162.5 to 325 mg should be given as an initial loading dose to achieve rapid and complete inhibition of platelet cyclooxygenase because lower doses (75 mg) may require 48 hours to reach maximal inhibition. Unfortunately, women are less likely to be prescribed aspirin after MI as docu-

Table 9-1 Evidence of Antiplatelet Drug Efficacy

Diagnosis	Duration of Treatment*	Events Avoided/ 1000 Patients
Primary prevention[†]	62	4
Secondary prevention[‡]		
Acute MI	1	38
History of MI	27	36
History of TIA or stroke	33	37
"High risk"[§]	16	23

MI = myocardial infarction; TIA = transient ischemic attack.
* Mean duration of scheduled antiplatelet therapy in antiplatelet trials.
[†] Trials enrolled men only.
[‡] Trials enrolled women and men; the results were similar for both sexes.
[§] Participants with unstable angina, stable angina, vascular surgery, angioplasty, atrial fibrillation, peripheral vascular disease, etc.
Data from Antiplatelet Trialists' Collaboration. Collaborative overview of randomized trials of antiplatelet treatment. Part 1: Prevention of death, myocardial infarction, and stroke by prolonged antiplatelet treatment. Br Med J. 1994; 30:81–106.

mented in the section on "Gender differences in the use of adjunctive medical therapy." The optimal duration of antiplatelet therapy is unclear because direct randomized comparisons of treatment duration have not been performed. In the absence of such data, it may be prudent to consider indefinite continuation of antiplatelet therapy unless a clear contraindication develops.

Primary Prevention

Presently, no randomized trial data exist on testing aspirin in the primary prevention of cardiovascular events in women. To our knowledge, only three prospective observational studies have explored the relationship between aspirin use and the subsequent development of cardiovascular disease in women, and the data are not entirely consistent (16–18). The Nurses Health Study examined this question in over 87,000 women followed for 6 years (16). Beginning in 1980, when the women were 34 to 59 years of age, information about regular aspirin use was obtained and updated every 2 years. A total of 240 MIs, 198 strokes, and 81 deaths from CAD were documented over the 6-year period of the study. Women who reported taking one to six aspirin tablets per week had a significantly reduced risk of MI (relative risk [RR] = 0.75; 95% confidence interval [CI], 0.58–0.99) compared with women who took no aspirin after controlling for coronary risk factors, alcohol intake, postmenopausal hormone use, and dietary fat. The reduction in risk of MI was apparent across all coronary risk factor strata, with particularly large reductions among current smokers and women with a history of hypertension or hypercholesterolemia. The benefit, however, was not seen in women younger than 50 years of age or in women of any age who took seven or more aspirin per week. There were also slight but insignificant reductions in risk for cardiovascular death, important vascular events, and total mortality in this category of aspirin consumption. Aspirin use was not related to risk of total, ischemic, and hemorrhagic stroke except among those who took 15 or more aspirins per week, where the relative risk of hemorrhagic stroke was not significantly increased.

On the other hand, two other prospective studies found no association between aspirin intake and risk of CAD in women (17,18). The American Cancer Society Study found no association between aspirin use and CAD deaths as ascertained by death certificates over 6 years of follow-up (17). In addition to the lack of verification of end points by medical records, the classification of aspirin status was crude (never, seldom, or often) and exposure status was not updated. All these factors would decrease the study's ability to find an association. The second study assessed the association between aspirin use (none, less than daily, and daily) and cardiovascular end points in an elderly population of 8881 women and 5106 men during 6 years of follow-up (18). The analyses were adjusted only for age, and aspirin status was not updated. No reduction in MI was found in women, although a statistically insignificant reduction was evident in men. The relative risks of ischemic heart disease seemed to be elevated in both women and men who took aspirin (1.39 and 1.46, respectively; $p < 0.05$ for both); but again, these relative risks were not controlled for coronary risk factor status and other potential confounders. It is possible that women who were at higher risk for ischemic heart disease were more likely to take aspirin in an attempt to lower that risk.

Only two randomized trials of aspirin in primary prevention have been completed, both among male physicians (19,20). In addition to a randomized trial of beta-carotene that will be discussed later in this chapter, the U.S. Physicians Health Study simultaneously tested 325 mg of aspirin taken on alternate days using a 2 x 2 factorial design in 22,071 men aged 40 to 84 years (19). The aspirin component of the trial was terminated early in 1988 primarily due to the emergence of a statistically extreme 44% reduction in the risk of MI ($p < 0.0001$). The benefit was apparent only in those who were 50 years of age and older. Overall, a statistically significant 18% reduction was observed for the combined end point of important cardiovascular events, but the effect on stroke and cardiovascular death remained inconclusive due to inadequate numbers of such end points. There was, however, a trend toward an increase in hemorrhagic stroke (RR = 2.14; 95% CI, 0.96–4.77; $p = 0.06$) in the aspirin group. The other primary prevention trial was conducted among 5139 British aged 50 to 75 years who were randomized to 500 mg of aspirin daily using an open design in which the controls were asked simply to avoid aspirin (20). After 6 years of treatment and follow-up, this trial found no difference for MI, stroke, or vascular death. Apart from the differences in design and aspirin dose, the smaller sample size limited the statistical power of this study compared with the U.S. study.

Despite the significant benefit on MI in the Physicians Health Study, the unclear effect on cardiovascular mortality and possible increase in hemorrhagic stroke complicates the decision about whether to use aspirin as primary prevention in men. It is even more unclear whether aspirin should be used as primary prevention in women due to the lack of randomized trial data. For this reason, the U.S. Preventive Services Task Force has recommended that low-dose aspirin should be considered for primary prevention of MI in men only. The critical issue underlying the need for direct trial data in women is the possibility that the benefit-to-risk ratio for prophylactic aspirin use in women may be less favorable. In comparison with men of the same age, women have lower rates of MI (11), which is the principal outcome that aspirin may prevent, and women have higher rates of hemorrhagic stroke (12), which may be increased by aspirin use. In the National Survey of Stroke, the age-adjusted incidence rate of hemorrhagic stroke was approximately 60% higher in women than for men (12). For this reason, definitive findings from large-scale primary prevention trials in women are crucial to formulate reliable treatment recommendations for women. The Women's Health Study is currently testing 100 mg of aspirin taken simultaneously with vitamin E every other day in a 2 x 2 factorial design among 40,000 female health professionals aged 45 years and older (21,22). The results of this trial will provide crucial information on the risks and benefits of low-dose aspirin in apparently healthy women and will be available within the next 5 years.

Antioxidants

Basic research has demonstrated that oxidation of lipids and oxidative injury to the vascular wall promote atherogenesis, abnormal vascular wall reactivity, and thrombus formation. Substantial laboratory, animal, and human data suggest that oxidation of low-density lipoprotein (LDL) cholesterol may play an important role in the initiation and propagation of atherosclerosis. Oxidized LDL has been shown to accelerate several steps in atherosclerosis, including endothelial cell damage and alteration in function (23,24), monocyte and macrophage recruitment (25), increased uptake of LDL by foam cells (26,27), alteration in vascular tone (28), as well as formation of auto-antibodies to LDL, which are found in patients with atherosclerosis (29). In addition to the oxidation of LDL, oxidant stress through generation of free radicals may directly damage arterial endothelium (30), promote thrombosis (31), and interfere with normal vasomotor regulation (32). Antioxidant vitamins presumably exert their effects through the prevention of oxidation. In vitro and in vivo studies have demonstrated inhibition of LDL oxidation by several natural antioxidants, including vitamin E (alpha-tocopherol), vitamin C (ascorbic acid), and possibly beta-carotene (33–36). Both vitamins E and C have been demonstrated to reduce or retard the progression of atherosclerotic lesions in animal models of atherosclerosis (37). However, the antioxidant properties of these vitamins are not the only mechanism by which they may reduce the development or progression of atherosclerosis. Both vitamins E and C may inhibit platelet aggregation (38,39), reduce blood pressure (40), and have favorable effects on coronary vasomotion (41,42). Vitamin C may improve the lipid profile (43,44) and decrease monocyte adhesion to endothelium (45), and it is inversely related to fibrinogen and other hemostatic factors (46,47).

Vitamin E

Observational Studies
Observational studies have found that people who consume large amounts of fruits and vegetables have lower rates of CAD; however, the strength of the

epidemiologic evidence differs for each of the antioxidant vitamins. These vitamins include vitamins E and C and beta-carotene, which are all naturally occurring and found in vitamin supplements. Of these three antioxidant vitamins, the observational data regarding vitamin E are the most consistent. Several large-scale cohort studies have investigated the relationship between vitamin E intake and CAD incidence. The largest observational study to examine this hypothesis—the Nurses Health Study (NHS)—examined in 1980 the association between the intake of antioxidant vitamins and subsequent cardiovascular disease in a cohort of more than 87,000 women aged 34 to 59 years who were free of angina, MI, stroke, and other cardiovascular disease (48). Dietary antioxidant intake and use of antioxidant vitamin supplements was ascertained through a semiquantitative food frequency questionnaire administered in 1980, and information on antioxidant supplements was updated biennially. During 8 years of follow-up, there were 552 incident cases of CAD, including 437 nonfatal MI and 115 coronary deaths. Women in the highest vitamin E quintile had a 34% lower risk of major coronary disease (i.e., nonfatal MI and fatal CAD) (p-trend < 0.001) compared with those in the lowest quintile after adjustment for age and smoking status. The benefit was largely confined to those consuming more than 100 IU of vitamin per day, an intake level that is attributable almost entirely to supplements rather than diet. When vitamin E intake from the diet and supplements were analyzed separately, an inverse association was apparent only for vitamin supplements. Women who took vitamin E supplements for short periods had little apparent benefit, but those who took them for more than 2 years had a 0.59 relative risk of major coronary disease (95% CI, 0.38–0.91) after adjustment for age, cardiac risk factors, exercise, alcohol intake, regular use of aspirin, postmenopausal hormone use, and intake of vitamin C and beta-carotene. Similar findings have been reported among men in the Health Professionals Follow-up Study [HPFS] (49).

In contrast to the Nurses Health Study, the Iowa Women's Health Study (a cohort of 34,486 postmenopausal women aged 55 to 69 years in 1986 who were free of known cardiovascular disease) reported an inverse association between vitamin E intake from diet and fatal CAD over 7 years of follow-up (50). Dietary vitamin E intake differs from supplements not only in the lower dose of vitamin E as previously mentioned but also in its composition. Dietary intake contains gamma- as well as alpha-tocopherol, whereas supplements are largely alpha-tocopherol. The association between dietary vitamin E intake and fatal CAD was strongest in the subgroup of 21,809 women who did not consume vitamin supplements. In this subgroup, women in the highest quintile of dietary intake of vitamin E had a 64% lower risk of CAD mortality than those in the lowest quintile of intake (p-trend $= 0.004$) after adjustment for potential confounders. It is possible that vitamin E derived from food is simply a marker for other dietary factors related to the risk of CAD, but the relationship persisted even after controlling for other dietary factors, such as linoleic acid, folate, fiber, and other antioxidant vitamins that are associated with the intake of vitamin E. These results are in agreement with a prospective study from Finland that also found a significant inverse association between dietary intake of vitamin E and coronary mortality among 2385 women 30 to 69 years of age over 14 years of follow-up (51). In further contrast to the findings in the NHS, use of vitamin E supplements was not associated with protection from fatal CAD (p-trend = 0.39) in this cohort.

In summary, the two largest observational studies in women, the NHS study and the Iowa Women's Health Study, reported apparently conflicting results. The NHS did not find a beneficial association between increasing dietary intake of vitamin E and the subsequent development of CAD, whereas the Iowa Women's Health Study found a strong inverse association. On the other hand, the Iowa Study did not find a beneficial association between the use of vitamin E supplements and CAD, whereas the NHS found a strong association. The reason for the discrepancies between the results of these two studies is not entirely clear. Differences in the study cohorts potentially could account for some of the discrepancy. The women in the Iowa Study were older and had more fatal CAD events and would have had more power to assess the effect of dietary vitamin E on this outcome. In addition, the outcome events also differed between the studies. The outcome used in the Iowa and Finnish studies was fatal CAD documented by death certificate alone in contrast to the combined end point of fatal and nonfatal CAD confirmed by medical records used in the NHS and HPFS. It is possible that the conflicting results could be due to a disparity in the treatment effects of dietary vitamin E on fatal and nonfatal end points. The disparate results of vitamin E supplements may be partially explained by the relatively few women who reported using high doses of supplements in the Iowa study compared with the NHS. Also, no information was available on duration of use in the Iowa study, and supplements were found to have an effect only after 2 years of use in the NHS. The conflicting results from these two large observational studies on dietary intake of vitamin E and intake of vitamin E supplements highlight the need for further observational studies and randomized trials examining this issue. Currently, several completed or ongoing randomized trials address the question of whether vitamin E supplements decrease CAD incidence; however, no current trials address whether dietary vitamin E decreases the risk of CAD.

Randomized Trials

The randomized trials, including vitamin E as primary and secondary prevention for CAD, have used vitamin E supplements. The completed and ongoing randomized trials of vitamin E are summarized in Table 9-2. Primary prevention trials have focused on populations at either low or high risk for

Table 9-2 Completed and Ongoing Randomized Clinical Trials of Vitamin E Alone or in Combination with Other Antioxidants

Trial Class and Name	Antioxidant (Dosage)	Study Participants	Duration	End Point	Relative Risk (95% CI)
Primary Prevention					
Chinese Cancer Prevention Trial (52)	Cocktail of vitamin E (30 mg/d), beta-carotene (15 mg/d), and selenium (50 mg/d)	29,584 women and men	5 years	Cerebrovascular mortality	0.90 (0.76–1.07)
ATBC (53)	Vitamin E (50 mg/d)	29,133 male smokers 50–69 years of age	6 years	Cardiovascular disease mortality	0.98 (0.89–1.08)
				Total mortality	1.02 (0.95–1.09)
Women's Health Study (50)	Vitamin E (600 IU every other day)	40,000 women > 45 years of age	7 years	MI, stroke, and death from cardiovascular disease	Ongoing
Secondary Prevention					
CHAOS (61)	Vitamin E (800 IU/d in 546 patients and 400 IU/d in 489 patients)	2002 patients with coronary artery disease on angiography	Median follow-up of 510 days	Nonfatal MI	0.23 (0.11–0.47)
				Cardiovascular death	1.18 (0.62–2.27)
				Combined end point of non-fatal MI and cardiovascular death	0.53 (0.34–0.83)
WACS (63)	Vitamin E (600 IU every other day)	8000 women with pre-existing cardiovascular disease or ≥ 3 coronary risk factors	6 years	MI, stroke, coronary revascularization, death from cardiovascular disease	Ongoing
HOPE (62)	Vitamin E (400 IU/d)	9000 women and men with previous MI, stroke, PVD, or diabetes		MI, stroke, death from cardiovascular disease	Ongoing
GISSI	Vitamin E (300 mg/d)	12,000 women and men with a recent history of MI (< 3 months)		Total mortality	Ongoing
HPS	Cocktail of vitamin E (600 IU/d), beta-carotene (20 mg/d), and vitamin C (50 mg/d)	20,000 women and men with previous angina, stroke, claudication, or diabetes		Total mortality	Ongoing

ATBC = Alpha-Tocopherol–Beta-Carotene Cancer Prevention Trial; CHAOS = Cambridge Heart Antioxidant Study; CI = confidence interval; GISSI = Groupo Italiano per lo Studio della Sopravvivenza nell'Infarcto Miocardio Acuto Prevention Trial; HOPE = Heart Outcomes Prevention Evaluation Study; HPS = Heart Protection Study; MI = myocardial infarction; PVD = peripheral vascular disease; WACS = Women's Antioxidant Cardiovascular Study; WHS = Women's Health Study.

CAD and its complications. At this time, none of the antioxidant vitamins including vitamin E has been shown to be beneficial as a primary prevention against CAD in randomized trials. The Chinese Cancer Prevention Trial randomized a poorly nourished population of 29,584 women and men to one of eight treatment arms comprised of various combinations of nine vitamins and minerals for 5 years. There was an apparent, though insignificant, reduction in cerebrovascular mortality (RR = 0.90 95% CI, 0.76–1.07) among those assigned a daily cocktail of beta-carotene (15 mg), vitamin E (30 mg), and selenium (50 mg) (52). The effects of individual micronutrients could not be assessed because of the cocktail design. In addition, CAD rates were too low in this population to assess the effect of this intervention on this end point. The Alpha-Tocopherol–Beta-Carotene (ATBC) Cancer Prevention Trial tested vitamin E and beta-carotene among 29,133 Finnish male smokers aged 50 to 69 years for an average treatment and follow-up period of 6 years (53). Participants were randomized in a 2 x 2 factorial design to 50 mg/d of alpha-tocopherol, 20 mg/d of beta-carotene, both active drugs, or both placebos. For vitamin E, there was no clear reduction in the risk of ischemic heart disease or ischemic stroke mortality; however, an increased risk of fatal hemorrhagic stroke (RR = 1.50; 95% CI, 1.03–2.20) was found but was insignificant after adjustment for multiple testing. In a subsequent report, the risk of developing angina was slightly lower among those assigned to vitamin E (RR = 0.91; 95% CI, 0.83–0.99). The apparent lack of benefit may be secondary to the relatively low dose of vitamin E given (54). The observational data from the NHS and HPFS discussed previously suggest that supplementation at higher doses ($\geq$ 100 IU) may be required to reduce the risk of heart disease (48,49).

The above trials do not address whether vitamin E may benefit patients with established cardiovascular disease or those at high risk for the development of cardiovascular disease. Similar to cholesterol lowering, the benefits of antioxidant vitamins may be greater in a population at high risk for subsequent cardiovascular disease morbidity and mortality and, therefore, may be more likely to outweigh the risks. Several small-scale trials have tested the effect of supplemental vitamin E among individuals with various forms of atherosclerotic disease, including claudication and angina. Three trials of vitamin E in the treatment of claudication revealed a clinical benefit over periods of 1 to 3 years (55–57), whereas the trials of angina pectoris had equivocal results with high doses of vitamin E (1600 and 3200 IU/d) (58,59). One recent small-scale trial tested the effect of vitamin E supplementation (400 IU) on restenosis rates following angioplasty in 100 patients. There was an insignificant 30% reduction in the risk of restenosis as measured by subsequent catheterization or exercise test (60). Both the small sample size and short duration of treatment may have limited the ability and the statistical power of these studies to detect small-to-moderate benefits.

In the recently reported Cambridge Heart Antioxidant Study (CHAOS), 2002 patients with angiographically proven CAD were assigned to either a placebo or supplemental vitamin E (546 patients were treated with 800 IU and 489 were treated with 400 IU after a protocol change) (61). Only 312 (15.6%) of the study participants were women, and the results were not reported by sex. After a median follow-up of 510 days, those assigned to vitamin E had a significantly lower risk of subsequent nonfatal MI (RR = 0.23, 95% CI, 0.11–0.47) and a combined end point of nonfatal MI and cardiovascular death (RR = 0.53; 95% CI, 0.34–0.83). However, there was also an insignificant excess of cardiovascular death (RR = 1.18; 95% CI, 0.62–2.27) and total mortality (3.5% vs. 2.7%; p = 0.31) among those assigned to vitamin E. The underlying mechanism for the disparity in the treatment effect between nonfatal MI and cardiovascular death is unclear.

In summary, observational studies have generally found inverse associations between high vitamin E intake (either through dietary or supplement sources) and CAD incidence or death. If this association proves to be causal, it is unclear what the optimal dose of vitamin E might be and whether this can be obtained through diet alone. In the NHS and HPFS, the optimal dose seemed to be greater than 100 IU/d, which would require vitamin supplements, whereas the Iowa Women's Health Study found that much lower doses obtained through dietary intake were associated with a decreased risk. It is also unclear what role the composition of the vitamin E (alpha- vs. gamma-tocopherol) plays and whether there exists a disparity of effect on fatal end points compared with nonfatal end points. The only completed randomized trial of vitamin E supplements in primary prevention in a well-nourished population was conducted in men and found no benefit of vitamin E on cardiovascular disease. This trial may have been limited by an inadequate dose of vitamin E, but the possible increase in hemorrhagic stroke among those assigned to this small dose does raise some concern. Despite the promising observational data, definitive conclusions on the efficacy of high-dose vitamin E supplements (< 100 IU/d) can not be made until results from randomized trials are available. The ongoing Women's Health Study is currently testing a higher dose of vitamin E (600 IU every other day) among 40,000 apparently healthy female health professionals aged 45 years and older in the primary prevention of cardiovascular disease and cancer (21,22). This study will provide important information on the risks and benefits of high-dose vitamin E supplements in the primary prevention of cardiovascular disease. It is prudent, therefore, to await the results of this trial before initiating therapy with high-dose supplements in apparently healthy women or men to prevent cardiovascular disease.

With regard to secondary prevention, although the results from the CHAOS trial are promising, the disparity in the treatment effects on cardiovascular disease death and non-fatal MI needs to be evaluated further in a larger trial before advocating widespread use of high-dose vitamin E supplements for the secondary prevention of cardiovascular disease. Currently, several secondary prevention trials are testing vitamin E alone or in combination with other antioxidants. The Heart Outcomes Prevention Evaluation (HOPE) Study is testing vitamin E among 9,000 men and women with previous MI, stroke, or known peripheral vascular disease (62), and the Gruppo Italiano per lo Studio della Sopravvivenza nell'Infarcto Miocardio (GISSI) study is conducting a nonblind trial of vitamin E among those with a recent MI. The Heart Protection Study is testing a cocktail of vitamin E, vitamin C, and beta-carotene in a factorial design among 20,000 individuals with coronary risk factors but who do not yet have known cardiovascular disease. However, this trial will be unable to test the individual effect of each of the antioxidant vitamins. The Women's Antioxidant Cardiovascular Study (WACS) is testing these antioxidant vitamins in a factorial design and therefore will be able to test the individual effects of vitamin E, vitamin C, and beta-carotene as secondary prevention of cardiovascular disease (63). The trial is being conducted among 8,000 female health professionals, age 40 years or older, who have either preexisting cardiovascular disease or at least three coronary risk factors for cardiovascular disease. The results of these trials will be the basis for future recommendations regarding the use of vitamin E supplements in the secondary prevention of cardiovascular disease.

Beta-Carotene

Observational Studies
Seven prospective cohort studies have examined the relationship between beta-carotene intake and cardiovascular disease. Five studies have found protective trends (49,64–67); however, only two (one of which included women) achieved statistical significance (49,64). The HPFS (which was composed entirely of men) found a lower risk of CAD associated with higher carotene intake only among current and former smokers (49). The Massachusetts Health Care Panel Study also found an inverse association between higher carotene intake from fruits and vegetables and total cardiovascular disease mortality among 1299 women and men aged 65 years and older (64). In the Nurses Health Study, a 22% reduction in the risk of CAD events was observed among women in the highest quintile of beta-carotene intake as compared with women in the lowest quintile; however, this risk reduction was no longer statistically significant after adjustment for vitamins E and C (67). The Iowa Women's Health Study did not find any protective association between beta-carotene intake and cardiovascular disease (50). Studies of serum carotenoids and beta-carotene have yielded similar inconclusive results (68). Two prospective studies in men found a decreased risk of ischemic heart dis-

ease in association with higher serum carotenoid concentrations (69,70a). In the Prospective Basel Study, low plasma concentrations of beta-carotene were associated with an increased risk of fatal CAD, and the risk was even higher if both vitamin C and beta-carotene concentrations were low (70a). In summary, the observational data support a trend toward a modest risk reduction associated with high dietary carotenoid intake (70b). The magnitude of the effect, however, seems less than that seen with vitamin E, with many of the risk reductions failing to reach statistical significance.

Randomized Trials

Beta-carotene has been tested extensively as primary prevention against CAD in randomized trials, but the results have been disappointing. The completed and ongoing randomized trials of beta-carotene are summarized in Table 9-3. In the previously described ATBC trial among 29,133 Finish male smokers, there was an insignificant increase in ischemic heart disease deaths (RR = 1.12; 95% CI, 1.00–1.25) (53) and no reduction in the risk of angina among those assigned to 20 mg/d of beta-carotene (54). Similar results were found with a combined treatment of beta-carotene (30 mg/d) and retinol (25,000 IU/d) in the Beta-Carotene and Retinol Efficacy Trial (CARET) among 18,314 men and women who were either smokers or had been exposed to asbestos (71). The latter trial was stopped after 4 years of treatment due to a projected inability to detect a benefit over the planned funding period and a trend toward increased lung cancer in the treatment group. Data on nonfatal cardiovascular disease events are not yet available, but a trend toward excess cardiovascular disease deaths (RR = 1.26; 95% CI, 0.99–1.61) and an increase in total mortality (RR = 1.18; 95% CI, 1.02–1.37) was reported. In the Physicians Health Study (PHS), we found no benefit or harm of 12 years of treatment with beta-carotene (50 mg on alternate days) among 22,071 U.S. male physicians (72). There were no differences in the risks of MI, cardiovascular disease death, stroke, or a composite of the three end points between treatment groups. These randomized trials provide clear evidence of no benefit of beta-carotene in the primary prevention of cardiovascular disease, despite previous promising observational data, and they underscore the importance of randomized trials of adequate size. In addition, two of these trials raise the possibility of harm in smokers, emphasizing the need for randomized trials even when agents are thought to be harmless.

Despite the clear lack of benefit in the primary prevention of cardiovascular disease, beta-carotene supplementation may be of benefit in the secondary prevention of cardiovascular disease for the same reasons noted above for vitamin E. Currently, no data exist from any randomized trials specifically designed to answer this question. We conducted a subgroup analysis within the PHS among 333 men who had a history of angina or a coronary revasculariza-

Table 9-3 Completed and Ongoing Randomized Clinical Trials of Beta-Carotene Alone or in Combination with Other Antioxidants

Trial Class and Name	Antioxidant (Dosage)	Study Participants	Duration	End Point	Relative Risk (95% CI)
Primary Prevention					
Chinese Cancer Prevention Trial (52)	Cocktail of vitamin E (30 mg/d), beta-carotene (15 mg/d), and selenium (50 mg/d)	29,584 women and men	5 years	Cerebrovascular mortality	0.90 (0.76–1.07)
ATBC (53)	Beta-carotene (20 mg/d)	29,133 male smokers, 50–69 years of age	6 years	Cardiovascular disease mortality	1.12 (1.00–1.25)
				Total mortality	1.08 (1.01–1.16)
CARET (71)	Beta-carotene (30 mg/d) and retinol (25,000 IU/d)	18,314 women and men who were smokers or had been exposed to asbestos	4 years	Cardiovascular disease mortality	1.26 (0.99–1.61)
				Total mortality	1.18 (1.02–1.37)
PHS (72)	Beta-carotene (50 mg on alternate days)	22,071 U.S. male physicians	12 years	Cardiovascular disease mortality	1.09 (0.93–1.27)
				MI	0.96 (0.84–1.09)
				Total mortality	1.02 (0.93–1.11)
Secondary Prevention					
PHS (72)	Beta-carotene (50 mg on alternate days)	333 men who had a history of angina or a coronary revascularization before random-ization in PHS	12 years	MI, stroke, death from cardiovas-cular disease	0.71 (0.47–1.07)
WACS (63)	Beta-carotene (600 IU every other day)	8000 women with pre-existing cardiovascular disease or ≥ 3 coronary risk factors	6 years	MI, stroke, coro-nary revascu-larization, death from cardiovas-cular disease	Ongoing
HPS	Cocktail of vitamin E (600 IU/d), beta-carotene (20 mg/d), and vitamin C (50 mg/d)	20,000 women and men with previous angina, stroke, claudica-tion, or diabetes		Total mortality	Ongoing

ATBC = Alpha-Tocopherol–Beta-Carotene Cancer Prevention Trial; CARET = Beta-Carotene and Retinol Effi-cacy Trial; CI = confidence interval; HPS = Heart Protection Study; MI = myocardial infarction; PHS = Physi-cians Health Study; WACS = Women's Antioxidant Cardiovascular Study.

tion procedure before randomization. Among subjects randomized to beta-carotene, a 54% reduction (RR = 0.46; 95% CI, 0.24–0.85) in the risk of major vascular events emerged after 5 years of follow-up (73); a persistent, although insignificant, 29% reduction (RR = 0.71 95% CI; 0.47–1.07) emerged after 12 years of follow-up (74). Although promising, this subgroup analysis will need to be confirmed in randomized trials of adequate size. Currently, the only randomized trial testing the individual effect of beta-carotene in the secondary prevention of cardiovascular disease is the previously described WACS trial among 8000 women with either pre-existing cardiovascular disease or at least three coronary risk factors for cardiovascular disease. WACS is currently testing beta-carotene (50 mg on alternate days) in a factorial design with vitamin E and vitamin C and therefore will provide important information on the individual effect of beta-carotene as secondary prevention against cardiovascular disease (63). The only other secondary prevention trial testing beta-carotene, the Heart Protection Study (HPS) among 20,000 individuals with coronary risk factors, is testing a cocktail of beta-carotene and vitamins E and C. Although unable to test the individual effect of beta-carotene, this trial will provide important information on the effectiveness of a combination of antioxidant vitamins in the secondary prevention of CAD. Currently, especially given the results of the primary prevention trials mentioned above, use of beta-carotene as secondary prevention against CAD is not recommended. Decisions regarding its effectiveness for this indication should await the results of these ongoing trials.

Vitamin C

Observational Studies

Although many studies have examined the relationship between vitamin C intake and the incidence of CAD, the results are inconsistent. Several studies have found an apparent protective effect from high vitamin C intake (66,75). The National Health and Nutrition Examination Survey I (NHANES I), a prospective study of 11,348 women and men, found that a daily intake of 50 mg of vitamin C was associated with a 42% reduction in the cardiovascular standardized mortality ratio (75). The association was observed for vitamin C from supplements but not from dietary sources; however, intake of other antioxidant vitamins was not controlled for in the analysis. Others studies, such as the Nurses Health Study (76), have found protective associations that were no longer significant after adjustment for intake of other vitamins. Two of these studies, the HPFS (49) and the Iowa Women's Health Study (50), found trends toward an increase in risk for vitamin C after multivariate adjustments were made. The lack of an association between vitamin C and CAD in these cohorts may have been due to the relatively high intake of vitamin C, with the mean in the lowest quintile above the recommended daily allowance.

Despite the conflicting observational data, a substantial amount of experimental data suggest that vitamin C may be of benefit in preventing atherosclerosis, particularly in smokers. Chronic smoking is associated with reduced plasma levels and increased consumption of vitamin C (77). Of all the antioxidants, vitamin C quenches oxidants in a hydrophilic environment (78) and may be particularly important in preventing cigarette smoke–induced free-radical formation and therefore LDL oxidation. Oral supplementation with vitamin C has been shown to reverse the increase in monocyte adhesion observed in smokers, which may be mediated through oxidized LDL (79). Specific interactions between smoking and vitamin C intake have not been reported in observational studies.

Randomized Trials

Supplementation with vitamin C has not been adequately tested in primary or secondary prevention trials. Currently, the only large-scale randomized trial to test vitamin C is the Chinese Cancer Prevention Trial mentioned previously. This trial found no benefit of a combination of 125 mg of vitamin C and 30 µg of molybdenum on cerebrovascular mortality among 29,584 poorly nourished men (47). As mentioned earlier, this trial did not have enough CAD end points to analyze this outcome. We are not aware of any ongoing trials that are testing vitamin C in primary prevention of CAD, and currently the observational data are conflicting and do not support its use for this indication. The only trials testing vitamin C are the two previously discussed secondary prevention trials, which are also testing beta-carotene. WACS is testing the individual effect of 500 mg/d of vitamin C in 8000 women, and the Heart Protection Study is testing a cocktail of vitamin C combined with vitamin E and beta-carotene. Recommendations regarding the use of vitamin C supplements in the secondary prevention of CAD will depend on the results of these ongoing trials.

Alcohol

Although the data are not entirely consistent, a large body of research suggests that moderate alcohol intake is associated with decreased risks of CAD events. The biological mechanisms underlying this association have not been fully explained, but favorable changes in lipids and hemostatic factors are thought to be partly responsible. A number of studies have demonstrated a strong positive association between alcohol consumption and high-density lipoprotein (HDL) cholesterol (80–82). In one case-control study that examined the interrelationship between alcohol intake, HDL cholesterol, and MI, the addition of HDL (or either of its subfractions to the multivariate model) substantially reduced the inverse association between alcohol intake and MI, providing support for the hypothesis that HDL cholesterol partially mediates this inverse association (83). This and other analyses adjusting for the influence of HDL cholesterol indicate that this variable accounts for approximately half the reduction in risk attributable to moderate alcohol intake (81,82).

Alcohol also has favorable effects on the fibrinolytic system, which could reduce coronary risk (84). Alcohol consumption has been inversely associated with fibrinogen levels (85) and directly associated with plasma concentrations of tissue-type plasminogen activator (t-PA) independent of HDL levels (86). Alcohol has been shown to increase endothelial cell production of t-PA in vitro (87,88) and to elevate both t-PA antigen and PAI-1 levels and increase morning t-PA activity in response to an evening ingestion (89). In addition to these favorable effects, however, alcohol consumption increases blood pressure and resultant hypertensive heart disease (90). Alcohol, at heavy levels, may cause cardiomyopathy (91) and may precipitate ventricular arrhythmias and sudden death (92).

Observational Epidemiologic Studies

Evidence that the inverse association between moderate alcohol consumption and CAD reflects a true protective effect of alcohol is provided by the consistency of the finding in large well-conducted studies in diverse populations and settings. In general, most prospective studies of alcohol consumption have found a U-shaped relationship with CAD deaths (93–99) and a more linear or L-shaped relationship (83,99,100) with nonfatal events. The largest study in women to examine the association between alcohol and CAD was the Nurses Health Study (99). In 1980, over 87,000 women aged 34 to 59 years without a history of MI, angina, stroke, or cancer completed a dietary questionnaire that assessed their consumption of beer, wine, and liquor. After 4 years of follow-up, a total of 164 nonfatal infarctions, 36 CAD deaths, 86 nonfatal strokes, and 34 fatal strokes were identified. In comparison to nondrinkers, women consuming 5 to 14 g of alcohol daily (3–9 drinks per week) had a statistically significant 40% lower risk of CAD. The women with the highest alcohol intake (≥ 25 g of alcohol per day) were at the lowest risk after multivariate adjustment (RR = 0.4; 95% CI, 0.2–0.9). However, because the level of alcohol in the cohort was generally moderate (> 98% of the drinkers reported consuming ≤ 45 g/d of alcohol [3–4 drinks per day]), this study's data do not contain evidence of the effects of heavy drinking on CAD risk. These findings are consistent with studies in men (93,95–97) and smaller studies in women (101). Alcohol intake was also associated with a decreased risk of ischemic stroke in this study, and although the number of cases was small, an increased risk of subarachnoid hemorrhage was seen (99). Wine was found to be slightly more protective in this study, but other studies have found other sources of alcohol to be more important (93,95). Thus, the overall epidemiologic evidence from studies in diverse population settings indicate an inverse association between moderate alcohol intake and CAD that is not specific to any type of alcoholic beverage.

Aside from the apparent beneficial effects on CAD, alcohol has many well-known adverse health effects at higher levels of consumption, including increased rates of certain cancers, cirrhosis, hemorrhagic stroke, and trauma (102). In fact, heavy alcohol consumption is the third leading preventable cause of mortality in the United States (103). Studies of the association between alcohol consumption and total mortality provide important information on the balance of these risks and benefits. Most studies evaluating total mortality in men have consistently reported a U- or J-shaped pattern, with moderate drinkers (1–9 drinks per week) at lowest risk due to an overwhelming lower risk of CAD mortality (104–107). Those individuals with higher consumption levels experience increased mortality from a variety of other causes. The results of these studies may not be directly applicable to women, because alcohol's risk to benefit ratio might differ in women as discussed previously for aspirin. Also as mentioned previously, women have a lower risk of CAD than men, which might reduce the likelihood of benefit. Women, too, seem to be more susceptible to alcoholic liver disease (108) and to ethanol-induced cardiomyopathy (109). Moreover, consumption of alcohol at the same moderate levels that are inversely associated with CAD risk has been associated with an increased risk of breast cancer in several studies (110–112).

The Nurses Health Study examined this risk-to-benefit ratio for alcohol in a subsequent analysis of total mortality after 12 years of follow-up (113). The initially collected information on alcohol intake in 1980 was updated in 1984 and 1986. Light-to-moderate drinking (1.5–29.9 g/d) was associated with a reduced risk of total mortality with a nadir of risk (RR = 0.83; 95% CI, 0.74–0.93) at approximately 1.5 to 4.9 g/d (1–3 drinks per week). The lower risk associated with light drinking principally was due to a lower risk of fatal cardiovascular disease. The women who consumed 30 g/d or more of alcohol (≥ 2 drinks per day) had a 19% increased risk of total mortality (95% CI, 0.02–0.38) primarily due to an increase in noncardiac deaths, such as breast cancer and cirrhosis. In a manner consistent with these competing effects, the apparent benefit associated with light-to-moderate drinking was greatest among women at greater risk for CAD and among those aged over 50 years with or without one or more risk factors for CAD. This result is tempered somewhat by the lower number of deaths among those younger than 50 years of age and those without cardiac risk factors, limiting the ability to detect an association. Among women without cardiac risk factors, however, the risk of total mortality associated with consumption of more than 30 g/d of alcohol was significantly higher than in those with cardiac risk factors (RR = 2.22 vs. 1.12; p = 0.04), and although the numbers were small, the results were also consistent with a higher risk among younger women. This finding cannot be explained by inadequate end points, and it suggests that the risk associated with moderate-to-heavy consumption of alcohol may be greater in younger women or in those without CAD risk factors. These findings with respect to age were consistent with another large cohort study involving women from Kaiser Permanente (104). This study also found that the reduction in cardiovascular mortality associated with light drinking was more pronounced in older people, whereas the increase in mortality risk associated with heavy drinking was more pronounced in younger people and in women in general.

As mentioned previously, observational studies are limited in their ability to prove causation because unmeasured and residual confounding by other lifestyle factors remains an alternative explanation for these findings. It is unlikely that randomized trials of alcohol will be performed given the complex reasons why people consume alcohol and the concern about inducing alcoholism in susceptible people who currently do not drink. Therefore, as physicians, we have to make recommendations to our patients based only on the observational data, despite their limitations. The weight of this evidence suggests that cardioprotective effects associated with light-to-moderate alcohol consumption seem to outweigh the adverse effects in women, especially among those at increased risk for CAD (age > 50 years, presence of CAD risk factors, or both). Whether moderate alcohol consumption is beneficial in younger women or those without CAD risk factors is less clear. In the Nurses Health Study, the nadir of cardiovascular risk occurred at one to three drinks per week, which is below the level of consumption associated with increased risks of breast cancer in that (111) and other studies (110); therefore, this level of consumption will probably be safe even for those who are not at risk for CAD. Women who choose to consume alcohol in light-to-moderate amounts need not be counseled to stop such behavior. The much more difficult question is whether women (either with or without CAD risk factors) who do not consume alcohol regularly should be advised to drink alcohol moderately for its cardioprotective effects. For such individuals, although the initiation of regular, light-to-moderate alcohol consumption might yield net health benefits, the potential for addiction and adverse psychologic and physiologic effects at slightly greater levels of consumption precludes any such general recommendation. It is clear, however, that heavy alcohol consumption is associated with an increase in all-cause mortality, and the public health message to curtail such use should be unequivocal. Recent assessment of primary care screening tests for alcohol use documents the benefit of the Alcohol Use Disorders Identification Test (AUDIT), a 10-question screen developed by the World Health Organization over the (AGE) or Self-Administered Alcoholism Screening Test (SAAST) in effectively screening ambulatory female and male patients of various ethnicities (114).

Summary

Interest in pharmacologic agents for the prevention of CAD in women has increased with the recognition of the magnitude of this public health problem in women. Observational data suggest that antioxidant vitamins, particularly vitamin E, aspirin, and moderate alcohol consumption (1–3 drinks per week) may be efficacious in the primary prevention of CAD in women. Although the observational data are promising, definitive findings from large-scale primary prevention trials in women are crucial to formulate reliable treatment recommendations for women. Currently, no direct randomized trial data exist on any of these agents in women, but the ongoing Women's Health Study is currently testing aspirin (100 mg every other day) simultaneously with vitamin E (600 IU every other day) in a 2 x 2 factorial design among 40,000 female health professionals aged 45 years and older. This study will provide important information on the risks and benefits of high-dose vitamin E supplements and low-dose aspirin in the primary prevention of cardiovascular disease in women; firm recommendations on whether to use these agents as primary prevention should await the results of this trial. Beta-carotene has been adequately tested in randomized trials. Based on the results of these trials, beta-carotene is not recommended as primary prevention, despite previous promising observational data.

With respect to secondary prevention, strong evidence supports the use of medium- to low-dose aspirin (75–325 mg) in women who have a previous history of cardiovascular disease (e.g., MI, stroke, TIAs, chronic stable angina, and peripheral vascular disease). Aspirin therapy in this setting reduces subsequent cardiac cardiovascular events and death; it should be used in all patients unless a serious contraindication exists. Furthermore, aspirin (165–325 mg) should be given acutely to all women with symptoms, electrocardiographic evidence, or both suggesting an acute MI or unstable angina. The data for vitamin E as secondary prevention are promising but also raise the concern that there may be a disparity in effect of vitamin E on fatal and nonfatal cardiac end points, because the benefit in the CHAOS trial was limited to nonfatal reinfarction. The results from several ongoing randomized trials will provide invaluable information as to whether vitamin E should be recommended as secondary prevention in all women with a history of cardiovascular disease. Currently, no randomized trial data exist on the use of vitamin C or beta-carotene as secondary prevention, but the ongoing WACS is currently testing these antioxidant vitamins in a factorial design as secondary prevention of cardiovascular disease in women.

Finally, low-to-moderate levels of alcohol consumption (1–14 drinks per week) are associated with lower risks of CAD in observational studies and may be effective as both primary and secondary prevention. This benefit must be balanced against the known risks of alcohol, most notably, breast cancer, cirrhosis, and the potential for addiction. Because it is unlikely that a randomized trial of alcohol will be performed, recommendations must be based on the available observational data and should be individualized after balancing the potential for the known risks and benefits in each patient. As would be expected, the benefit seems greater in those over 50 years of age and in those with CAD risk factors who are at higher risk for a CAD end point. The optimum level of consumption is unknown, but the maximal benefit on CAD mortality occurred at approximately one to three drinks per week in a large observational study of women. Reassuringly, this level of consumption was associated with a reduction in total mortality and was not associated with an increased risk of breast cancer; therefore, this level of consumption is probably safe for most women. Caution must be exercised, however, when recommending alcohol as a cardioprotective agent, because the potential for addiction and abuse exists even in those without a family history of alcoholism.

REFERENCES

1. **American Heart Association.** Heart and Stroke Facts: 1995 Statistical Supplement. Dallas: American Heart Association; 1994.

2. **Rich-Edwards JW, Manson JE, Hennekens CH, Buring JE.** The primary prevention of coronary artery disease in women. N Engl J Med. 1995;332:1758–66.

3. **Kannel WB, Abott RD.** Incidence and prognosis of myocardial infarction in women: the Framingham study. In: Eaker ED, Packard B, Wenger NK, Clarkson TB, Tyroler HA, eds. Coronary Artery Disease in Women. New York: Haymarket-Doyma; 1987: 208–14.

4. **Pinsky JL, Jette AM, Branch LG, et al.** The Framingham Disability Study: relationship of various coronary artery disease manifestations to disability in older persons living in the community. Am J Public Health. 1990;80:1363–7.

5. **O'Brien JR.** Effects of salicylates on human platelets. Lancet. 1968;1:779–83.

6. **Moncada S, Vane JR.** Arachidonic acid metabolites and the interaction between platelets and blood-vessel walls. N Engl J Med. 1979;300:1142–7.

7. **Patrono C, Ciabattoni G, Patrignani P, et al.** Clinical pharmacology of platelet cyclooxygenase inhibition. Circulation. 1985;72:1177–84.

8. **Masotti G, Galanti G, Poggesi L, et al.** Differential inhibition of prostaglandin production and platelet aggregation by aspirin. Lancet. 1979;2:1213–7.

9. **Ridker PM, Cushman M, Stampfer MJ, et al.** Inflammation, aspirin, and the risk of cardiovascular disease in apparently healthy men. N Engl J Med. 1997;336:973–9.

10. **Ho PC, Triggs EJ, Bourne DWA, Heazlewood VJ.** The effects of age and sex on the disposition of acetylsalicylic acid and its metabolites. Br J Clin Pharmacol. 1985;19:675–84.

11. **Centers for Disease Control and Prevention.** Coronary artery disease incidence by sex. MMWR. 1992;41:526–9.

12. **Robins M, Baum HM.** The National Survey of Stroke: Incidence. Stroke. 1981;12: 145–7.

13. **Antiplatelet Trialists' Collaboration.** Secondary prevention of vascular disease by prolonged antiplatelet therapy. Br Med J. 1988;296:320–321.

14. **ISIS-2 (Second International Study of Infarct Survival) Collaborative Group.** Randomized trial of intravenous streptokinase, oral aspirin, both, or neither among 17,187 cases of suspected acute myocardial infarction: ISIS-2. Lancet. 1988;2:349–60.

15. **Antiplatelet Trialists' Collaboration.** Collaborative overview of randomized trials of antiplatelet treatment. Part 1: Prevention of death, myocardial infarction, and stroke by prolonged antiplatelet treatment. Br Med J. 1994; 30:81–106.

16. **Manson JE, Stampfer MJ, Colditz GA, et al.** A prospective study of aspirin use and primary prevention of cardiovascular disease in women. JAMA. 1994;266:521–7.

17. **Hammond EC, Garfinkel L.** Aspirin and coronary artery disease: findings of a prospective study. Br Med J. 1975;2:269–71.

18. **Paganini-Hil A, Chao A, Ross RK, Henderson BE.** Aspirin use and chronic diseases: a cohort of the elderly. Br Med J. 1989;299:1247–50.

19. **Steering Committee of the Physicians' Health Study Research Group.** Final report on the aspirin component of the ongoing Physicians' Health Study. N Engl J Med. 1989;321:129–35.

20. **Peto R, Gray R, Collins R, et al.** A randomized trial of prophylactic daily aspirin in British male doctors. Br Med J. 1988;296:313–6.

21. **Women's Health Study Research Group.** The Women's Health Study: rationale and background. J Myocardial Ischemia. 1992;4:30–40.

22. **Women's Health Study Research Group.** The Women's Health Study: summary of study design. J Myocardial Ischemia. 1992;4:27–9.

23. **Hessler JR, Morel DW, James LJ, Chisolm GM.** Lipoprotein oxidation and lipoprotein-induced cytotoxicity. Arteriosclerosis. 1983;3:215–22.

24. **Yagi K.** Increased serum lipid peroxides initiate atherogenesis. Bioessays. 1984;1: 58–60.

25. **Quinn MT, Parthasarathy S, Steinberg D.** Endothelial cell-derived chemotactic activity for mouse peritoneal macrophages and the effects of modified forms of low density lipoprotein. Proc Natl Acad Sci USA. 1985;82:5949–53.

26. **Fogelman AM, Schechter I, Hokom M, et al.** Malondialdehyde alteration of low-density lipoproteins leads to cholesterol ester accumulation in human monocyte macrophages. Proc Natl Acad Sci USA. 1980;77:2214–8.

27. **Goldstein JL, Ho YK, Basu SK, Brown MS.** Binding site on macrophages that mediates uptake and degradation of acetylated low-density lipoprotein, producing massive cholesterol deposition. Proc Natl Acad Sci USA. 1979;76:333–7.

28. **Kugiyama K, Kerns SA, Morisett JD, et al.** Impairment of endothelium-dependent arterial relaxation by lysolecithin in modified low-density lipoproteins. Nature. 1990; 344:160–2.

29. **Salonen T, Yla-Herttuala S, Yamamoto R, et al.** Autoantibody against oxidized LDL and progression of carotid atherosclerosis. Lancet. 1992;839:883–7.

30. **Beckman JS, Beckman TW, Chen J, et al.** Apparent hydroxyl radical production by peroxynitrate: implications for endothelial injury from nitric oxide and superoxide. Proc Natl Acad Sci USA. 1990;87:1620–4.

31. **Marcus AJ, Silk ST, Safier LB, Ullman HL.** Superoxide production and reducing activity in human platelets. J Clin Invest. 1977;59:149–58.

32. **Saran M, Michael C, Bors W.** Reaction of NO with O_2: implications for the action of endothelium-derived relaxing factor (EDRF). Free Radic Res Commun. 1990;10:221–6.

33. **Esterbauer H, Gebicki J, Puhl H, Jurgens G.** The role of lipid peroxidation and antioxidants in oxidative modification of LDL. Free Radical Biol Med. 1992;13:341–90.

34. **Jailal I, Norkus E, Cristol L, Grundy SM.** Beta-carotene inhibits the oxidative modification of low-density lipoprotein. Biochim Biophys Acta. 1991;1086:134–8.

35. **Harats D, Ben-Naim M, Dabach Y, et al.** Effect of vitamin C and E supplementation on susceptibility of plasma lipoproteins to peroxidation induced by acute smoking. Atherosclerosis. 1990;85:47–54.

36. **Esterbauer H, Dieber-Rotheneder M, Striegl G, Waeg G.** Role of vitamin E in preventing the oxidation of low-density lipoprotein. Am J Clin Nutr. 1991;53:314–21s.

37. **Verlangieri AJ, Bush M.** Effects of D-alpha-tocopherol supplementation on experimentally induced primate atherosclerosis. J Am Coll Nutr. 1983;38:631–9.

38. **Steiner M.** Influence of vitamin E on platelet function in man. J Am Coll Nutr. 1991;10:466–73.

39. **Cordova C, Musca A, Viola F, et al.** Influence of ascorbic acid on platelet aggregation in vitro and in vivo. Atherosclerosis. 1982;41:15–9.

40. **Stamler J, Ruth KJ, Liu K, Shekkele RB.** Dietary antioxidants and blood pressure in the Western Electric Study [Abstract]. Tampa, FL: 34th Annual Conference on Cardiovascular Epidemiology and Prevention; 1993.

41. **Levine GN, Frei B, Koulouris SN, et al.** Ascorbic acid reverses endothelial vasomotor dysfunction in patients with coronary artery disease. Circulation. 1996;93:1107–13.

42. **Keaney JF Jr, Gaziano JM, Xu A, et al.** Dietary antioxidants preserve endothelium-dependent vessel relaxation in cholesterol-fed rabbits. Proc Natl Acad Sci USA. 1993;90:11880–4.

43. **Ginter E, Cerna O, Budlovsky J, et al.** Effect of ascorbic acid on plasma cholesterol in humans in a long-term experiment. Int J Vit Nutr Res. 1977;47:123–34.

44. **Trout DL.** Vitamin C and cardiovascular risk factors. Am J Clin Nutr. 1991;53:322–5S.

45. **Weber C, Wolfgang E, Weber K, Weber P.** Increased adhesiveness of isolated monocytes to endothelium is prevented by vitamin C intake in smokers. Circulation. 1996;1993:1488–92.

46. **Bordia A, Verma SK.** Effects of vitamin C on blood lipids, fibrinolytic activity, and platelet aggregation in coronary artery disease patients. Clin Cardiol. 1985;552–4.

47. **Khaw KT, Woodhouse P.** Interrelation of vitamin C, infection, haemostatic factors, and cardiovascular disease. BMJ. 1995;310:1559–63.

48. **Stampfer MJ, Hennekens CH, Manson JE, et al.** Vitamin E consumption and the risk of coronary disease in women. N Engl J Med. 1993;328:1444–9.

49. **Rimm EB, Stampfer MJ, Ascherio A, et al.** Vitamin E consumption and the risk of coronary artery disease among men. N Engl J Med. 1993;328:1450–6.

50. **Kushi LH, Folsom AR, Prineas RJ, et al.** Dietary antioxidant vitamins and death from coronary artery disease in postmenopausal women. N Engl J Med. 1996;18:1156-62.

51. **Knekt P, Reunanen A, Jarvinen R, et al.** Antioxidant vitamin intake and coronary mortality in a longitudinal population study. Am J Epidemiol. 1994;139:1180–9.

52. **Blot WJ, Li JY, Taylor PR, et al.** Nutrition intervention trials in Linxian, China: supplementation with specific vitamin/mineral combinations, cancer incidence, and disease specific mortality in the general population. J Natl Cancer Inst. 1993;85: 1483–92.

53. **The Alpha-Tocopherol–Beta-Carotene Cancer Prevention Study Group.** The effect of vitamin E and beta-carotene on the incidence of lung cancer and other cancers in male smokers. N Engl J Med. 1994;330:1029–35.

54. **Rapola JM, Virtamo J, Haukka JK, et al.** Effect of vitamin E and beta-carotene on the incidence of angina pectoris: a randomized, double-blind, controlled trial. JAMA. 1996;275:693–8.

55. **Livingston PD, Jones C.** Treatment of intermittent claudication with vitamin E. Lancet. 1958;2:602–4.

56. **Williams HTG, Fenna D, MacBeth RA.** Alpha-tocopherol in the treatment of intermittent claudication. Surg Gyn Obstetrics. 1971;132:662–6.

57. **Haeger K.** Long-time treatment of intermittent claudication with Vitamin E. Am J Clin Nutr. 1974;27:1179–81.

58. **Anderson TW.** Vitamin E in angina pectoris. Can Med Assoc J. 1974;110:401–6.

59. **Gillilan RE, Mandell B, Warbasse JR.** Quantitative evaluation of Vitamin E in the treatment of angina pectoris. Am Heart J. 1977;93:444–9.

60. **Demaio SJ, King SB III, Lembo NJ, et al.** Vitamin E supplementation, plasma lipids, and incidence of restenosis after percutaneous transluminal angioplasty (PTCA). J Am Coll Nutr 1992;11:131–8.

61. **Stephens NG, Parsons A, Schofield PM, et al.** Randomized controlled trial of vitamin E in patients with coronary disease: Cambridge Heart Antioxidant Study (CHAOS). Lancet. 1996;347:781–6.

62. **HOPE Study Investigators.** The HOPE (Heart Outcomes Prevention Evaluation) study: the design of a large simple randomized trial of an angiotensin-converting enzyme (ramipril) and vitamin E for patients at high risk for cardiovascular events. Can J Cardiol. 1996;12:127–37.

63. **Manson JE, Gaziano JM, Spelsberg A, et al.** A secondary prevention trial of antioxidant vitamins and cardiovascular disease in women: rationale, design, and methods. Am J Epidemiol. 1995;5:260–9.

64. **Gaziano JM, Manson JE, Branch LG, et al.** A prospective study of the consumption of carotenoids in fruits and vegetables and decreased cardiovascular mortality in the elderly. Ann Epidemiol. 1995;5:255–60.

65. **Pandey DK, Shekelle R, Selwyn BJ, et al.** Dietary vitamin C and beta-carotene and risk of death in middle-aged men: the Western Electric Study. Am J Epidemiol. 1995;5:255–60.

66. **Knekt P, Reunanen A, Jarvinen R, et al.** Antioxidant vitamin intake and coronary mortality in a longitudinal population study. Am J Epidemiol. 1994;139:1180–9.

67. **Manson JE, Stampfer MJ, Willett WC, et al.** A prospective study of antioxidant vitamins and the incidence of coronary artery disease in women [Abstract]. Circulation. 1991;84(Suppl II):546.

68. **Jha P, Flather M, Lonn E, et al.** The antioxidant vitamins and cardiovascular disease: a critical review of the epidemiologic and clinical trial data. Ann Intern Med. 1995; 123:860–72.

69. **Morris DL, Kritchevsky SB, Davis CE.** Serum carotenoids and coronary artery disease: the Lipid Research Clinics Coronary Primary Prevention Trial and Follow-up Study. JAMA. 1994;272:1439–41.

70a. **Salonen JT, Salonen R, Pentilla I, et al.** Serum fatty acids, apolipoproteins, selenium, vitamin antioxidants, and the risk of death from coronary artery disease. Am J Cardiol. 1985;56:226–31.

70b. **Stein JH, McBride PE.** Hyperhomocysteinemia and atherosclerotic vascular disease: pathophysiology, screening, and treatment. Arch Intern Med 1998;158:1301–6.

71. **Omenn GS, Goodman GE, Thornquist MD, et al.** Effects of a combination of beta-carotene and vitamin A on lung cancer and cardiovascular disease. N Engl J Med. 1996;334:1150–5.

72. **Hennekens CH, Buring JE, Manson JE, et al.** Lack of effect of long term supplementation with beta-carotene on the incidence of malignant neoplasms and cardiovascular disease. N Engl J Med. 1996;334:1145–9.

73. **Gaziano JM, Manson JE, Ridker PM, et al.** Beta-carotene therapy for chronic stable angina. Circulation. 1990;82(Suppl III):202.

74. **Gaziano JM, Manson JE, Ridker PM, et al.** Beta-carotene therapy for chronic stable angina. Circulation. In press.

75. **Enstrom JE, Kanim LE, Klein MA.** Vitamin C intake and mortality among a sample of United States population. Epidemiology. 1992;3:194–202.

76. **Manson JE, Stampfer MJ, Willett WC, et al.** A prospective study of vitamin C and incidence of coronary artery disease in women [Abstract]. Circulation. 1992;85:865.

77. **Cross CE, Halliwell B.** Nutrition and human disease: how much extra vitamin C might smokers need? [Letter]. Lancet. 1993;341:1091.

78. **Frei B, England M, Ames B.** Ascorbate is an outstanding antioxidant in human blood plasma. Proc Natl Acad Sci USA. 1989;86:6377–81.

79. **Weber C, Erl W, Weber K, Weber PC.** Increased adhesiveness of isolated monocytes to endothelium is prevented by vitamin C intake in smokers. Circulation. 1996;93: 1488–92.

80. **Hulley SB, Gordon S.** Alcohol and high-density lipoprotein cholesterol: causal inference from diverse study designs. Circulation. 1981;64(Suppl III):57–63.

81. **Suh I, Shaten BJ, Cutler JA, Kuller LH.** Alcohol use and mortality from coronary artery disease: the role of high-density lipoprotein cholesterol. The Multiple Risk Factor Intervention Trial Research Group. Ann Intern Med. 1992;116:881–7.

82. **Langer RD, Criqui MH, Reed DM.** Lipoproteins and blood pressure as biological pathways for effect of moderate alcohol consumption on coronary artery disease. Circulation. 1992;85:910–5.

83. **Gaziano JM, Buring JE, Breslow JL, et al.** Moderate alcohol intake, increased levels of high-density lipoprotein, and its subfractions, and decreased risk of myocardial infarction. N Engl J Med. 1993;329:1829–34.

84. **Meade TW, Chakrabati R, Haines AP, et al.** Characteristics affecting fibrinolytic activity and plasma fibrinogen concentrations. Br Med J. 1979;1:153–6.

85. **Folsom AR, Wu KK, Davis CE, et al.** Population correlates of plasma fibrinogen and factor VII, putative cardiovascular risk factors. Atherosclerosis. 1991;91:191–205.

86. **Ridker PM, Vaughan DE, Stampfer MJ, et al.** Association of moderate alcohol consumption and plasma concentration of endogenous tissue-type plasminogen activator. JAMA. 1994;272:929–33.

87. **Laug WE.** Ethyl alcohol enhances plasminogen activator secretion by endothelial cells. JAMA. 1983;250:772–76.

88. **Smokovitis A, Kokolis N, Ploumis T.** Enhancement of plasminogen activator activity in the gastric wall after chronic ethanol consumption. Alcohol. 1991;8:17–20.

89. **Hendricks HFJ, Veenstra J, Velthuis te Wierik EJM, et al.** Effect of moderate-dose of alcohol with evening meal on fibrinolytic factors. BMJ. 1994;308:1003–6.

90. **MacMahon S.** Alcohol consumption and hypertension. Hypertension. 1987;9:111–121.

91. **Rubin E.** Alcoholic myopathy in heart and skeletal muscle. N Engl J Med. 1979;301: 28–33.

92. **Wannamethee G, Shaper AG.** Alcohol and sudden death. Br Heart J. 1992;68:443–8.

93. **Yano K, Rhoads GG, Kagan A.** Coffee, alcohol, and risk of coronary artery disease among Japanese men living in Hawaii. N Engl J Med. 1977;297:405–9.

94. **Freedman LA, Kimball AW.** Coronary artery disease mortality and alcohol consumption in Framingham. Am J Epidemiol. 1986;124:481–9.

95. **Rimm EB, Giovannucci EL, Willett WC, et al.** Prospective study of alcohol consumption and risk of coronary disease in men. Lancet. 1991;303:211–6.

96. **Boffetti P, Garfinkel L.** Alcohol drinking and mortality among men enrolled in an American Cancer Society prospective study. Epidemiology. 1990;1:342–8.

97. **Klatsky AL, Armstrong MA, Friedman GD.** Risk of cardiovascular mortality in alcohol drinkers, ex-drinkers, and nondrinkers. Am J Cardiol. 1990;66:1237–42.

99. **Stampfer MJ, Colditz GA, Willett WC, et al.** A prospective study moderate alcohol consumption and the risk of coronary disease and stroke in women. N Engl J Med. 1988;319:267–73.

100. **Maclure M.** Demonstration of deductive meta-analysis: ethanol intake and myocardial infarction. Epidemiol Rev. 1993;15:328–51.

101. **Cullen KJ, Knuiman MW, Ward NJ.** Alcohol and mortality in Busselton, Western Australia. Am J Epidemiol. 1993;137:242–8.

102. **National Institute on Alcohol Abuse and Alcoholism.** Eighth Special Report to the U.S. Congress on Alcohol and Health. Rockville, MD: U.S. Department of Health and Human Services; 1993.

103. **McGinnis JM, Foege WH.** Actual causes of death in the United States. JAMA. 1993; 270:2707–12.

104. **Klatsky AL, Armstrong MA, Friedman GD.** Alcohol and mortality. Ann Int Med. 1992;117:646–54.

105. **Doll R, Peto R, Hall E, et al.** Mortality in relation to consumption of alcohol: 13 years' observations on male British doctors. BMJ. 1994; 308:302–6.

106. **Gronbaek M, Deis A, Sorenson TIA, et al.** Influence of sex, age, body mass index, and smoking. BMJ. 1994;308:302–6.

107. **Camargo CA, Hennekens CH, Gaziano JM, et al.** Prospective study of moderate alcohol consumption and mortality in U.S. male physicians. Arch Int Med. 1997;157: 79–85.

108. **Norton R, Batey R, Dwyer T, Macmahon S.** Alcohol consumption and the risk of alcoholic cirrhosis in women. BMJ. 1987;295:80–2.

109. **Urbano-Marquez A, Estruch R, Fernandez-Sola J, et al.** The greater risk of alcoholic cardiomyopathy and myopathy in women compared to men. JAMA. 1995;274:149–54.

110. **Longnecker MP.** Alcoholic beverage consumption in relation to risk of breast cancer: meta-analysis and review. Cancer Causes Control. 1994;5:73–82.

111. **Willett WC, Stampfer MJ, Colditz GA, et al.** Moderate alcohol consumption and the risk of breast cancer. N Engl J Med. 1987;316:1174–80.

112. **Schatzkin A, Jones DY, Hoover RN, et al.** Alcohol consumption and breast cancer in the Epidemiologic Follow-Up Study of the First National Health and Nutrition Examination Survey. N Engl J Med. 1987;316:1169–73.

113. **Fuchs CS, Stampfer MJ, Colditz GA, et al.** Alcohol consumption and mortality among women. N Engl J Med. 1995;332:1245–50.

114. **Steinbauer JR, Carter SB, Holzer CE, Volk RJ.** Ethnic and sex bias in primary care screening tests for alcohol use disorders. Ann Intern Med. 1998;129:353–62.

CHAPTER 10

Hormone Replacement Therapy and the Prevention of Coronary Artery Disease

ROGER S. BLUMENTHAL, MD

TRUDY L. BUSH, PHD, MHS

Cardiovascular diseases, including coronary artery disease (CAD) and stroke, are the major causes of death in the United States, accounting for approximately half of all deaths that occur in women (1). Each year, over twice as many women die from CAD than die from all cancers combined. CAD also is associated with serious morbidities, including disabilities, that affect quality of life, particularly in the later years. Furthermore, CAD accounts for a high proportion of health care costs in women as well as in men.

Menopause is a significant physiologic transition in a woman's life that may be viewed as a time of accelerated biologic aging. Before menopause, the occurrence of CAD is rare; however, after menopause (a time of increased age and reduction of endogenous ovarian hormones) CAD becomes more common. The role of endogenous hormones in the pathogenesis of CAD has not been well described, although the high levels of circulating estrogens found in the premenopausal woman are thought to be protective.

The current evidence for a protective association between postmenopausal hormone replacement therapy (HRT) or estrogen replacement therapy (ERT) and CAD in women comes almost exclusively from observational studies rather than from clinical trials. Thus, this evidence is thought by many to be preliminary at best. Similarly, trials are pending for newer agents.

This chapter reviews the epidemiologic studies that have examined the effects of HRT on CAD risk in women, assesses whether the evidence from these studies meets the epidemiologic criteria for a causal association, explores in some detail the potential biologic mechanisms by which HRT may protect against CAD, and examines in brief the overall benefits and risks of HRT.

Epidemiologic Studies

Over the past 25 years, a relatively large number of published studies have addressed the question of whether HRT affects the risk of heart disease. Reports included in this chapter were selected from the published literature if they 1) included menopausal women who were at risk of CAD, 2) assessed HRT, 3) had a major cardiovascular disease as an outcome, and 4) presented unadjusted or age-adjusted risk estimates only. A total of 33 published studies that met these criteria was found.

The studies reviewed here are organized by basic study design because designs are ranked by the likelihood of biases to influence the results (e.g., clinical trials are least likely to be biased). The amount of confidence in a finding from any single study is a function of several factors but particularly the study design, procedural integrity, and sample size.

Review of Study Types

Experimental Studies

There are two basic types of epidemiologic studies: experimental and observational. Experimental studies are interventional studies or clinical trials in which participants are assigned to a therapeutic regimen and followed for a period of time for the occurrence of outcome(s). The most rigorous type of trial is that which has been randomized (i.e., assignment to therapy is conducted in an unbiased manner), placebo controlled (i.e., a sham-treated comparison group is present), and double blinded (i.e., neither investigator nor participant is aware of actual treatment assignment). Results from these randomized, placebo-controlled, double-blinded clinical trials provide the highest confidence level, because 1) there is an unbiased selection to the intervention, 2) individuals are followed prospectively, and 3) outcomes are (usually) determined by investigators who are unaware of the treatment status of the participant. However, clinical trials are costly, particularly in prevention trials; thus, the number of human prevention trials is relatively limited due to the high costs of this approach.

Observational Studies

Observational studies are those in which no intervention is done. There are four major subtypes of observational studies: prospective (or cohort), clinical cross-sectional, case controlled, and uncontrolled or population controlled. These are listed in a hierarchical order, i.e., prospective studies are considered the best because exposure (in this case, HRT) is assessed before the outcome.

Prospective (Cohort) Studies

Prospective (cohort) studies differ from randomized clinical trials in one key area—assignment to therapy is by self-selection and thus may be biased.

Clinical Cross-Sectional Studies

Clinical cross-sectional studies are similar to case-control studies in which individuals initially are defined as "diseased" or "nondiseased" (cases or controls) and the exposure is assessed at the same time. An example of this study design is an angiographic study in which women referred for this procedure are divided into two groups based on the results of their angiograms. Those with coronary artery occlusion(s) are the diseased group, and those with no evident disease are the nondiseased comparison group. The prevalence of HRT use in each group is then assessed and compared. Clinical cross-sectional studies are robust because the disease is defined anatomically and the cases and controls come from the same clinical population. The major limitation is that exposure status is not assessed before diagnosis.

Case-Control Studies

Case-control studies, in which HRT use in women who have clinical CAD (cases) is compared with HRT use in women who do not have CAD (controls), provide useful information. These studies, however, are more likely to be biased because women are already ill when the exposure is assessed, and those who are sick may be more or less likely to recall an exposure than those who are well. Furthermore, the possibility of including nonrepresentative cases and controls can seriously bias the risk estimate. Because of these limitations, case-control studies are viewed as less reliable than prospective studies.

Uncontrolled or Population-Controlled Studies

Uncontrolled or population-controlled studies are those in which the experience of a group of patients is compared with the experience of the population in general. For example, the death rate of HRT users in one clinical practice would be compared with the death rate of all women in the state. Although it provides some information, this design is the least well controlled and thus the least reliable of all the study designs.

Overview of Studies

Although estrogens have been used clinically for over 50 years, there is only one randomized clinical trial of HRT in women with CAD as the end point (2).

In this small trial, 84 pairs of women matched for age and medical condition were randomly assigned to HRT or placebo. The patients were long-term residents of a chronic disease hospital in New York City and were treated and followed for 10 years. This trial was small, and the results were not statistically significant; however, the risk estimate for myocardial infarction (MI) in HRT users compared with nonusers was 0.3. Several large clinical trials are underway in the United States (Heart and Estrogen/Progestin Replacement Study [HERS] and Women's Health Initiative [WHI]) that will test the hypothesis that estrogen use protects against the development of CAD. HERS results are reviewed in a Postscript; WHI results are not expected for years.

Fourteen prospective studies, ranging in size from very small (3) to the very large Nurses Health Study (4), are presented in Table 10-1 (3–17). The median risk estimate is 0.6, and six of these 14 risk ratios are statistically significant. Only one prospective study, the Framingham study, found a insignificant increased risk of cardiovascular disease among estrogen users (14,15). Another report from Framingham found a slight decrease in CAD occurrence in HRT users (18).

The clinical cross-sectional studies are presented in Table 10-2 (19–22). All of these studies showed significantly less atherosclerosis in HRT users compared with non-HRT users when CAD was defined anatomically. The magnitude of the reduction in coronary lesions ranged from 50% to 63% among hormone users.

Overall, 10 published case-control studies (23–32) have examined the association of HRT with CAD (Table 10-3), ranging in size from very small (17 cases) (32) to moderately large (336 cases) (24). Most of these studies reported

Table 10-1 Prospective Studies of Postmenopausal Hormone Use and Coronary Artery Disease

Study	Relative Risk
Lafferty et al (3)	0.16*
Stampfer et al (4)	0.30*
Hammond et al (5)	0.33*
Bush et al (6)	0.34*
Potocki (7)	0.47
Henderson et al (8)	0.54*
Petitti et al (9)	0.60
Wolf et al (10)	0.66
van der Giezen et al (11)	0.67
Folsom et al (12)	0.74
Falkeborn et al (13)	0.81*
Boysen et al (14)	0.81
Criqui et al (15)	0.81
Wilson et al (16,17)	1.94

*$p < 0.05$.

Table 10-2 Clinical Cross-Sectional Studies of Postmenopausal Hormone Use and Coronary Artery Disease

Study	Risk Estimate ($p < 0.05$)
Gruchow et al. (19)	0.37
Sullivan et al. (20)	0.44
McFarland et al. (21)	0.50
Manolio et al. (22)	*

*Estrogen users had significantly thinner carotid intima.

Table 10-3 Case-Control Studies of Postmenopausal Hormone Use and Coronary Artery Disease

Study	Risk Estimate
Talbott et al (23)	0.34
Rosenberg et al (24)	0.47
Beard et al (25)	0.55
Psaty et al (26)	0.69
Avila et al (27)	0.70
Adam et al (28)	0.79
Szklo et al (29)	0.83
Rosenberg et al (30)	1.05
La Vecchia et al (31)	1.62*
Jick et al (32)	7.50*

*$p < 0.05$.

a reduction of 20% or more in the risk of CAD in women using HRT; however, none of these results was statistically significant. Furthermore, two reports actually found an increased risk of MI among women taking hormones (31,32).

The three published population-controlled studies all showed statistically significant reductions in the risk of CAD, ranging from 50% to 70%. Two of these studies were from the United States (33,34) and one was from Great Britain (35).

If the risk estimates in these 33 published studies are weighted for study type and study size, an overall summary risk can be estimated. This summary risk estimate is 0.5—a 50% reduction in the risk of CAD in women using hormones. This degree of reduction (~50%) has also been reported with more sophisticated approaches (36,37).

Epidemiologic Criteria for Causality

Although many believe that a causal association cannot be demonstrated in the absence of a clinical trial, it is difficult, expensive, and sometimes unethical to conduct randomized, double-blinded, placebo-controlled clinical trials.

Because of this situation, a set of criteria has been proposed that, if met, would provide sufficient evidence of a causal association in the absence of experimental (clinical trial) data (38). An example of assessing causality using epidemiologic data and reasoning is associating lung cancer with cigarette smoking. Given the quality, quantity, and biological plausibility of data on smoking and lung cancer risk, nearly all scientists conclude that smoking causes lung cancer. This conclusion, however, is based on implicit reasoning using epidemiologic criteria for causality rather than on clinical trial evidence. This same logical process can be used to assess the relationship of HRT to CAD in women. The six criteria for causality are as follows:

1. Consistency of the association
2. Proper time sequence
3. Dose-response association
4. Strength of the association
5. Change in risk with change in exposure
6. Biological plausibility

The association of HRT with CAD in women by these causal criteria is reviewed below (39).

Consistency of the Association

This first criterion requires that most of the data be consistent. One way to assess consistency is to examine the association over time, across geographic areas, or with different methods or populations. Some degree of reduction in CAD in women using HRT has been reported in each decade since the 1960s. Furthermore, a reduction in CAD risk is seen with a variety of endpoints, including nonfatal and fatal MI, stroke, coronary stenosis, fatal heart disease, sudden death, and all cardiovascular disease. Reductions in CAD risk among HRT users are seen also in disparate geographic areas, including Poland, England, New Zealand, Israel, Germany, Canada, and various states in the United States. There is also a consistent relationship across different age groups, i.e., HRT users in their sixth, seventh, eighth, and ninth decades had reductions in CAD. Based on these findings, it seems that the association between HRT and CAD meets the first criterion for causality.

Proper Time Sequence

This criterion requires that the exposure occur before the outcome. In the one clinical trial and all of the prospective studies, HRT use preceded the occurrence of CAD.

Dose-Response Association

Few studies assessed the issue of whether the dose of HRT was associated with a differential risk of disease. Only four studies addressed the possibility of a dose-response effect; three found no association between increasing dose of HRT and protection against CAD. However, one study (the Leisure World Study) found that 1.25 mg of conjugated estrogens was superior to 0.625 mg (8). Given this limited information, no conclusions can be made about this criterion.

Strength of Association

To fulfill this criterion, the strength of the association between HRT and CAD must be substantial and clinically meaningful. Approximately two thirds of the studies presented here have found the risk of CAD in HRT users to be less than 0.5. This represents an approximate 50% reduction in the risk of developing CAD, the leading cause of mortality (and morbidity) in women.

Change in Risk with Change in Exposure

This uniquely important criterion is met when a change in risk occurs with a change in the exposure (i.e., smoking cessation leads to a reduction in risk of lung cancer). Three of these studies have assessed whether current HRT users had lower risks of CAD than women who had ever used HRT. The results of all three studies found that current users have a lower risk of CAD than ever users; thus, this criterion is fulfilled.

Biological Plausibility

The exact biological mechanisms by which HRT may influence the development or progression of CAD are not fully known and represent one of the most exciting areas in cardiovascular research. Protective mechanisms probably involve several different pathways, including favorable effects on plasma lipids, modulation of vascular reactivity (40,41), antioxidant effects, and favorable effects on the coagulation system (42). It has been estimated mathematically that 25% to 50% of the beneficial effects of HRT for CAD protection could result from beneficial alterations in lipoprotein levels (43); therefore, the criterion of biological plausibility is met.

With one exception (i.e., dose-response association), the estrogen–CAD association seems to meet the epidemiologic criteria for causality. The hypothesis that HRT prevents CAD now must be considered serious enough to be documented, because the quantitative evaluations of the published literature suggest that estrogen use is associated with a reduction of approximately 50% in cardiovascular disease occurrence, and a qualitative evaluation suggests that estrogen use is causally associated with the reduction of CAD.

Hormones and Secondary Prevention of Coronary Artery Disease

Most studies that have evaluated the effect of HRT on CAD are studies of primary prevention. However, seven reports have assessed the effect of HRT on the occurrence of cardiovascular death and future CAD events in women who have CAD (44–50); also, two studies have shown prospectively that HRT use is associated with a significant reduction in carotid plaque size (51) and carotid intimal thickness (52). The seven studies of secondary prevention all show that in women with established disease HRT reduces the risk of death and future events by approximately 50% to 90% (Table 10-4). This degree of reduction in risk is marked and has been seen rarely with any therapeutic intervention. This also suggests that estrogens influence the risk of subsequent CAD through powerful nonlipid mechanisms, probably resulting in a stabilized vascular system that is resistant to spasm. This hypothesis is plausible, given that estrogens have long been used effectively to treat peri- and post-menopausal hot flashes and flushes (vasomotor instability). These results further suggest the additional hypothesis that the primary prevention of CAD with HRT may be mediated more likely through lipoprotein changes, whereas the secondary prevention of CAD with HRT may be mediated in large part through a stabilized vascular system. Regression trials of HRT in women with documented coronary lesions are underway in the United States (53).

Table 10-4 Studies of Postmenopausal Hormone Use and Secondary Prevention of Coronary Artery Disease

Study	Reduction	Events
Brett et al (44)	47%	CAD death
Newton et al (45)	50%	CAD death
Nachtigall et al (46)	74%	CAD death
Bush et al (47)	82%	CAD death
Henderson et al (48)	66%	CAD death
Cooperative Study Group (49)	82%	Death, stroke, or retinal infarction
Sullivan et al (50)	90%	Death

CAD = coronary artery disease.

Estrogen and Progestin Use

The effects of adding progestins to an estrogen regimen have not been well studied. Although some investigators have suggested that this combination of HRT is superior to estrogen only (54), others are less optimistic. The full effect of progestins is not known, because they may negate or overwhelm the effect of estrogen on many biologic systems and may have adverse effects not mediated through estrogen receptors. However, with the notable exception of high-density lipoprotein (HDL) cholesterol levels, results from PEPI have shown that progestin has no adverse effects of major CAD risk factors, including low-density lipoprotein (LDL) cholesterol, fibrinogen, and lipoprotein(a) (Lp[a]) levels (55).

Nevertheless, issues about progestins remain important. All progestins have androgenic effects that administered alone decrease HDL cholesterol levels, increase LDL cholesterol levels, and increase glucose intolerance. Recently, Rosano and colleagues (56) have shown that progestins have a negative influence on blood flow. These and possibly other effects may result in an unfavorable cardiovascular risk profile.

Some direct information exists about cardiovascular risk in women using estrogen/progestin compounds (13,26). Both these reports show no attenuation of estrogen's protective effects on CAD risk with the addition of a progestin. However, caution is necessary, because some women who are prescribed progestins do not use progestins since animal data suggest adverse effects in CAD occurrence. Furthermore, evidence from women using oral contraceptives suggests that the rate of arterial disease increases with the increase in progestin content of oral contraceptives (57).

Biological Mechanisms

Lipid Effects

Total and LDL cholesterol levels rise with age and probably with menopause. Estrogen deficiency is associated with a fall in the number of hepatic LDL receptors, possibly leading to decreased clearance of LDL cholesterol from plasma. There is also a shift in LDL particle size from large, buoyant particles to smaller, denser, more atherogenic LDL particles (58).

The use of ERT has a number of favorable effects on the lipoprotein profile. It increases HDL cholesterol and apoA-I levels and reduces LDL cholesterol and Lp(a) levels. Recent clinical trials report that unopposed estrogen use (ERT) raises the HDL cholesterol level by approximately 10% to 15% and that ERT or estrogen with a progestin (HRT) lowers LDL cholesterol levels by a similar amount. Estrogen replacement therapy lowers LDL cholesterol levels by accelerating LDL catabolism, probably by increasing the density of LDL receptors in the liver (59). It also increases very-low-density lipoprotein (VLDL) cholesterol and triglyceride levels, but whether this effect is deleterious in certain women with elevated triglyceride levels is unclear. This rise in the larger, more buoyant VLDL particles due to HRT does not seem to be associated with an increase in CAD risk.

A low HDL cholesterol level is a more potent predictor of CAD risk in women than in men (60,61). Women with HDL cholesterol levels below 35 mg/dL have twice the number of CAD events as men with similar levels (62). The increase in HDL cholesterol levels with HRT is thought to be due to an increase in particles containing apoA-I; these particles stimulate cholesterol efflux from peripheral cells and are inversely correlated with CAD (63). Estrogen suppresses hepatic lipase activity, thus reducing conversion of HDL_2 cholesterol to HDL_3 cholesterol.

Coronary artery disease risk is predicted by Lp(a) in a variety of different populations (64). This lipoprotein has structural features of plasminogen and LDL, and may be atherogenic and thrombogenic. Individuals with an elevated level of plasma Lp(a) have impaired endothelium-dependent vasomotor responses (65). Concentrations of Lp(a) are higher in postmenopausal women, suggesting a link between Lp(a) and circulating estrogen levels (66). Although ERT decreases Lp(a) levels, this specific effect may be attenuated by concomitant progestin therapy. It has been reported that the greater the androgenic potency of the progestin, the greater the attenuation of estrogen's favorable effects on Lp(a) and HDL (67). However, data from the PEPI trial, in which less androgenic progestins were used, show no deleterious effects of progestins on Lp(a) levels (68).

The effect of transdermal estrogens on plasma lipids is attenuated compared with oral estrogens; transdermal preparations are associated with only modest beneficial changes in HDL and LDL cholesterol levels. Transdermal estrogen has little effect on total and LDL cholesterol levels, but unlike oral estrogens it does not significantly increase triglycerides. In theory, transdermal estrogen administration mimics ovarian estrogen secretion more closely. By avoiding the enterohepatic metabolism, transdermal estradiol does not seem to increase hepatic coagulation proteins.

The PEPI trial demonstrated that HRT lowered LDL cholesterol levels 10% to 15% even with the addition of a progestin (55). The estrogen-only arm had the most favorable effect on HDL cholesterol levels, whereas the use of micronized progesterone had the least attenuation of the estrogen-induced increase of HDL cholesterol levels. The high rate of endometrial hyperplasia (~10% per year in the unopposed estrogen arm) leads most physicians to prescribe HRT rather than ERT in postmenopausal women with a uterus.

Antioxidant Effects

Oxidized LDL cholesterol plays a key role in atherogenesis. In addition, the in vitro susceptibility of LDL cholesterol to oxidation has been associated with the severity of coronary atherosclerosis (69). This may be significant because estrogen has been shown to have antioxidant effects. A supraphysiologic concentration of 17-β estradiol inhibits LDL cholesterol oxidation and cholesterol ester formation in cultured macrophages (70) and protects cultured endothelial cells from the cytotoxic effects of oxidized LDL cholesterol (71). Native HDL cholesterol protects LDL cholesterol from oxidation and mediates reverse cholesterol transport, in which cholesterol is removed from the vessel wall and is returned to the liver. It has been estimated that, in the presence of HDL cholesterol and estrogen, LDL cholesterol oxidation is reduced by 50% (72).

In vitro studies demonstrate that estrogen inhibits LDL cholesterol oxidation (73). It was recently reported that the time of onset of LDL cholesterol oxidation increased after an infusion of 17-β estradiol or after 3 weeks of transdermal administration. This indicates that concentrations achieved with therapeutic doses of ERT are sufficient to alter favorably LDL cholesterol susceptibility to oxidation (74). However, modulation of endothelial function by inhibition of LDL cholesterol oxidation is unlikely to explain the rapid in vivo vasomotor effects observed with estrogen administration.

Coagulation System Effects

Estrogen's effects on fibrinolytic activity may account partially for the reduced incidence of CAD observed in women using HRT. The risk of CAD has been associated with increased factor VII and fibrinogen levels (75). In the Atherosclerosis Risk in Communities Study, women using HRT had lower fibrinogen levels than non-HRT users. Although women using ERT had higher factor VII levels than non-HRT users, this elevation was attenuated in women on combined HRT. In the PEPI trial, ERT and HRT both lowered fibrinogen levels by approximately 10% (55).

Plasminogen activator inhibitor-1 (PAI-1) is the primary inhibitor of tissue plasminogen activator (tPA); its highest values are in the early morning. High estrogen levels are associated with lower PAI-1 levels and greater fibrinolytic activity (76). Of note, postmenopausal women on ERT have lower levels of PAI-1 and higher levels of tPA in serum than women not treated with ERT. In addition, women taking combined HRT have higher levels of PAI-1 than women on ERT. This suggests that progestin may attenuate the some of the fibrinolytic effects of estrogen (77).

Plasma triglyceride levels are increased by ERT; hypertriglyceridemia may be associated with hypercoagulability in certain groups of individuals. The mechanisms for this association may involve elevated concentrations of factors VII and Xa (78) as well as increased cellular expression of factor III (tissue factor), which is highly thrombogenic (79).

A number of studies have shown variations in human vascular responses related to sex hormone levels. Hashimoto and colleagues (80) reported variations in flow- and nitroglycerin-mediated brachial vasodilation throughout the menstrual cycle. Moreover, a recent study indicated that HRT seems to lower selectively peak PAI-1 in the morning, attenuating the diurnal pattern of hypercoagulability. These observations hold true for both ERT and HRT, despite a rise in triglycerides (76). The authors speculated that HRT may attenuate the circadian rhythm of atherothrombotic factors and thus may protect women from excess CAD events that occur in the morning (80).

Vasoreactivity Effects

Estrogen favorably modulates vascular reactivity in ovariectomized Cynomolgus monkeys (81) and in postmenopausal women (41). The acute administration of estrogen in these studies has been postulated to have favorable effects on nitric oxide (82) and cyclic GMP (83). Favorable effects on vasoreactivity are important because attenuation of vasoconstriction may lead to reduced myocardial ischemia and perhaps fewer episodes of plaque rupture. Abnormal coronary vasoreactivity has been implicated in the pathogenesis of unstable angina, acute MI, and sudden death.

Estrogen seems to alter favorably arterial myocyte electrical properties (84). This results in vasodilatation and may be mediated by an estrogen-induced increase in vascular smooth muscle cell potassium conductance. Other studies report that 17-β estradiol favorably affects prostaglandin biosynthetic activity, leading to a direct vascular relaxant effect (85).

Estrogen acutely blocks endothelin-1–mediated vasoconstriction (86) and seems to have a calcium-antagonist effect (87). Sudhir and colleagues (88) have demonstrated that estrogen causes acute vasodilation by inhibition of vascular smooth muscle cell calcium channels and by favorably affecting adenosine triphosphate–sensitive potassium channels.

Animal studies show that immediate and long-term administrations of estrogen are associated with favorable changes in coronary vasoreactivity (40). Although supraphysiologic doses of estrogen may dilate the coronary conductance vessels, there does seem to be a favorable effect on the microcirculation, even if there is not dilatation of the epicardial vessels. Studies in ovariectomized monkeys that were fed an atherogenic diet showed that although estrogen did not affect the caliber of atherosclerotic conductance arteries or administration of estrogen attenuated abnormal vasomotor responses to acetylcholine (ACh) infusion (89).

A variety of elegant investigations have shown that immediate administration of estrogen to postmenopausal women results in vasodilation of coronary resistance and brachial arteries. Intravenous administration of a single pharmacologic dose of 35 mg of ethinyl estradiol in postmenopausal women not on HRT has been shown to increase coronary blood flow immediately, decrease coronary resistance, and attenuate abnormal coronary vasomotor responses to ACh (41). Attenuation of inappropriate constriction of coronary-resistant arteries may be an important mechanism of estrogen's cardioprotective effects.

Other studies show that 17-β estradiol favorably modulates the response to ACh in women referred for coronary angiography (82,90). Recent work indicates that long-term ERT significantly attenuates the response of human coronary arteries to the immediate vasomotor effects of a 35-mg dose of ethinyl estradiol. This response may be caused by long-term estrogen-induced coronary flow augmentation (91). Alternatively, coronary arteries may develop vasomotor tolerance to ERT administered on a long-term basis.

Glucose Metabolism and Body Composition Effects

Studies of the effects of ERT on glucose metabolism have yielded contradictory results. Synthetic estrogens and progestins in oral contraceptive preparations tend to impair glucose tolerance, whereas long-term use of conjugated estrogens may modestly improve glucose tolerance. Some evidence exists that estrogens may reduce the insulin resistance associated with obesity. Age-related increases in body fat, especially in the abdominal region, seem to be reduced by HRT, without adverse effects on muscle mass (92,93).

Estrogen and Men

Supraphysiologic estrogen administration in men is associated with an increased cardiovascular event rate (94,95). Male MI survivors treated with 5 mg/d of conjugated estrogens had a higher incidence of repeat MI as well as higher frequency of pulmonary embolism and thrombophlebitis compared with those on placebo. Of note, MI survivors treated with 2.5 mg/d showed no difference from those treated with placebo. It should be emphasized that the dosage of 2.5 mg/d is approximately four times higher than that which is usually prescribed for postmenopausal women!

Collins and colleagues (82) reported that acute administration of 17-β estradiol does not influence coronary tone in men (82). However, one component of conjugated estrogens, 17-α-dihydroequilenin, has potent vasodilator properties that prevent paradoxical ACh-induced coronary vasoconstriction in male Rhesus monkeys (96). Specific components of conjugated estrogens may have vasoactive properties in men. A longer duration of estrogen exposure in men may also be needed before vascular effects are seen.

Several small studies indicate that intravenous estrogen may have favorable acute coronary vasomotor effects in men (97). This suggests that non-feminizing estrogenic compounds, such as phytoestrogens, may have possible clinical applications in men with CAD. Animal studies have shown that soy phytoestrogens have favorable coronary vasodilator properties in monkeys (98). The anti-atherosclerotic and lipid-lowering effects of nonfeminizing estrogens need to be investigated in future trials.

The drug raloxifene is the first of a series of selective estrogen-receptor modulators that are now in clinical trials (99). Raloxifene is now in trials to test its efficacy for osteoporosis treatment and also its potential cardioprotective effects. These so-called "designer" estrogens potentially could have favorable effects on bone and vascular tissue, without affecting breast or uterine tissue (100).

Estrogen Receptors

Recent data show a positive correlation between estrogen receptor (ER) expression and the absence of atherosclerosis in human coronary arteries (101). The transcriptional regulation of target genes by estrogen would require binding of a ligand to an intracellular receptor, leading to a sequence of events that would result in the modulation of gene expression. Functional ERs have been identified in many tissues, including vascular smooth muscle cells (102). A recent study confirmed the presence of ERs in endothelial cells (103). This suggests that endothelial cells constitutively possess the potential for transcriptional regulation of target genes by estrogen. The finding of ERs in both human and bovine endothelial cells suggests conservation of estrogen responsiveness in endothelium and a common mechanism for estrogen regulation of endothelial function (103).

Estrogen and Thrombosis

Recently, studies from three groups of researchers showed that women using HRT were more likely than non-HRT users to experience deep vein thrombosis or pulmonary emboli, although the overall risk is small (104–106). Users of HRT had two to four times the risk of developing clots as non-HRT users. The authors of one of the studies estimated that the threefold increase in risk would account for only 16 cases of thrombosis per 100,000 women in any given year. For pulmonary emboli, five cases per 100,000 women could be attributed to HRT. Of these data, however, only those corresponding to pulmonary emboli are persuasive, because diagnosis of deep vein thrombosis is often dependent on knowledge of estrogen use.

Estrogen Replacement Therapy: Benefits and Risks

Concern still remains as to whether the benefits of ERT outweigh the known risks, and this concern is emphasized because some investigators do not agree that estrogen use is causally associated with a reduction in CAD. Instead, some physicians argue that selection bias to estrogen use, rather than estrogen use per se, accounts for much of the protective effect observed. In other words, healthier women are more likely to take HRT than less healthy women; therefore, estrogen users are protected not because of the estrogens but because they were healthier initially.

Selection bias cannot be ruled out in any observational study, i.e., women who take estrogen may do better because of some factors associated with their taking the drug rather than the drug itself. Although a clinical trial is considered necessary to fully address this issue, subgroup analysis can provide insights into whether selection bias exists, and, if so, how much of the effect may be due to it. Several studies have addressed this issue of selection bias indirectly, and the results suggest that any selection biases for hormone use do not markedly influence the magnitude of the protection afforded estrogen users (6,20,47).

There are questions, however, about the effect of administration route on cardioprotection. No data exist on the effects of non-oral estrogens on CAD per se. Furthermore, compared with oral agents, lipid and lipoprotein changes with non-oral estrogens are either absent or diminished (107,108); thus, it cannot be assumed that the cardioprotective and other metabolic effects are similar to those seen with oral estrogen.

Two important risks are associated with unopposed estrogen therapy: the documented increased risk of uterine cancer and a perceived increased risk of breast cancer. Uterine cancer occurs in 2 per 1000 postmenopausal women per year (109). After 2 to 4 years of unopposed estrogen use, that rate is increased three to five times; furthermore, the risk is also dose and duration dependent and persists for several years after therapy is halted (110,111). Estrogen-associated endometrial cancer, however, tends to be a small, well differentiated, low grade, early stage disease that is treatable and has no adverse effect on mortality (112–115).

The evidence on HRT and breast cancer risk is equivocal at best. Although some studies show an increased risk, others show no effect or protection. Reasons for an association between HRT and breast cancer can be hypothesized because estrogen stimulates mitoses in breast cells and has been shown to promote breast tumors in rats. It may also be indirectly associated with a variety of risk factors for breast cancer, including early menarche, late age at first pregnancy, late age at menopause, and early oophorectomy. However, androgens and other ovarian hormones (specifically dihydroepiandrosterone [DHEA]) have been linked to breast cancer occurrence (116).

Several meta-analyses have been published that have attempted to examine the estrogen–breast cancer association (37,117,118). Overall, these summary reports suggest virtually no increase in breast cancer incidence among women who have ever used HRT (relative risk [RR] = 1.1) but a slight increase in long-term (10+ years) users (RR ≈ 1.4). However, survivorship after the diagnosis of breast cancer in women who have used HRT is markedly improved compared with women who had never used estrogens (15,48,119,120). Overall, these data should be relatively reassuring because breast cancer does not seem to be markedly increased among HRT users. Furthermore, because investigators have been looking for an estrogen–breast cancer link for decades, the lack of convincing and compelling evidence should be reassuring as well.

Summary

Despite the impressive epidemiologic data on the cardioprotective effects of estrogen, many areas of uncertainty exist. We do not know the optimal dose of HRT for postmenopausal women, and we have few data about the cardioprotective effects of transdermal estrogen use. Furthermore, most of the existing data examine women who started unopposed estrogen therapy at the time of menopause and who continued therapy for the next 5 to 15 years. Thus, the observational data are limited, particularly with regard to different dose effects, different routes of administration, effects at older ages, and effects with the use of concurrent progestins.

Most of the data on HRT in the United States is based on use with conjugated equine estrogens, which contain at least ten active compounds in varying proportions. Whether all estrogen preparations have similar cardioprotective effects is unknown. Furthermore, HRT users tend to have healthier lifestyles than non-HRT users and may be more adherent with physician advice. These are major potential confounding factors in the interpretation of the magnitude of risk reduction seen in the observational data.

Although we await the results of ongoing randomized trials, such as HERS (121) and WHI (122), we agree with the recommendations of the American College of Physicians–American Society of Internal Medicine and the National Cholesterol Education Program that HRT be considered in women at high risk of CAD. We would go beyond those recommendations to suggest strongly that HRT be considered for women either with documented CAD or at risk of CAD. This latter recommendation is based on the epidemiologic and biologic evidence to date, which supports a causal association between HRT and CAD and offers multiple and highly plausible biologic mechanisms by which HRT could influence CAD risk.

Postscript

The Heart and Estrogen/Progestin Replacement Study (HERS) was published in August 1998 (121). It was designed to examine the effectiveness of estrogen/progestin therapy in preventing coronary events. Previous observational studies, such as the Nurses Health Study, indicated that women who "self-selected" to take HRT had a 50% lower risk of subsequent CAD. The benefit associated with HRT use (most of the data were from women taking unopposed estrogen) appeared to be even greater in those women with established CAD.

HERS was the first randomized, double-blind, placebo-controlled trial of HRT. It enrolled 2763 women with an average age of 67 at 18 different academic medical centers. All participants had documented CAD, were less than 80 years of age, and had never undergone a hysterectomy. Only continuous-combined HRT was used. The primary outcome was the occurrence of the combined end point of CAD death and nonfatal MI.

To the surprise of most HERS investigators, HRT did not prevent coronary events over an average follow-up of 4 years. There were 172 CAD events in the HRT group and 176 in the placebo group. During the first year of the trial, there were 57 events in the HRT group and 38 in the placebo group (relative hazard [RH] = 1.52). During the first 4 months of the trial, RH was 2.3, whereas RH was 1.5 during the second 4 months. Thus, it appears that HRT may have a prothrombotic effect in a small group of "susceptible" women.

In years 4 and 5, however, there were 33 events in the CAD group and 49 in the placebo group (RH = 0.67). Thus, there was a clear trend for benefit if women tolerated the therapy for 2 years without an intercurrent event. The HERS investigators have not been able to find a common factor or constellation of factors that would identify the women at increased risk for an early CAD event. One could speculate that these "susceptible" women may have had a thrombogenic profile because of the presence of factor V Leiden, the presence of the PI.A2 allele of the glycoprotein IIb/IIIa gene, elevated homocysteine levels, or a grouping of other risk factors. However, it will be very hard to test these hypotheses, because a significant number of the women who sustained the early CAD events are no longer alive.

Hormone replacement therapy did significantly raise the risk of venous thromboembolism by nearly threefold (34 vs. 12 events) and the risk of gallbladder disease by about 40% (84 vs. 62 events). However, because of the clear trend for benefit in terms of CAD events over the final 2 years of the trial, we have asked the participants to stay on their original therapeutic assignments. Women assigned to placebo have been asked not to start HRT or a selective estrogen receptor modulator (SERM), and women assigned to HRT have been asked to continue it. We will follow these women for at least 2 more, and probably 4 more, years.

The power of the trial to detect a cardioprotective effect of HRT was limited by several factors. The event rate, expected to be 5% per year, was only 3.3%. The average duration of follow-up was 6.5 months shorter than planned, because most of the participants were recruited at the end of the 18-month recruitment period. Moreover, there was an 18% crossover rate from HRT to placebo by the end of the first year, whereas a 5% rate was expected. In addition, there was a 1.7% crossover rate from placebo to HRT per year, whereas a 1% rate had been assumed. These factors diminished the statistical power of HERS to detect a benefit for HRT. Of note, in an analysis of those women who were compliant with the treatment, there was a 13% decrease in events that was not statistically significant.

Another possible explanation for the neutral outcome of HERS is that progestin may attenuate the cardioprotective effects of estrogen. Medroxyprogesterone acetate has been shown to attenuate the beneficial effects of estrogen on coronary vasoreactivity and plaque size in cynomolgus monkeys. Perhaps a less androgenic progestin may have led to better clinical outcomes.

Many smaller randomized trials of the effect of HRT on coronary vasoreactivity and atherosclerosis progression will be issuing results over the next few years. Unfortunately, none looks at overall clinical events. These trials will be scrutinized closely to see if there is a suggestion of early hazard and late benefit with HRT. The HRT arm of the Women's Health Initiative (WHI) involves 27,500 women, but its results are not expected until 2005.

The estrogen-CAD hypothesis has been battered but not disproved. We await the follow-up event data on the HERS subjects and the reports of other studies using different HRT regimens to help us determine which women will have significant cardioprotective effects from HRT and which women may be susceptible to its potential thrombogenic effects. Only future research will ultimately prove or disprove the estrogen-CAD hypothesis.

REFERENCES

1. **National Center for Health Statistics.** Vital Statistics of the United States, 1986. Vol. II: Mortality, Part A. US Government Printing Office: Washington, DC. DHHS pub. no. 88-1122; 1988.

2. **Nachtigall LE, Nachtigall RH, Nachtigall RD, et al.** Estrogen replacement therapy. Part II: A prospective study in the relationship to carcinoma and cardiovascular and metabolic problems. Obstet Gynecol. 1979;54:74–9.

3. **Lafferty FW, Helmuth DO.** Post-menopausal estrogen replacement: the prevention of osteoporosis and systemic effects. Maturitas. 1985;7:147–59.

4. **Stampfer MJ, Willett WC, Colditz GA, et al.** A prospective study of post-menopausal estrogen therapy and coronary heart disease. N Engl J Med. 1986;313:1044–9.

5. **Hammond CB, Jelovsek FR, Lee KL, et al.** Effects of long-term estrogen replacement therapy. Part I: Metabolic effects. Am J Obstet Gynecol. 1979;133:525–36.

6. **Bush, TL, Barrett-Connor E, Cowan LD, et al.** Cardiovascular mortality and non-contraceptive estrogen use in women: results from the Lipid Research Clinics Program follow-up study. Circulation. 1987;75:1102–9.

7. **Potocki J.** Wplyw leczenia estrogenami na niewydolnose wiencowa u kobiet po menopauzie. Pol Tyg Lek. 1971;216:1812–5.

8. **Henderson BE, Paganini-Hill A, Ross RK.** Estrogen replacement therapy and protection from acute myocardial infarction. Am J Obstet Gynecol. 1988;159:312–7.

9. **Petitti DB, Perlman JA, Sidney S.** Noncontraceptive estrogens and mortality: long-term follow-up of women in the Walnut Creek Study. Obstet Gynecol. 1987;70:289–93.

10. **Wolf PH, Madans JH, Finucane FF, et al.** Reduction of cardiovascular disease-related mortality among postmenopausal women who use hormones: evidence from a national cohort. Am J Obstet Gynecol. 1991;164:489–94.

11. **van der Giezen AM, Schopman-Geurts van Kessel JG, Schouten EG, et al.** Systolic blood pressure and cardiovascular mortality among 13,740 Dutch women. Prev Med. 1990;19:456–65.

12. **Folsom AR, Mink PJ, Sellers TA, et al.** Hormonal replacement therapy and morbidity and mortality in a prospective study of postmenopausal women. Am J Publ Health. 1995;85:1128–32.

13. **Falkeborn M, Perrson I, Adami HO, et al.** The risk of acute myocardial infarction after oestrogen and oestrogen-progestogen replacement. Br J Obstet Gynecol. 1992;99: 821–8.

14. **Boysen G, Nyboe J, Appleyard M, et al.** Stroke incidence and risk factors for stroke in Copenhagen, Denmark. Stroke. 1988;19:1345–53.

15. **Criqui MH, Suwarez L, Barrett-Connor E, et al.** Postmenopausal estrogen use and mortality. Am J Epidemiol. 1988;128:606–14.

16. **Wilson PWF, Garrison RJ, Castelli WP.** Postmenopausal estrogen use and heart disease [Letter]. N Engl J Med. 1986;315:135.

17. **Wilson PWF, Garrison RJ, Castelli WP.** Postmenopausal estrogen use, cigarette smoking, and cardiovascular morbidity in women over 50: the Framingham Study. N Engl J Med. 1985;313:1038–43.

18. **Eaker ED, Castelli WP.** Coronary heart disease and its risk factors among women in the Framingham Study. In: Eaker ED, Packard B, Wenger N, eds. Coronary Heart Disease in Women. New York: Haymarket Doyma; 1987:122–30.

19. **Gruchow HW, Anderson AJ, Barboriak JJ, et al.** Postmenopausal use of estrogen and occlusion of coronary arteries. Am Heart J. 1988;115:954–63.

20. **Sullivan JM, Vander Zwaag R, Lemp GF, et al.** Postmenopausal estrogen use and coronary atherosclerosis. Ann Intern Med. 1988;108:358–63.

21. **McFarland KF, Boniface ME, Hornung CA, et al.** Risk factors and noncontraceptive estrogen use in women with and without coronary disease. Am Heart J. 1989;117: 1209–14.

22. **Manolio T, Furberg CD, Shemanski L, et al.** Associations of postmenopausal estrogen use with cardiovascular disease and its risk factors in older women. Circulation. 1993;88:2163–71.

23. **Talbott E. Kuller LH, Detre K, et al.** Biologic and psychosocial risk factors of sudden death from coronary disease in white women. Am J Cardiol. 1977;39:858–64.

24. **Rosenberg L, Armstrong B, Jick H.** Myocardial infarction and estrogen therapy in post-menopausal women. N Engl J Med. 1976;294:1256–9.

25. **Beard CM, Kottke TE, Annegers JS, et al.** The Rochester Coronary Heart Disease project: effect of cigarette smoking, hypertension diabetes, and steroidal estrogen use on coronary heart disease among 40- to 59-year-old women, 1960–82. Mayo Clin Proc. 1989;64:1471–80.

26. **Psaty BM, Heckbert AR, Atkins D, et al.** The risk of myocardial infarction associated with the combined use of estrogens and progestins in postmenopausal women. Arch Intern Med. 1994;154:1333–9.

27. **Avila MH, Walker AM, Jick H.** Use of replacement estrogens and the risk of myocardial infarction. Epidemiology. 1990;1:128–33.

28. **Adam S, Williams V, Vessey MP.** Cardiovascular disease and hormone replacement treatment: a pilot case-control study. BMJ. 1981;282:122–8.

29. **Szklo M, Tonascia J, Gordis L, et al.** Estrogen use and myocardial infarction risk: a case-control study. Prev Med. 1984;13:510–6.

30. **Rosenberg L, Slone D, Shapiro S, et al.** Noncontraceptive estrogens and myocardial infarction in young women. JAMA. 1980;244:399–42.

31. **La Vecchia C, Franceschi S, Decarli A, et al.** Risk factors for myocardial infarction in young women. Am J Epidemiol. 1987;125:832–43.

32. **Jick H, Dinan B, Rothman K.** Noncontraceptive estrogens and nonfatal myocardial infarction. JAMA. 1978;239:1407–8.

33. **MacMahon B.** Cardiovascular disease and non-contraceptive oestrogen therapy. In Oliver MF, ed. Coronary Heart Disease in Young Women. Edinburgh: Churchill Livingstone; 1978:197–207.

34. **Burch JC, Byrd BF Jr, Vaughn WK.** The effects of long-term estrogen on hysterectomized women. Am J Obstet Gynecol. 1974;118:778–82.

35. **Hunt K, Vessey M, McPherson K.** Mortality in a cohort of long-term users of hormone replacement therapy: an updated analysis. Br J Obstet Gynaecol. 1990;97:1080–6.

36. **Stampfer MJ, Colditz GA.** Estrogen replacement therapy and coronary heart disease: a quantitative assessment of the epidemiologic evidence. Prev Med. 1991;20:47–63.

37. **Grady D, Rubin SM, Petitti DB, et al.** Hormone therapy to prevent disease and prolong life in postmenopausal women. Ann Intern Med. 1992;117:1016–37

38. **Mausner JS, Kramer S.** Epidemiology: An Introductory Text. Philadelphia: WB Saunders; 1985:185–7.

39. **Bush TL.** Noncontraceptive estrogen use and risk of cardiovascular disease: an overview and critque of the literature. In: Menopause: Biologic and Clinical Consequences of Ovarian Failure—Evaluation and Management. Korenman SG, ed; Norwell, MA: Serona Symposium; 1990.

40. **Williams JK, Adams MR, Klopfenstein HS.** Estrogen modulates responses of atherosclerotic cornary arteries. Circulation. 1990;81:1680–7.

41. **Reis SE, Gloth ST, Blumenthal RS, et al.** Ethinyl estradiol acutely attenuates abnormal coronary vasomotor responses to acetylcholine in postmenopausal women. Circulation. 1994;89:52–60.

42. **Nabulsi AA, Folsom AR, White A, et al.** Association of hormone replacement therapy with various cardiovascular risk factors in postmenopausal women. N Engl J Med. 1993;2328:1069–75.

43. **Barrett-Connor E, Bush TL.** Estrogen and coronary heart disease in women. JAMA. 1991;265:1861–7.

44. **Brett KM, Madans JH.** Long-term survival after coronary heart disease: comparisons between men and women in a national sample. Ann Epidemiol. 1995;5:25–32.

45. **Newton KM.** Estrogen replacement therapy and prognosis after first myocardial infarction [Abstract]. San Diego: AHA Meeting; 1995.

46. **Nachtigall M, Smilen SW, Nachtigall RD, et al.** Incidence of breast cancer in a 22-year study of women receiving estrogen-progestin replacement therapy. Obstet Gynecol. 1992;80:827–30.

47. **Bush TL.** Long-term effect of estrogen use on cardiovascular death in women. Orlando, FL: AHA Meeting; 1991.

48. **Henderson BE, Paganini-Hill A, Ross RK.** Decreased mortality in users of estrogen replacement therapy. Arch Intern Med. 1991;151:75–8.

49. **The American-Canadian Cooperative Study Group.** Persantine Aspirin Trial in cerebral ischemia. Part III: Risk factors for stroke. Stroke. 1986;17:12–18.

50. **Sullivan JM, Vander Zwaag R, Hughes JP, et al.** Estrogen replacement and coronary artery disease: effect on survival in postmenopausal women. Arch Intern Med. 1990; 150:2557–62.

51. **Akkad A, Hartshorne T, Bell PR, al-Azzawi F.** Carotid plaque regression on oestrogen replacement: a pilot study. Eur J Vasc Endovasc Surg. 1996;11:347–8.

52. **Espeland M, et al.** Estrogen replacement therapy and progression of intimal-medial thickness in the carotid arteries of postmenopausal women: ACAPS investigators. Am J Epidemiol. 1995;142:1011–9.

53. **Pepine CJ, Lewis JF, Limacher MC, Handberg E.** Ongoing studies on ischemic heart disease in women. J Myocardial Ischemia. 1995;7:290–2.

54. **Wood H, Wang-Cheng R, Nattinger AB.** Postmenopausal hormone replacement: are two hormones better than one? J Gen Intern Med. 1993;8:451–8.

55. **Postmenopausal Estrogen/Progestin Interventions Trial Writing Group.** Effects of estrogen or estrogen/progestin regimens on heart disease risk factors in postmenopausal women. JAMA. 1995;273:199–208.

56. **Rosano GMC, Sarrel PM, Chierchia SL, et al.** Medroxyprogesterone but not natural progesterone reverses the beneficial effect of estradiol 17-beta upon exercise-induced myocardial ischemia [Abstract]. Circulation. 1996;94:18.

57. **Kay C.** Progestogens and arterial disease: evidence from the Royal College of General Practitioners study. Am J Obstet Gynecol. 1982;142:762–5.

58. **Campos H, McNamara JR, Wilson PWF, et al.** Differences in low-density lipoprotein subfractions and apolipoproteins in premenopausal and postmenopasual womenl J Clinical Endocrinol Metab. 1988;67:30–5.

59. **Ma PTS, Yamamoto T, Goldstein JL, et al.** Increased mRNA for low-density lipoprotein receptor in livers of rabbits treated with 17-alpha ethinyl estradiol. Proc Natl Acad Sci U S A. 1986;83:792–6.

60. **Jacobs DR, Mebane IL, Bangdiwala SI, et al.** High-density lipoprotein cholesterol as a predictor of cardiovascular disease mortality in men and women: the followup study of the Lipid Research Clinics Prevalence Study. Am J Epidem. 1990;131:32–47.

61. **Bass KM, Newschaffer CJ, Klag MJ, Bush TL.** Plasma lipoprotein levels as predictors of cardiovascular death in women. Arch Intern Med. 1993;153:2209–16.

62. **Gordon T, Castelli WP, Hjortland MC, et al.** High-density lipoprotein as a protective factor against coronary heart disease. Am J Med. 1977;62:707–14.

63. **OíBrien T, Nguyen TT, Hallaway BJ, et al.** The role of lipoprotein A-I and lipoprotein A-I/A-II in predicting coronary artery disease. Arterioscl Thromb Vasc Biol. 1995; 15:228–31.

64. **Mahe VM, Brown BF.** Lp(a) and coronary heart disease. Curr Opin Lipidol. 1995;6: 229–35.

65. **Tsurumi Y, Nagashima H, Ichikawa K, et al.** Influence of plasma Lp(a) levels on coronary vasomotor response to acetylcholine. J Am Coll Cardiol. 1995;26:1242–50.

66. **Kim CJ, Jang HC, Cho DH, Min YK.** Effects of hormone replacement therapy on lipoprotein(a) and lipids in postmenopausal women. Arterioscler Thromb Vasc Biol. 1994;14:275–81.

67. **Kim CJ, Min YK, Ryu WS, et al.** Effect of hormone replacement therapy on Lp(a) and lipid levels in postmenopausal women: influence of various progestogens and duration of therapy. Arch Intern Med. 1996;156:1693–700.

68. **Espeland MA.** Personal communication.

69. **Regnstrom J, Nilsson J, Tronvall P, et al.** Susceptibility to low-density lipoprotein oxidation and coronary atherosclerosis in man. Lancet. 1992;339:1183–6.

70. **Rifci VA, Khachadurian AK.** The inhibition of low-density lipoprotein oxidation by 17-beta estradiol. Metabolism. 1992;41:1110–4.

71. **Negre-Salvayre A, Pieraggi MT, Mabile L, et al.** Protective effect of 17-beta estradiol against the cytotoxicity of minimally oxidized LDL to cultured bovine aortic endothelial cells. Atherosclerosis. 1993;99:207–17.

72. **Banka CL.** High density lipoprotein and lipoprotein oxidation. Curr Opin Lipidol. 1996;7:139–42.

73. **Subbian MTR.** J Endocrin Metab. 1993;77:1095–7.

74. **Sack MN, Rader DJ, Cannon RO III.** Oestrogen and inhibition of oxidation of low-density lipoproteins in postmenopausal women. Lancet. 1994;343:269–70.

75. **Meade TW, Mellows S, Brozovic M, et al.** Haemostatic function and ischaemic heart disease: principal results of the Northwick Park heart study. Lancet. 1986;2:533–7.

76. **Katz RJ, Hsia J, Walker P, et al.** Effects of hormone replacement therapy on the circadian pattern of atherothrombotic risk factors. Am J Cardiol. 1996;78:876–80.

77. **Gebara O, Mittleman M, Sutherland O, et al.** Association between increased estrogen status and increased fibrinolytic potential in the Framingham Offspring Study. Circulation. 1995;91:1952–8.

78. **Mitropoulos KA.** Hypercoagulability and factor VII in hypertriglyceridemia. Semin Thromb Hemost. 1988;14:246–52.

79. **Levy GA, Schwartz BS, Curtiss LK, et al.** Plasma lipoprotein induction and supression of the generation of cellular procoagulant activity in-vitro. J Clin Invest. 1981; 67:1614–22.

80. **Hashimoto M, Akishita M, Eto Me, et al.** Modulation of endothelium-dependent flow-mediated dilation of the brachial artery by sex and menstrual cycle. Circulation. 1995;92:341–5.

81. **Williams JK, Honore EK, Washburn SA, Clarkson TB.** Effects of hormone replacement therapy on reactivity of atherosclerotic coronary arteries in cynomolgus monkeys. J Am Coll Cardiol. 1994;24:1757–61.

82. **Collins P, Rosano G, Sarrel PM, et al.** Estrogen attenuates acetylcholine-induced coronary arterial constriction in women but not in men with coronary heart disese. Circulation. 1995;92:24–30.

83. **Weiner CP, Lizasoain I, Baylis SA, et al.** Induction of calcium-dependent nitric oxide synthases by sex hormnes. Proc Natl Acad Sci U S A. 1994;91:5212–6.

84. **Harder DR, Coulson PB.** Estrogen receptors and effects of estrogen on membrane electrical properties of coronary vascular smooth muscle. J Cell Physiol. 1979;100: 375–82.

85. **Chang WC, Nakao J, Orimo H, Murota SI.** Stimulation of prostacyclin biosynthetic activity by estradiol in rat aortic smooth muscle cells in culture. Biochim Biophys Acta. 1980;619:107–18.

86. **Jiang C, Sarrel PM, Poole-Wilson PA, Collins P.** Acute effect of 17-beta estradiol on rabbit coronary artery contractile repsonses to endothelin-1. Am J Physiol. 1992;263: H271–5.

87. **Jiang C, Sarrel PM, Lindsay DC, et al.** Endothelium-independent relaxation of rabbit coronary arteries by 17-beta estradiol in vitro. Br J Pharmacol. 1991;104:1033–7.

88. **Sudhir K, Chou TM, Mullen WL, et al.** Mechanism of estrogen-induced vasodilatation: in vivo studies in canine coronary conductance and resistance arteries. J Am Coll Cardiol. 1995;26:807–14.

89. **Williams JK, Adams MR, Herrington DM, Clarkson TB.** Short-term administration of estrogen and vascular responses of atherosclerotic coronary arteries. J Am Coll Cardiol. 1992;20:452–7.

90. **Gilligan DM, Quyyumi AA, Cannon RO III.** Effects of physiological levels of estrogen on coronary vasomotor function in postmenopausal women. Circulation. 1994;89: 2541–51.

91. **Blumenthal RS, Brinker JA, Resar JR, et al.** Chronic estrogen therpary abolishes acute estrogen-induced coronary flow augmentation in postmenopausal women. Am Heart J. 1997;133:323-8.

92. **Folsom AR, Kaye SA, Sellers TA, et al.** Body fat distribution and 5-year risk of death in older women. JAMA. 1993;269:483–7.

93. **Poehlman ET, Toth MJ, Gardner AW.** Changes in energy balance and body composition at menopause: a controlled longitudinal study. Ann Intern Med. 1995;123:673–5.

94. **Coronary Drug Project Research Group.** The coronary drug project: initial findings leading to modifications of its research protocol. JAMA. 1970;214:1303–13.

95. **Coronary Drug Project Research Group.** The coronary drug project: findings leading to discontinuation of the 2.5 mg/d estrogen group. JAMA. 1973;226:652–7.

96. **Washburn SA, Honore EK, Cline JM, et al.** Effects of 17-alpha-dihydroequilenin sulfate on atherosclerotic male and female Rhesus monkeys. Am J Obstet Gynecol. 1996; 175:341–51.

97. **Blumenthal RS, Heldman AW, Brinker JA, et al.** Acute effects of conjugated estrogens on coronary blood flow response to acetylcholine in men. Am J Cardiol. 1997;80:1021-4.

98. **Honore EK, Williams JK, Anthony MS.** Enhancement of coronary vasodilation by soy phytoestrogens and genistein [Abstract]. Circulation. 1995;92:349.

99. **Black LJ, Sato M, Rowley ER, et al.** Raloxifene (LY13948 HC1) prevents bone loss and reduces serum cholesterol without causing uterine hypertrophy in ovariectomized rats. J Clin Invest. 1994;93:63–9.

100. **Kauffman RF, Bryant HU.** Selective estrogen receptor modulators. Drug News Perspect. 1995;8:531–9.

101. **Losordo DW, Kearney M, Kim EA, et al.** Variable expression of the estrogen receptor in normal and atherosclerotic coronary arteries of premenopausal women. Circulation. 1994;89:1501–10.

102. **Karas RH, Patterson BL, Mendelsohn ME.** Human vascular smooth muscle cells contain functional estrogen receptor. Circulation. 1994;89:1943–50.

103. **Venkov CD, Rankin AB, Vaughan DE.** Identification of authentic estrogen receptor in cultured endothelial cells. Circulation. 1996;94:727–33.

104. **Daly E, Vessey MP, Hawkins MM, et al.** Increased risk of venous thromboembolism in hormone replacement therapy users. Lancet. 1996;348:977–80.

105. **Jick H, Derby LF, Myers MW, et al.** Risk of hospital admission for idiopathic venous thromboembolism among users of postmenopausal estrogens. Lancet. 1996;348: 981–3.

106. **Grodstein F, Stampfer MJ, Goldhaber SZ, et al.** A prospective study of exogenous hormones and risk of pulmonary embolism in women. Lancet. 1996;348:983–7.

107. **Bush TL, Miller V.** Effects of pharmacologic agents used during menopause: impact on lipids and lipoproteins. In: Mishell D, ed. Menopause, Physiology, and Pharmacology. Chicago: Year Book Medical Publications; 1987:187–208.

108. **Jensen J, Riis BJ, Strom V.** Long-term effects of percutaneous estrogens and oral progesterone on serum lipoproteins in postmenopausal women. Am J Obstet Gynecol. 1987;156:66–71.

109. **Miller BA, Ries LAG, Hankey BF, et al (eds).** Cancer Statistics Review: 1973–89. Washington, DC: National Cancer Institute. NIH pub. no. 92-2789; 1992.

110. **Shapiro S, Kelly JP, Rosenberg L.** Risk of localized and widespread endometrial cancer in relation to recent and discontinued use of conjugated estrogens. N Engl J Med 1985;313:969–72.

111. **Grady D, Gebretsadik T, Kerlikowske K, et al.** Hormone replacement therapy and endometrial cancer risk: a meta-analysis. Obstet Gynecol. 1995;85:304–13.

112. **Collins J, Donner A, Allen LH, et al.** Oestrogen use and survival in endometrial cancer. Lancet. 1980;3:961–4.

113. **Elwood JM, Boyes DA.** Clinical and pathological features and survival of endometrial cancer patients in relation to prior use of estrogens. Gynecol Oncol. 1980;10:173–87.

114. **Underwood PB, Miller C, Kreutner, Joyner CA, Lutz MH.** Endometrial carcinoma: the effect of estrogens. Gynecol Oncol. 1978;8:60–73.

115. **Robboy SJ, Bradley R.** Changing trends and rognostic features in endometrial cancer associated with exogenous estrogen therapy. Obstet Gynecol. 1979;54:269–77.

116. **Gordon G, Bush T, Helzlsouer K, et al.** Relationship of serum levels of dihydro-epiandrosterone and dihydroepiandrosterone sulfate to the risk of developing postmenopausal breast cancer. Cancer Res. 1990;59:3859–62.

117. **Dupont WD, Page DL.** Menopausal estrogen replacement therapy and breast cancer. Arch Intern Med. 1991;151:67–72.

118. **Steinberg KK, Thacker SB, Smith JC.** A meta-analysis of the effect of estrogen replacement therapy on the risk of breast cancer. JAMA. 1991;265:1985–90.

119. **Bergkvist L, Adami HO, Persson I, et al.** The risk of breast cancer after estrogen and estrogen-progestin replacement. N Engl J Med. 1989;321:293–7.

120. **Bergkvist L, Adami HO, Persson I, et al.** Prognosis after breast cancer diagnosis in women exposed to estrogen and estrogen-progesterone replace-ment therapy. Am J Epidemiol. 1989;130:221–8.

121. **Hulley S, Grady D, Bush T, et al.** Randomized trial of estrogen plus progestin for secondary prevention of coronary heart disease in postmenopausal women. JAMA. 1998; 280:605–13.

122. **Lindsay R, Bush TL, Grady D, et al.** Therapeutic controversy: estrogen replacement in menopause. J Clin Endocrinol Metab. 1996;81:3829–38.

CHAPTER 11

Hormone Replacement Therapy: Practical Prescribing

KEVIN C. FLEMING, MD

MARY P. EVANS, MD

JONATHAN M. EVANS, MD

Hormone replacement therapy (HRT) is a therapy of increasing importance for tens of millions of perimenopausal and postmenopausal women. New indications and pharmacologic treatments are evolving. Nevertheless, hormone therapy may be underprescribed as a result of confusion about its indications, contraindications, risks, and benefits, as well as uncertainty among physicians about management of common side effects. Only 25% of postmenopausal women have ever taken estrogen. Of those prescribed estrogen, 20% never fill the prescription and another 20% discontinue therapy within 9 months (1), largely because of their concerns about side effects. In this chapter, the indications and contraindications for HRT are reviewed, and useful dosing regimens and common side effects and strategies to prevent or manage them are discussed.

Indications for Hormone Replacement Therapy

Cardiovascular Disease

Postmenopausal HRT may have some beneficial effects on cardiovascular health. It is associated in epidemiologic studies with a lower risk of initial myocardial infarction and stroke (2,3). (A detailed review of the potential effects of postmenopausal HRT on the cardiovascular system is in Chapter 10.)

Osteoporosis

Hormone replacement therapy in postmenopausal women is recommended for the prevention and treatment of osteoporosis. The most rapid loss of bone mass occurs in the years immediately after menopause. However, women who start HRT at menopause and then stop after 5 or 10 years of use suffer a similar accelerated decline in bone density. Much, but not all, of the protective effect of HRT on bone is lost in the 10 or 15 years after cessation of estrogen therapy. This therapy, then, is most effective when initiated at menopause and continued indefinitely. Nevertheless, a beneficial effect is still seen in women in their seventies receiving HRT for the first time. Women who do not initiate HRT until their sixties or seventies can still experience a 5% to 10% increase in bone mass in the spine and hip, which may represent up to a 50% reduction in fracture risk (4–6). When considering HRT for an older woman, it is important to bear in mind that approximately two thirds of osteoporotic hip fractures occur after the age of 75. These fractures are disabling and result in at least temporary nursing home placement for many sufferers. Costs associated with hip fractures in the United States approach $10 billion annually.

Vaginal Atrophy, Urinary Incontinence, and Infections

Hormone replacement therapy can improve the elasticity, moisture, and thickness of vaginal, perineal, and periurethral tissues, thus ameliorating symptoms of vaginal dryness, dyspareunia, and urinary incontinence (7,8). Recurrent vaginal and urinary tract infections may also result from hypoestrogenic vaginal atrophy and in turn cause changes in vaginal pH and alteration in vaginal flora. Atrophy of the urethra and the trigone of the bladder, both estrogen-responsive tissues, can result in urinary urgency symptoms and incontinence. Stress incontinence may result from hypoestrogenic effects on tissue supporting the urinary bladder and urethra, most notably the posterior urethrovesical junction. These symptoms may be alleviated more rapidly by the use of topically applied (intravaginal) estrogen preparations than by oral administration. Topical preparations can be discontinued after 6 to 12 months of oral estrogen.

Hot Flushes and Mood Changes

Hormone replacement therapy is used to alleviate vasomotor symptoms and mood alterations associated with decreasing hormonal levels around the time of the menopause (9–11). Vasomotor or "hot" flushes occur in about 10% of perimenopausal women, affecting up to 50% around the cessation of menses.

Box 11-1 Causes of Hot Flushes

Estrogen deficiency
Medications (calcitonin, corticotropin-releasing hormone,
    disulfiram, niacin, nifedipine, nitroglycerin, vancomycin)
Alcohol use and withdrawal states
Monosodium glutamate (MSG)
Diabetic insulin reaction
Psychogenic (anxiety, panic disorder)
Hyperthyroidism
Pheochromocytoma
Carcinoid tumors
Leukemia
Pancreatic tumors
Tuberculosis
Medullary thyroid carcinoma

One in five women still will be having symptoms 4 years after menopause. It is important to recognize that not all hot flushes are due to estrogen deficiency (Box 11-1). Although there is no direct correlation between symptoms and a particular estrogen level, persistent hot flushes despite an adequate estrogen regimen may be psychogenic in origin (blood estradiol levels are 40 to 150 pg/mL on standard HRT doses). However, some clinicians empirically increase the estrogen dose (to 0.9 or 1.25 mg of conjugated estrogens) in an attempt to alleviate symptoms, allowing 6 weeks between dosage adjustments. Hypoestrogenism is not associated with any specific psychiatric disorder such as depression. However, limited evidence suggests that estrogen therapy may improve psychological function (12) and depression symptoms (13).

Dementia

Estrogen use is associated with a lower incidence of Alzheimer disease and an older age of dementia onset in epidemiologic studies. The association is strongest among those using HRT for longer durations (14). Several mechanisms have been proposed, including estrogen effects on neurotransmitters or neurite growth, amyloid deposition, apolipoprotein E levels, cerebral blood flow, and glucose utilization. As a result, estrogen use has been advocated by some physicians for those women with a higher risk of dementia (e.g., family history) and in those already diagnosed with Alzheimer disease in hopes of slowing its progression.

Contraindications to Hormone Replacement Therapy

Absolute and relative contraindications for HRT (Box 11-2) are discussed in the following sections.

Absolute Contraindications

Unexplained Vaginal Bleeding

As a result of the decline in ovarian function, the perimenopausal endometrium demonstrates less predictable monthly shedding, producing prolonged, frequent, or excessive menses in some women. However, uterine myomas, endometrial hyperplasia, or carcinoma may also present in this manner. Uterine cancer may be stimulated by estrogen. Because uterine cancer typically presents with abnormal vaginal bleeding, chronic estrogen therapy is never recommended when the cause of vaginal bleeding is unknown. Endometrial biopsy is indicated for diagnosis when there is abnormal irregular bleeding perimenopausally and when bleeding occurs postmenopausally in subjects not on estrogen supplementation. Postmenopausal bleeding while on HRT is discussed below.

Box 11-2 Contraindications to Hormone Replacement Therapy

Absolute
>   Undiagnosed abnormal vaginal bleeding
>   Known or suspected pregnancy
>   Known or suspected breast cancer
>   Known or suspected endometrial cancer
>   Active venous thrombosis or thromboembolic disorder

Currently debated
>   History of breast cancer
>   History of endometrial cancer

Relative
>   Uterine leiomyomata
>   Endometriosis
>   History of migraine
>   History of pregnancy or OCP-related thrombosis
>   History of cholelithiasis
>   Liver disease
>   Hypertriglyceridemia
>   Severe hypertension

Known or Suspected Pregnancy

The transitional time before menopause can be measured in months to years and is marked by a dramatic decline in fecundity. In addition, menses may be irregular as a consequence of anovulatory cycles. Pregnancy is still possible, however. Standard HRT is not effective as a contraceptive, and these doses may not be sufficient to regulate menses in premenopausal women. Oral contraceptives are preferred for treatment of irregular menses in perimenopausal women and are a safe method of contraception for nonsmoking women in their forties.

History of (or Suspected) Breast Cancer

Breast cancer cells may be stimulated by estrogen. Estrogen should therefore never be used if breast cancer is suspected. The use of estrogen in patients with a history of estrogen-sensitive tumors such as breast carcinoma is currently the subject of ongoing study and debate (15). Nevertheless, until further data are available, one should continue to consider estrogen to be contraindicated in this setting. Hormone replacement is not contraindicated in cervical, epithelial, ovarian, vulvar, or vaginal carcinomas (16). However, tamoxifen can be used for its osteoporosis and cardiovascular protective effects after the diagnosis of breast cancer.

A complete discussion of the risk of breast cancer caused by HRT in patients without historical or suspected malignancy is beyond the scope of this chapter. However, a recent reanalysis of all available epidemiologic studies of HRT and breast cancer is important to consider when discussing the benefits and adverse effects of HRT with patients. The risk of having breast cancer diagnosed is somewhat increased in women using HRT for 5 years or longer, and the risk increases the longer estrogen is used (Table 11-1). This effect essentially disappears within 5 years of stopping HRT, with no significant excess breast cancers found among these women, regardless of previous duration of estrogen use (17). Breast cancers diagnosed among HRT users tend to be less clinically advanced than those found in women who have never used estrogen (17). Because these data are observational rather than based on controlled clinical trials, the additional risk should be viewed as a possibility rather than a certainty (18). Such trials are forthcoming and will likely provide more definitive answers.

History of (or Suspected) Endometrial Cancer

Although prescription of estrogen replacement therapy (ERT) to patients with a past history of endometrial cancer remains somewhat controversial, many gynecologic oncologists are now recommending ERT to patients with stage I, low-grade endometrial adenocarcinoma who have undergone definitive surgical therapy (hysterectomy). Such patients are at low risk for disease recur-

Table 11-1 Breast Cancer and Hormone Replacement Therapy*

Hormone Replacement Therapy	Cumulative Incidence of Breast Cancer
Example: Women Aged 50 to 70 Years	
Never	45 cases per 1000 women (baseline)
5 years	2 extra cases (CI 1-3)
10 years	6 extra cases (CI 3-9)
15 years	12 extra cases (CI 5-20)
Example: Women Aged 70 Years	
Never	63 cases per 1000
20 years	75 cases per 1000
Underwent HRT for 20 years, then none for 5 years	Essentially 63 cases per 1000

*Modified data from Collaborative Group on Hormonal Factors in Breast Cancer. Breast cancer and hormone replacement therapy: collaborative reanalysis of data from 51 epidemiologic studies of 52,705 women with breast cancer and 108,411 women without breast cancer. Lancet. 1997;350:1047-59.

rence, and ERT is often initiated during the postoperative period (16,19–21). A 1996 study reviewed the outcomes of 123 women treated for stage I and stage II endometrial cancer, 62 of whom received ERT after cancer treatment. Death rates from recurrence of endometrial cancer were similar whether or not estrogen was taken (22). The decreased morbidity and mortality with long-term use from osteoporosis and perhaps atherosclerosis may outweigh the possible risk of endometrial carcinoma recurrence from ERT.

Active Thromboembolic Disease

Estrogen replacement stimulates hepatic production of coagulation factors and increases fibrinolytic activity. Oral contraceptive pills (OCPs) induce increases in factor VII coagulant activity and fibrinogen concentrations but reduce levels of antithrombin. Early forms of oral contraceptives contained high doses of estrogen and were associated with an increased risk of venous thromboembolism (VTE). This effect appears to be dose-related, however. In the PEPI trial, postmenopausal women given placebo showed increased fibrinogen levels, but these concentrations remained stable in women taking various HRT regimens. Previous studies have reported that standard doses of postmenopausal estrogen preparations have not been shown to cause an increased risk of thrombosis (23); however, both the number and size of these studies are small.

Recent larger studies of postmenopausal women receiving HRT have found that the risk of idiopathic VTE is about two to four times higher among current users of replacement estrogen than among nonusers. The number of additional cases appears to be about one in 5000 users per year. The increased risk is reported to be highest in the first year of exposure to estrogen, even if given for short-term use. However, no appreciable increase in risk of VTE among past users of OCPs or HRT was found. In addition, there was no significant difference in risk between users of oral and transdermal HRT, nor between users of unopposed estrogen and combined regimens. Nevertheless, idiopathic VTE was rare in the study populations, and the increased risk was felt to cause little excess morbidity (24–26).

The many other risks and benefits of HRT are more significant than the small risk of VTE for most women. Initiation of HRT during active VTE is contraindicated. Subjects who develop thrombotic disease while on HRT are advised to discontinue estrogen. There appears to be no residual effect of postmenopausal HRT on risk for VTE after discontinuation of its use. Individuals with risk factors for VTE, such as previous VTE, family history, morbid obesity, or immobilization, warrant special concern when considering HRT.

Active Liver Disease

As a result of the hepatic metabolism of estrogen, and estrogenic induction of coagulation factors produced in the liver, OCPs and HRT should be avoided during active liver disease.

Relative Contraindications

Uterine Leiomyomata

Menopause commonly results in regression of the size of uterine leiomyomata. Fibroid tumors of the uterus may be stimulated to grow by replacement doses of estrogen (27). Hormone replacement therapy can be delayed for 3 to 12 months after menopause to allow involution to occur. Even so, patients with submucosal leiomyomata may experience irregular or heavy bleeding with estrogen therapy. Women with a history of fibroids who are going to initiate HRT should be alert for symptoms that can result from fibroid enlargement, such as abnormal uterine bleeding, low abdominal and pelvic pain, dyspareunia, and urinary frequency or retention. Periodic pelvic examinations of the asymptomatic female to monitor fibroid size are prudent as well. Fibroid enlargement after menopause is cause for concern, and specialty evaluation is recommended.

Postmenopausal bleeding may occur as a result of uterine leiomyomata, but significant pathology must be excluded by endometrial sampling. Dilation and curettage (D&C) may have a therapeutic effect on abnormal uterine bleeding caused by fibroids and allow a menopausal woman to avoid surgery. Hysterectomy is the definitive surgical management of uterine leiomyomata causing more severe or recurrent symptoms. In selected cases, myomectomy may be performed to preserve the uterus. Leiomyomata recurs in at least 15%

to 30% of cases, however, and multiple myomectomies carry significant additional risks (blood loss, adhesions, infection, ischemia).

Endometriosis

Most women with symptomatic endometriosis experience a resolution of their disease with menopause, and it is rare for endometriosis to first appear after menopause. Although estrogen stimulates the growth of endometrial implants, the dose of estrogen in HRT appears to be insufficient to maintain the disease (28). Therefore, HRT is safe in postmenopausal women with a history of endometriosis. Close follow-up for symptom recurrence after initiation of HRT is prudent. Rarely, individuals with more severe symptoms may require definitive surgery before initiating estrogen replacement. Hormone replacement therapy has been used successfully in women who have undergone hysterectomy and oophorectomy because of severe endometriosis (29).

History of Migraine Headaches

Migraine and other vascular headaches frequently cease at the time of the menopause and may rarely recur with estrogen supplementation. Women with a history of migraine headaches may benefit from a daily continuous HRT regimen, bypassing the cyclic changes in hormone levels that may serve to trigger vascular headaches. Often these patients tolerate the transdermal route better than they do oral medications, because the serum levels appear to be more constant (9,10). If a woman with no previous history of headaches develops them while on HRT, other diagnoses should also be considered.

History of Pregnancy-Related or Oral Contraceptive–Related Thrombosis

Given the recent studies reporting an increased risk for idiopathic VTE with estrogen use (see above), individuals with a previous episode of estrogen-related VTE appear to be at some increased risk for recurrent venous thrombosis with HRT. The studies cited herein excluded persons with previous VTE, however, so the absolute risk of estrogen supplementation in these women remains unclear. The benefits of HRT must be weighed against the risks of venous thrombosis and its attendant morbidities, including pulmonary embolism and the postphlebitic syndrome.

History of Cholelithiasis

Hormone replacement therapy elevates the cholesterol fraction of bile, leading to an increase in the rate of formation of gallstones in about 20% of patients. As a result, there is a 1.5- to 2-fold increase in the incidence of cholelithiasis. Although this has not clearly been shown to translate into a similar increase in the incidence of cholecystitis, at-risk patients could use transdermal estrogen, which does not increase bile cholesterol saturation.

Routine periodic screening blood tests for liver and biliary function are not recommended for women taking HRT. Careful monitoring for suggestive signs and symptoms is sufficient for the diagnosis of gall bladder disease in this population.

Chronic Liver Disease

Impaired hepatic metabolism can result in significantly elevated levels of circulating estrogen. Reduced dosages of orally administered estrogen or, alternatively, vaginal or transdermal estrogen may allow some patients with chronic hepatic dysfunction to use HRT. Short-term and chronic alcohol intake (without evidence of hepatic dysfunction) have been shown to increase blood levels of estrogen up to three-fold in women on HRT (30). Although the clinical implications for this finding are unclear, caution is advised when women with high alcohol intake are prescribed estrogen. Periodic laboratory assessment of liver function tests in these patients is prudent.

Hypertriglyceridemia

Oral estradiol and conjugated estrogens may increase serum triglycerides. Conversely, estrogens given by transdermal or vaginal routes may reduce triglyceride levels (31). This is attenuated by the addition of progesterone, because both oral and nonoral regimens of cyclic-combined HRT regimens reduce triglycerides. Nevertheless, the clinical significance of these triglyceride changes is unclear given that the cardioprotective effect of estrogen is by no means limited to its improvement on the lipid profile.

Severe Hypertension

Most users of HRT experience either a modest decline in blood pressure or no change at all. Rarely, individuals may suffer an idiosyncratic response to estrogen that results in significant blood pressure elevation. There are no data allowing one to predict those at risk for this reaction, including presence or severity of pre-existing hypertension. Therefore, blood pressure should be monitored after initiation of estrogen therapy. Hormone replacement therapy is safe in normotensive and hypertensive women after menopause (32). Given the potential benefits of estrogen, it would seem that hypertensive women may be appropriately targeted for HRT, rather than excluded from it.

Malignant Melanoma

Cutaneous malignant melanoma (CMM) is often listed among absolute or relative contraindications to HRT. However, there is no evidence that estrogen supplementation, either OCPs or HRT, has a role in the etiology of CMM. Indeed, women with CMM present with thinner lesions, have lesions at different anatomic sites, and have a more favorable prognosis than do men. Moreover, true estrogen receptors have not been demonstrated in primary or metastatic CMM, which suggests that hormonal factors play only a limited role, if any (33–35). Therefore, patients with a history of CMM should not be excluded from HRT.

Initial Screening and Assessment

At a minimum, HRT should be initiated in conjunction with a review of gynecologic history, recent related symptoms, physical examination including breast and pelvic examination, and screening mammography to rule out occult breast carcinoma. A lifestyle review of smoking and alcohol habits as well as exercise and diet regimens (with special attention to calcium intake) is also important. Other laboratory tests, such as liver function tests and serum lipid profile, can be performed at the discretion of the physician. As with other medications, the potential risks, benefits, alternatives, and choices of regimens, as well as common expected side effects, should be discussed with the patient before commencement of therapy.

When Should Hormone Replacement Therapy Be Started?

As a result of decreasing estrogen and progesterone production, most women experience some degree of menstrual irregularity for the 6 to 8 years before the cessation of menses. There is tremendous individual variability, however. This transitional time may be characterized by irregular menses and altered flow, which can be variably light or heavy. The majority of women enter menopause between the ages of 45 and 55 years, with a median age of 51. The age of menopause is unrelated to the age of menarche, parity, or oral contraceptive use. Family history of timing of menopause may be helpful, although not always predictive. Smoking lowers the age of menopause by about two years (36). Late menopause increases the risk for endometrial cancer, presumably as a result of prolonged cumulative exposure to estrogen.

Oral contraceptives are effective treatment for dysfunctional uterine bleeding caused by physiologic perimenopausal oligo-ovulation and are approved by the Food and Drug Administration for this indication. In nonsmokers, OCPs can be safely used until the time of menopause. Oral contraceptive pills can effectively prevent endometrial hyperplasia, decrease the occurrence of functional ovarian cysts, and delay or avoid operative procedures such as D&C or hysterectomy. Low-dose OCPs also provide approximately four to five times the bioavailable dose of common postmenopausal estrogen replacement. This supplies a significant estrogen boost perimenopausally and decreases the rate of postmenopausal bone loss (37–39). Postmenopausal women who begin estrogen therapy earlier and continue estrogen longer have a lower risk of hip fracture than women who begin HRT later in life or discontinue therapy after a shorter interval (5).

Hormone replacement therapy should be offered to eligible and interested postmenopausal women at or shortly after the menopause or at the time of oophorectomy in premenopausal women. Hormone replacement therapy can be initiated for short-term symptom management (e.g., hot flushes, vaginal atrophy, mood changes) or long-term prevention. Women who wish to begin estrogen therapy must agree to periodic monitoring, including breast examinations, mammograms, and routine health assessments (blood pressure checks and appropriate physical examination).

Recently, women are considering initiation of hormonal therapy long after menopause for prevention of coronary artery disease (CAD), osteoporosis, and dementia. Although age alone is not a reliable predictor for the presence of illness, in general the burden of disease increases with advancing age. A woman at age 80 has an additional life expectancy of nearly ten years, during which time her risks of hip fracture and CAD are highest.

Nevertheless, HRT has been found to have a beneficial effect on hip fracture prevention even among women who first began estrogen therapy in their seventies (5). In addition, HRT has been shown in observational studies to dramatically decrease the incidence of CAD, and more accurate prospective studies are in progress. The first prospective study available focused on secondary prevention of CAD and did not find overall CAD benefit but a trend towards benefit over 4 years of follow-up (40). Finally, the beneficial effect of HRT in the prevention of Alzheimer disease has recently been demonstrated as well. For these reasons, there is no particular age beyond which HRT is currently not recommended. The risk of estrogen therapy on breast cancer among women in their eighties and beyond has never been studied, however.

Prescribing Strategies

The ideal dose of estrogen is one that will maximally retard bone loss, improve cardiovascular health, and alleviate vasomotor symptoms and genitourinary atrophy, while at the same time having the fewest side effects or risks. Virtually all studies that demonstrated long-term benefits of HRT used a dose of estrogen equivalent to 0.625 mg of Premarin (or higher). Consequently, this is typically the standard dose, or lowest starting dose, because the efficacy of lower doses in reducing cardiovascular risk and preventing osteoporosis has not been well studied. Younger women who experience surgical menopause may initially require a higher estrogen dose to control vasomotor symptoms. An initial dose of 0.9 or 1.25 mg Premarin per day is usually sufficient for women who are less than 50 years old. On the other hand, many elderly women may not tolerate even the equivalent of 0.625 mg Premarin. Consequently, in some instances lower doses must of necessity be used (e.g., 0.3 mg Premarin, sufficient for some antiosteoporosis effect). The ideal dose of progestin is sufficient to protect the endometrium from endometrial hyperplasia and carcinoma but low enough to avoid negative effects on serum lipids and side effects such as depression, weight gain, and irritability. The ideal dose of either drug, however, may vary from patient to patient. Equivalent doses of different brands of estrogen and progestin are shown in Box 11-3.

When using estrogen, it is also necessary to include a progestin therapy to prevent endometrial hyperplasia and endometrial carcinoma. The risk of endometrial cancer is effectively eliminated when progestins are added to estrogen regimens. A daily dose of 2.5 mg progestin for combined-continuous HRT, or 10 mg progestin taken for at least 10 days per month in sequential regimens, is required to achieve this risk reduction (41,42). Progestins are not necessary nor are they recommended for women whose uterus has been surgically removed. Previously, it was felt that a protective effect against breast carcinoma was gained by adding progestin; recent studies have refuted this, however (43).

A primary goal of any HRT regimen is to achieve amenorrhea, because continued withdrawal bleeding is intolerable to many postmenopausal women and contributes to poor compliance. The numerous strategies for administering estrogen and progesterone offer varied treatment options in terms of bleeding patterns. The most common regimens are "continuous-combined" and "cyclic-combined" (Box 11-4). There are two advantages to

---

Box 11-3 Equivalent Hormone Dosages

Equivalent dosages of estrogen preparations
   Conjugated equine estrogens (Premarin) 0.625 mg
   Micronized estradiol (Estrace) 1.0 mg
   Piperazine estrone sulfate (Ogen) 0.625 mg
   Transdermal estradiol
      Estraderm 0.05 mg, changed twice weekly
      Climara 0.05 mg, applied once per week
   Esterified estrogens (Estratabs) 0.625 mg

Equivalent dosages of progestin
   Medroxyprogesterone acetate (Provera) 2.5 to 5 mg
   Norethindrone acetate (Norlutate) 1.0 to 2.5 mg

continuous-combined therapy. Compliance may be improved because many patients find it easier to remember to take one or two pills every day than to adjust their medications depending upon the day or week of the month. In addition, the continuous progesterone stimulation renders the endometrium atrophic, and with time the likelihood of breakthrough bleeding is reduced.

In one study, more than 80% of patients had no bleeding at the end of 1 year on continuous-combined therapy (44). However, when the number achieving amenorrhea includes those who dropped out of the study, this figure drops to between 45% and 55%. Indeed, it has been reported that less than half of women still bleeding after 6 to 8 months of treatment achieved amenorrhea at 12 months (45,46).

Menstrual periods induced by cyclic-combined HRT are often similar in volume to those found in the normal premenopausal population and greater than those in women on OCPs. Nearly 85% of women receiving sequential progestin will experience withdrawal bleeding for as long as HRT is prescribed; only a minority (usually older women) ever develop amenorrhea (47).

Box 11-4 Common Hormone Replacement Regimens

Continuous-combined estrogen and progestin
1. Premarin 0.625 mg or Estrace 1.0 mg, every day of month
   and
   Provera 2.5 mg, every day of month
2. Prempro, combined therapy in a single tablet
   Conjugated estrogens 0.625 mg with medroxyprogesterone acetate 2.5 mg

Cyclic-combined estrogen and progestin
1. Premarin 0.625 mg or Estrace 1.0 mg daily
   and
   Provera 5 to 10 mg, days 1 to 14
2. Premarin 0.625 mg, days 1 to 25 or
   Estrace 1.0 mg, days 1 to 25
   and
   Provera 5 to 10 mg, days 13 to 25
3. Premphase, combined therapy in a single tablet
   Conjugated estrogens 0.625 mg, days 1 to 14, then conjugated estrogens
   0.625 mg and medroxyprogesterone acetate 5 mg, days 14 to 28

Long-cycle therapy
   Climara 0.05 mg, applied once per week, administered cyclically (3 weeks on,
   1 week off), discontinue or taper dose every 3 to 6 months

---

For this reason, noncompliance is even more common among users of sequential HRT programs.

Another method of HRT administration, though not widely used, is one in which estrogen is given continuously but progesterone is given in a 3-day-on and 3-day-off schedule (or for 5 days a week, in some regimens) (48,49). Symptom control and endometrial protection were demonstrated with this "interrupted" progestin regimen, and the lower bleeding rates may improve compliance.

Long-cycle HRT is advocated by some to reduce the frequency of withdrawal bleeds. Daily estrogen for 3 months is followed by 10 days of a progesterone compound in the fourth cycle (50,51). Four- and six-month regimens have also been described. Although this method may promote less frequent withdrawal bleeding, the incidence and volume of bleeding can be quite significant. In addition, long-cycle HRT may be insufficient to prevent endometrial atrophy. Recent data strongly suggest that progestin in sequential estrogen-progestin replacement therapy needs to be given for at least 10 days per month to effectively eliminate any increased risk of endometrial cancer (41,42). Therefore, long-cycle HRT is not recommended.

Other Routes of Estrogen Administration

Transdermal estradiol is a newer but popular route of estrogen administration. Potential advantages of this method include minimal hepatic first pass effect and potentially lesser adverse effects on thrombosis. It is believed by some that continuous transdermal administration mimics ovarian function more closely. Transdermally administered estrogen may be better tolerated than oral estrogen in patients with nausea or occasional migraine headaches.

Vaginally administered estrogen cream is another alternative to oral therapy. Conjugated equine estrogen cream, 0.3 mg per day, or estradiol cream, 0.2 mg per day, can be administered at bedtime with a vaginal applicator that resembles a tampon. This route may be a good choice for a patient whose symptoms are primarily genitourinary in origin, such as vaginal dryness and dyspareunia due to atrophic vaginitis. Approximately 25% of the intravaginal dose is absorbed systemically, the amount absorbed being directly related to the dose administered. However, peak serum levels are lower than with orally administered estrogen, and absorption is too variable to be acceptable for prevention of cardiovascular disease and osteoporosis (42,52). Nevertheless, because of this systemic effect, the patient with an intact uterus theoretically still requires the addition of progestogen to prevent endometrial hyperplasia and carcinoma. This has never been formally studied, however.

When To Start, When To Stop

In general, menopause can be clinically defined as 6 months of amenorrhea. In the absence of abnormal vaginal bleeding, commencing HRT somewhere near this time is acceptable. It is reasonable to consider HRT when a woman complains of vasomotor symptoms or vaginal dryness yet is still experiencing occasional menses.

If there is uncertainty as to whether a patient's symptoms are caused by menopause, especially in younger patients in whom menopause would be considered less likely, an elevated level of serum follicular stimulating hormone can be helpful in confirming ovarian failure before initiating HRT. Follicular stimulating hormone levels greater than 40 mIU/mL can be considered postmenopausal. Because bone density declines after age of 35, and the rate of decline accelerates in the first 5 years after menopause, it is important to introduce HRT as early after menopause as possible, rather than waiting until osteoporosis is established. For that reason, it seems prudent and cost-effective to omit routine serial bone densitometry testing which documents bone loss over time in favor of beginning ERT in eligible patients.

Bone densitometry can help identify subnormal bone mass in women with additional risk factors for osteoporosis, such as a positive family history, tobacco abuse, immobilization, previous fractures, or loss of height. Some women who are undecided whether to pursue HRT may be persuaded to do so if bone densitometry indicates that bone loss has already occurred. Because of the expense, however, routine densitometry studies are recommended only when the test results will alter treatment decisions.

The question sometimes arises as to whether women who are many years postmenopausal should receive HRT and how long HRT should be continued. While the greatest reduction in hip fracture rates occurs in women who began HRT soon after menopause, women over 70 years old still continue to benefit (5,9). Therefore, it may be appropriate to continue HRT indefinitely, particularly in women who already have osteoporosis.

When Should Endometrial Sampling Be Performed?

Endometrial sampling is indicated to rule out endometrial cancer or precancerous conditions. Some gynecologists have advocated routinely sampling the endometrium of all patients before initiating HRT (10,53). Because endometrial cancer typically presents with abnormal bleeding, we advocate sampling only if abnormal bleeding occurs. In the setting of combined cyclic HRT, abnormal bleeding is defined as bleeding that occurs at a time of the cycle other than at the cessation of the progesterone compound.

Regular withdrawal bleeding at the time of the progesterone administration
is expected, especially in women who are newly menopausal. Withdrawal
bleeding is usually not associated with endometrial hyperplasia or carcinoma (54). Spotting that occurs in a patient using continuous combined
hormonal replacement is more difficult to evaluate and may therefore require endometrial sampling to rule out neoplasia. If the biopsy shows normal or atrophic tissue, observation alone is justified. If irregular spotting
continues, however, repeat biopsy, D&C, or hysteroscopic evaluation may be
considered.

Management of Postmenopausal Bleeding

In women who have not undergone hysterectomy, the single most cited reason for discontinuing HRT is postmenopausal bleeding (Box 11-5). This
problem is especially common in women who have only recently reached
menopause. One can be reasonably sure that bleeding occurring at the time

---

**Box 11-5 Postmenopausal Bleeding in Patients Receiving Hormone
Replacement Therapy**

Evaluation
1. Common in recent menopause. Bleeding during progestational withdrawal
   in a cyclic-combined regimen is expected. Endometrial sampling is usually
   not necessary.
2. Irregular bleeding requires endometrial sampling.
3. Higher-risk patients (obesity, hypertension, diabetes, nulliparity, early
   menarche, late menopause) should have endometrial sampling regardless
   of timing.
Management
1. Switch from a cyclic-combined to a continuous-combined regimen. Increase the dose of progestogen by 2.5 mg until amenorrhea or intolerable
   side effects occur.
2. If biopsy shows endometrial hyperplasia without atypia, increase the dose
   or duration of progestin (e.g., cyclic progestin, 10 mg per day, for 14 days of
   the month for 6 months). After 6 months, the endometrium should be resampled for resolution of the hyperplasia.
3. If biopsy shows endometrial hyperplasia with atypia, there is an increased
   risk of carcinoma and a D&C is indicated.

of progestational withdrawal in a cyclic-combined regimen is caused by hormonal stimulation of the endometrium (54). Some patients will tolerate regular withdrawal bleeding if they are reassured that it is expected in cyclic-combined therapy. In the absence of abnormal uterine bleeding, endometrial sampling is generally not necessary if the patient is on continuous-combined HRT.

However, bleeding that occurs irregularly through the cycle should be evaluated by endometrial sampling, using either office techniques or surgical D&C. Patients with other risk factors for endometrial cancer (obesity, hypertension, diabetes mellitus, nulliparity, early menarche, or late menopause) should undergo endometrial sampling for abnormal postmenopausal bleeding regardless of timing of bleeding.

Bleeding during continuous-combined HRT occurs in at least 40% of users during the first 6 months of therapy and persists in some for more than 12 months. Such bleeding is usually light, often just scant spotting, but even this can be intolerable for many older women, especially after experiencing the amenorrheic state. Although there are no established criteria defining "abnormal" bleeding among women receiving continuous-combined HRT, endometrial assessment should be considered for bleeding occurring after the first 6 months of therapy or if bleeding reappears after amenorrhea had been established (47). Ultrasound and/or endometrial tissue sampling are sufficient for diagnosis.

The goal of medical management of postmenopausal bleeding is to induce endometrial atrophy and subsequent amenorrhea. This can be accomplished in a number of ways: often, switching from a cyclic-combined to a continuous-combined regimen will induce amenorrhea. Approximately 80% of patients become amenorrheic on this type of regimen (44). Another option is to increase the dose of progestogen incrementally by 2.5 mg until either amenorrhea or side effects intervene. In an attempt to prevent bleeding from occurring upon initiation of continuous-combined HRT, temporary use of higher-dose progestin (e.g., Provera 5 mg daily instead of 2.5 mg daily) for the first month may be used for 2 to 4 weeks before beginning estrogen replacement.

If endometrial sampling reveals endometrial hyperplasia without atypia, addition of more progestin is indicated (Table 11-2). This can be accomplished by increasing either the dose or the duration of progestin therapy. A cyclic progestin administered 10 mg per day for 14 days of the month for 6 months should be sufficient to induce endometrial atrophy and reverse the hyperplasia. After 6 months, the endometrium should be resampled to demonstrate resolution of the hyperplasia. When endometrial sampling shows endometrial hyperplasia with atypia, there is an increased risk of underlying endometrial carcinoma and a formal surgical D&C is indicated.

Table 11-2 Progestin Effects on Endometrial Hyperplasia

Hormone Regimen	Endometrial Hyperplasia Incidence at 18 Months, %	Endometrial Cancer Odds Ratio*
Unopposed estrogen	30	2.17
Estrogen plus progestin for 7 d/mo	4	1.87
Estrogen plus progestin for 10 d/mo	2	1.07
Estrogen plus progestin for 12 d/mo	0	...
Estrogen plus progestin daily	<1	1.07

*Per 5-year use of hormone regimen.
Data from Collaborative Group on Hormonal Factors in Breast Cancer. Breast cancer and hormone replacement therapy: collaborative reanalysis of data from 51 epidemiologic studies of 52,705 women with breast cancer and 108,411 women without breast cancer. Lancet. 1997;350:1047-59; and Sagraves R. Estrogen therapy for postmenopausal symptoms and prevention of osteoporosis. J Clin Pharmacol. 1995;35(suppl):2S-10S.

Side Effects of Hormone Replacement Therapy

The side effects of HRT and their treatment are discussed in the following sections (Box 11-6).

Estrogen-Related Side Effects

Nausea

Nausea associated with HRT is often self-limited and usually resolves within the first 2 months of therapy. This side effect may be diminished by taking the medication with food and at bedtime. Some patients who experience nausea on ERT may find the transdermal patch easier to tolerate. Some patients may tolerate one brand or formulation of estrogen better than another. Because most of the estrogen-related side effects are dose related, dose reduction may ultimately be necessary for some women, particularly women of advanced age or lower body weight.

Breast Tenderness

Breast tenderness is usually caused by the estrogen component and often responds to dose reduction. One strategy is to give estrogen on Monday through Friday each week or days 1 to 25 of the month, giving the patient an "estrogen break." If these changes do not bring relief, sometimes switching to a different progestin is helpful (see Box 11-6). Limiting caffeine intake is important in preventing breast tenderness caused by fibrocystic breast changes. Some patients find relief with the addition of a mild diuretic (e.g., hydrochloro-

---

Box 11-6 Treatment of Side Effects of Hormone Replacement Therapy

Nausea

Often self-limited.

Take medication with food or at bedtime.

Consider different brand, lower dose, or transdermal patch.

Breast tenderness

Use the lowest effective estrogen dose. Give an "estrogen break": administer Monday through Friday each week or days 1 to 25 of the month.

Switch to a different progestin.

Limit caffeine intake.

Brief use of 25 to 50 mg hydrochlorothiazide per day.

Consider underlying breast disease.

Migraine headaches

A relative contraindication to HRT. The transdermal patch is often better tolerated. New onset headaches should be investigated.

Mood swings

Switch to a different progestin or decrease the intermittent dose from 10 to 5 mg daily. Consider continuous 2.5 mg daily dose.

Abdominal bloating

Switch to a different progestin.

Try hydrochlorothiazide 25 mg/d during the last few days of progestogen therapy.

Rash, skin irritation, itching

Rotate the site of application.

Apply on the buttock or thigh.

Apply a fresh patch after swimming.

Allow the patch to air-dry briefly before applying.

---

thiazide, 25 to 50 mg per day, for 5 to 7 days). It is important also to consider underlying breast disease in the management of breast tenderness.

Headaches

See Relative Contraindications.

Progestational Side Effects

Mood Alterations

Mood swings, especially those noted during the progestational administration in cyclic regimens, can sometimes be alleviated by switching to a different progestin or by decreasing the dose from 10 to 5 mg per day. Some patients may tolerate a 2.5 mg dose administered daily throughout the month better than 5 or 10 mg taken intermittently.

Bloating

Abdominal bloating is another common side effect related to progestins. Some patients may tolerate one progestin formulation better than another, whereas others may benefit from the addition of a mild diuretic (e.g., hydrochlorothiazide 25 mg/d), during the last few days of progestin therapy.

Rashes Associated with Patch Use

Transdermal estrogen administration may result in localized skin irritation and itching at the patch site. Rotating the site of application from one dose to the next minimizes this side effect. Some patients find they have less skin sensitivity on the buttock or thigh areas than on the abdomen. Patients who swim or bathe in hot tubs may develop a rash related to the accumulation of moisture behind the patch. These patients should be instructed to apply a fresh patch after swimming. The patch itself is packaged in a foil envelope with isopropyl alcohol added as a preservative. The alcohol sometimes contributes to skin irritation, which may be alleviated by allowing the patch to air-dry for a minute after removing it from the packaging and before applying it to the skin. The effect of newer, stickier adhesives on these symptoms remains unclear.

Unopposed Estrogen Replacement Therapy

Patients should be discouraged from taking unopposed ERT if the uterus has not been surgically removed. However, some patients cannot tolerate progestins. In patients who still wish to take estrogens yet are unable to take progestins, careful attention must be paid to bleeding episodes. In this setting, endometrial sampling is recommended annually and at any time bleeding occurs. Use of a uterine ultrasound on an annual basis is advocated by some to reduce discomfort and avoid negative curettages, especially among older women with cervical stenosis. In postmenopausal women, an endometrial thickness of less than 4 mm is highly unlikely to be neoplastic and does not warrant histologic sampling. Histologic assessment can thus be limited to women found by ultrasound to have an endometrium that is thicker than 4 mm (55).

Alternatives to Estrogen

There are several alternatives available for those patients in whom estrogen therapy is contraindicated. Hot flashes can often be managed by administration of clonidine 0.1 to 0.2 mg bid. Androgen compounds are also sometimes used to alleviate hot flashes, decrease breast tenderness, and increase libido in postmenopausal women. Provera therapy, 10 to 40 mg per day, can also relieve hot flashes in patients for whom ERT is contraindicated. Megestrol acetate (Megace), a progestational agent, has been shown to prevent or improve symptoms of estrogen deprivation in patients with breast cancer (56).

Indications for Referral to a Gynecologist

Consideration should be given to referring any patient who experiences unexplained vaginal bleeding at a time other than with progestational withdrawal for endometrial sampling by either office techniques or formal D&C. Office endometrial sampling is most often performed by gynecologists.

The patient who experiences HRT side effects that are not alleviated by the techniques given above may also benefit from a referral to a gynecologist or a reproductive endocrinologist with expertise in managing menopausal patients.

Final Considerations

When considering HRT, additional issues that may be overlooked in the management of postmenopausal patients are the importance of weight-bearing exercise, smoking cessation, calcium supplementation, and a well-balanced diet. Calcium intake should total at least 1000 mg per day in postmenopausal women on ERT and 1500 mg per day in women not on ERT.

Hormone replacement therapy is indicated for the prevention and treatment of CAD, osteoporosis, and Alzheimer dementia. However, only women agreeing to regular follow-up are candidates for HRT. Women using HRT should be carefully monitored and evaluated for possible adverse events. Procedures should include regular screening mammography, breast examination and, for some, surveillance for endometrial cancer.

REFERENCES

1. **Ravnikar VA.** Compliance with hormone therapy. Am J Obstet Gynecol. 1987;156: 1332-4.
2. **Falkeborn M, Persson I, Terént A, et al.** Hormone replacement therapy and the risk of stroke: follow-up of a population-based cohort in Sweden. Arch Intern Med. 1993; 153:1201-9.
3. **Finucane FF, Madans JH, Bush TL, et al.** Decreased risk of stroke among postmenopausal hormone users: results from a national cohort. Arch Intern Med. 1993; 153:73-9.

4. **Lindsay R, Thome JF:** Estrogen treatment of patients with established osteoporosis. Obstet Gynecol. 1990;76:290.

5. **Cauley JA, Seeley DG, Ensrud K, et al.** Estrogen replacement therapy and fractures in older women. Ann Intern Med. 1995;122:9-16.

6. Effects of hormone therapy on bone mineral density: results from the Postmenopausal Estrogen/Progestin Interventions (PEPI) trial. JAMA. 1996;276:1389-96.

7. **Raz R, Stamm WE.** A controlled trial of intravaginal estriol in postmenopausal women with recurrent urinary tract infection. N Engl J Med. 1993;329:753.

8. **Bhattia NN, Bergman A, Karram MM.** Effects of estrogen on urethral function in women with urinary incontinence. Obstet Gynecol. 1989;160:176.

9. **Lufkin EG, Carpenter PC, Ory SJ, et al.** Estrogen replacement therapy: current recommendations. Mayo Clin Proc. 1988;63:453-60.

10. **Kempers RD.** Postmenopausal hormone replacement therapy: cyclic and continuous. Postgrad Obstet Gynecol. 1990;10:1-6.

11. **Greendale GA, Judd HL.** The menopause: health implications and clinical management. J Am Geriatr Soc. 1993;41:426-36.

12. **Ditkoff EC, Crary WG, Cristo M, Lobo RA.** Estrogen improves psychological function in asymptomatic postmenopausal women. Obstet Gynecol. 1991;78:991-5.

13. **Grady D, Rubin SM, Petitti DB, et al.** Hormone therapy to prevent disease and prolong life in postmenopausal women. Ann Intern Med. 1992;117:1016-37.

14. **Paganini-Hill A, Henderson VW.** Estrogen replacement therapy and risk of Alzheimer's disease. Arch Intern Med. 1996;156:2213.

15. **Cobleigh MA, Berris RF, et al.** Estrogen replacement therapy in breast cancer survivors: a time for change. JAMA. 1994;272:540-5.

16. **Buller RE.** Hormone replacement therapy following gynecologic cancer. Postgrad Obstet Gynecol. 1993;13:1-6.

17. **Collaborative Group on Hormonal Factors in Breast Cancer.** Breast cancer and hormone replacement therapy: collaborative reanalysis of data from 51 epidemiologic studies of 52,705 women with breast cancer and 108,411 women without breast cancer. Lancet. 1997;350:1047-59.

18. **LaCroix AZ, Burke W.** Breast cancer and hormone replacement therapy [Commentary]. Lancet. 1997;350:1042-3.

19. **Creasman WT, Henderson D, Hinshaw W, Clarke-Pearson DL.** Estrogen replacement therapy in the patient treated for endometrial cancer. Obstet Gynecol. 1986;67:326-30.

20. **Baker D.** Estrogen replacement therapy in patients with previous endometrial carcinoma. Comp Ther. 1990;16:28-35.

21. **Lee RB, Burke TW, Park RC.** Estrogen replacement therapy following treatment for stage I endometrial carcinoma. Gynecol Oncol. 1990;36:189-91.

22. **Chapman JA, DiSaia PJ, Osann K, et al.** Estrogen replacement in surgical stage I and II endometrial cancer survivors. Am J Obstet Gynecol. 1996;175:1195-200.

23. **Lowe GDO, Greer IA, et al.** Risk of and prophylaxis for venous thromboemoblism in hospital patients. Baillieres Clini Obstet Gynaecol. 1996;10:567-74.

24. **Daly E, Vessey MP, Hawkins MM, et al.** Risk of venous thromboembolism in users of hormone replacement therapy. Lancet. 1996;348:977-80.

25. **Jick H, Derby LE, Myers MW, et al.** Risk of hospital admission for idiopathic venous thromboembolism among users of postmenopausal estrogens. Lancet. 1996;348:981-3.

26. **Grodstein F, Stampfer MJ, Goldhaber SZ, et al.** Prospective study of exogenous hormones and risk of pulmonary embolism in women. Lancet. 1996;348:983-7.

27. **Frigo P, Eppel W, Asseryanis E, et al.** The effects of hormone substitution in depot form on the uterus in a group of 50 perimenopausal women: a vaginosonographic study. Maturitas. 1995;21:221-5.

28. **Wingfield M, Healy D.** Endometriosis: medical therapy. Baillieres Clini Obstet Gynaecol. 1993;813-38.

29. **Whitehead M.** Treatment for menopausal and postmenopausal problems: present and future. Baillieres Clini Obstet Gynaecol. 1996;10:515-30.

30. **Ginsburg ES, Mello NK, Mendelson JH, et al.** Effects of alcohol ingestion on estrogens in postmenopausal women. JAMA. 1996;276:1747-51.

31. **Crook D, Cust MP, Gangar KF, et al.** Comparison of transdermal and oral estrogen/progestin replacement therapy: effects on serum lipids and lipoproteins. Am J Obstet Gynecol. 1992;166:950-5.

32. **Lip GY, Beevers M, Churchill D, Beevers DG.** Hormone replacement therapy and blood pressure in hypertensive women. J Hum Hypertens. 1994;8:491-4.

33. **Jatoi I, Gore ME.** Sex, pregnancy, hormones, and melanoma. BMJ. 1993;307:2-3.

34. **Hartge P, Tucker MA, Shields JA, et al.** Case-control study of female hormones and eye melanoma. Cancer Res. 1989;49:4622-5.

35. **Franceschi S, Barón AE, La Vecchia C.** The influence of female hormones on malignant melanoma. Tumori. 1990;76:439-49.

36. **Writing Group for the PEPI Trial.** Effects of estrogen or estrogen/progestin regimens on heart disease risk factors in postmenopausal women. JAMA. 1995;273:199.

37. **Walmer DK.** Hormonal therapy in the perimenopausal woman. Postgrad Obstet Gynecol. 1994;14:1-6.

38. **Lindsay R, Tohme J, Kanders B.** The effect of oral contraceptive use on vertebral bone mass in pre- and post-menopausal women. Contraception. 1986;34:333-40.

39. **Enzelsberger H, Metka M, Heytmanek G, et al.** Influence of oral contraceptive use on bone density in climacteric women. Maturitas. 1988;9:375-8.

40. **Hulley S, Grady D, Bush T, et al.** Randomized trial of estrogen plus progestin for secondary prevention of coronary heart disease in postmenopausal women. JAMA. 1998; 280:605-13.

41. **Pike MC, Peters RK, Cozen W, et al.** Estrogen-progestin replacement therapy and endometrial cancer. J Natl Cancer Inst. 1997;89:1110-6.

42. **Witt DM, Lousberg TR.** Controversies surrounding estrogen use in postmenopausal women. Ann Pharmacother. 1997;31:745-55.

43. **Persson I, Yuen J, Bergkvist L, et al.** Combined estrogen-progestogen replacement and breast cancer risk. Lancet. 1992;340:1044.

44. **Weinstein L, Bewtra C, Gallagher JC.** Evaluation of a continuous combined low-dose regimen of estrogen-progestin for treatment of the menopausal patient. Am J Obstet Gynecol. 1990;162:1534-42.

45. **Flowers CE Jr, Wilborn WH, Hyde BM.** Mechanisms of uterine bleeding in postmenopausal patients receiving estrogen alone or with a progestin. Obstet Gynecol. 1983;61:135-43.

46. **Whitehead MI, Townsend PT, Pryse-Davies J, et al.** Effects of estrogens and progestins on the biochemistry and the morphology of the postmenopausal endometrium. N Engl J Med. 1981;305:1599-605.

47. **Spencer CP, Cooper AJ, Whitehead MI.** Management of abnormal bleeding in women receiving hormone replacement therapy. BMJ. 1997;315:37-42.

48. **Mishell DR, Shoupe D, et al.** Postmenopausal hormone replacement therapy with a combination estrogen-progestin regimen for 5 days per week. Baillieres Clini Obstet Gynaecol. 1996;10:351-5.

49. **Casper RF, MacLusky NJ, et al.** Rationale for estrogen with interrupted progestin as a new low-dose hormonal replacement therapy. J Soc Gynecol Invest. 1996;3:225-34.

50. **Ettinger B.** Cyclic hormone replacement therapy using quarterly progestin. Obstet Gynecol. 1994;83:693.

51. Menopause Management. July/August 1994;12-32.

52. **Baker VL.** Alternatives to oral estrogen replacement. Obstet Gynecol North Am. 1994;21:271-97.

53. **Chambers JT, Chambers SK.** Endometrial sampling: when? where? why? with what? Clin Obstet Gynecol. 1992;35:28-39.

54. **Padwick ML, Pryse-Davies J, Whitehead MI.** A sample method for determining the optimal dosage of progestin in postmenopausal women receiving estrogens. N Engl J Med. 1986;315:930-4.

55. **Agarwal SK, Judd HL.** Menopause. In: Bardin CW, ed. Current Therapy in Endocrinology and Metabolism. 6th Ed. St. Louis: Mosby; 1997;624-29.

56. **Loprinski CL, Michalak JC, Quella SK, et al.** Megestrol acetate for the prevention of hot flashes. New Engl J Med. 1994;331:347-52.

Diagnosis

CHAPTER 12

Differential Diagnosis of Chest Pain

PAULA A. JOHNSON, MD, MPH

Chest pain syndromes are among the most common patient symptoms for both the internist and cardiologist. Sixteen percent of the 2717 healthy relatives in the Framingham cohort complained of chest pain (1). The evaluation of chest pain is critical because of the possibility of misdiagnosis. The outcome may be fatal when ischemic pain, a dissecting aortic aneurysm, or severe pulmonary problems such as pulmonary embolism are not promptly diagnosed and treated. The appropriate evaluation of chest pain syndromes must account for gender-specific data regarding risk factors for type of presentation and artery disease entities including coronary artery disease (CAD). This chapter focuses on the differential diagnosis of chest pain in women, with emphasis on nonischemic etiologies that may be particularly important in the female population.

Typical angina is described classically as a pressure-type chest pain that is mainly substernal and radiates to the left arm, neck, and/or jaw. The discomfort is usually precipitated by exercise and resolves with rest within several minutes (2,3). Unfortunately, this constellation of symptoms is neither highly sensitive nor specific. In the Coronary Artery Surgery Study (CASS), for example, women with a history defined as *definite angina* had a prevalence of CAD at coronary angiography of 72%, whereas only 36% of women with *probable angina* and 6% with *nonspecific chest pain* had CAD defined by angiography (4). This association has held true in a number of other studies (5-7). Additional data should be evaluated when considering the diagnosis of angina, including associated symptoms, risk factors (e.g., patient's menopausal status), and basic testing (e.g., electrocardiogram). (Angina is further characterized in Chapter 15.) The challenge lies in the ability to appropriately risk-stratify women patients with chest pain.

Through the Multicenter Chest Pain Study, a prospective study evaluating patients with acute chest pain presenting to the emergency department, Lee et al were able to identify a combination of factors that placed patients into a low-risk category for acute myocardial infarction (AMI) (8). Low-risk patients were more likely to have pain that was described as sharp, stabbing, pleuritic, positional, or reproduced by chest wall palpation and were likely not to have a history of angina or myocardial infarction. Suprisingly, pain described as a pressure-like sensation was as predictive of AMI as pain described as burning or similar to indigestion. Because AMI occurs significantly less frequently in women in whom the "classic" symptoms are present, interpretation of these symptoms is not as straightforward for women as for men (9). To complicate matters further, women with AMI are more likely to have neck and shoulder pain, nausea, vomiting, fatigue, or dyspnea as presenting symptoms (10,11). Women who have chronic stable angina also tend to have more atypical characteristics such as pain with emotional or mental stress or pain during sleep (12).

Douglas and Ginsburg recently presented a scheme for placing female patients into high, medium, and low risk groups for CAD according to the presence of a series of risk factors that consider gender (13). Major determinants of CAD in women include typical angina pectoris, postmenopausal status without hormone replacement, diabetes mellitus, and peripheral vascular disease. Intermediate determinants include hypertension, smoking, and lipoprotein abnormalities, especially low high-density lipoprotein (HDL). Minor determinants of CAD include age greater than 65 years, obesity, sedentary lifestyle, and family history. Women who are at the highest risk of having CAD (>80%) will have two or more major determinants or one major and at least one intermediate or minor determinant. Women at moderate risk for CAD (20%-80%) will have one major determinant or multiple intermediate and minor determinants. Finally, those at low likelihood for CAD (<20%) will have no major determinants and one or no intermediate or two or fewer minor determinants. This schema may assist the physician in stratifying the female patient with chest pain into the appropriate risk group. The remainder of this chapter addresses the differential diagnosis of patients who fall into the group in whom the probability of CAD is moderate or low or in whom exercise stress testing has placed CAD low in the differential diagnosis.

Differential Diagnosis of Nonischemic Chest Pain

Nonischemic chest pain can be described in two ways: by etiology or by the location of the pain. It may be more useful to think of chest pain in terms of the site of origin, because that most similarly mimics the way we take a history and how we begin to formulate a differential diagnosis. Figure 12-1 shows the organs of the chest and abdomen that can be associated with chest pain. A full description of every disorder causing pain in the chest and the surrounding areas is beyond the scope of this chapter. Those entities that present most similarly to ischemic pain will be discussed in detail by organ system.

Cardiac Causes

Mitral Valve Prolapse

Mitral valve prolapse is more common in women than men by approximately a 2:1 ratio (14). It may be primary or secondary. The most common underlying primary etiologies are Marfan syndrome and types I and III Ehlers-Danlos syndrome. Secondary mitral valve prolapse is rare.

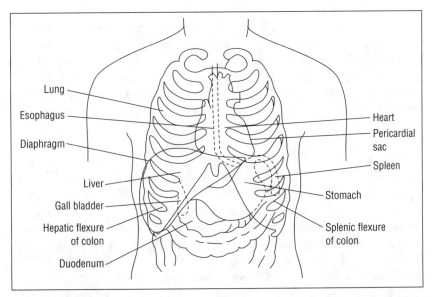

Figure 12-1 Diagrammatic representation of the organs of the chest and abdomen that can be associated with chest pain. Note particularly the close anatomical relationships between many of the organs. (Adapted from Miller AJ. Diagnosis of Chest Pain. New York: Raven Press;1998:174.)

The entity of mitral valve prolapse is commonly purported to be associated with atypical chest pain and several additional symptoms such as dyspnea and anxiety. This has been debated in the literature, and population-based studies have not supported the association of mitral valve prolapse and chest pain (14,15). The Framingham Heart Study data, evaluating the offspring of the original Framingham cohort, did not indicate any increase in the presence of chest pain in the 7% of patients with echocardiographically proven mitral valve prolapse when compared with the unaffected population (1). Because mitral valve prolapse is felt to be inherited, Devereux et al compared first-degree relatives with the disorder to those relatives who were unaffected (15). They found no difference in the prevalence of atypical chest pain in the affected and unaffected relatives. Patients with more severe mitral valve prolapse, associated with significant mitral regurgitation, may be more likely to experience symptoms of chest pain, but this hypothesis has not been well studied.

Chest Pain and Normal Coronary Arteries

Patients with chest pain and normal coronary arteries can fall into several categories. The evaluation of each of these groups of patients will depend on the individual patient's risk factor profile and the nature of the symptoms. It is recognized that chest pain with normal coronary arteries is a phenomenon more common in women. It is important to determine if patients have symptoms that are typical of angina and whether they have ischemia during exercise testing. The entity of anginal chest pain and normal epicardial arteries has been termed *syndrome X* (16). Most of these patients are women. Insulin resistance has been reported in a series of patients with chest pain and normal coronary arteries (17). Coronary artery spasm can also cause ischemic chest pain without obvious disease of the epicardial arteries.

Patients who have normal coronary arteries, typical anginal chest pain, and who may experience ischemia during exercise testing usually have an excellent prognosis (18). Up to 25% of these patients may develop some decrease in left ventricular function (19). The pathophysiology of this disorder is not known. Data suggest that these patients have a lower pain threshold in response to forearm ischemia. In addition, adenosine may be released in response to microvascular contraction, leading to stimulation of pain receptors (17,20). The roles of insulin resistance and microvascular constriction in the development of left ventricular dysfunction are not clear.

In patients with evidence of ischemia, management includes traditional anti-ischemic medications to control symptoms. Small studies have shown that estrogen replacement in postmenopausal women (21,22) and imipramine (23) have resulted in a decrease in the frequency of chest pain. An important goal in this population is to control symptoms so that quality of life does not suffer.

Aortic Dissection

Aortic dissection can present with symptoms of chest pain that is usually characterized as "tearing," "ripping," or "splitting" (24). The pain is usually sudden and severe at the onset. Aortic dissections that involve the proximal aorta (ascending aorta and aortic arch) are usually associated with chest pain, whereas those involving the descending aorta are usually characterized by back pain (24,25). Although aortic dissection is more common in men than women, with a 3:1 male-to-female predominance, 50% of aortic dissections in women under the age of 40 occurs during pregnancy (26). Risk factors for aortic dissection during pregnancy include hypertension, Marfan syndrome, trauma, coarctation of the aorta, bicuspid aortic valve, advanced age, multiparity, and Ehler-Danlos type IV syndrome. When aortic dissection occurs during pregnancy, it is usually during the third trimester. Sixty-three percent of dissections are not associated with any of these factors (27-29).

Expanding proximal aortic aneurysms may also cause chest pain. Aortic aneurysms are usually found in an older age group (postmenopausal) who are at higher risk for atherosclerosis.

Other Cardiac Causes of Chest Pain

Other cardiac causes of chest pain include pericarditis and cardiomyopathy (hypertrophic or dilated). Pericarditis is characterized by pleuritic and positional chest pain. These etiologies are not particulary more common in women, except in patients who have autoimmune diseases such as systemic lupus erythematosus (30-32).

Pulmonary Causes

Chest pain is the most frequent presenting symptom that occurs with pulmonary embolism (33). In a study of 387 patients with pulmonary embolism in the Urokinase-Streptokinase Pulmonary Embolism Trial, 88% had chest pain and 74% described their chest pain as pleuritic (34). Frequently, patients will also present with a complaint of dyspnea and have tachypnea and tachycardia on physical examination. Pulmonary infarction, usually due to smaller, distal pulmonary emboli, is also associated with severe pleuritic chest pain (35).

Risk factors for pulmonary embolism that are either specific to women or more common in women include the use of oral contraceptives, pregnancy, and a history of systemic lupus erythematosus with or without antiphospho-lipid syndrome.

Primary pulmonary hypertension is an uncommon disease that affects women more often than men. Data from the Mayo Clinic and from a national registry show that women comprise between 63% and 73% of patients with primary pulmonary hypertension (36,37). The mean age of diagnosis is the mid-thirties. Common presenting symptoms include exertional dyspnea and chest pain (38). The chest pain associated with primary pulmonary hypertension can be caused by ischemia of the right ventricle (39).

Gastrointestinal Causes

Esophageal Disorders

Esophageal disorders are probably the most common cause of nonischemic chest pain that can mimic true angina. It is estimated that up to 50% of patients with normal coronary arteries and chest pain may have esophageal disorders (40-42). These patients can experience continued, recurrent pain leading to increased resource utilization (43). It is important to recognize that the prevalence of both esophageal dysfunction and CAD increases with age, and that it is not unusual for both to exist together (44). This may be especially important in women, because they develop CAD at an older age than men. The most likely esophageal disorders to mimic ischemic chest pain are esophageal reflux and esophageal motility disorders. The motility disorders consist of achalasia, nutcracker esophagus, diffuse esophageal spasm, and hypertensive lower esophageal sphincter. The disorders of the esophagus can be very difficult to discern from true anginal pain because they both can respond to nitrates and calcium channel blockers. In addition, for patients with reflux, an infusion of acid into the esophagus can lower the threshold for angina. Reflux is often associated with a hiatus hernia. This disorder can be diagnosed with a barium study.

Esophageal motility abnormalities and their relationship to retrosternal chest pain are somewhat controversial. Achalasia is the best-described esophageal motility disorder. Early achalasia may be associated with substernal chest pain, whereas later symptoms are characterized more by dysphagia (43). Achalasia can be diagnosed radiographically. Nutcracker esophagus has received much attention, especially since the advent of manometry. High-amplitude peristaltic pressures in the distal esophagus characterize the disorder. Although the relationship between high amplitude contractions and chest pain is not always seen, somewhere between 25% and 50% of patients with noncardiac chest pain have these contractions on manometry (45–47).

Certain characteristics of esophageal pain may help to distinguish it from anginal pain (Table 12-1). Testing for esophageal disorders may include basic radiologic studies such as a barium swallow to rule out achalasia and/or an upper gastrointestinal series to rule out a hiatus hernia. In addition, esophageal pH monitoring can be performed to assist in the diagnosis of reflux. Other testing includes esophageal manometry to identify motility disorders (especially nutcracker esophagus), esophageal sphincter abnormalities, and diffuse esophageal spasm. Finally, provocative tests use pharmacologic agents to provoke symptoms or pressure abnormalities. These provocative tests include acid perfusion (Bernstein), ergonovine, edrophonium, and bethanechol.

It is important to differentiate between reflux and an esophageal motility disorder. Some of the therapies for a motility disorder, such as calcium channel blocking agents, may exacerbate reflux. If gastroesophageal reflux is a significant concern, a trial of therapy aimed at controlling acid secretion should be given (43,48).

Table 12-1 Similarities and Differences Between Esophageal and Cardiac Pain.

	Similarities of Cardiac and Esophageal Pain	Distinguishing Features of Esophageal Pain
Location	Mid or lower retrosternal. May be a severe epigastric pain with radiation up to neck.	High epigastric, behind xiphoid process or in low retrosternal area.
Nature	Heaviness, squeezing, tightness, or burning. Can be associated with weakness, diaphoresis, and anxiety.	Often burning or perceived as spasm. Heartburn is frequent association. Can be associated with increased salivation. Dysphagia occurs.
Radiation	Upward toward throat. May radiate to left neck, shoulder, or arm.	Tends to ascend but not radiate to left side. Radiation to both shoulders and/or arms is less frequent. When pain begins in lower retrosternal area it often radiates down to epigastrium.
Precipitants	Angina is more likely with physical activity after eating.	After eating certain foods—alchohol, coffee, spices. Less likely to be brought on by exertion. Can be precipitated by change in posture, e.g., by lying down.
Duration	Can last a short duration (2 to 10 minutes).	May last hours; may wax and wane.
Relieving factors	May be relieved or eased by nitroglycerin, standing, and relaxing.	

Adapted from Miller AJ. Diagnosis of Chest Pain. New York: Raven Press; 1988:74–6.

Musculoskeletal Causes

Pain and tenderness on palpitation of the costochondral or chondrosternal joints is a common cause of chest pain. The syndrome described by Titze in 1921 is characterized by swelling of the costal cartilages and local pain and tenderness of the anterior chest wall (49). In a prospective study of patients presenting with chest pain to the emergency department, women comprised 69% of the patients with costochondritis (50). The treatment of choice for costochondritis is an anti-inflammatory agent.

Psychological Causes

Panic Disorder

There is a growing body of evidence that panic disorder may be associated with chest pain syndromes in patients who have angiographically normal coronary arteries (51–53). Panic disorder is common, affecting between 1% and 2% of the U.S. population (54). This disorder may affect up to 30% of patients with chest pain and normal coronary angiograms (54). The diagnosis of panic disorder is made via a structured interview and should meet the psychiatric definition as detailed in DSM-IV (55). The usefulness of laboratory challenge studies, such as the lactate challenge test and the carbon dioxide challenge (in which the patient breathes in 35% carbon dioxide), has not been fully determined.

Katon et al evaluated 74 patients with chest pain who were referred for coronary angiography. Interestingly, 43% of the 28 patients with normal angiograms were found to have panic disorder compared with only 5% of the 46 patients who had significant coronary atherosclerosis on angiography (56). The patients with panic disorder more frequently had autonomic symptoms associated with chest pain such as tachycardia, dyspnea, and dizziness. They were also more likely to have atypical chest pain. Similarly, Beitman et al found that of 74 patients with atypical or nonanginal chest pain and a normal electrocardiogram, exercise treadmill test, or coronary angiography, 58% had panic disorder (57). Yingling et al studied 334 patients with acute chest pain who presented to the emergency department of an urban teaching hospital. Patients were interviewed by telephone within 48 hours of their visit. The authors found a prevalence of panic disorder in 17.5% and depression in 23% of the population. Of these patients, greater than 50% of those who met the criteria for panic disorder or depression visited the emergency department more than one time in the previous year with a complaint of chest pain (52).

These findings may have important implications for treatment. If a patient has panic disorder, the more traditional treatments for nonischemic chest pain will not be effective. Resolution of symptoms will only occur by treating the disorder directly (58). It is known that patients with chest pain and normal coronary angiography suffer ongoing disability. It appears that patients with panic disorder suffer a more severe disability and have worse health status (59,60). (For further discussion of panic attacks, see Chapter 20.)

Summary

Careful history and mutual assessment may often clarify the etiology of a woman's chest pain. Esophageal symptoms most often mimic angina. Avoiding misdiagnosis of potentially treatable conditions is essential.

REFERENCES

1. **Savage DD, Devereux RB, Garrison RJ, et al.** Miltral valve prolapse in the general population. 2. Clinical features: the Framingham Study. Am Heart J. 1983;106:577-81.

2. **Rutherford JD.** Chronic ischemic heart disease. In: Braunwald E. Heart Disease: A Textbook of Cardiovascular Medicine. 4th ed. Philadelphia: WB Saunders; 1992:1292-1364.

3. **Braunwald E.** The history. In: Braunwald E. Heart Disease: A Textbook of Cardiovascular Medicine. 4th ed. Philadelphia: WB Saunders; 1992.

4. **Chaitman BR, Bourassa MG, Davis K, et al.** Angiographic prevalence of high-risk coronary artery disease in patient subsets (CASS). Circulation. 1981;64:360-7.

5. **Weiner DA, Ryan TJ, McCabe CH, et al.** Exercise stress testing: correlations among history of angina, ST-segment response and prevalence of coronary/artery disease in the Coronary Artery Surgery Study (CASS). N Engl J Med. 1979;301:230-5.

6. **Melin JA, Wijins W, Vanbutsele RJ, et al.** Alternative diagnostic strategies for coronary artery disease in women: demonstration of the usefulness and efficiency of probability analysis. Circulation. 1985;71:535-42.

7. **Chaitman BR, Lam J, et al.** Noninvasive diagnosis of coronary heart disease in women. In: Eaker ED, Wenger NK, et al., eds. Coronary Heart Disease in Women. New York: Haymarket Doyma; 1987;222.

8. **Lee TH, Cook EF, Weisberg M, et al.** Acute chest pain in the emergency room: identification and examination of low-risk patients. Arch Intern Med. 1985;145:65-9.

9. **Cunningham MA, Lee TH, Cook EF, et al.** The effect of gender on the probability of myocardial infarction among emergency department patients with acute chest pain: a report from the Multicenter Chest Pain Study Group. J Gen Intern Med. 1989;4:392-8.

10. **Maynard C.** Treatment of women with acute MI: new findings from the MITI registry. Myocardial Ischemia. 1992;4:27-37.

11. **Willich SN, Lewis M, Arntz R, et al.** Unexplained gender differences in clinical symptoms of acute myocardial infarction. J Am Coll Cardiol. 1993;21:238A.

12. **Pepine CJ, Abrams J, Marks RG, et al.** Characteristics of a contemporary population with angina pectoris: TIDES investigators. Am J Cardiol. 1994;74:226-31.

13. **Douglas PS, Ginsburg GS.** The evaluation of chest pain in women [see Comments]. N Engl J Med. 1996;334:1311-5.

14. **Levy D, Savage D.** Prevalence and clinical features of mitral valve prolapse. Am Heart J. 1987;113:1281-90.

15. **Devereux RB, Kramer-Fox R, Kligfield P.** Mitral valve prolapse: causes, clinical manifestations, and management. Ann Intern Med. 1989;111:305-17.

16. **Kemp HG Jr, Vokonas PS, Cohn PF, Gorlin R.** The anginal syndrome associated with normal coronary arteriograms: report of a six-year experience. Am J Med. 1973;54: 735-42.

17. **Cannon RO 3rd, Epstein SE.** Pathophysiological dilemma of syndrome X. Circulation. 1992;85:883-92.

18. **Lichtlen PR, Bargheer K, Wenzlaff P.** Long-term prognosis of patients with angina-like chest pain and normal coronary angiographic findings. J Am Coll Cardiol. 1995;25:1013-8.

19. **Alpert MA.** The continuing conundrum of syndrome X: further evidence of heterogeneity [Editorial; Comment]. J Am Coll Cardiol. 1995;25:1318-20.

20. **Cannon RO 3rd, Quyyumi AA, Schenke WH, et al.** Abnormal cardiac sensitivity in patients with chest pain and normal coronary arteries. J Am Coll Cardiol. 1990;16: 1359-66.

21. **Rosano GM, Lefroy D, et al.** 17-beta-Estradiol therapy lessens angina in postmenopausal women with Syndrome X. J Am Coll Cardiol. 1996;28:1500-5.

22. **Collins P.** Hormone replacement therapy and syndrome X. Br J Obstet Gynaecol. 1996;103:68-72.

23. **Cannon RO 3rd.** The sensitive heart: a syndrome of abnormal cardiac pain perception. JAMA. 1995;273:883-7.

24. **Crawford E.** The diagnosis and management of aortic dissection. JAMA. 1990;264: 2537-41.

25. **DeSanctis RW, Doroghazi RM, Austen WG, Buckley MJ.** Aortic dissection. N Engl J Med. 1987;317:1060-7.

26. **Pumphrey CW, Fay T, Weir I.** Aortic dissection during pregnancy. Br Heart J. 1986;55:106-8.

27. **Williams GB, Gott VL, Brawley RK, et al.** Aortic disease associated with pregnancy. J Vasc Surg. 1988;8:470-5.

28. **Konishi YT, Tatsuta N, Kumada K, et al.** Dissecting aneurysm during pregnancy and the puerperium. Jpn Circ J. 1980;44:726-33.

29. **Snir E, Levinsky L, Salamon J, et al.** Dissecting aortic aneurysm in pregnant women without Marfan disease. Surg Gynecol Obstet. 1988;167:463-465.

30. **Bulkley BH, Roberts WC.** The heart in systemic lupus erythematosus and the changes induced in it by corticosteroid therapy: a study of 36 necropsy patients. Am J Med. 1975;58:243-64.

31. **Leung WH, Wong KL, Lau CP, et al.** Cardiac abnormalities in systemic lupus erythematosus: a prospective M-mode, cross-sectional and Doppler echocardiographic study. Int J Cardiol. 1990;27:367-75.

32. **Murai K, Oku H, Takeuchi K, et al.** Alterations in myocardial systolic and diastolic function in patients with active systemic lupus erythematosus. Am Heart J. 1987;113: 966-71.

33. **Goldhaber S.** Strategies for diagnosis. In: Goldhaber SZ, ed. Pulmonary Embolism and Deep Venous Thrombosis. Philadelphia: WB Saunders; 1985.

34. **Bell WR, Simon TL, DeMets DL.** The clinical features of submassive and massive pulmonary emboli. Am J Med. 1977;52:355-60.

35. **Tsao MS, Schraufnagel D, Wang NS.** Pathogenesis of pulmonary infarction. Am J Med. 1982;72:599-606.

36. **Fuster V, Steele PM, Edwards WD, et al.** Primary pulmonary hypertension: natural history and the importance of thrombosis. Circulation. 1984;70:580-7.

37. **Rich S, Dantzker DR, Ayres SM, et al.** Primary pulmonary hypertension: a national prospective study. Ann Intern Med. 1987;107:216-23.

38. **Rubin LJ.** Pathology and pathophysiology of primary pulmonary hypertension. Am J Cardiol. 1995;75:51A-54A.

39. **Ross RS.** Right ventricular hypertension as a cause of precordial pain. Am Heart J. 1961;61:134-5.

40. **DeMeester TR, O'Sullivan GC, Bermudez G, et al.** Esophageal function in patients with angina-type chest pain and normal coronary angiograms. Ann Surg. 1982;196: 488-98.

41. **Kline M, Chesne R, Sturdevant RA, McCallum RW.** Esophageal disease in patients with angina-like chest pain. Am J Gastroenterol. 1981;75:116-23.

42. **Davies HA, Jones DB, Rhodes J.** "Esophageal angina" as the cause of chest pain. JAMA. 1982;248:2274-8.

43. **Richter JE, Bradley LA, Castell DO.** Esophageal chest pain: current controversies in pathogenesis, diagnosis, and therapy. Ann Intern Med. 1989;110:66-78.

44. **Svensson O, Stenport G, Tibbling L, Wranne B.** Oesophageal function and coronary angiogram in patients with disabling chest pain. Acta Med Scand. 1978;204:173-8.

45. **Traube M, Albibi R, McCallum RW.** High-amplitude peristaltic esophageal contractions associated with chest pain. JAMA. 1983;250:2655-9.

46. **Orr WC, Robinson MG.** Hypertensive peristalsis in the pathogenesis of chest pain: further exploration of the "nutcracker" esophagus. Am J Gastroenterol. 1982;77:604-7.

47. **Katz PO, Dalton CB, Richter JE, et al.** Esophageal testing in patients with noncardiac chest pain or dysphasia: results of three years' experience with 1161 patients. Ann Intern Med. 1987;106:593-7.

48. **Fass R, Fennerty MB, Ofman JJ, et al.** The clinical and economic value of a short course of omeprazole in patients with noncardiac chest pain. Gastroenterology. 1998; 115:42-9.

49. **Epstein SE, Gerber LH, Borer JS.** Chest wall syndrome: a common cause of unexpected cardiac pain. JAMA. 1979;241:2793-7.

50. **Disla E, Rhim HR, Reddy A, et al.** Costochondritis: a prospective analysis in an emergency department setting. Arch Intern Med. 1994;154:2466-9.

51. **Raymond C.** Chest pain not always what is seems; panic disorder may be cause in some. JAMA. 1989;261:1101-2.

52. **Yingling KW, Wuslin LR, Arnold LM, Rouan GW.** Estimated prevalences of panic disorder and depression among consecutive patients seen in an emergency department with acute chest pain. J Gen Intern Med. 1993;8:231-5.

53. **Katon WJ.** Chest pain, cardiac disease, and panic disorder. J Clin Psychiatry. 1990;51: 27-30.

54. **Beitman BD.** Panic disorder in patients with angiographically normal coronary arteries. Am J Med. 1992;92:5A-33S.

55. **American Psychiatric Association.** Diagnostic and Statistical Manual of Mental Disorders. 4th ed. Washington, DC: American Psychiatric Association; 1994.

56. **Katon WJ, Hall ML, Russo J, et al.** Chest pain: the relationship of psychiatric illness to coronary arteriography results. Am J Med. 1988;84:1-9.

57. **Beitman BD, Basha I, Flaker G, et al.** Atypical or nonanginal chest pain: panic disorder or coronary artery disease? Arch Intern Med. 1987;147:1548-52.

58. **Nagy LM, Krystal JH, Charney DS, et al.** Long-term outcome of panic disorder after short-term imipramine and behavioral group treatment: 2.9 year naturalistic follow-up study. J Clin Psychopharmacol. 1993;13:16-24.

59. **Bass C, Wade C.** Chest pain with normal coronary arteries: a comparative study of psychiatric and social morbidity. Psychol Med. 1984;14:51-61.

60. **Ockene IS, Shay MJ, Alperts JS, et al.** Unexplained chest pain in patients with normal coronary arteriograms: a follow-up study of functional status. N Engl J Med. 1980;303:1249-52.

CHAPTER 13

Noninvasive Testing Techniques for Diagnosis and Prognosis

LESLEE J. SHAW, PHD
ERIC D. PETERSON, MD, MPH
LYNNE L. JOHNSON, MD

Many physicians perceive that electrocardiographic and scintigraphic tests may be less sensitive and unreliable in women than in men. Under-representation of women in the published literature of clinical and noninvasive diagnostic tests has contributed to this perception (1). Published reports have excluded women when the inclusion criteria were limited to typical anginal symptoms or to referral populations. A review of the literature on noninvasive testing reveals limited representation of women (Table 13-1) (2). The fewest number of women were included in exercise electrocardiography reports (8%), and the greatest number of women were included in myocardial-perfusion imaging reports (27%). The absolute numbers of women represented in the 64 reports is small, ranging from 32 women with exercise electrocardiography to 230 women with radionuclide ventricular function imaging. Few reports have included end-point data by gender (3,4). More recently, studies have focused on the diagnostic and prognostic accuracy of noninvasive imaging in women.

Assessing Pretest Clinical Risk

For women, coronary disease incidence lags 10 years behind that of men but increases after the onset of menopause (5). Certain risk factors, including age

Table 13-1 Representation of Women in Published Studies of Noninvasive Testing of Coronary Artery Disease*

Stress Noninvasive Modalities	No. of Reports	No. of Total Patients	No. of Women	No. of Women per Trial Range	Average No. of Women per Trial
Electrocardiography	22	26,254	1980 (8%)	0–272	32
Myocardial perfusion imaging	21	8621	2311 (27%)	0–275	110
Ventricular function imaging	5	3375	827 (25%)	12–674	230
Echocardiography	16	2615	573 (22%)	0–123	56

* Including peer-review journals with sufficient documentation on patient inclusion criteria, greater than 80% follow-up, and/or cardiac catheterization end-point data.

and diabetes, are associated with a higher mortality for coronary artery disease (CAD) in women compared with men (6,7). All-cause and cardiovascular mortality is threefold higher for diabetic women compared with diabetic men (8). Recent studies from Framingham have indicated that mild glucose intolerance is a risk factor for women but not for men. This effect may partially explain why obesity seems to be a significant risk factor for coronary disease in women (9,10). Hypertension is more prevalent in women than in men. Cigarette smoking is associated with a similar increased risk of CAD in women and men (5,11).

When assessing risk for CAD in women, hormonal status must also be taken into consideration. In epidemiologic studies, postmenopausal women receiving estrogen replacement have a 40% to 50% lower relative risk of ischemic heart disease when compared with women not receiving hormonal replacement therapy (12–14). However, recent results from the prospective HERS study noted an increase in thromboembolic complications with hormone replacement therapy (15a).

It has been shown repeatedly that more women present to their primary care physician with atypical chest pain symptoms that occur more frequently at rest or at times of nonexertion (15b). In addition, chest pain presentation in women may be mixed (exhibiting typical and atypical components), although typical anginal symptoms have been repeatedly shown to be a powerful diagnostic and prognostic risk marker (16–19). Despite the differing symptom presentation, important chest pain characteristics that should be documented include 1) location of pain; 2) chest pain quality; 3) duration of symptoms; 4) any precipitating events; 5) radiation to extremities or other locations; 6) associated dyspnea, diaphoresis, or nausea; and 7) how the symptoms are relieved. Clinicians should also consider noncardiac reasons for symptoms, including gastrointestinal, musculoskeletal, pulmonary, or psychiatric disorders for all patients presenting with chest pain symptoms (20).

Following the initial clinical assessment, physicians must integrate clinical history and risk factor information into an impression of the patient's pretest probability of coronary disease and survival. Integrated predictive models based on clinical history and physical examination parameters have been developed (7,16–18,21,22). These models can aid in predicting the risk of significant CAD. Figure 13-1 is a nomogram for predicting significant CAD based on age and clinical characteristics (16).

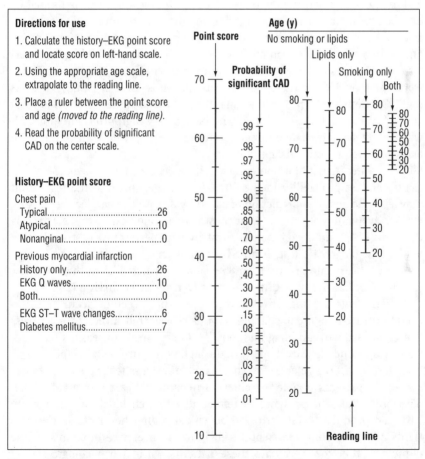

Figure 13-1 Nomogram for estimating the likelihood of significant coronary artery disease in women. CAD = coronary artery disease; EKG = electrocardiogram findings. (Adapted from Pryor DB, Harrell FE, Lee KL, et al. Estimating the likelihood of significant coronary artery disease. Am J Med. 1983;75:771–80.)

Use of Noninvasive Testing To Enhance Pretest Risk Estimates

A primary objective of noninvasive testing for detection of myocardial ischemia is to identify those patients who potentially will benefit from further medical or surgical intervention, with increased likelihood for survival and reduction of anginal symptoms. The greatest value to both the patient and the referring physician will come from a test that either excludes the possibility of flow-limiting CAD (giving some prognostic estimate for event-free survival over a certain period of time) or establishes the presence of coronary disease (giving some indication of the extent and severity of disease).

Based on Bayesian theory, the predictive accuracy of a test is limited by disease prevalence. When pretest risk is low, an abnormal test will not result in a substantial improvement in diagnostic or prognostic prediction. For example, in a recent report on 4672 patients with chest pain undergoing exercise treadmill testing, post-test probability estimates for disease and survival were less than 15% in the cohort of patients whose pretest clinical risk was low (23). Conversely, proceeding directly to cardiac catheterization is most cost-effective for women and men who have a very high probability for CAD with severe symptoms. Additional noninvasive testing will be helpful only in assessing their functional capacity.

The greatest benefit for noninvasive testing occurs in intermediate-risk patients (pretest probability in the 20%–70% range), because the test result may alter the post-test prediction of coronary disease and cardiac events (24). For the evaluation of patients with chest pain and normal resting electrocardiogram (EKG), the recommended strategy is to perform EKG stress testing as the first diagnostic test. If no ST-segment changes exist and the patient achieves a heart rate greater than 85% of age predicted, then there is a low likelihood of flow-limiting CAD that can adversely affect survival (23).

Patients with resting EKG abnormalities that preclude accurate interpretation of ST-segment changes should be referred directly for a stress test combined with an imaging modality. For a variety of reasons (e.g., advanced age and debility and musculoskeletal, neurologic, or peripheral vascular disease), a referral for pharmacologic stress testing should be reserved for patients unable to achieve a maximum heart rate greater than 85% predicted. The presence of left bundle branch block on the resting EKG can produce septal perfusion defects at higher heart rates; these patients can have abnormal septal wall motion on echocardiograms. Some clinicians, therefore, evaluate these patients with pharmacologic stress-perfusion imaging. Other clinicians proceed directly to catheterization if indicated by the clinical setting.

Diagnostic models that predict significant and extensive CAD as well as cardiac survival from stress testing have been developed from a catheterized population (16–18). These models have been validated in two populations with suspected CAD: a managed care population (Medica Health Plan) and an international patient cohort (25). A synthesis of these models demonstrates that gender is an independent predictor of coronary disease, even after adjustment for a variety of clinical risk markers. Separate predictive nomograms, therefore, have been developed to predict the likelihood of disease in women and men (16). Additional predictors of coronary disease and survival include type of angina, history of previous myocardial infarction (MI), age, and the presence of risk factors. For both women and men with known CAD, stress imaging modalities are the noninvasive modality of choice to evaluate the functional significance of known anatomic lesions and to identify patients who need interventional procedures.

Stress Electrocardiography

Exercise-induced ST depression has been reported to have lower diagnostic accuracy in women than in men. Barolsky and colleagues (26) reported a reduced specificity for exercise testing in women. Conversely, Hlatky and colleagues (27) found that only sensitivity (but not the specificity) of exercise testing was reduced in women. Finally, Shaw and colleagues (28) found that the presence of greater degrees of ST-segment depression (> 2 mm) was equally predictive of cardiac death or MI in women and men. The general consensus from this literature is that the presence of a diagnostic ST-segment depression greater than 1 mm during or immediately following exercise has diminished predictive accuracy in women (especially for younger women) compared with men.

Integrating additional hemodynamic and functional parameters with ST-segment changes can enhance predictive estimates (22–25). Okin and Kligfield (29) found that the ST-segment depression/heart rate index improved specificity and sensitivity for the diagnosis of coronary disease in women. Mark and colleagues (30) developed a treadmill exercise score that includes duration of exercise, ST-segment deviation, and presence of angina during the exercise examination and categorizes patients into low-, moderate-, and high-risk groups. In a recent report of 1617 symptomatic women, 5-year cardiac death rates were 2%, 6%, and 13% for low-, intermediate-, and high-risk women, respectively (Table 13-2) (31). In these same risk groups, 75% of 24 high-risk women had either proximal left anterior descending stenoses or multivessel coronary disease. Conversely, 69% of low-risk women had no

Table 13-2 Frequency of 5-Year Cardiac Survival and Coronary Disease Subsets for the Duke Treadmill Score in 1617 Women*

Duke Treadmill Score[†]	5-Year Death Rate	No Stenosis (≥ 85%)	1 VD (≥ 75%)	2 VD or Proximal LAD	2 VD with LAD or 3 VD
Low risk (400; 35%)	1.8% (7)	69% (277)	23% (89)	4.3% (17)	4.3% (17)
Moderate risk (1198; 62%)	5.5% (66)	48% (574)	29% (346)	8.4% (102)	15% (176)
High risk (24; 3%)	13% (3)	4.2% (1)	21% (5)	8.3% (2)	67% (16)

LAD = left anterior descending; VD = vessel disease(s).
* Patients were assigned anatomic extent classification from most to least extensive disease.
[†] Duke Treadmill Score = Exercise Time – (5 × ST deviation) – (4 × exercise angina [0 = none, 1 = nonlimiting, 2 = exercise limiting]). From this score, low risk equals a score of ≥ 5, moderate risk scores range from –10 to +4, and high risk scores are ≤ –11.
Adapted from Kesler KL, O'Brien JE, Peterson ED, et al. Examining the prognostic accuracy of exercise treadmill testing in 1617 symptomatic women. Circulation. 1996;94:565.

coronary stenosis less than 75%. A nomogram for estimating the 2-year survival is presented in Table 13-3. Treadmill EKG should be considered initially for women with low-to-intermediate likelihood for disease and normal resting EKG. Achieving predicted maximum heart rate levels in women may be aided by the use of more "gentle" protocols that increase by 1 to 2 METs per stage (e.g., the Cornell protocol) (29).

Recent studies have reported that hormone replacement therapy may result in either an increase or decrease in positive EKG changes with exercise testing (32,33). A lower rate of ST-segment changes with exercise and improvements in exercise duration may result from the documented effects of estradiol to potentiate endothelium-dependent maximal vasodilatation. A higher rate of ST-segment changes may be explained by the digoxin-like effect of estrogen, resulting in a greater frequency of exertional ST-segment depression. All of these reports, however, are observational and should not be considered conclusive. The likelihood of a false-positive EKG, however, is highly dependent on age, with premenopausal women having the greatest frequency of nonobstructive coronary disease (32,33).

Stress Perfusion Imaging

Imaging the relative myocardial uptake of a radiotracer that distributes according to regional myocardial blood flow improves the diagnostic accuracy for CAD detection. It has also improved the accuracy for prognostic assess-

Table 13-3 Treadmill Exercise Test Nomogram Predicting Survival in 1617 Symptomatic Women

Duke Treadmill Score*	Points	Points	2-Year Survival
−45	100	73	0.60
−40	92	68	0.70
−35	85	62	0.80
−30	77	52	0.90
−25	69	43	0.95
−20	62	36	0.97
−15	54	30	0.98
−10	46	21	0.99
−5	38		
0	31		
5	23		
10	15		
15	8		
20	0		

* Duke Treadmill Score = Exercise Time − (5 × ST deviation) − (4 × exercise angina [0 = none, 1 = nonlimiting, 2 = exercise limiting]). From this score, low risk equals a score of ≥ 5, moderate risk scores range from −10 to +4, and high risk scores are ≤ −11.
Adapted from Kesler KL, O'Brien JE, Peterson ED, et al. Examining the prognostic accuracy of exercise treadmill testing in 1617 symptomatic women. Circulation. 1996;94:565.

ment over conventional exercise EKG and the prognostic assessment in certain pretest risk subsets (34,35). Soft-tissue attenuation artifacts are frequently created in the anterior and anterolateral segments by breast tissue (36). Although these artifacts occur frequently, especially when T1-201 is used, experienced readers feel confident that they can "read around" them without compromising the test's diagnostic accuracy (37). The diagnositc accuracy of SPECT imaging was recently reported in 7024 women. The rate of significant CAD was 7%, 76%, 79%, and 98%, respectively, for those with a normal, mildly abnormal, moderately abnormal, or severely abnormal scan (38a). Furthermore, diagnostic certainty may be enhanced with nuclear imaging for women with a strongly positive exercise EKG. In a small series of 52 women with a strongly positive exercise EKG, no CAD was noted in 76% of patients with a normal perfusion scan (38b).

Recently, the Economics of Noninvasive Diagnosis Multicenter Study Group reported on the prognostic value of stress-induced ischemia in 3402 women and 5009 men, all of whom were referred for myocardial-perfusion imaging with stable chest pain symptoms (38c). In this report, mortality associated with an anterior-wall perfusion defect was similar by gender to that of

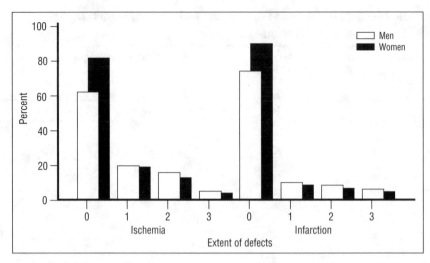

Figure 13-2 Prevalence of ischemic and infarcted defects in 3402 women and 4500 men with stable chest pain symptoms. 0 = no vascular territories with defects; 1 = one vascular territory with a defect; 2 = two vascular territories with defects, and 3 = three vascular territories with defects; p = 0.0001 for both ischemia and infarction. (Adapted from Marwick TH, Lauer MS, Shaw LJ, et al. Myocardial perfusion imaging predicts cardiac mortality in women. Circulation. 1996;94:1–13.)

an inferior- or lateral-wall perfusion defect. Although the extent of perfusion abnormalities was less in women (Fig. 13-2), the number of perfusion defects was equally effective in stratifying risk for women and men (Fig. 13-3). The majority of these patients underwent perfusion imaging using the radiotracer technetium-99m sestamibi, which has better imaging properties than thallium, including less scatter and attenuation of emitted photons. Taillefer et al recently reported a 25% increase in test specificity with technetium-99m sestamibi over T1-201 imaging in women (39). Because of the relatively short physical half-life of technetium-99m (6 h), a high enough dose of the technetium-99m–labeled perfusion tracers can be administered to permit gating of the ECG signal during acquisition. The resulting images allow for assessment of both perfusion and global and regional left ventricular function. The dynamic display of the gated images is similar to a low-resolution cine-MRI scan. The "cine" display of the gated images helps the reader differentiate between soft-tissue attenuation artifact due to breast tissue and a fixed anterior-wall perfusion defect. In the case of the former, the anterior-wall motion and wall thickening would be normal, whereas in the latter there would likely be some degree of anterior-wall dyssynergy (39). Recent advances in gamma-camera design should improve the diagnostic accuracy of perfusion imaging in both women and men. Several vendors have developed hardware and soft-

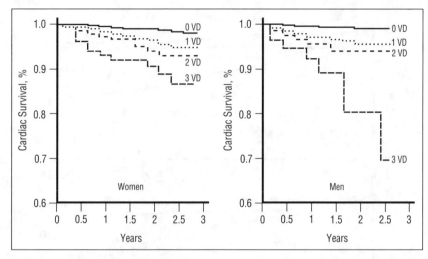

Figure 13-3 Kaplan–Meier cardiac survival by the number of ischemic perfusion vascular territories for women and men with stable chest pain syndromes. Overall, cardiac survival is high for women and men with no areas of ischemia on their perfusion scan. 0–3 VD = 0–3 vascular territory defect areas. (Adapted from Marwick TH, Lauer MS, Shaw LJ, et al. Myocardial perfusion imaging predicts cardiac mortality in women. Circulation. 1996;94: 1–13.)

ware that corrects for attenuation. Preliminary reports of clinical trials suggest that attenuation-correction algorithms work fairly well to correct for soft-tissue attenuation artifacts (40,41).

A high-risk clinical and noninvasive coronary risk scoring system based on gender, clinical parameters, stress EKG results, and stress perfusion imaging results has been developed for patients with suspected coronary disease (42). Risk is defined at three levels:

1. *Low Risk*—no resting EKG ST–T changes, left ventricular hypertrophy, or insulin-requiring diabetes

2. *Moderate Risk*—any resting EKG ST–T changes, left ventricular hypertrophy, or non–insulin-requiring diabetes

3. *High Risk*—a) reversible stress perfusion defect plus diabetes, b) insulin-requiring diabetes in a women, and c) reversible perfusion defect plus any two of the clinical or EKG descriptors (except diabetes)

The hard-event–free survival is depicted in Figure 13-4 for the 349 women from whom this score was derived. From the Economics of Noninvasive Diagnosis study group, a subset of 3402 symptomatic women who underwent initial stress myocardial perfusion imaging was identified and a nomogram

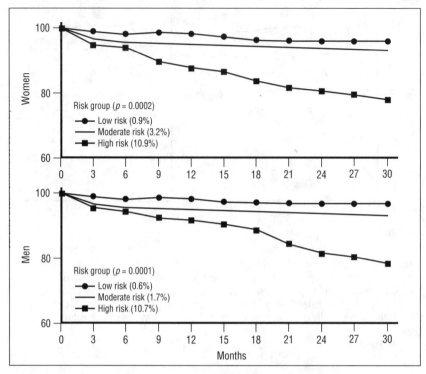

Figure 13-4 Cardiac-event–free survival for women and men by hazard risk group. *Low risk* is defined as the absence of resting EKG nonspecific ST–T wave changes, left ventricular hypertrophy, or insulin-requiring diabetes. *Moderate risk* is defined as any resting EKG ST–T wave changes, left ventricular hypertrophy, or non–insulin-requiring diabetes. *High risk* is defined by 1) a reversible perfusion defect plus diabetes, 2) insulin-requiring diabetes in a woman, and 3) a reversible perfusion defect plus any two of the clinical or EKG descriptors (except diabetes). For women, event-free survival ranged from 0.9% to 10.9% for low- to high-risk groups. For men, event-free survival ranged from 0.6% to 10.7%. (Adapted from Shaw LJ, Miller DD, Gillespie KN, et al. A gender-specific clinical and noninvasive coronary risk scoring system for patients with suspected coronary artery disease. Clin Performance Quality Health Care. 1995;3:209–17.)

including diabetes was developed to predict cardiac death at 2.5 ± 1.5 years (Table 13-4) (38c).

Stress Echocardiography

Stress echocardiography also offers improved exercise test accuracy compared with standard exercise testing. The sensitivity of echocardiographic detection of significant CAD in women has been reported in several studies to

Table 13-4 Clinical and Stress Nuclear Imaging Nomogram Predicting Cardiac Survival in 3402 Women with Stable Chest Pain*

Age	Points	Clinical History	Points	Nuclear Results	Points	Points	2-Year Survival*
20	0	Diabetes	50	Reversible	15	100	1.000
30	17	Hypertension	70	defect		150	0.990
40	33	CHF	70	Fixed defect	80	175	0.980
50	50	Prior MI	45			200	0.975
60	66					225	0.970
70	83					250	0.950
80	100					275	0.925
						300	0.900
						325	0.850
						350	0.800
						375	0.750
						400	0.650
						425	0.550
						450	0.500

CHF = congestive heart failure; MI = myocardial infarction.
* Predictions of cardiac survival are at 2.5 ± 1.5 years in 3402 women with stable chest pain from a multicenter registry.

exceed 75% (43–46). Stress echocardiography additionally provides evaluation of systolic and diastolic function, valvular function, and chamber size. This is particularly advantageous in the evaluation of the symptomatic mitral valve prolapse patient. Limitations of stress echocardiography include obese patients or those with lung disease, because it may be difficult to obtain an adequate acoustic window (10%–15% of patients) (47). Use of newer contrast agents have been shown to enhance the diagnostic accuracy of patients who were previously nondiagnostic, result in improved visualization of all myocardial segments, and enhance the Doppler signal. Although only one agent is now available for use in the United States (Optison), a number of agents are currently in phase III development whose results seem promising for this previously nondiagnostic cohort of patients.

The accuracy of stress echocardiography has been reported to be similar to stress perfusion modalities with a sensitivity of 86% and a specificity of 79% in a recent meta-analysis of 296 women (48). In 161 lower risk women without a previous Q-wave MI, investigators from the Cleveland Clinic evaluated the accuracy of stress echocardiography and found the specificity of exercise echocardiography to be 80% compared with 44% for exercise EKG ($p = 0.05$) (49). The accuracy of detecting worsening ventricular-wall dyssynergy is less in the presence of a resting-wall motion abnormality (46). Another recent se-

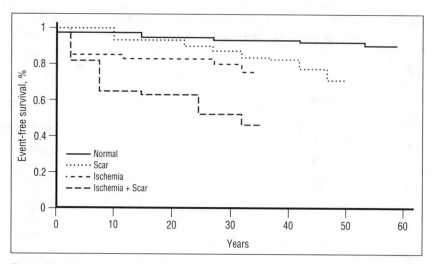

Figure 13-5 Event-free survival for 508 women with normal results on exercise echocardiogram, ischemia, infarction, and ischemia with infarction. (Adapted from Heupler S, Mehta R, Lobo A, Leung D, Marwick TH. Prognostic implications of exercise echocardiography in women with known or suspected coronary artery disease. J Am Coll Cardiol. 1997;30:414–20.)

ries from this investigative group reported on the prognostic value of exercise echocardiography in 508 women (Fig. 13-5). With nearly 4 years of follow-up, a Cox proportional hazards model revealed that a history of known CAD (odds ratio = 6.6) and echocardiographic ischemia (odds ratio = 4.3) were the two greatest predictors of outcome (50).

It can be a difficult decision-making process to select the best noninvasive test for an individual patient. A meta-analysis of exercise echocardiography and nuclear exercise (thallium or technetium) studies published between January 1990 and October 1997 included a total of 44 studies with 2456 patients. Patients after MI, percutaneous transluminal coronary angioplasty (PTCA), or coronary artery bypass graft or with recent unstable angina were excluded from this report. The prevalence of CAD was 69%, and women comprised 34% of the subjects. Gender was not a significant predictor of stress testing outcome. Overall, exercise echocardiography had a sensitivity of 85% and a specificity of 77%, whereas nuclear exercise studies had a sensitivity of 87% and a specificity of 64%. These modalities provided better discrimination than stress EKG (51a). From the Mayo Clinic, the diagnostic accuracy has been reported in a large cohort of 1714 women and 1965 men with observed sensitivity and specificity of 78% and 40%, respectively (similar rates by gender). Corrections for verification bias improved test specificity to 83% to 86% (51b).

As a diagnostic tool, stress echocardiography has not been in existence as long as nuclear imaging; therefore, the diagnostic evidence is not as well developed. The American Society of Echocardiography is funding an outcomes project to further evaluate the prognostic significance of stress echocardiography. Ultimately, the physician's decision on whether to use stress echocardiography or nuclear imaging may depend most on local expertise.

Pharmacologic Stress Testing

Noninvasive tests using pharmacologic agents (e.g., dipyridamole, adenosine, dobutamine) are employed in patients who are unable to perform adequate exercise for a variety of reasons, including musculoskeletal diseases, neurologic disorders, vascular diseases, and general debility. Because this functionally impaired population is largely composed of elderly patients (at least half of whom are women) (44), pharmacologic stress imaging is probably the most frequently used noninvasive test to diagnose and assess severity of CAD in elderly women. The imaging modality used in combination with the pharmacologic stressor can be either perfusion imaging or echocardiography, with appropriate selection of the pharmacologic agent as discussed below.

The major mechanism of action of a vasodilator drug (e.g., dipyridamole or adenosine) is through increases in coronary blood flow, which can identify vascular beds with reduced blood-flow reserve that result from flow-limiting coronary artery stenoses. In the presence of severe stenoses and collateral supply to the distal bed, true ischemia (or imbalance between supply and demand) can be provoked through a coronary "steal" phenomenon, but this situation probably does not occur commonly in clinical practice. Heterogeneity of blood flow alone (without ischemia) can be identified best using technology that images perfusion.

The overall diagnostic accuracy of dipyridamole or adenosine stress-perfusion imaging has been shown to be similar to the accuracy of treadmill stress-perfusion imaging (45,46). In addition, a similar diagnostic accuracy of vasodilator stress-perfusion imaging in women and men was reported in 114 patients undergoing dipyridamole–thallium-201 myocardial-perfusion imaging (49). A recent study has shown a similar diagnostic accuracy of dipyridamole-perfusion imaging for detecting multivessel disease in women and men (52). A recent report using adenosine SPECT in 130 women revealed a nearly linear relationship with the probability of severe multivessel CAD to the extent and severity of stress-induced defects (53a). Although the patient cohort sizes in pharmacologic stress studies published to date are small, there have been attempts to assess the predictive value of pharmacologic stress testing in women. A recent series reported by Hendel and colleagues (53b) comprised 567 vascular surgery patients, including 33% women, and showed that the predictive value of transient perfusion defects was similar in both genders. Amanullah and colleagues (54) reported the results of pharmacologic stress testing using adenosine in 201 women. The diagnostic accuracy was high both for detecting disease and identifying individual coronary stenoses in a variety of subsets of pretest risk patients. Finally, consecutive female patients unable to exercise and referred for adenosine stress perfusion at a university-affiliated community hospital in a major urban area were followed for a mean of 26 months (55). Women with a normal scan had a low risk of MI or cardiac death; with abnormal scans the annual risk of MI increased from 0.9% to 7.5% for mild-to-severe abnormalities. Similarly the risk of cardiac death ranged from 2.4% to 3.5% for mild to severely abnormal scans.

Very obese women should undergo a 2-day protocol whenever possible to maximize image quality. In this protocol, two injections of a technetium-based myocardial-perfusion imaging agent are made both at rest and at peak stress on two separate days. This protocol allows for the administration of sufficiently high doses of a radiopharmaceutical to optimize myocardial counts.

One major contraindication to dipyridamole is recent asthma, because dipyridamole (and less likely adenosine) can induce a severe asthma attack. In these patients, dobutamine is the pharmacologic stress agent of choice. By increasing contractility, dobutamine increases myocardial oxygen demand. Dobutamine (56–59) is the echocardiographic pharmacologic stressor of choice in the United States. Dobutamine echocardiography is a commonly performed procedure (~500,000 patients annually), and two recent reports (3000 patients) have noted a very low side-effect profile with dobutamine and a low rate of serious adverse events (60,61a). No cardiac events were noted in women undergoing dobutamine sestamibi SPECT (over 23 months' follow-up) who had normal perfusion results (61b). In an upcoming report by Lewis and colleagues, the diagnostic accuracy of dobutamine stress echocardiography was reported in 92 low-risk women. The sensitivity and specificity for obstructive disease in this symptomatic group were 40% and 81%, respectively (61c).

Electron Beam Computed Tomography

Coronary artery calcification found on electron beam computed tomography (EBCT) has been studied as a subclinical marker for atherosclerosis (62–65). Gender differences might be expected because estrogen retards the development of atherosclerotic lesions and the calcified necrotic core found on ultrafast CT occurs late in the disease (66). Conflicting results have been reported in studies comparing EBCT with angiography. Cardiac risk factors and age were incrementally associated with coronary artery calcification, but CAD was not confirmed on angiography in one study of 865 women and men (67). In contrast, DeVries and colleagues (68a) studied 70 women and 70 men with both procedures; in individuals aged less than 60 years, the sensitivity of coronary calcium for the detection of coronary disease was lower in women than in men (50% and 87%, respectively). Results from three series revealed a sensitivity and specificity for significant CAD of 69% and 67%, respectively, for women (68a–68c). Of concern is the lower disease prevalence and advanced age of presentation for women that may result in test specificities approaching 50% (68a–68c). As calcium scores increase with age, it may be that prediction of coronary disease by EBCT becomes less precise with age. It is clear that additional evidence is needed to evaluate test performance of EBCT as compared with other modalities. The American College of Cardiology is currently evaluating the role of EBCT and will publish a position paper in 1999.

Gender Bias in Diagnostic Referral Patterns

Recent reports have suggested that women are referred less often for cardiac procedures, including noninvasive testing, cardiac catheterization, PTCA, and coronary artery bypass surgery (28,69–71). Mark and colleagues (72) examined whether women undergoing exercise testing for evaluation of angina were less likely than men to be referred for catheterization. In agreement with previous studies, these investigators found that women were referred less often for catheterization than men and that these lower rates of catheterization in women were accounted for by lower pre- and post-noninvasive test estimates of disease made by their referring physicians. Shaw and colleagues (28) found that the rate of catheterization was twofold higher in men compared with women, even after adjustment for multiple clinical variables. Because men were referred more often for diagnostic procedures, they had higher rates of revascularization procedures, and during 2 years of follow-up, the women had higher rates of cardiac death and nonfatal MI. In a subsequent report by Shaw and colleagues (73), older women had the lowest rate of subsequent diagnostic and interventional follow-up testing. Despite marked differences in outcome and follow-up between younger women and men (< 65 years of age), older women had a higher survival rate than older men and a lower rate of diagnostic follow-up through 2-year follow-up. In a more recent study from the database at Cedars Sinai Medical Center in Los Angeles, men were referred to catheterization following stress-perfusion imaging more frequently than women, but when stratified by the amount of abnormally perfused myocardium in the setting of severe ischemia, women were referred to catheterization more frequently than men. Due to the higher rate of hard events in the female cohort, this higher rate of referrals was appropriate (74).

There is evidence that gender bias in referral to catheterization may vary in different sections of the United States. Travin and colleagues found no such gender bias in referral to either catheterization or PTCA in several hospitals in New England (75). It seems, therefore, that accurate assessment of baseline clinical risk is an important determinant of referral for invasive and interventional procedures, and this is the salient step in determining appropriate care and enhanced outcomes, especially for women less than 65 years of age.

Deciding When To Refer a Woman to Cardiac Catheterization

There are documented advantages to the selective use of noninvasive testing before referral to catheterization in those women at low-to-intermediate cardiac risk, especially because the performance of cardiac catheterization has a direct influence on the rate of coronary bypass surgery and angioplasty (76). From a recent multicenter registry (77), the rate of coronary revascularization was 50% lower for women who were required to have provocable ischemia on stress-perfusion imaging or to have high-risk clinical symptoms before cardiac catheterization compared with those who were directly referred to cardiac catheterization. At 2-year follow up, the END study reported on 4638 women with the same event rate for both groups; therefore, the selective use of noninvasive testing minimized the normal catheterization rate and maximized the diagnostic yield from angiography.

Normal Coronary Arteries in Symptomatic Women

Despite the astuteness of a good clinician, a significant proportion of women presenting with chest pain symptoms and abnormal noninvasive testing (~33%–50%) will undergo coronary angiography and will be found to have unobstructed coronary arteries (78,79). Explanations for these findings include abnormalities of vascular endothelium involving either the large epicardial coronary vessels or the microvasculature. Acetylcholine, which is an endothelial-dependent vasodilator, has been shown on angiography to cause vasoconstriction in vessels with abnormal endothelium resulting from atherosclerosis of even a very mild degree (80). Estrogen affects the response to endothelial-dependent vasodilators. In an experimental study, primates who had had their ovaries removed were fed atherosclerotic diets; their coronary arteries constricted in response to acetylcholine before estrogen administration but dilated after estrogen administration (81). There is increasing clinical evidence that vasomotor instability associated with the perimenopausal period is also characterized by abnormal endothelial responses in peripheral vessels and possibly also in the coronary circulation (82,83). Further work in this area is needed, but it is likely that some chest pain syndromes occurring in perimenopausal women may be due to endothelial dysfunction in the setting of estrogen withdrawal and may respond to estrogen replacement therapy.

The diagnosis of syndrome X or "microvascular angina" is made more often in women than in men and may be defined as *abnormal coronary flow reserve*. The pathology is in the microcirculation and, rather than a fixed obstructive disease, abnormal vasomotion may be partially or totally responsible for producing this syndrome (84). In a preliminary report by Rosano and colleagues (33), ovarian hormone deficiency was associated with the onset of syndrome X in female patients. In a recent report from Duke University, Shaw and colleagues (85) evaluated 979 patients (52% women) with normal or insignificant CAD with anginal symptoms who underwent exercise electrocardiography, radionuclide angiography, or myocardial-perfusion imaging. The presence of stress-induced ischemia occurred in 33% of patients. In this report, evidence of ischemia on exercise testing was associated with a higher rate of MI (at 4 years) in women but not in men, yet survival was exceedingly high.

Cost-Effective Care for Women

The cost of noninvasive testing techniques varies widely, with exercise ECG being the least expensive. The cost of other tests may be as much as seven- to eight-fold higher than exercise ECG. Some of the financial components of nuclear imaging techniques include costs for radiopharmaceuticals, a gamma-camera, a technologist, and physician time. Of these, the single largest component is the initial investment for the camera and computer system. For echocardiography, the equipment costs are lower, but physician-time costs are higher than for other imaging techniques.

If a noninvasive test results in an efficient diagnosis and treatment, the initial cost may be less of a question. In a recent report by Marwick and colleagues (78) on 161 women, a stepwise diagnostic test strategy that included initial exercise electrocardiography followed by stress echocardiography for those with an abnormal or indeterminate study was less costly than routine use of angiography or exercise echocardiography alone. Thus, one also should consider the total cost associated with pursuing a given diagnostic strategy including "down-stream" medical costs resulting from the impact of test results on subsequent patient management. For example, if there is a high percentage of false-positive results for patients undergoing a particular noninvasive test who are then referred for cardiac catheterization, then the financial "cost" associated with the noninvasive test is high. Conversely, if there is a high percentage of false-negative results of a particular noninvasive test, then many patients may be admitted for subsequent cardiac events as a result of poor detection of at-risk patients. To estimate this potential impact in clinical practice, Pryor and colleagues (17) identified a cohort of 324 patients presenting with chest pain who were at low risk (i.e., survival rate > 97%). Among low-risk patients, the authors found that all underwent some form of additional noninvasive testing, with 25% ultimately proceeding to cardiac catheterization, for a total diagnostic cost of $509 per patient. There was an exceedingly low event rate in this patient population (0.4% annual cardiac death rate); thus, considerable savings may have been accrued had physicians determined the likelihood for coronary disease before referring very-low-risk patients for tests that might give false-positive results and lead to even more invasive procedures.

In a recent report by Miller and colleagues (77), the total diagnostic and follow-up costs of care were compared between two matched cohorts of symptomatic women undergoing one of two diagnostic strategies: 1) initial stress-perfusion imaging followed by cardiac catheterization for patients with provocable ischemia or those at clinically high risk, or 2) proceeding directly to cardiac catheterization. This study included 4638 symptomatic women who were followed for 3 years following their initial diagnostic test. A more selective use of cardiac catheterization resulted in a substantially lower cost of care (30%–40%). The clinical outcomes for the two groups was similar over the ensuing 2 years. Most of the difference in cost of care was the result of a substantially higher rate of PTCA (nearly twofold higher) for the women who went directly to cardiac catheterization.

In the aforementioned Multicenter Registry (77) most patients underwent technetium-99m sestamibi imaging that resulted in cost-effective care for symptomatic women. Recently, a decision model study comparing the cost effectiveness of exercise echocardiography, nuclear imaging, and treadmill testing was performed (86). The marginal cost effectiveness per quality-adjusted life-years revealed that stress echocardiography resulted in improved outcomes and lower cost when compared with stress EKG or T1-201 imaging for women with chest pain syndromes. Improved image quality with technetium-99m sestamibi has shown enhanced cost efficiency for testing at-risk women (77).

Summary

The selection of the first noninvasive diagnostic test depends on the woman's age, symptoms, risk-factor profile, body habitus, and functional capacity. Current clinical history nomograms may be used to guide the initial choice of a noninvasive screening test. If a woman is at low risk (i.e., has ≤ 15% probability of coronary disease), then usually no additional diagnostic testing is warranted.

If a woman's probability of coronary disease exceeds 85% and she is symptomatic, then a more aggressive work-up, including diagnostic cardiac catheterization, should be considered. In intermediate patients, routine noninvasive testing is the most beneficial in determining subsequent patient management.

In intermediate-risk women, if the resting EKG is normal, a routine treadmill stress test is an appropriate screening test, and if the stress EKG is indeterminate or of intermediate risk, then a noninvasive stress-imaging test (either stress perfusion or stress echocardiogram) is indicated. Work-up for noncardiac causes of chest pain syndrome should also be pursued. For a woman of any age with diabetes, a stress-imaging test should be performed as the first "screening" diagnostic test. Very elderly women or those with musculoskeletal, neurologic disorders, or arthritis should undergo pharmacologic stress testing. For stress echocardiography, the use of a contrast agent with obese women or those with a poor acoustic window should be considered. For nuclear imaging, the radiopharmaceutical agent of choice is a technetium-based–perfusion imaging agent; tomographic imaging with either gating or attenuation correction will maximize the diagnostic yield. At this time few data are available to warrant the use of technetium-99m tetrofosmin but do favor the use of technetium-99m sestamibi as an imaging agent. Very obese women should undergo a 2-day nuclear protocol whenever possible to maximize image quality. Any woman with a high-risk noninvasive test should undergo cardiac catheterization and revascularization if a suitable candidate. Because availability and quality of imaging technologies may be limited by local expertise, this should be considered when referring a woman for evaluation.

REFERENCES

1. **Maynard C, Selker HP, Beshansky JR, et al.** The exclusion of women from clinical trials of thrombolytic therapy: implications for developing the thrombolytic predictive instrument database. Med Dec Making. 1995;15:38–43.

2. **Johnson LL.** Sex specific issues relating to nuclear cardiology. J Nucl Cardiol 1995;2: 339–48.

3. **Chae SC, Heo J, Iskandrian AS, et al.** Identification of extensive coronary disease in women by exercise single-photon emission computed tomographic (SPECT) thallium imaging. J Am Coll Cardiol. 1993;21:1305–11.

4. **Travin MI, Rama PR, Athur AL, et al.** The relationship of gender to the use of prognostic value of stress technetium-99m fraction analysis during multistage exercise [Abstract]. J Nucl Med. 1994;232:60A.

5. **Lerner DJ, Kannel WB.** Patterns of coronary heart disease morbidity and mortality in the sexes: a 26-year follow-up of the Framingham population. Am Heart J. 1986;111: 383–90.

6. **Fetters JK, Peterson ED, Shaw LJ, et al.** Sex-specific differences in coronary artery disease risk factors, evaluation, and treatment: have they been adequately evaluated? Am Heart J. 1996;131:796–813.

7. **Anderson KM, Wilson PW, Odell PM, Kannel WB.** An updated coronary risk profile: a statement for angiography. Circulation. 1991;83:356–62.

8. **Barrett-Connor EL, Cohn BA, Wingard DL, Edelstein SL.** Why is diabetes mellitus a stronger risk factor for fatal ischemic heart disease in women than in men? JAMA. 1991;265:627–31.

9. **Manson JE, Colditz GA, Stampfer MJ, et al.** A prospective study of obesity and risk of coronary heart disease in women. N Engl J Med. 1990;322:882–9.

10. **Hubert HB, Feinleib M, McNamara PM, Castelli WP.** Obesity as an independent risk factor for cardiovascular disease: a 26-year follow-up of participants in the Framingham heart study. Circulation. 1983;67:968–77.

11. **Fiore MC, Novotny TE, Pierce JP, et al.** Trends in cigarette smoking in the United States: the changing influence of gender and race. JAMA. 1989;261:49–55.

12. **Stampfer MJ, Colditz GA, Willett WC, et al.** Postmenopausal estrogen therapy and cardiovascular disease: 10-year follow-up from the Nurse's Health Study. N Engl J Med. 1991;325:756–62.

13. **Sullivan JM, Vander Zwaag R, Hughes JP, et al.** Estrogen replacement and coronary artery disease: effect on survival in postmenopausal women. Arch Intern Med. 1990; 150:2557–62.

14. **Grady D.** Hormone therapy and the risk of cancer. In: Wenger NK, Speroft L, Packard B, Eds. Cardiovascular Health and Disease in Women: Proceedings of an NHLBI Conference. Greenwich, CT: Le Jacq Communications; 1993:199–211.

15a. **Hulley S, Grady D, Bush T, et al.** Randomized trial of estrogen plus progestin for secondary prevention of coronary heart disease in postmenopausal women. Heart and Estrogen/progestin Replacement Study (HERS) Research Group. JAMA. 1998;280:605-13.

15b. **Douglas PS, Ginsburg GS.** The evaluation of chest pain in women. N Engl J Med. 1996;334:1311–6.

16. **Pryor DB, Harrell FE Jr, Lee KL, et al.** Estimating the likelihood of significant coronary artery disease. Am J Med. 1983;75:771–80.

17. **Pryor DB, Shaw L, Harrell FE, et al.** Estimating the likelihood of severe coronary artery disease. Am J Med. 1991;90:553–62.

18. **Pryor DB, Shaw L, McCants CB, et al.** Value of the history and physical in identifying patients at increased risk for coronary artery disease. Ann Intern Med. 1993;118: 81–90.

19. **Chaitman BR, Bourassa MG, Davis K, et al.** Angiographic prevalence of high-risk coronary artery disease in patient subsets. Circulation. 1981;64:360–7.

20. **Peterson ED, Shaw LJ, Oddone E.** An empirical approach to evaluation of chest pain in women. J Clin Outcomes. 1996;2:9–23.

21. **Weiner DA, Ryan TJ, McCabe CH, et al.** Exercise stress testing correlations among history of angina, ST segment response, and prevalence of CAD in the Coronary Artery Surgery Study (CASS). N Engl J Med. 1979;301:230–5.

22. **Vlietstra R, Frye R, Kronmal R, et al.** Risk factors and angiographic coronary artery disease: a report from the Coronary Artery Surgery Study (CASS). Circulation 1980; 62:254–61.

23. **Shaw LJ, Peterson ED, Shaw LK, et al.** Use of a prognostic treadmill score in identifying diagnostic coronary disease subgroups. Circulation. 1998;98:1622-30.

24. **Diamond GA, Forrester JS.** Analysis of probability as an aid in the clinical diagnosis of coronary artery disease. N Engl J Med. 1979;300:1350–8.

25. **Gray D, Hampton JR, Shaw LK, et al.** Successful international application of a predictive model of coronary disease. Circulation. 1992;86:41.

26. **Barolsky SM, Gilbert CA, Faruqui A, et al.** Differences in electrocardiographic responses to exercise of women and men: a non-Bayesian factor. Circulation. 1979;60:1021–7.

27. **Hlatky MA, Pryor DB, Harrell FE Jr, et al.** Factors affecting sensitivity and specificity of exercise electrocardiography: multivariable analysis. Am J Med. 1984;77:64–71.

28. **Shaw LJ, Miller DD, Romeis JC, et al.** Gender differences in the noninvasive evaluation and management of patients with suspected coronary artery disease. Ann Intern Med. 1994;120:559–66.

29. **Okin P, Kligfield P.** Gender-specific criteria and performance of the exercise electrocardiogram. Circulation. 1995;92:1209–16.

30. **Mark DB, Shaw L, Harrell FE Jr, et al.** Prognostic value of a treadmill exercise score in outpatients with suspected coronary artery disease. N Engl J Med. 1991;325:849–53.

31. **Kesler KL, O'Brien JE, Peterson ED, et al.** Examining the prognostic accuracy of exercise treadmill testing in 1617 symptomatic women. Circulation. 1996;94:565.

32. **Barrett-Connor E, Wilcosky T, Wallace RB, Heiss G.** Resting and exercise electrocardiographic abnormalities associated with sex hormone use in women: the Lipid Research Clinics Program Prevalence Study. Am J Epidemiol. 1986;123:81–8.

33. **Rosano GMC, Sarrel PM, Poole-Wilson PA, Collins P.** Beneficial effect of oestrogen on exercise-induced myocardial ischaemia in women with coronary artery disease. Lancet. 1993;342:133–6.

34. **Morise AP, Diamond GA, Detrano R, Bobbio M.** Incremental value of exercise electrocardiography and thallium-201 testing in men and women for the presence and extent of coronary artery disease. Am Heart J. 1995;130:267–76.

35. **Marie PY, Danchin N, Durand JF, et al.** Long-term prediction of major ischemic events by exercise thallium-201 single-photon emission computed tomography. J Am Coll Cardiol. 1995;26:879–86.

36. **Wackers FJT.** Diagnostic pitfalls of myocardial perfusion imaging in women. J Myocardial Ischemia. 1992;4:10.

37. **Desmaris RL, Kaul S, Watson DD, Beller GA.** Do false positive thallium-201 scans lead to unnecessary catheterization? Outcome of patients with perfusion defects on quantitative planar thallium-201 scintigraphy. J Am Coll Cardiol. 1993;21:1058–63.

38a. **Shaw LJ, Hachamovitch R, Lewin HC, et al.** Diagnostic and prognostic risk stratification in 7024 women undergoing SPECT imaging. J Nucl Med. 1998;39:115P.

38b. **He ZX, Dakik HA, Vaduganathan P, et al.** Clinical and angiographic significance of a normal thallium-201 tomographic study in patients with a strongly positive exercise electrocardiogram. Am J Cardiol. 1996;78:638-41.

38c. **Marwick TH, Lauer MS, Shaw LJ, et al.** Myocardial perfusion imaging predicts cardiac mortality in women. Circulation. 1996;94:1–13.

39. **Taillefer R, DePuey EG, Udleson J, et al.** Comparative diagnostic accuracy of thallium-201 and Tc-99m sestamibi (perfusion and gated SPECT) in detecting coronary artery disease in women. J Am Coll Cardiol. 1997;29:69–77.

40. **Ficaro EP, Shreve PD, Kritzman JN, et al.** Evaluation of attenuation corrected cardiac SPECT perfusion imaging in women. Circulation. 1996;84:1–13.

41. **Hendel RC, Berman DS, Follansbee WP, et al.** Effects of attenuation corrected SPECT myocardial perfusion imaging on diagnostic accuracy: results of a multicenter trial. Circulation. 1996;94:303.

42. **Shaw LJ, Miller DD, Gillespie KN, et al.** A gender-specific clinical and noninvasive coronary risk scoring system for patients with suspected coronary artery disease. Clin Performance Quality Health Care 1995;3:209–17.

43. **Marwick TH, Anderson T, Williams MJ, Haluska B, Melin JA, et al.** Exercise echocardiography is an accurate and cost-efficient technique for detection of coronary artery disease in women. J Am Coll Cardiol. 1995;26:335–41.

44. **Shaw L, Chaitman BR, Hilton TC, et al.** Prognostic value of dipyridamole thallium-201 imaging in elderly patients. J Am Coll Cardiol. 1992;19:1390–8.

45. **Beller GA.** Pharmacologic stress imaging. JAMA. 1991;265:633–8.

46. **Nishimura S, Mahmarian JJ, Boyce TM, Verani MS.** Equivalence between adenosine and exercise thallium-201 myocardial tomography: a multicenter, prospective, crossover trail. J Am Coll Cardiol. 1992;265–75.

47. **Hsiah A, Jollis JG, Kesler KL, et al.** Prognostic value of transthoracic echo in the Duke Cardiovascular Disease Database. Circulation. 1996;94:27.

48. **Kwok Y, Kim C, Grady D, et al.** The accuracy of exercise tests for detecting coronary artery disease in women. Am J Cardiol. In press.

49. **Kong BA, Shaw L, Miller DD, Chaitman BR.** Comparison of accuracy for detecting coronary artery disease and side-effect profile of dipyridamole thallium-201 myocardial perfusion imaging in women versus men. Am J Cardiol. 1992;70:168–73.

50. **Heupler S, Mehta R, Lobo A, et al.** Prognostic implications of exercise echocardiography in women with known or suspected coronary artery disease. J Am Coll Cardiol. 1997;30: 414–20.

51a. **Fleischmann KE, Hunink MGM, Kuntz KM, Douglas PS.** Exercise echocardiography or exercise SPECT imaging? A meta-analysis of diagnostic test performance. JAMA. 1998:280:913–20.

51b. **Roger VL, Pellikka PA, Bell MR, et al.** Sex and verification bias: impact on the diagnostic value of exercise echocardiography. Circulation. 1997;95:405–10.

52. **Katz MS, Moulton AW, Travin MI, Johnson LL.** Accuracy of SPECT perfusion imaging to diagnose multivessel disease in women as compared to men [Abstract]. J Am Coll Cardiol. 1996:27:968.

53a. **Amanullah AM, Berman DS, Hachamovitch R, et al.** Identification of severe or extensive coronary artery disease in women by adenosine technetium-99m sestamibi SPECT. Am J Cardiol. 1997;80:132-7.

53b. **Hendel RC, Chen MH, Litalien GJ, et al.** Sex differences in perioperative and long-term cardiac event-free survival in vascular surgery patients: an analysis of clinical and scintigraphic variables. Circulation. 1995;91:1044–51.

54. **Amanullah AM, Kiat H, Friedman JD, Berman DS.** Adenosine technetium-99m sestamibi myocardial perfusion SPECT in women: diagnostic efficacy in detection of coronary artery disease. J Am Coll Cardiol 1996;27:803–9.

55. **Amanullah AM, Berman DS, Erel J, et al.** Incremental prognostic value of adenosine myocardial perfusion single-photon emission computed tomography in women with suspected coronary artery disease. Am J Cardiol. 1998:82:725–30.

56. **Martin TW, Seaworth JF, Johns JP, et al.** Comparison of adenosine, dipyridamole, and dobutamine in stress echocardiography. Ann Intern Med. 1992;116:190–3.

57. **Dagianti A, Penco M, Agati L, et al.** Stress echocardiography: comparison of exercise, dipyridamole and dobutamine in detecting and predicting the extent of coronary artery disease. J Am Coll Cardiol. 1995;26:18–25.

58. **Ostojic M, Picano E, Beleslin B, et al.** Dipyridamole-dobutamine echocardiography: a novel test for the detection of milder forms of coronary artery disease. J Am Coll Cardiol. 1994;23:1115–22.

59. **Severi S, Picano E, Michelassi C, et al.** Diagnostic and prognostic value of dipyridamole echocardiography in patients with suspected coronary artery disease: comparison with exercise electrocardiography. Circulation. 1994;89:1160–73.

60. **Secknus MA, Marwick TH.** Evolution of dobutamine stress echocardiography protocols and indications: safety and side effects in 3011 studies over 5 years. J Am Coll Cardiol. 1997;29:1234–40.

61a. **Mertes H, Sawada SG, Ryan T, et al.** Symptoms, adverse effects, and complications associated with dobutamine stress echocardiography. Circulation. 1993;88:15–19.

61b. **Geletjinse ML, Elhenoy A, van Domburg RT, et al.** Prognostic significance of normal dobutamine-atropine stress sestamibi scintigraphy in women with chest pain. Am J Cardiol. 1996;77:1057-61.

61c. **Lewis JF, Lin L, McGorray S, et al.** Dobutamine stress echocardiography in women with chest pain: pilot phase data from NHLBI Women's Ischemia Syndrome Evaluation (WISE). J Am Coll Cardiol. In press.

62. **Breen JF, Sheedy PF II, Schwartz RS, et al.** Coronary artery calcification detected with ultrafast CT as an indication of coronary artery disease. Radiology. 1992;185:435–9.

63. **Simons DB, Schwartz RS, Edwards WD, et al.** Noninvasive definition of anatomic coronary artery disease by ultrafast computed tomographic screening: a quantitative pathologic comparison study. J Am Coll Cardiol. 1992;20:1118–26.

64. **Khan A, Mond DJ, Kallman CE, et al.** Computed tomography of normal and calcified coronary arteries. J Thorac Imaging. 1994;9:1–7.

65. **Fiorino AS.** Electron-beam computed tomography, coronary artery calcium, and the evaluation of patients with coronary artery disease. Ann Intern Med. 1998;128:839–47.

66. **Stary HC, Chandler AB, Dinsmore RE, et al.** A definition of advanced types of atherosclerotic lesions and a histological classification of atherosclerosis. Circulation. 1995;92:1355–74.

67. **Wong ND, Vo A, Abrahamson D, et al.** Detection of coronary artery calcium by ultrafast computed tomography and its relation to clinical evidence of coronary artery disease. Am J Cardiol. 1994;73:223–7.

68a. **DeVries S, Wolfkiel C, Fusman B, et al.** Influence of age and gender on the presence of coronary calcium detected by ultrafast computed tomography. J Am Coll Cardiol. 1995;25:76–82.

68b. **Rumberger JA, Sheedy PF 3rd, Breen JF, Schwartz RS.** Coronary calcium, as determined by electron beam computed tomography, and coronary disease on arteriogram: effect of patient's sex on diagnosis. Circulation. 1995;91:1363-7.

68c. **Detrano R, Hsiai T, Wang S, et al.** Prognostic value of coronary calcification and angiographic stenoses in patients undergoing coronary angiography. J Am Coll Cardiol. 1996;27:285-90.

69. **Shaw LJ, Califf RM.** Should women be treated differently than men? A meta-analysis of randomized trials of acute and secondary prevention. Circulation. 1995;92:674.

70. **Tobin JN, Wassertheil-Smoller S, Wexler JP, et al.** Sex bias in considering coronary bypass surgery. Ann Intern Med. 1987;107:19–25.

71. **Ayanian JZ, Epstein AM.** Differences in the use of procedures between women and men hospitalized for coronary heart disease. N Engl J Med. 1991;325:221–5.

72. **Mark DB, Shaw L, Delong ER, et al.** Absence of sex bias in the referral of patients for cardiac catheterization. N Engl J Med. 1994;330:1101–6.

73. **Shaw LJ, Miller DD, Romeis JC, et al.** Prognostic value of noninvasive risk stratification and coronary revascularization in nonelderly and elderly patients referred for evaluation of clinically suspected coronary artery disease. J Am Geriatr Soc. 1996;44:1–8.

74. **Hachamovitch R, Berman DS, Kiat H, et al.** Gender-related differences in clinical management after exercise nuclear testing. J Am Coll Cardiol. 1995;26:1457–64.

75. **Travin MI, Duca MD, Kline GM, et al.** The relationship of gender to the prognostic value of stress Tc-99m sestamibi SPECT imaging. J Nucl Med. 1996;37:14.

76. **Kuhn EM, Hartz AJ, Baras M.** Correlation of rates of coronary artery bypass surgery, angioplasty, and cardiac catheterization in 305 large communities for persons age 65 and older. Health Serv Res. 1995;30:425–36.

77. **Miller DD, Taillefer R, Heller GV, Shaw LJ.** Cost analysis of stress myocardial perfusion imaging in 4638 women with stable angina: comparison to a strategy of direct coronary angiography. J Nucl Med. 1996;37:68.

78. **Marwick TH, Anderson T, Williams MJ, et al.** Exercise echocardiography is an accurate and cost-efficient technique for detection of coronary artery disease in women. J Am Coll Cardiol. 1995;26:335–41.

79. **Chaitman BR, Bourassa MG, Davis K, et al.** Angiographic prevalence of high-risk coronary artery disease in patient subsets (CASS). Circulation. 1981,64:360–7.

80. **Welch CC, Proudfit WL, Sheldon WC.** Coronary arteriographic findings in 1000 women under age 50. Am J Cardiol. 1975;35:211–5.

81. **Vita JA, Treasure CB, Yeung AC, et al.** Patients with evidence of coronary endothelial dysfunction as assessed by acetylcholine infusion demonstrate marked increased in sensitivity to constrictor effects of catecholamines. Circulation. 1992;85:1390–7.

82. **Williams JK, Adams MR, Herrington DM, Clarkson TB.** Short-term administration of estrogen and vascular responses of atherosclerotic coronary arteries. J Am Coll Cardiol. 1992;20:452–7.

83. **Gilligan D, Badar D, Panza J, et al.** Acute vascular effects of estrogen in postmenopausal women. Circulation. 1994;90:786–91.

84. **Sarrel PM, Lindsay D, Rosano GMC, Poole-Wilson PA.** Angina and normal coronary arteries in women: gynecologic findings. Am J Obstet Gynecol. 1992;167:467–72.

85. **Shaw LJ, Kesler K, Peterson ED, et al.** Long-term prognostic implications of abnormal stress electrocardiographic or myocardial perfusion scintigraphic measures in patients with angiographically insignificant coronary artery disease [Abstract]. J Am Coll Cardiol. 1996;27:78A.

86. **Redberg RF.** Diagnostic testing for coronary artery disease in women and gender differences in referral for revascularization. Cardiol Clin. 1998;16:67-77.

CHAPTER 14

Influence of Gender on the Referral of Patients to and from Coronary Angiography

THOMAS H. MARWICK, MD, PHD
D. DOUGLAS MILLER, MD

In contrast to U.S. men, the reduction of cardiovascular disease mortality in U.S. women over the last 20 years has remained relatively static (1). Several factors may have contributed to these patterns. First, the onset of coronary artery disease (CAD) in women is approximately a decade later than in men (2); thus, age or comorbidities may be important contributors to mortality. Second, the older age of presentation in women may influence the suitability of the patient for intervention. Finally, some data suggest that women and men with known or suspected coronary disease are treated differently (3). Coronary angiography has maintained a central role in the decision-making process about coronary disease, and the selection of patients for angiography and the management of patients following angiography are critical decision points in patient management. Studying these patient-management decisions may therefore elucidate the extent to which gender influences the treatment of coronary disease.

The evaluation of gender-specific differences in the evaluation and treatment of coronary disease is complex. As discussed by Fetters and colleagues (4), two concepts have a critical impact on the relationship between gender and patient outcomes. First, the covariables of gender (e.g., age, comorbidity) and differences in physician responses to the same clinical presentations in women and men may influence outcome as much as biologic differences due to gender alone. Application of regression analysis to identify the relative contributions of these variables requires that sufficient numbers of patients be studied. The sec-

ond critical factor that influences assessment of the influence of gender on outcome is statistical power. Because of the modest effects of most treatments on
patient outcome, large populations are needed to separate the effects of gender
on outcome. This poses problems in respect to feasibility for future studies as
well as in limiting retrospective analysis of existing data because of the relatively sparse representation of women in previous studies. The latter has occurred because women of child-bearing age and older individuals (among
whom women are disproportionately represented) have been excluded (5).

The limitations of past research and current practice in the care of female
patients with known and suspected coronary disease are addressed in this chapter. Due to the deficiencies of the existing data, many of the aspects discussed
in this section involve some conjecture. To highlight differences, we describe
conventional indications, current referral patterns, and recommendations for
practice for each of the following topics: known or suspected CAD, unstable
angina, myocardial infarction (MI), and referral for coronary artery bypass graft
surgery or angioplasty. Medical therapy is discussed in several other chapters.

Influence of Gender on Referral to Angiography

Known or Suspected Coronary Artery Disease

Conventional Indications for Coronary Angiography
Patients with known or suspected coronary disease are referred for angiography either to confirm the diagnosis of coronary disease (in patients with or
without anginal symptoms), to assess the risk of cardiac events, or to help
plan treatment (6). The common preludes to angiography in each case are
anginal symptoms and positive stress test responses.

Symptom Status
The symptoms of coronary disease in women and men seem to be quite different. Atypical chest pain is more common in women than in men, reflecting a
higher prevalence of nonischemic chest pain due to mitral valve prolapse or
microvascular disease (7). The direct referral of patients with typical anginal
symptoms for coronary angiography is probably the most cost-effective approach to the identification of coronary disease in high-probability patients
(8), although stress testing may be of value in these patients to guide therapy.
However, even in women with typical angina, the prevalence of angiographically verified coronary disease is less in women than in men (9). In the Coronary Artery Surgery Study (CASS) study, 62% of women with typical angina
had coronary disease compared with 40% of women with probable angina and
4% of women with nonischemic pain (10). Rest pain is more common in

chronic stable angina in women than in men (11). Finally, in addition to the different symptom profile of women compared with men and the different relationship between symptoms and angiographic findings, the response of physicians to symptoms in women may be different based on the patient's presentation style (12). Therefore, although the first presentation of coronary disease in women is often chest pain, this symptom is a nonspecific finding. The real or perceived unreliability of symptom status in women may influence the physician's decision to perform coronary angiography.

Stress Testing

In general, patients most commonly proceed to angiography following the finding of a positive stress test. The accuracy of the common stress testing modalities seem to be somewhat different in women compared with men. (Although this has been discussed in a separate chapter, no chapter on angiography on women can ignore this issue, because the reliability of the stress testing data have a direct impact on the preparedness of the physician to refer patients to angiography based on these data.) Gender may influence the development of ST-segment changes with exercise from a young age (13). Exercise testing offers less incremental value to clinical data in women than in men (14), and problems have been described with respect to the sensitivity (15–17) and specificity (18–20) of exercise testing in women. Thus, although the data are fragmented and derived from relatively small studies, many physicians remain anxious about the use of the standard exercise electrocardiography (ECG) for the evaluation of chest pain in women.

Noninvasive stress imaging approaches are not without their problems in women as well. The accuracy of stress myocardial perfusion imaging may be affected by problems with sensitivity (21–23) and specificity (19,24). Sensitivity may be compromised by the performance of submaximal exercise, the failure to detect ischemia resulting from the smaller size of the female heart (25), and the challenges posed by the spatial resolution of the imaging techniques. Specificity may be compromised by breast attenuation artifacts (26). Both of these problems seem to have been reduced by the use of newer technetium-99m–labeled radionuclides (e.g., isonitriles) and the widespread use of single-photon–emission computed tomography (SPECT). Stress echocardiography seems to be specific in women (27–30), but the impact of submaximal exercise on sensitivity remains a problem. More sophisticated approaches in identifying women who are likely to exercise submaximally before testing are important in selecting appropriate patients for pharmacologic stress.

Current Referral Patterns of Women and Men to Angiography

Studies that have investigated the presence of a gender-based bias in the selection of patients with angina for angiography are summarized in Table 14-1.

Table 14-1 Frequency of Coronary Angiography by Gender in Patients with Chronic Coronary Artery Disease

Author	Study Group	No. of Patients	Percentage of Women	Catheterization Rate in Women (in Men)	Relative Risk in Men (vs. Women)
Tobin (31)	Chronic CAD	390	35%	5% (34%)	6.50
Chae (21)	Chronic CAD, stress positive	840	47%	34% (45%)	—
Morise (32)	Chronic CAD, stress	1980	44%	24% (21%)	—
Shaw (33)	Abnormal GXT	840	47%	34% (45%)	—
Morise (32)	Chronic CAD	1980	44%	24% (21%)	—
Gregor (34)	Chronic CAD	9737	33%	18% (24%)	—
Ayanian (35)	Chronic CAD (Massachusetts)	49,623	43%	16% (28%)	1.28
	Chronic CAD (Maryland)	33,159	46%	18% (29%)	1.15
Kee (36,37)	Chronic CAD	24,179	37%	3% (7%)	2.10
D'Hoore (38)	Chronic CAD	33,940	34%	—	1.47

GXT = graded exercise test.

These studies show some heterogeneity, although the proportion of women and men studied after stress testing was similar only in the 1980 patients reported by Morise and colleagues (32). Studies that have incorporated a multivariate analysis to adjust for the contribution of comorbidity to the relationship between gender, stress testing, and referral for angiography are of most interest and are discussed further.

Shaw and colleagues (33) examined the frequency of subsequent coronary disease evaluation and revascularization in 840 middle-aged patients (47% of whom were women) with stable symptoms, undergoing exercise testing for suspected coronary disease. Additional testing (usually angiography) was performed in 62% of men but in only 38% of women ($p = 0.002$); in a multivariate model, male gender was associated with increased likelihood of follow-up testing (relative risk [RR], 1.9; 95% confidence interval [CI], 1.6–6.0; $p = 0.005$) as were positive stress test results (including ST-segment depression and thallium defects), anti-anginal therapy, and care by a cardiologist. These data are concordant with a previous series of 390 patients undergoing nuclear medicine studies (31) among whom 40% of men but only 4% of women with positive studies were referred for coronary angiography. In the latter series, multiple logistic regression identified gender, positive stress test results, symptoms status, and age to be independent predictors of the likelihood of angiography. Both studies contrast with the outcome of 130 women and 280 men in a study reported by Mark and colleagues (39); although women were less commonly referred for angiography than men (18% and 27%, respectively; p = 0.03), this was accounted for by their lower pretest probability of coronary disease and lower rate of positive exercise test results. Moreover, comparison of the physicians' estimates of disease probability showed that they overestimated rather than underestimated the actual prevalence of disease.

Recent data obtained using stress imaging techniques have not identified gender bias in the treatment of patients after these tests. A study of 1318 women and 2351 men undergoing exercise thallium SPECT at the Cleveland Clinic showed no evidence of gender bias in the selection of patients for coronary angiography (40). Although women were less likely than men to undergo angiography (6% and 14%, respectively; $p < 0.001$), this reflected the fact that women had as lower prevalence of abnormal thallium imaging than men (8% and 29%, respectively; $p < 0.001$). In logistic regression analyses, women were as likely as men to be referred for coronary angiography (RR, 1.00; 95% CI, 0.75–1.34). Similarly, in a study of 1074 women and 2137 men undergoing exercise dual-isotope SPECT at Cedars-Sinai Medical Center, angiography was more commonly performed in men than women (10.6% and 7.1%, respectively; $p < 0.001$), but after stratification by the amount of malperfused myocardium, the angiography rate was similar (41). These data reflect the high level of confidence in the results of SPECT at institutions with large-volume nuclear laboratories.

Recommendations for the Selection of Women and Men for Angiography

Coronary angiography is recommended for diagnostic purposes in patients with a high probability of coronary disease on clinical grounds and in those with positive noninvasive tests, especially if considered at high risk of subsequent cardiac events (6). Nonetheless, in many series, 40% to 50% of women undergoing angiography have no significant coronary disease (42). Unfortunately, obtaining a normal coronary angiogram has little or no therapeutic value in allaying the patient's concerns or in reducing their subsequent presentations with ongoing pain (43,44).

There may be a gender bias toward less frequent angiography in women with a positive stress test, which likely reflects a lower clinician confidence in the results of the stress test. On the basis of the above review, this seems to be more the case with exercise ECG testing than stress imaging techniques. In an environment in which there is increasing impetus to investigate patients in a cost-effective fashion, attempts will be made to reduce the number of patients undergoing angiography with no significant coronary disease. This may eventually be attained by selection of women for angiography based on the results of stress-imaging tests rather than symptom status and exercise ECG results. At present, however, insufficient data exist to alter the indications for angiography based on patient gender.

Unstable Angina

Unstable angina is composed of a heterogeneous group of conditions characterized by anginal chest pain at rest. Some of these patients have obstructive coronary disease at subsequent angiography, others have mild coronary stenoses (which present acutely due to coronary spasm or thrombus formation on ruptured atherosclerotic plaques), and a portion have noncardiac chest pain or microvascular disease.

Conventional Management
The usual management of intermediate- to high-risk patients with unstable angina involves intravenous heparin and nitrates (45). Patients whose symptoms resolve with medical therapy should undergo risk stratification, usually with predischarge stress testing, although the contribution of noncardiac presentations and non–flow-limiting coronary disease to this patient group often renders these tests negative. Coronary angiography and intervention usually are performed in those who fail to stabilize with medical therapy or in those judged to be at high risk based on their clinical course or results of noninvasive testing that suggest multivessel disease (6).

Current Referral Patterns of Women and Men to Angiography
The influence of gender on the performance of angiography in patients hospitalized for coronary disease was reported in 1991 by Ayanian and colleagues (35). This study examined the use of coronary angiography and revascularization in nearly 83,000 patients being discharged from hospitals in Massachusetts and Maryland. After adjustment for age, principal and secondary diagnoses, race, and insurance data, the odds of undergoing angiography in Massachusetts and Maryland were higher in men than in women (28% and 15%, respectively). The reason for this discrepancy was not apparent from this study (in particular, the impact of exercise testing and imaging were not studied), and the consequences of these differences on outcome were not addressed. Interestingly, the greater probability of angiography in men caused a similar increment in the performance of revascularization in men. Thus, to the extent that women and men are treated differently, the main influence is in the recognition of coronary disease in women. Once a women had MI or cardiac catheterization (which signaled the presence of disease), no difference in the treatment of women and men was seen, which is consistent with the phenomenon of the "Yentl" syndrome (46).

Recommendations for the Selection of Women and Men for Angiography
The diagnosis and treatment of patients with unstable angina should correspond to the NIH-AHCPR guidelines discussed above (45), unless a biologic justification for gender-based treatment becomes apparent. Coronary angiography should be performed in those patients who fail to respond to medical therapy and in patients considered to be at high risk. The latter may be influenced by the evaluation of clinical symptoms and the accuracy of exercise testing in women, and the importance of stress imaging approaches to the clinical decision-making process may increase in the future.

Myocardial Infarction

Following MI, the risk of mortality after discharge is greater in women than in men (47,48), even after controlling for age. This statistic highlights the need for careful risk stratification in women following MI.

Conventional Management
Patients presenting with acute MI should undergo thrombolytic therapy unless specific contraindications are present (49) or unless primary angioplasty can be administered without delay. The role of gender in selecting patients for lytic therapy is discussed elsewhere, but it seems that both sexes enjoy a mortality benefit from this therapy (50), although this may be less in women than in men (51), even after adjustment for baseline differences such as older age at the time of infarction. Patients with ongoing or recurrent ischemia following lytic therapy or with a complicated course should proceed to angiography, and they may benefit from rescue angioplasty to establish vessel patency (49).

Stress tests are routinely used for the risk stratification of patients after stabilization post-MI. After thrombolysis, patients are generally at low risk for subsequent events (52) and benefit less from risk stratification than those in whom thrombolysis has not been performed. Decisions must be made about the timing of risk stratification (during or at the end of the hospital course or late in recovery) and the nature of the stress (pharmacologic or exercise-related). The benefit of predischarge testing is that many patients prone to subsequent events suffer these within the first few weeks of MI. Submaximal exercise testing received some notoriety for early risk stratification a decade ago, but maximal symptom-limited studies offer an assessment of functional capacity and yield ischemic responses nearly twice as often as submaximal tests (53,54). If stress testing demonstrates ischemia (particularly in the setting of reduced ventricular function) or if the ischemia is extensive, then angiography is justified.

Current Referral Patterns of Women and Men to Angiography

Several studies have examined the role of gender in the referral of patients to coronary angiography following MI (Table 14-2). In a sub-study of the SAVE trial, Steingart and colleagues (61) followed 389 women and 1842 men with left ventricular dysfunction after MI. As was described in patients with stable chronic coronary disease, women were less likely to have undergone angiography *before* their index MI, although the prevalence of angina in women and men was similar and women complained of worse functional disability. Previous coronary angiography had been performed in 58% of men with a previous infarction compared with 44% of women; however, at the time of the index infarction, women and men were equally likely to undergo cardiac catheterization and revascularization. Very likely, these results were biased by the fact that patients were required by the study to undergo angiography and revascularization if they had symptoms or signs of ischemia after their index infarction. Also, some selection bias was provoked by the fact that more women than men were excluded from entry to the study because catheterization was not performed in spite of ongoing clinical ischemia.

Similar findings were reported by Chiriboga and colleagues (58) in 4762 patients with MI, 39% of whom were women. Twelve percent of men and 8% of women underwent angiography, yielding an odds ratio of 1.46 (95% CI, 1.18–1.80). In a study by Kostis and colleagues (56) involving over 42,000 patients in New Jersey, the frequency of angiography following MI was 32% in men and 18% in women with an odds ratio of 1.39 (95% CI, 1.32–1.47) favoring the performance of angiography in men. In the Medicare population, Udvarhelyi and colleagues (55) found a 28% frequency of angiography in men compared with 18% in women in over 218,000 patients with an odds ratio of 1.22.

Table 14-2 Frequency of Coronary Angiography by Gender in Patients After Myocardial Infarction

Author	Study Group	No. of Patients	Percentage of Women	Catheterization Rate in Women (in Men)	Relative Risk in Men (vs. Women)
Udvarhelyi (55)	Post-MI	218,427	50%	18% (28%)	1.22
Kostis (56)	Post-MI	42,595	24%	18% (32%)	1.39
Krumholz (57)	Post-MI	2473	45%	22% (34%)	1.01
Chiriboga (58)	Post-MI	4762	39%	8% (12%)	1.46
Dellborg (59)	Post-MI	1515	33%	0.2% (1.9%)	—
Maynard (60)	Post-MI	4891	34%	40% (58%)	—
Steingart (61)	Post-MI	2231	17%	15% (27%)	1.87

The only study contradicting these data was reported by Krumholz and colleagues (57) in 2473 patients, 45% of whom were women. The frequency of angiography was 22% in women and 34% in men, with an odds ratio of 1.01 (95% CI, 0.89–1.33). In this study, after correction for age, gender was not an independent predictor of angiography rates between women and men.

The decision to proceed to angiography following MI may be influenced by a number of covariables other than gender. What first might seem to be gender bias may represent good clinical judgment if female gender is correlated with other variables that increase the risk of surgery. Avoidance of angiography may be responsible for a lower prevalence of coronary interventions following MI; this is discussed in the next section.

Recommendations for the Selection of Women and Men for Angiography
On the basis of existing data, women and men should undergo angiography following MI if they fail to respond to initial therapy, are hemodynamically unstable, or are believed to be at high risk for cardiac complications (based on clinical or noninvasive data). The major exclusions are situations in which there is a reason to avoid angiography and revascularization because of age or comorbidity.

Factors Influencing Referral from Angiography

Although coronary angiography is used commonly as the standard method for coronary disease documentation (with a 50%, 70%, or 75% diameter stenosis cut-off), the correlation between lesion severity and physiologic significance is weak (62). Therefore, unless stenosis severity is very tight (e.g., a 90% proximal left main lesion) or the patient is clearly symptomatic (e.g., a 60% stenosis in a patient with clear anginal symptoms in a post-menopausal patient), angiography may not be used in isolation to decide about the plan of therapy. In asymptomatic patients or in individuals whose symptoms are atypical, the decision to proceed with intervention should be based on the identification of inducible myocardial ischemia by functional tests. Therefore, again, differences in the decisions to undergo intervention may be biased by gender-based differences in the accuracy and results of noninvasive testing.

Referral for Coronary Bypass Surgery

Factors Influencing Referral Patterns of Women and Men to Revascularization Surgery
At the time of their initial presentation of coronary disease, women are older, have more frequent comorbidity (e.g., hypertension, diabetes), and tend to be

more unstable (4). It is not surprising, therefore, that several studies indicate that women have a higher cardiac surgical mortality than men (63,64). Moreover, although perioperative death is twice as common in women (65), this is probably because women are sent for surgery later than men (63). Thus, higher morbidity and mortality of women with coronary surgery may not only support the physician's decision against bypass surgery but may also be a consequence of delayed intervention.

The clinical course in women and men after coronary surgery may be different. Women have less adequate control of angina following surgery, and the frequency of graft occlusion is greater than that seen in men (66), probably reflecting the small size of the grafted vessels as well as the atherogenic milieu. In the Bypass Angioplasty Revascularization Investigation (BARI)—a randomized trial of symptomatic patients with multivessel disease—women who were randomly selected to undergo CABG surgery rather than PTCA had higher rates of postprocedure Q-wave MI and congestive heart failure or pulmonary edema (67). When adjusted for age, however, long-term survival is similar for women and men (68,69).

Current Referral Patterns of Women and Men to Revascularization Surgery

Data summarizing the influence of gender of performance on coronary bypass surgery are given in Table 14-3. The frequency of coronary bypass surgery is less in women than in men. This is explained mainly by a lower frequency of angiography, because after a patient is identified as having coronary disease, women and men are treated the same (67). On the issue of women and men being treated differently, Laskey and colleagues (69) pointed out that the decision to refer patients for coronary revascularization as opposed to medical management is based largely on the nature and severity of symptoms, the relationship of symptoms to the likelihood of coronary disease, the risk of death from MI, and the risk-benefit ratio of each strategy. The presence of comorbidity is very important in selection of patients for coronary intervention. Furthermore, rather than indicating bias, nonreferral may represent good clinical judgment by avoiding surgery in situations that either present a greater risk to the patient or are less likely to benefit the patient.

Indeed, when such variables are taken in account in a study from Duke University, no gender bias was apparent. Bickell and colleagues (71) examined nearly 6000 patients with angiographically documented coronary disease from the Duke database. In their experience, no significant difference was found between women and men regarding referral for surgery (44% and 46%, respectively). In patients at low risk for cardiac death, male referral for surgery predominated, with an odds ratio of 1.23 (95% CI, 1.05–1.58). In the high risk group, however, the odds ratio was 0.84 (95% CI, 0.68–1.04). Rather than having an inappropriately low frequency of surgery, these findings sug-

Table 14-3 Frequency of Coronary Revascularization by Gender in Patients with Coronary Artery Disease

Author	Study Group	No. of Patients	Percentage of Women	PTCA Rate in Women (in Men)	CABG Rate in Women (in Men)	RR of PTCA in Men (vs. Women)	RR of CABG in Men (vs. Women)
Kuykendall (70)	Chronic CAD	31,657	28%	—	32% (33%)	0.92	—
Bickell (71)	All catheterization patients	5795	19%	—	44% (46%)		1.23 (low risk) 0.84 (high risk)
Sullivan (42)	Chronic CAD	886	23%	26% (16%)	12% (43%)	—	—
Shaw (33)	Abn GXT	840	47%	2.0% (4.9%)*	2.0% (4.9%)*	—	—
Ayanian (35)	Chronic CAD (Massachusetts)	49,623	43%	7% (16%)*	7% (16%)*	1.31*	1.31*
	Chronic CAD (Maryland)	33,159	46%	7% (14%)*	7% (14%)*	1.40*	1.40*
D'Hoore (38)	Chronic CAD	33,940	34%	—	—	1.38*	1.38*

CABG = coronary artery bypass graft; PTCA = percutaneous transluminal coronary angioplasty; RR = relative risk.
* Reflects combined revascularization (PTCA and CABG).

gest that the performance of surgery in women was appropriate and men tended to be more commonly sent for inappropriate surgery in low-risk situations. Such experience, however, may not be uniform. For example, in the SAVE study, women were less likely to have undergone revascularization even though they reported more cardiac disability than men (61).

Recommendations for the Selection of Women and Men for Revascularization Surgery

In women and men, coronary bypass surgery is indicated for the treatment of patients with 1) stable angina, 2) unstable angina and MI unresponsive to medical and percutaneous interventions, 3) prognostically important coronary disease (left main or multivessel disease with impaired left ventricular function), and 4) acute complications of or recurrent restenosis from coronary angioplasty (72). The decision to refer the patient for surgery needs to be modulated by other factors that influence the risk of the procedure and the likelihood of successful outcome, including the age of the patient, the presence of comorbidity, and the suitability of the vessels for bypass grafting. On the basis of current data (notwithstanding the latter points), the referral rate of women for coronary bypass surgery should be generally similar to that of men.

Coronary Angioplasty

The initial studies of coronary angioplasty suggested that the procedure was less effective in women than in men. In the NHLBI registry, women were three times more likely to die following angioplasty (73), and as with surgery these findings were influenced by the greater age, comorbidity, and unstable symptom status of the patient. However, in the more modern angioplasty era, the efficacy of the procedure seems to be similar in women and men (74), and the rate of restenosis is also similar. In the BARI trial, women randomly selected to undergo angioplasty had more successful dilations of intended lesions than men and a lower mortality (67). (Trials comparing primary angioplasty and thrombolytic treatment after MI are discussed in Chapter 18.)

There seems to be less bias in the selection of women for angioplasty than bypass surgery (Table 14-4). Studies showing an odds ratio of less than 1.00 may reflect a referral pattern of women towards angioplasty because of concerns about the complication rate of surgery. In many instances (e.g., the elderly female patient with suitable stenoses), this may reflect good clinical judgment rather than referral bias.

Medical Therapy

Women and men with chronic stable coronary disease that is not prognostically significant generally are treated medically; however, the efficacy of medical therapy in chronic stable angina has not been studied according to gender (see Chapter 15). Large studies have documented the efficacy of antiplatelet agents, beta-blockers, angiotensin-converting enzyme inhibitors, and thrombolytics in reducing mortality and morbidity following MI. (For more detailed discussion of gender-specific data, see Chapters 16 and 21.)

Thrombolytic Therapy
Generally, in the current era, thrombolysis is performed before angiography. Of the studies involving lytic therapy, 20% to 25% of patients enrolled are women (4). This under-representation probably reflects the selection criteria for trials to exclude elderly patients (many of whom are women) or women of child-bearing age. However, even after adjustment for comorbidities, Maynard and colleagues (60) reported that women were less likely to be selected for thrombolytic therapy than men. Although women benefit from thrombolytic therapy, this benefit is less than what is seen in men, and this is not com-

Table 14-4 Frequency of Coronary Revascularization by Gender in Patients After Myocardial Infarction

Author	Study Group	No. of Patients	Percentage of Women	PTCA Rate in Women (in Men)	CABG Rate in Women (in Men)	RR of PTCA in Men (vs. Women)	RR of CABG in Men (vs. Women)
Udvarhelyi (55)	Post-MI	218,427	50%	22% (21%)	27% (32%)	0.94	1.15
Krumholz (57)	Post-MI	2473 (?)	45%	51% (55%)	16% (21%)	0.86	1.54
Chiriboga (58)	Post-MI	4762 (?)	39%	1.0% (3.4%)	1.1% (1.5%)	2.48	1.02
Kostis (56)	Post-MI	42,595	24%	3.5% (6.9%)	6.0% (10.4%)	—	—
Maynard (60)	Post-MI	4891	34%	14% (22%)	8% (11%)	—	—
	MI/Post-catheterization			36% (38%)	20% (18%)	—	—
Steingart (61)	Post-MI	2231	17%	—	6% (13%)	—	1.84
	MI/Post-catheterization			—	38% (46%)	—	NS
Johnstone (75)	Post-MI (LV dysfunction)	2568	20%	—	24% (30%)	—	—
	Post-MI	4215	13%	—	28% (41%)	—	—

CABG = coronary artery bypass graft; LV = left ventricular; NS = not significant; PTCA = percutaneous transluminal coronary angioplasty; RR = relative risk.

pletely explained by adjustment for covariables (51). For example, in GUSTO I, the mortality of women was 15% greater than men. The complication rates of thrombolytic therapy seem to be similar in women and men, although the risk of intracranial hemorrhage in women seems to be greater than that anticipated from the usual risk factors of bleeding (76).

Few data are available to suggest that women and men should be treated differently with lytic agents. The higher risk of intracranial bleeding, however, may make primary infarct-vessel angioplasty a more attractive option, particularly in older women. This technique is subject to clinical availability shortly after presentation.

Aspirin and Beta-Blockers

The efficacy of primary prevention with aspirin in women has been studied in the Nurses Health Study; aspirin reduced the risk of subsequent coronary events in 32% of women (77), an efficacy similar to men. In a meta-analysis of secondary postinfarct studies, the use of aspirin in women reduced the risk of vascular events by 33% (78).

In the ISIS-2 subgroup analysis, low-dose aspirin was of equal efficacy in women and men (79). Thus, the efficacy of aspirin following infarction seems to be similar in women and men. The Women's Health Study should eventually identify the efficacy of aspirin in patients with risk factors but without coronary disease.

Beta-blockers reduce mortality from MI by approximately 30% in women (80). In one community-based study, women and men were equally likely to be treated with thrombolytics or beta-blockers (81). (For other studies in which women were less likely to receive beta-blockers, see Chapter 16.)

Summary

Women have been under-represented in studies relating to the diagnosis and treatment of coronary disease. The frequency of angiography and intervention is less in women than in men, but whether this has been due to gender bias or age and comorbidity is contested. Few data exist to justify different treatment of women and men with either acute or chronic coronary disease. As always, good clinical judgment—accounting for factors other than gender—should be used in the selection of patients for invasive procedures.

REFERENCES

1. **American Heart Association.** Heart and Stroke Facts: 1996 Statistical Supplement. Dallas: American Heart Association; 1996.
2. **Lerner DJ, Kannel WB.** Patterns of coronary heart disease morbidity and mortality in the sexes: a 26-year follow-up of the Framingham population. Am Heart J. 1986;111:383–90.
3. **Chandra NC, Zeigelstein RC, Rogers WJ, et al.** Observations of the treatment of women in the United States with myocardial infarction: a report from the national registry of myocardial infarction. Arch Intern Med. 1998;158:981–8.
4. **Fetters JK, Peterson ED, Shaw LJ, et al.** Sex-specific differences in coronary artery disease risk factors, evaluation and treatment: have they been adequately evaluated? Am Heart J. 1996;131:796–813.
5. **Wenger NK, Speroff L, Packard B.** Cardiovascular health and disease in women. N Engl J Med. 1993;329:247–56.
6. **Ross J, Brandenburg RO, Dinsmore RE, et al.** Guidelines for coronary angiography: a report of the American College of Cardiology/American Heart Association task force on assessment of diagnostic and therapeutic cardiovascular procedures. J Am Coll Cardiol. 1987;10:935–50.
7. **Douglas PS, Ginsburg GS.** The evaluation of chest pain in women. N Engl J Med. 1996;334:1311–5.

8. **Patterson RE, Eisner RL, Horowitz SF.** Comparison of cost-effectiveness and utility of exercise ECG, single-photon-emission computed tomography, positron-emission tomography, and coronary angiography for diagnosis of coronary artery disease. Circulation. 1995;91:54–65.

9. **Diamond GA, Forrester JS.** Analysis of probability as an aid in the clinical diagnosis of coronary artery disease. N Engl J Med. 1979;300:1350–8.

10. **Weiner DA, Ryan TJ, McCabe CH, et al.** Exercise stress testing: correlations among history of angina, ST-segment response, and prevalence of coronary artery disease in the Coronary Artery Surgery Study (CASS). N Engl J Med. 1979;301:230–5.

11. **Pepine CJ, Adams J, Marks RG, et al.** Characteristics of a contemporary population with angina pectoris. Am J Cardiol. 1994;74:226–31.

12. **Birdwell BG, Herbers JE, Kroenke K.** Evaluating chest pain: the patient's presentation style alters the physician's diagnostic approach. Arch Intern Med. 1993;153: 1991–5.

13. **James FW.** Exercise ECG test in children. In: Chung EK (ed). Exercise Electrocardiography: A Practical Approach. 2nd ed. Baltimore: Williams & Wilkins; 1997:132

14. **Goldman L, Cook EF, Mitchell N, et al.** Incremental value of the exercise test for diagnosing the presence or absence of coronary disease. Circulation. 1982;66:945–53.

15. **Hlatky MA, Pryor DB, Harrell FE, et al.** Factors affecting sensitivity and specificity of exercise electrocardiography: multivariable analysis. Am J Med. 1984;77:64–71.

16. **Sketch MH, Mohiuddin SM, Lynch JD, et al.** Significant sex differences in the correlation of electrocardiographic exercise testing and coronary arteriograms. Am J Cardiol. 1975;36:169–73.

17. **Linhart JW, Laws JG, Satinsky JD.** Maximum treadmill exercise electrocardiography in female patients. Circulation. 1974;50:1173–8.

18. **Barolsky SM, Gilbert CA, Faruqui A, et al.** Differences in electrocardiographic response to exercise of women and men: a non-Bayesian factor. Circulation. 1979;60: 1021–7.

19. **Hung J, Chaitman BR, Lam J, et al.** Noninvasive diagnostic test choices for the evaluation of coronary artery disease in women: a multivariate comparison of cardiac fluoroscopy, exercise electrocardiography, and exercise thallium myocardial perfusion scintigraphy. J Am Coll Cardiol. 1984;4:8–16.

20. **Guiteras P, Chaitman BR, Waters DD, et al.** Diagnostic accuracy of exercise ECG lead systems in clinical subsets of women. Circulation. 1982;65:1465–74.

21. **Chae SC, Heo J, Iskandrian AS, et al.** Identification of extensive coronary artery disease in women by exercise single-photon-emission computed tomographic (SPECT) thallium imaging. J Am Coll Cardiol. 1993;21:1305–11.

22. **Friedman TD, Greene AC, Iskandrian AS, et al.** Exercise thallium-201 myocardial scintigraphy in women: correlation with coronary arteriography. Am J Cardiol. 1982;49:1632–7.

23. **Melin JA, Wijns W, Vanbutsele RJ, et al.** Alternative diagnostic strategies for coronary artery disease in women: demonstration of the usefulness and efficiency of probability analysis. Circulation. 1985;71:535–42.

24. **Kong BA, Shaw L, Miller DD, Chaitman BR.** Comparison of accuracy for detecting coronary artery disease and side-effect profile of dipyridamole thallium-201 myocardial perfusion imaging in women versus men. Am J Cardiol. 1992;70:168–73.

25. **Hansen CL, Crabbe D, Rubin S.** Lower diagnostic accuracy of thallium-201 SPECT myocardial perfusion imaging in women: an effect of smaller chamber size. J Am Coll Cardiol. 1996;28:1214–9.

26. **Stolzenberg J, Kaminsky J.** Overlying breast as cause of false-positive thallium scans. Clin Nucl Med. 1978;3:229.

27. **Williams MJ, Marwick TH, O'Gorman D, Foale RA.** Comparison of exercise echocardiography with an exercise score to diagnose coronary artery disease in women. Am J Cardiol. 1994;74:435–8.

28. **Masini M, Picano E, Lattanzi F, et al.** High-dose dipyridamole echocardiography test in women: correlation with exercise electrocardiography test and coronary arteriography. J Am Coll Cardiol. 1988;12:682–5.

29. **Sawada SG, Ryan T, Fineberg NS, et al.** Exercise echocardiographic detection of coronary artery disease in women. J Am Coll Cardiol. 1989;14:1440–7.

30. **Marwick TH, Anderson T, Williams MJ, et al.** Exercise echocardiography is an accurate and cost-efficient technique for the detection of coronary artery disease in women. J Am Coll Cardiol. 1995;26:335–41.

31. **Tobin JN, Wassertheil-Smoller S, Wexler JP, et al.** Sex bias in considering coronary bypass surgery. Ann Intern Med. 1987;107:19–25.

32. **Morise AP, Singh P, Duval R.** Correlation of reported exercise test results with recommendations for coronary angiography in men and women with suspected coronary artery disease. Am J Cardiol. 1994;75:180–7.

33. **Shaw LJ, Miller DD, Romeis JC, et al.** Gender differences in the noninvasive evaluation and management of patients with suspected coronary artery disease. Ann Intern Med. 1994;120:559–66.

34. **Gregor RD, Bata I, Eastwood BJ, et al.** Gender differences in the presentation, treatment, and short-term mortality of acute chest pain. Clin Invest Med. 1994;17:551–62.

35. **Ayanian JZ, Epstein AM.** Differences in the use of procedures between women and men hospitalized for coronary heart disease. N Engl J Med. 1991;325:221–5.

36. **Kee F.** Gender bias in treatment for coronary heart disease: fact or fallacy? Q J Med. 1995;88:587–96.

37. **Kee F, Gaffney B, Currie S, O'Reilly D.** Access to coronary catheterization: fair shares for all? BMJ. 1993;307:1305–7.

38. **D'Hoore W, Sicote C, Tilquin C.** Sex bias in the management of coronary artery disease in Quebec. Am J Public Health. 1994;84:1013–15.

39. **Mark DB, Shaw LK, DeLong ER, et al.** Absence of sex bias in the referral of patients for cardiac catheterization. N Engl J Med. 1994;330:1101–6.

40. **Lauer MS, Pashkow FJ, Snader CE, et al.** Gender and referral for coronary angiography after treadmill thallium testing. Am J Cardiol. 1996;78:278–83.

41. **Hachamovitch R, Berman DS, Kiat H, et al.** Gender-related differences in clinical management after exercise nuclear testing. J Am Coll Cardiol. 1995;26:1457–64.

42. **Sullivan AK, Holdright DR, Wright CA, et al.** Chest pain in women: clinical, investigative, and prognostic features. BMJ. 1994;308:883–6.

43. **Isner JM, Salem DN, Banas JS, Levine HJ.** Long-term clinical course of patients with normal coronary arteriography: follow-up study of 121 patients with normal or nearly normal coronary arteriograms. Am Heart J. 1981;102:645–53.

44. **Waxler EB, Kimbiris D, Dreifus LS.** The fate of women with normal coronary arteriograms and chest pain resembling angina pectoris. Am J Cardiol. 1971;28:25–32.

45. **Braunwald E, Mark DB, Jones RH, et al.** Unstable Angina: Diagnosis and Treatment. Rockville, MD: U.S. Department of Health and Human Services; 1994.

46. **Healy B.** The Yentl syndrome. N Engl J Med. 1991;325:274–6.

47. **Dittrich HC, Gilpin E, Nicod P, et al.** Acute myocardial infarction in women: influence of gender on mortality and prognostic variables. Am J Cardiol. 1988;62:1–7.

48. **Greenland P, Reicher-Reiss H, Goldbourt U, et al.** In-hospital and 1-year mortality in 1524 women after myocardial infarction. Circulation. 1991;83:484–91.

49. **Ryan TJ, Anderson JL, Antman EM, et al.** ACC/AHA guidelines for the management of patients with acute myocardial infarction: a report of the American College of Cardiology/American Heart Association task force on practice guidelines. J Am Coll Cardiol. 1996;28:1328–428.

50. **Fibrinolytic Therapy Trialists Collaborative Group.** Indications for fibrinolytic therapy in suspected acute myocardial infarction: collaborative overview of early mortality and major morbidity results from all randomized trials of more than 1000 patients. Lancet. 1994;343:311–22.

51. **Lincoff AM, Califf RM, Ellis SG, et al.** Thrombolytic therapy for women with myocardial infarction: is there a gender gap? J Am Coll Cardiol. 1993;22:1780–7.

52. **Newby LK, Califf RM, Guerci A, et al.** Early discharge in the thrombolytic era: an analysis of criteria for uncomplicated infarction from the Global Utilization of Streptokinase and tPA for occluded coronary arteries (GUSTO) trial. J Am Coll Cardiol. 1996;27:625–32.

53. **Juneau M, Colles P, Theroux P, et al.** Symptom-limited versus low-level exercise testing before hospital discharge after myocardial infarction. J Am Coll Cardiol. 1992;20:927–33.

54. **Senaratne MP, Hsu LA, Rossall RE, Kappagoda CT.** Exercise testing after myocardial infarction: relative values of the low-level predischarge and the postdischarge exercise test. J Am Coll Cardiol. 1988;12:1416–22.

55. **Udvarhelyi IS, Gatsonis C, Epstein A, et al.** Acute myocardial infarction in the Medicare population: process of care and clinical outcomes. JAMA. 1992;268:2530–6.

56. **Kostis J, Wilson A, O'Dowd K, et al.** Sex differences in the management and long-term outcome of acute myocardial infarction. Circulation. 1994;90:1715–30.

57. **Krumholz HM, Douglas PS, Lauer MS, Pasternak RC.** Selection of patients for coronary angiography and coronary revascularization early after myocardial infarction: is there evidence for a gender bias? Ann Intern Med. 1992;116:785–90.

58. **Chiriboga D, Yarzebski J, Goldberg R, et al.** A community-wide perspective of gender differences and temporal trends in the use of diagnostic and revascularization procedures for acute myocardial infarction. Am J Cardiol. 1993;71:268–73.

59. **Dellborg M, Swedberg K.** Acute myocardial infarction: difference in the treatment between men and women. Qual Assur Health Care. 1993;5:261–5.

60. **Maynard C, Althouse R, Cequeira M, et al.** Underutilization of thrombolytic therapy in eligible women with acute myocardial infarction. Am J Cardiol. 1991;68:529–30.

61. **Steingart RM, Packer M, Hamm P, et al.** Sex differences in the management of coronary artery disease: Survival and Ventricular Enlargement Investigators. N Engl J Med. 1991;325:226–30.

62. **White CW, Wright CB, Doty DB, et al.** Does visual interpretation of the coronary arteriogram predict the physiologic importance of a coronary stenosis? N Engl J Med. 1984;310:819–24.

63. **Loop FD, Golding LR, MacMillan JP, et al.** Coronary artery surgery in women compared with men: analyses of risks and long-term results. J Am Coll Cardiol. 1983;1: 383–90.

64. **Hannan EL, Bernard HR, Kilburn HC, O'Donnell JF.** Gender differences in mortality rates for coronary artery bypass surgery. Am Heart J. 1992;123:866–72.

65. **Davis K.** Coronary artery bypass surgery in women. In: Eaker ED, Packard B, Wenger NK, et al (eds). Coronary Heart Disease in Women. New York: Haymarket Doyma; 1987:247–50.

66. **Douglas JS, King SB, Jones EL, et al.** Reduced efficacy of coronary bypass surgery in women. Circulation. 1981;64(suppl II):11–6.

67. **Jacobs AK, Kelsey SF, Brooks MM, et al.** Better outcome for women compared to men undergoing coronary revascularization: a report from the Bypass Angioplasty Revascularization Investigation (BARI). Circulation. 1998;98:1279–85.

68. **Eaker ED, Kronmal R, Kennedy JW, Davis K.** Comparison of the long-term post-surgical survival of women and men in the Coronary Artery Surgery Study (CASS). Am Heart J. 1989;117:171–81.

69. **Laskey WK.** Gender differences in the management of coronary artery disease: bias or good clinical judgment? Ann Intern Med. 1992;116:869–71.

70. **Kuykendall D, Johnstone ML.** Administrative databases, case-mix adjustments, and hospital resource use: the appropriateness of controlling patient characteristics. J Clin Epidemiol. 1995;48:423–30.

71. **Bickell NA, Pieper KS, Lee KL, et al.** Referral patterns for coronary artery disease treatment: gender bias or good clinical judgment? Ann Intern Med. 1992;116:791–7.

72. **Kirklin JW, Akins CW, Blackstone EH, et al.** Guidelines and indications for coronary artery bypass graft surgery. J Am Coll Cardiol. 1991;17:543–89.

73. **Kent KM, Bentivoglio LG, Block PC, et al.** Percutaneous transluminal coronary angioplasty: report from the registry of the National Heart, Lung, and Blood Institute. Am J Cardiol. 1982;49:2011–20.

74. **Bell MR, Holmes DR, Berger PB, et al.** The changing in-hospital mortality of women undergoing percutaneous transluminal coronary angioplasty. JAMA. 1993;269: 2091–5.

75. **Johnstone D, Limacher M, Rousseau M, et al.** Clinical characteristics of patients in Studies of Left Ventricular Dysfunction (SOLVD). Am J Cardiol. 1992;70:894–900.

76. **Gruppo Italiano per lo Studio della Sopravivenza nell'Infarcto Miocardico.** GISSI-2: a multifactorial trial of alteplase versus streptokinase and heparin versus no heparin among 12,490 patients with myocardial infarction. Lancet. 1990;336:65–71.

77. **Manson JE, Stampfer MJ, Colditz GA, et al.** A prospective study of aspirin use and primary prevention of cardiovascular disease in women. JAMA. 1991;266:521–7.

78. **Antiplatelet Triallists' Collaboration.** Collaborative overview of randomized trials of antiplatelet therapy. Part II: Maintenance of vascular graft or arterial patency by antiplatelet therapy. BMJ. 1994;308:159–68.

79. **Second International Study of Infarct Survival (ISIS) Collaborative Group.** Randomized trial of intravenous streptokinase, oral aspirin, both, or neither among 17,187 cases of suspected acute myocardial infarction (ISIS-2). Lancet. 1988;2:349–60.

80. **First International Study of Infarct Survival (ISIS) Collaborative Group.** Randomized trial of intravenous atenolol among 16,027 cases of suspected acute myocardial infarction (ISIS-1). Lancet. 1986;2:57–66.

81. **Pagley PR, Yarzebski J, Goldberg R, et al.** Gender differences in the treatment of patients with acute myocardial infarction: a multihospital, community-based perspective. Arch Intern Med. 1993;153:625–9.

Management

CHAPTER 15

Angina Pectoris

MICHELLE DEL VALLE, MD

WILLIAM H. FRISHMAN, MD

PAMELA CHARNEY, MD

Effort-induced angina pectoris has been defined as an uncomfortable feeling in the chest most often associated with atheromatous narrowing of one or more coronary arteries (1). This feeling was first described in 1772 as "a sense of strangling and anxiety" (2). Since then, understanding of the pathophysiology and epidemiology of angina has increased, as have improvements in management, which are reviewed in this chapter. (Unstable angina is discussed in Chapters 14 and 16.)

Angina is a common diagnosis partly because the prevalence of angina increases with age, and the population is aging. Although most patients with angina do not die from complications of coronary artery disease (CAD), more than half report limitations during daily activities (2); therefore, it is important to both 1) identify women with angina at high risk for adverse events and 2) optimize symptom control. Whenever possible, women and men are compared with regard to the differences and similarities in their clinical presentations, diagnostic evaluations, and treatment approaches.

Definition and Pathophysiology

Angina occurs when there is an imbalance between myocardial perfusion and the oxygen needs of the myocardium; the resulting chest discomfort may be associated with transient left ventricular dysfunction. A small proportion of women may also present with angina pectoris and normal coronary arteries, a condition labeled as "syndrome X" (2). The symptoms of chest pain in women are often atypical and may be dismissed by clinicians, especially in younger women in which the prevalence of CAD is low. The important features of angina chest discomfort are its location, relationship to exercise, character, and duration.

Location of Discomfort

Discomfort is typically described as originating in the retrosternal area, but it frequently radiates across the precardium, up the neck, and down the ulnar surface of the left arm or down both arms. Frequently the pain can start in one of these other areas and later spread to the midsternal area. Angina pain occurring above the mandible or below the epigastrium is rare (1). The chest discomfort may be associated with or even overshadowed by dyspnea, fatigue, lightheadedness, and mild epigastric discomfort.

Characteristics of Discomfort

Terms used to describe angina include heaviness, pressure, squeezing, crushing, or a strangling sensation. The pain may vary in its intensity from a mild localized discomfort to severe pain. Other descriptions of chest pain that are atypical of angina pectoris include pinpricks, pins and needles, pain relieved by changes in position, or constant pain that lasts for hours (1,2).

Duration of Discomfort

Typical angina begins gradually during exercise and usually is relieved within 3 minutes of rest. The discomfort may last up to 10 minutes or even longer after very strenuous exercise or emotional duress. Chest pain lasting for more than 30 minutes may suggest an acute myocardial infarction (MI). Angina episodes related to syndrome X frequently are longer in duration and less consistent in their relation to exercise than those in patients with atherosclerotic CAD (1,2).

Relation of Angina to Exercise

Angina pectoris is typically induced by cardiac exertion related to the increased myocardial oxygen demands that result from exercise or other stressors; it is relieved by rest. Emotional stress may be another provocative stimulus for angina. Angina occurring at rest suggests coronary artery vasospasm, an arrhythmia, or unstable angina (1,2). Box 15-1 shows various classifications of angina pectoris based on functional capacity (3).

Box 15-1 Various Classifications of Angina Pectoris Based on Functional Capacity

Class I

NYHA functional classification

Individuals have cardiac disease but without resulting limitations of physical activity. Ordinary physical activity does not cause undue fatigue, palpitations, dyspnea, or anginal pain.

CCS functional classification

Ordinary physical activity (e.g., walking, climbing stairs) does not cause angina. Individuals experience angina with strenuous or rapid or prolonged exertion at work or recreation.

Specific activity scale

Individuals can perform to completion any activity requiring ≤7 metabolic equivalents, i.e., they can carry 24 lb up eight steps, carry objects that weigh 80 lb, do outdoor work (e.g., shovel snow, spade soil), do recreational activities (e.g., skiing, basketball, squash, handball, jogging, or walking 5 mph).

Class II

NYHA functional classification

Individuals have cardiac disease, resulting in slight limitation of physical activity. Individuals are comfortable at rest.

Ordinary physical activity results in fatigue, palpitations, dyspnea, or anginal pain.

CCS functional classification

Individuals experience a slight limitation of ordinary activities (e.g., walking or climbing stairs rapidly; walking uphill; walking or climbing stairs after meals, in the cold, in the wind, when under emotional stress, or only during the few hours after awakening; walking more than two blocks on level ground; climbing more than one flight of ordinary stairs at a normal pace and under normal conditions).

Specific activity scale

Individuals can perform to completion any activity requiring ≥ 5 metabolic equivalents but cannot and do not perform to completion activities requiring ≥ 7 metabolic equivalents (e.g., rake, weed, roller skate, work in the garden, dance the fox trot, walk at 4 mph on level ground, have sexual intercourse without stopping).

Class III

NYHA functional classification

Individuals have cardiac disease that results in marked limitation of physical activity. Individuals are comfortable at rest.

Less-than-ordinary physical activity causes fatigue, palpitation, dyspnea, or anginal pain.

Continued

Box 15-1 Various Classifications of Angina Pectoris Based on Functional Capacity (*Continued*)

CCS functional classification

Individuals experience marked limitation of ordinary physical activity (e.g., walking one or two blocks on level ground, climbing more than one flight of stairs under normal conditions).

Specific activity scale

Individuals can perform to completion any activity requiring ≥ 2 metabolic equivalents but cannot and do not perform to completion any activities requiring ≥ 5 metabolic equivalents (e.g., shower without stopping, strip and make bed, clean windows, walk 2.5 mph, bowl, play golf, dress without stopping).

Class IV

NYHA functional classification

Individuals have cardiac disease that results in an inability to carry on any physical activity without discomfort.

Symptoms of cardiac insufficiency or of the anginal syndrome may be present even at rest.

If any physical activity is undertaken, discomfort is increased.

CCS functional classification

Individuals display an inability to carry on any physical activity without discomfort.

Anginal syndrome may be present at rest.

Specific activity scale

Individuals cannot or do not perform to completion activities requiring ≥ 2 metabolic equivalents.

Individuals cannot carry out activities listed above under Class III, Specific activity scale).

CCS = Canadian Cardiovascular Society; NYHA = New York Heart Association.

Adapted from Goldman L, Hashimoto B, Cook EF, Loscalzo A. Comparative reproducibility and validity of systems for assessing cardiovascular functional class: advantages of a new specific activity scale. Circulation. 1981;64:1228.

As discussed in Chapter 12, symptoms suggestive of angina have both cardiac and noncardiac causes. Cardiac causes of chest pain unrelated to CAD include syndrome X, severe pulmonary hypertension, pulmonary embolus, pericarditis, aortic stenosis, hypertrophic cardiomyopathy, mitral valve prolapse, and arrhythmia. Noncardiac causes include gastroesophageal reflux, peptic ulcer disease, pneumonia, cholelithiasis, musculoskeletal disorder, and anxiety states. The pretest likelihood of having CAD in female and male patients with typical and atypical angina pain (2) is shown in Table 15-1.

Table 15-1 Pretest Likelihood of Coronary Artery Disease in Symptomatic Patients According to Age and Sex

Age (y)	Typical Angina		Atypical Angina		Nonanginal Chest Pain	
	Women	Men	Women	Men	Women	Men
30–39	25.8 ± 6.6	69.7 ± 3.2	4.2 ± 1.3	21.8 ± 2.4	0.8 ± 0.3	5.2 ± 0.8
40–49	55.2 ± 6.5	87.3 ± 1.0	13.3 ± 2.9	46.1 ± 1.8	2.8 ± 0.7	14.1 ± 1.3
50–59	79.4 ± 2.4	92.0 ± 0.6	32.4 ± 3.0	58.9 ± 1.5	8.4 ± 1.2	21.5 ± 1.7
60–69	90.1 ± 1.0	94.3 ± 0.4	54.4 ± 2.4	67.1 ± 1.3	18.6 ± 1.9	28.1 ± 1.9

Adapted from Recommendations of the Task Force of the European Society of Cardiology: Management of stable angina pectoris. Eur Heart J. 1997;18:398.

Epidemiology: Impact of Gender, Age, and Race

Data from the Framingham study have revealed that the most common presentation of CAD in women is angina pectoris that occurs an average of 10 years later than in men (4). By 75 years of age, angina is more common in women. In comparison, men often present with MI as their first manifestation of CAD. Thus, it is not surprising that most studies focusing on middle-age populations in countries where CAD is common (despite varying data-collection methods) demonstrate that angina is less prevalent in women than in men by approximately 50%.

When older populations are studied, the prevalence of angina approaches parity for women and men (2,5). The exact age at which this occurs depends on the population studied. Some report that after 75 years of age, the diagnosis of angina occurs more frequently with approximately the same rate in women and men (2,5). The multicenter Cardiovascular Health Study (reviewed in Table 15-2) found that parity occurred after 85 years of age (6).

In the Framingham study, the prevalence of obstructive CAD was seen less commonly in women with angina pectoris than in men (4). For both women and men, there is a greater risk of CAD if angina symptoms are typical rather than atypical, with the lowest incidence of CAD in patients having nonanginal chest pain (2) (see Table 15-1). The prevalence of angina has not been adequately studied by race.

In the Asymptomatic Cardiac Ischemic Pilot (ACIP) trial, we compared the demography and clinical outcomes of women and men of similar age with stable angina pectoris (7). Subjects needed a positive stress electrocardiography (ECG) examination, evidence of obstructive CAD on angiography, and evidence of silent myocardial ischemia on a 48-hour ambulatory ECG to enter this trial. Qualified subjects were then randomly placed into two medical treatment arms and one surgical treatment arm. One of the medical treatment arms used anti-anginal drug therapies titrated to relieve only symptoms; the second treatment arm used anti-anginal drug therapies to relieve both symptoms and

Table 15-2 Cardiovascular Health Study: Prevalence of Angina by Sex and Age, 1989 to 1990

Age	65–69 y	70–74 y	75–79 y	80–84 y	≥ 85 y
Women	(n = 1134)	(n = 892)	(n = 589)	(n = 242)	(n = 89)
Definite	8.0	9.3	12.2	12.8	13.5
Unreported	4.3	5.3	6.1	5.4	11.2
Possible	1.4	1.2	1.4	0.8	0.0
Total	13.7	15.8	19.7	19.0	24.7
Men	(n = 698)	(n = 724)	(n = 472)	(n = 253)	(n = 103)
Definite	14.7	14.7	17.8	17.4	9.7
Unreported	5.5	6.1	7.0	8.7	14.6
Possible	0.9	0.8	0.0	1.2	1.9
Total	21.1	21.6	24.8	27.3	26.2

Adapted from Mittlemark MB, Psaty BM, Rautaharju PM, et al. Prevalence of cardiovascular disease among older adults: the Cardiovascular Health Study. Am J Epidemiol. 1993;137:311–7.

silent ischemia on the ambulatory ECG. For the surgical treatment arm, subjects were treated either with coronary angioplasty or coronary bypass surgery, depending on the severity of the obstructive CAD on angiography (8).

In ACIP, there were many more men than women randomly selected for the study. Although the mean ages were the same, women had more risk factors for CAD than men (7), including a higher prevalence of diabetes and hypertension (Table 15-3). In contrast, men had more obstructive CAD than women (7). Similar findings were noted in a large retrospective experience from Emory that compared women and men with CAD (9). In ACIP, despite having more CAD, men could perform better on the treadmill than women; however, both groups demonstrated similar amounts of ischemia on the ambulatory ECG examination. Women had higher left ventricular ejection fractions than men (7).

Prognosis

Chronic stable angina is associated with a relatively good prognosis in the majority of patients, with an annual mortality rate of 2% to 3% and a similar, new nonfatal MI rate (2,10). Women with angina tend to have a better prognosis than men with angina (11,12), yet black women generally have a higher mortality rate from CAD than white women. In fact, in black women aged 35 to 39 years, CAD is the leading cause of death (13–15).

Because in the Framingham study (11) women with angina (n = 319) were less likely to have obstructive disease and were only slightly older (64 vs. 61 y), it is not surprising that their risk of death or MI was lower than men with

Table 15-3 Baseline Characteristics by Gender from the Asymptomatic Cardiac Ischemia Pilot (ACIP) Trial

	Women (n = 79)		Men (n = 479)		p*
	No.	%	No.	%	
Age	60.6 ± 9.1		61.6 ± 8.2		0.350
Race					
White	60	76.0	418	87.3	0.008
Non-white	19	24.0	61	12.7	
History					
Angina†	61	77.2	330	68.9	0.140
Previous MI	32	40.5	194	40.5	1.000
Diabetes	19	24.0	71	14.8	0.400
Heart failure	5	6.3	11	2.3	0.500
Peripheral vascular disease	8	10.1	30	6.3	0.390
Hypertension	41	51.9	168	35.1	0.004
Current smoker	13	16.7	77	16.2	0.930
Ever smoked	39	49.4	327	68.3	0.001
Previous PTCA, CABG, or both	20	25.3	106	22.1	0.530
Family history of CAD‡	41	51.9	190	39.7	0.040
Examination					
Systolic pressure (mm Hg)	141.0 ± 20.2		138.4 ± 19.3		0.1600
Diastolic pressure (mm Hg)	77.5 ± 9.5		79.7 ± 10.0		0.0700
Number of vessels with stenosis ≥ 50% mean ± SD	1.80 ± 0.08		2.2 ± 0.8		0.0002
QV AECG					
AECG ischemic episodes	4.4 ± 4.3		5.0 ± 5.2		0.36
AECG duration of ischemic episodes	35.7 ± 53.8		44.1 ± 58.6		0.23
QV ETT					
Total exercise time on ETT	5.7 ± 2.2		7.0 ± 3.3		0.0007
Maximum ST depression on ETT	2.1 ± 0.8		2.5 ± 1.0		0.0030

* p value from chi-square test, Mantel–Haenszel test of trend, or student's t-test.
† Angina ≤ 6 wk of entry or on QV ETT or other stress test or with ischemic episode on QV AECG.
‡ Family history of CAD < 55 y of age.
AECG = ambulatory electrocardiogram; CABG = coronary artery bypass graft ; CAD = coronary artery disease; ETT = exercise tolerance test; MI = myocardial infarction; PTCA = percutaneous transluminal coronary angioplasty; QV = qualifying visit; SD = standard deviation.
Adapted from Frishman WH, Gomberg-Maitland M, Hirsch H, et al. Differences between male and female patients with regard to baseline demographics and clinical outcomes in the Asymptomatic Cardiac Ischemia Pilot (ACIP) Trial. Clin Cardiol. 1998;21:184–90.

angina ($n = 291$). Similar outcomes were found in a longitudinal study from the Mayo Clinic in Rochester, Minnesota, in which women and men were followed after an initial diagnosis of CAD was made between 1960 and 1979. Women with angina ($n = 529$) were compared with men with angina ($n = 504$). Women were older than men (mean age 67 and 60 y, respectively) and smoked less often. Rates of diabetes and hypertension were similar for both groups (12). The 10-year survival of women after a new diagnosis of angina was 70.4% compared with 59.2% for men (relative risk [RR], 0.45; 95% CI, 0.37–0.55). Although the risk of subsequent MI or cardiac death was also less for women (RR 0.47; 95% CI, 0.42–0.58), the risk increased with age more rapidly for women than men.

The prognosis in angina high-risk subgroups with three-vessel disease and left main CAD with and without left ventricular dysfunction is less benign (2). In the evaluation of patients with new-onset or chronic stable angina, it is important to identify these high-risk subgroups, which may benefit from coronary revascularization procedures more than from medical therapy. The medical prognosis of stable angina pectoris may be improved with the use of beta-blockers, aggressive lipid-lowering therapy and aspirin.

Diagnostic Evaluation

Initial evaluation includes a careful history of symptoms and assessment of their impact on daily functioning. After a complete physical examination, a noninvasive diagnostic evaluation is performed to definitively establish CAD as the most likely cause for angina pectoris. This evaluation also helps to quantify the severity of ischemic heart disease and assess other causes of angina pectoris (e.g., aortic stenosis, hypertrophic cardiomyopathy). (More in-depth discussion of noninvasive testing can be found in Chapter 13.)

Resting Electrocardiography

The first part of any noninvasive evaluation is the resting ECG. Findings can be normal or show an infarct pattern or an ischemic repolarization pattern suggestive of underlying CAD (2). Women with suspected CAD show a higher prevalence of ECG repolarization abnormalities than men in both the ACIP and Coronary Artery Surgery Study (CASS) trials (7,16).

Electrocardiography Stress Testing

The diagnostic value of stress testing is lower in women than in men because of the lower prevalence of CAD, especially in younger women with chest pain (Table 15-4) (2). Women more commonly have a false-positive stress ECG (38%–67%) than men (7%–44%) related to a lower pretest likelihood of disease in younger women (17). Some of these repolarization abnormalities with exercise may be caused by estrogen (18). In women over 50 years of age, the likelihood increases that an abnormal stress ECG is predictive of CAD (2). A negative exercise test has a similar specificity for demonstrating the absence of coronary disease in both women and men.

Table 15-4 Coronary Artery Disease Post-Test Likelihood (%) Based on Age, Sex, Symptom Classification, and Exercise-Induced Electrocardiographic ST-Segment Depression

Age (y)	ST Depression (mV)	Typical Angina		Atypical Angina		Nonanginal Chest Pain		Asymptomatic	
		Women	Men	Women	Men	Women	Men	Women	Men
30–39	0.00–0.04	7	25	1	6	< 1	1	< 1	< 1
	0.05–0.09	24	68	4	21	1	5	4	2
	0.10–0.14	42	83	9	38	2	10	< 1	4
	0.15–0.19	59	91	15	55	3	19	1	7
	0.20–0.24	79	96	33	76	8	39	3	18
	> 0.25	93	99	63	92	24	68	11	43
40–49	0.00–0.04	22	61	3	19	1	4	< 1	1
	0.05–0.09	53	86	12	44	3	13	1	5
	0.10–0.14	72	94	25	64	6	26	2	11
	0.15–0.19	84	97	39	78	11	41	4	20
	0.20–0.24	93	99	63	91	24	65	10	39
	> 0.25	98	> 99	86	97	53	87	28	69
50–59	0.00–0.04	47	73	10	25	2	6	1	2
	0.05–0.09	78	91	31	57	8	20	3	9
	0.10–0.14	89	96	50	75	16	37	7	19
	0.15–0.19	94	98	67	86	28	53	12	31
	0.20–0.24	98	99	84	94	50	75	27	54
	> 0.25	99	> 99	95	98	78	91	56	81
60–69	0.00–0.04	69	79	21	32	5	8	2	3
	0.05–0.09	90	94	52	65	17	26	7	11
	0.10–0.14	95	97	72	81	33	45	15	23
	0.15–0.19	98	99	83	89	49	62	25	37
	0.20–0.24	99	99	93	96	72	81	47	61
	> 0.25	99	> 99	98	99	90	94	76	85

Adapted from Recommendations of the Task Force of the European Society of Cardiology: Management of stable angina pectoris. Eur Heart J. 1997;18:398.

Ambulatory 24-Hour Electrocardiography

In predicting the presence or absence of CAD, the specificity and sensitivity of the ST-segment abnormalities obtained with ambulatory ECG monitoring are lower than that seen with the stress ECG (2). In ACIP, women with positive stress ECG demonstrated as much ambulatory ECG ischemia as seen with men (7), but with less CAD present in women (*see* Table 15-3). For the most part, those subjects with strongly positive ECG stress tests will show the most ambulatory ischemia, and subjects with negative stress tests will show little ambulatory ischemia (19). The ambulatory ECG for diagnosis, therefore, provides little additional information beyond that obtained from the stress ECG, except for the detection of rest ischemia.

Myocardial Perfusion Scintigraphy

The advent of radionuclide perfusion imaging during stress testing or after inotropic stress has increased the sensitivity of the noninvasive evaluation of CAD in women (2,20). In addition, women who cannot exercise can receive vasodilators (e.g., dipyridamole, adenosine) to enhance perfusion in areas where the coronary supply is normal to augment the difference from abnormal areas (21). (Stress testing is discussed in detail in Chapter 13.)

In brief, it has been shown that thallium-201 perfusion scintigraphy with exercise is less sensitive in detecting CAD in women than in men, with an increased false-positive rate in women attributed to attenuation artifacts in breast soft tissue (22). The false-positive results are caused by increased attenuation and low-energy scatter. Higher energy radionuclides, such as technetium-99m sestamibi also have been studied in women. Amanullah and colleagues (23) studied the accuracy of adenosine technetium-99m sestamibi in detecting CAD and found this radionuclide to be a highly reliable agent in perfusion scintigraphy, with the overall sensitivity, specificity, and predictive accuracy to be 93%, 78%, and 88%, respectively. Studies also have compared the sensitivity and specificity of thallium-201 with technetium-99m sestamibi SPECT (single-photon–emission computed tomography) imaging in detecting CAD in women (24,25). The overall sensitivity was similar for thalium-201 and technetium-99m sestamibi (75% and 71.9%, respectively) (24). Specificity was found to be higher with technetium-99m sestamibi (24,25).

The diagnostic accuracy of radionuclide myocardial perfusion scintigraphy is affected by the patient population, the heart-rate response, the type of imaging acquisition, and the degree of soft tissue attenuation artifact. Therefore, the type of stress test (e.g., exercise vs. drug), the type of tracer, and the imaging protocol are important.

Iskandrian (26) recommends that the ideal radionuclide tracer have a high extraction fraction at high flow rates. The highest extraction fraction is achieved by teboroxime, thallium sestamibi, and tetrofosmin. The greatest impact on myocardial flow is achieved by adenosine, dipyridamole, dobutamine, and exercise.

Stress Echocardiography

Another noninvasive modality for the detection of CAD is stress echocardiography using dobutamine, arbutamine, or similar substances (2,21). Echocardiographic images are compared before and during the stress. A normal myocardial image shows an increase of wall motion and wall thickening during stress, whereas ischemia is recognized by reduced regional wall thickening of the ventricle and transient contractile abnormalities. Stress ECG appears to be as accurate as perfusion scintigraphy for detecting or ruling out CAD (2). Stress ECG with dobutamine is becoming the test of first choice in patients who are unable to exercise; however, its value is limited in those patients in whom good ECG images cannot be obtained.

Coronary Angiography

The question was first raised in 1987 when Tobin and colleagues (27) reported that the referral pattern for cardiac catheterization after abnormal radionuclide scans was 4% for women compared with 40% for men ($p < 0.001$). Gender differences remained after adjusting for age, MI, chest pain characteristics, and test results. Other studies have also documented lower rates of angiography in women than in men after positive stress tests (28–30).

Steingart and colleagues (30) explained the lower rate of angiography performance in women as follows:

1. Many women with angina do not have coronary disease. If they do, it is usually nonobstructive. This is true of studies in younger age groups.

2. Women in older age groups have a higher incidence of CAD. They may not be referred for coronary angiography because they are more likely to experience vascular and renal complications secondary to age and smaller body size. However, the complications of MI, stroke, and death are similar in women and men.

As discussed elsewhere, coronary angiography can be considered 1) in women with abnormal stress test results, 2) in those who have a high suspicion of disease because of an increased number of risk factors for CAD (24), or 3) in those whose noninvasive testing results are unsatisfactory or inconclusive (Table 15-5) (24). (A detailed review of the indications for coronary angiography appears in Chapter 14.)

Clinical Recommendations

General Management

Patients with stable angina pectoris related to CAD and syndrome X have good medical prognoses, and specific nonpharmacologic approaches should be used (Boxes 15-2 and 15-3). The most important risk factor is tobacco exposure. Smoking should be strongly discouraged, and patients should be warned to avoid second-hand smoke. Nicotine replacement therapies (e.g.,

Table 15-5 Use of Diagnostic Tests in Women with Chest Pain

Likelihood of CAD	Initial Test	Subsequent Test
Low (< 20%) No major and ≤ 1 intermediate or ≤ 2 minor determinants*	None indicated	None indicated
Moderate (20%–80%) 1 major or multiple intermediate and minor determinants	Routine ETT Negative Inconclusive Positive Imaging ETT Negative Inconclusive Positive	None indicated Further testing indicated; selection must be individualized Imaging test or catheterization None indicated Catheterization Catheterization
High (> 80%) ≥ 2 major or 1 major plus > 1 intermediate and minor determinants	Routine ETT Negative Inconclusive Positive Imaging ETT	None indicated; observe patient carefully Catheterization Catheterization None indicated

* Major determinants of CAD in women with chest pain include typical angina pectoris, postmenopausal
status without hormone replacement, diabetes mellitus, and peripheral vascular disease. Intermediate determinants include hypertension, smoking, lipoprotein abnormalities, especially low HDL cholesterol levels.
Minor determinants include age > 65 years, obesity (especially central obesity), sedentary lifestyle, family
history of CAD, other risk factors for CAD (e.g., psychosocial, hemostatic).
CAD = coronary artery disease; ETT = exercise tolerance test; HDL = high-density lipoprotein.
Adapted from Douglas PS, Ginsburg GS. The evaluation of chest pain in women. N Engl J Med. 1996;334:
1311.

patches, gum) seem to be effective in both women and men as part of a
smoke-ending program (31,32). No contraindication to nicotine replacement
therapy seems to exist in patients with stable angina pectoris (33a). (For a
more detailed discussion of smoking, see Chapter 2.)

Anemia and infection should be treated, because both conditions will increase
myocardial oxygen demands; a low hematocrit in anemia will also decrease oxygen supply. A diagnostic search should be made to rule out the presence of thyroid disorders, which are more common in women than in men. Specific
infections may even be associated with an increased prevalence of CAD (33b).

Hypertension and diabetes need to be treated vigorously with diet (*see* Drug
Therapy section for medical treatments). A low-fat diet rich in vegetables,
fruit, fish, and poultry should be prescribed, and weight reduction should be
encouraged in overweight individuals. Alcohol in moderation may be beneficial (34). The safety of anti-obesity drugs has not been determined in patients
with angina pectoris, and their use should be discouraged for now (35).

Box 15-2 Medical Approach to Women with Coronary Artery Disease and Angina Pectoris

---

Nonpharmacologic

  Weight control (role of anti-obesity drugs in patients with CAD unknown)

  Low fat diet (20%–22% of daily food calories as fat; 33% can be polyunsaturated fat)

  Diet high in fiber and vegetables

  Salt restriction if CHF is present

  Diabetic diet if hyperglycemia is present

  Smoking cessation (nicotine-replacement treatments are useful in women)

  Alcohol in moderation (< 1 oz of alcohol daily)

Pharmacologic

  Risk-factor control

  Lipid-lowering therapy with diet to reduce LDL cholesterol below 100 mg %

  Aspirin 75–160 mg/d, if tolerated

  Vitamin E 400 IU/d

  Folate 5 mg/d

  Pharmacologic control of systolic and diastolic hypertension

  Pharmacologic and diet control of hyperglycemia

  Antianxiety and antidepressant medication as needed (no data are available on SSRIs in women with angina, although they are probably the preferred drug for depression in women with CAD)

  Anti-anginal agents

  Beta-adrenergic blockers

  Nitrates

  Calcium-channel blockers

  Combinations of above

  ? Estrogens (improve vasomotor function)

  ? Lipid-lowering therapies (improve vasomotor function)

CAD = coronary artery disease; CHF = congestive heart failure; LDL = low-density lipoprotein; SSRIs = selective serotonin-reuptake inhibitors.

Regular isotonic exercise has been shown to benefit women in the prevention of cardiovascular events. Patients with angina pectoris should be encouraged to be as active as possible within the limits of their symptoms (36).

Finally, patients with angina are often anxious, depressed, or both. Anxiolytic agents may be used, and selective serotonin-reuptake inhibitors may be helpful in treating depression, even though no good evidence demonstrates their safety in patients with angina pectoris (37).

Box 15-3 Medical Treatment of Syndrome X

Nitrates
Calcium-channel blockers
? Estrogens

Drug Therapy

The pharmacologic approach to treating women with chronic stable angina pectoris involves both the prevention of the complications of atherosclerotic heart disease and the relief of chest pain symptoms. Some therapies are for prevention; others are used for both prophylaxis and treatment of chest pain episodes (Table 15-6).

Aspirin

In female and male patients with angina pectoris, there is a 33% reduction in vascular events with aspirin (38,39). Aspirin is absorbed more rapidly in women than men; therefore, aspirin's bioavailability may be higher in women (40,41). Women may also have a decreased antiplatelet effect with aspirin (42,43). Earlier studies suggested that women benefited less than men (26,44,45) regarding the clinical endpoints of MI and stroke; however, the Nurses Health Study demonstrated a reduction in MIs with aspirin use in women (46). Other studies have revealed benefits of aspirin use in high-risk women who are older and who have a previous history of MI (47,48). Although no study has specifically examined the morbidity and mortality effects of aspirin in women with angina pectoris, syndrome X, or both, women of all ages with angina pectoris should receive 75 to 160 mg/d of aspirin unless there are major contraindications to its use. (Further discussion on the effects of aspirin can be found in other chapters.)

Lipid-Lowering Therapy

Elevated cholesterol, low-density lipoprotein (LDL) cholesterol and triglyceride levels, and low high-density lipoprotein (HDL) cholesterol levels are predictors of CAD in women. These abnormalities seem to be less important in premenopausal women in whom it is suggested that estrogen interferes with the uptake of LDL-cholesterol by the arterial wall. In postmenopausal women, levels of LDL-cholesterol and HDL-cholesterol are higher than in age-matched men, and the Bronx Longitudinal Aging Study did confirm an increased risk of LDL-cholesterol for CAD in older women (49). Other studies have shown an increased risk for CAD in postmenopausal women with low HDL-cholesterol levels and high triglyceride, apolipoprotein A, and lipoprotein(a) levels (50).

Table 15-6 Selected Cardiovascular Medications and Gender Issues

Drug	Evidence for Efficacy in Women	Considerations When Treating Women
Aspirin	Primary prevention: U.S. Nurses Cohort shows decreased incidence of MI*	Women have higher rate of hemorrhagic stroke than men
	Women's Health Study in progress*	Physician's Health Study showed increased risk of bleeding on aspirin
	Women's Health Initiative in progress*	Increased risk of bleeding at term in pregnancy
		Present in breast milk
	Secondary CAD prevention: decreases reinfarction[†]	
Hypolipidemic agents		
Colestipol	No effect on primary prevention[†]	
Clofibrate	Effective in secondary prevention in women[†]	
Probucol	Effective in women	
HMG-CoA reductase inhibitors	Primary and secondary prevention: possible efficacy for women[†]	Gastrointestinal side effects more common in women
	Decreases cholesterol and slows plaque progression without respect to gender*	
Agents that affect blood pressure		
Beta-blockers	Antihypertension: effective in preventing MI, CVA, death in women[†]	Present in breast milk
	Post-MI: decreases mortality	
Thiazide diuretics	Decreased CVA, MI, death[†]	Decreased urinary calcium excretion
		Women have greater increase in risk of gout, acute pulmonary edema, and allergic interstitial pneumonitis
		Excreted in breast milk
ACE inhibitors	Post-MI: decreased mortality[†]	Cough is 2–3 times greater in women
	CHF: decreased mortality[†]	Increased fetal abnormalities possible
		Present in breast milk
Angiotensin-II receptor blockers	Edema may be more common in women	Increased fetal abnormalities possible
Calcium-channel blockers	Increased risk of MI in women[†]	Present in breast milk
		Verapamil clearance may be greater in women than men
	Increased effect of amlodipine in women in reducing blood pressure[†]	
Clonidine	No data about efficacy in women	Inability to achieve orgasm
		Possible decreased craving for tobacco more common in women

Continued

* Studies of efficacy in women.
[†] Studies of efficacy in both men and women, with analysis by gender.

Table 15-6 Selected Cardiovascular Medications and Gender Issues (*Continued*)

Drug	Evidence for Efficacy in Women	Considerations When Treating Women
Agents that affect blood pressure (*continued*)		
Guanethidine		Orthostatic hypotension more common in women
Nitrates	Decreased mortality after MI[†]	Potential for difference in metabolism in women
Conjugated estrogens	Increased HDL cholesterol decreases total cholesterol and lipoprotein[*] Post-MI: not effective[*]	Need for progestins in women with intact uterus to prevent endometrial abnormalities
Nicotine preparations	Gum equally effective in women[†] Patch effective in women[†]	Gum may suppress weight gain, probably safe in pregnancy
Anti-arrhythmia agents		
Procainamide	No gender-specific data available	Drug-induced SLE more common in women
Quinidine	No gender-specific data available	Torsades more common in women Clearance may be faster in women Present in breast milk

[*] Studies of efficacy in women.
[†] Studies of efficacy in both men and women, with analysis by gender.
ACE = angiotensin-converting enzyme; CAD = coronary artery disease; CHF = congestive heart failure; CVA = cerebrovascular accident; HDL = high-density lipoprotein; MI = myocardial infarction; SLE = systemic lupus erythematosus.
Adapted from Charney P, Meyer BR, Frishman WH, et al. Gender, race and genetic issues in cardiovascular pharmacotherapy. In: Frishman WH, Sonnenblick EH. Cardiovascular Pharmacotherapeutics. New York: McGraw-Hill; 1997:1350–1.

Studies using various HMG-CoA reductase inhibitors have demonstrated similar reductions in total cholesterol and LDL-cholesterol when comparing women and men with hypercholesterolemia (51–55). Studies in women have also shown a slowing of coronary artery plaque progression on repeat angiographic studies, and a reduction in cardiovascular events in women has been observed in a study of patients with angina pectoris, MI, or both who had hypercholesterolemia (52–55).

Studies with bile acid resins have shown no beneficial effects on the primary prevention of coronary artery events in women; fibric acid derivatives have been shown to be effective in secondary prevention; and probucol, although effective, has been shown to induce cardiac electrophysiologic abnormalities, specifically in women (56). (Further discussion of these agents can be found in Chapters 4 and 21.)

Based on the available information, women with angina pectoris should have their LDL-cholesterol reduced below 100 mg. The National Cholesterol Education Program Guidelines recommend estrogens as first-line lipid-lowering therapy in women; however, their effects on cholesterol and LDL-cholesterol are much more modest than with the HMG-CoA reductase inhibitors, which now should be considered as the first-line lipid-lowering drug therapy for women (57).

Antihypertensive Treatment

Combined systolic and diastolic hypertension and isolated systolic hypertension are powerful predictors of CAD in both women and men (58). Systolic hypertension is also an aggravator of angina pectoris because of its effect on raising myocardial oxygen demands by increasing ventricular wall stress. Hypertension-induced left ventricular hypertrophy also may cause angina pectoris without concomitant large-vessel CAD (59). Coronary vasodilator reserve has been shown to be impaired in patients with left ventricular hypertrophy, most likely due to medial thickening of the microvasculature of the myocardium (59). Also, the hypertrophy of individual myocytes without a parallel increase in the coronary microvasculature could result in a supply-demand imbalance and the development of anginal symptoms (59). Treatment of hypertension, therefore, is imperative in women with angina pectoris. Beta-adrenergic blockers as first-line therapy and calcium antagonists as alternative or additional treatment are ideal agents because both drugs lower blood pressure while relieving anginal symptoms (60). Around-the-clock nitrates are not useful for chronic blood pressure control because of pharmacologic tolerance. Additional blood pressure-lowering treatments without direct anti-anginal activity include diuretics, angiotensin-converting–enzyme (ACE) inhibitors, angiotensin-II–receptor blockers, and clonidine. The best treatment for left ventricular hypertrophy is not known, and the Antihypertensive and Lipid-Lowering Treatment to Prevent Heart Attack Trial (ALLHAT) is currently investigating in both women and men how different blood pressure-lowering drugs affect cardiovascular disease end points (61).

The diastolic goal of lowering blood pressure has been explored in the Hypertension Optimal Treatment Trial (HOT), a clinical trial including 18,970 patients from 26 countries (62). Participants were randomly selected to receive treatment to reach a target diastolic blood pressure of less than 90, 85, or 80 mm Hg by use of initial therapy with 5 mg of felodipine followed by an ACE inhibitor or a beta-blocker. Overall, lowering diastolic blood pressure to less than 85 mm Hg decreased the rate of cardiovascular complications, without additional benefit or risk. When diastolic blood pressure fell to less than 80 mm

Hg, there was the simultaneous achievement of a systolic blood pressure below 140 mm Hg. A subgroup analysis of the diabetic patients revealed a trend for less cardiovascular events when the diastolic goal was less than 80 mm Hg.

Treatment of Congestive Heart Failure

Angina pectoris can be aggravated in patients with systolic dysfunction because left ventricular dilatation increases wall stress and myocardial oxygen demands. Attempts should be made to minimize ventricular dilatation with diuretics and vasodilators. Beta-blockers can be used for treatment of angina and congestive heart failure in patients with stable stage II to III NYHA (New York Heart Association) congestive heart failure (63,64).

Treatment of Diabetes

Diabetes mellitus is a powerful determinant of CAD risk in women, and every attempt should be made to control hyperglycemia by both nonpharmacologic and pharmacologic means. No specific study, however, has analyzed the effects of glycemic control in women with angina pectoris.

Hormone Replacement

The evidence that estrogen (with and without progestin) may protect against CAD and its complications is evolving (65). The ongoing Women's Health Initiative will provide information in the general postmenopausal population. The Hormone Estrogen/Progestin Replacement Study (HERS) in women with known CAD is discussed in other chapters.

Estrogen does affect favorably plasma lipids and lipoproteins, and its direct effects on the vasculature may protect against coronary ischemic events. Estrogen therapy may also have a direct anti-anginal benefit on both symptoms and exercise tolerance (66,67). With evidence from HERS, however, it is not reasonable to recommend hormone-replacement therapy to postmenopausal women with angina pectoris for prevention of coronary morbidity and mortality unless they are receiving this treatment for other indications (e.g., osteoporosis) (68). Hormone replacement may be useful in patients with syndrome X, in which reduced coronary artery vasodilator reserve and endothelial cell dysfunction in blood vessels have been described (see Box 15-3) (69). (The assessment of women before initiation of therapy is reviewed in Chapter 10.)

Antioxidants and Folate

The theoretical benefits of supplementary antioxidant therapy have not been confirmed in definitive prospective clinical trials; however, the available evidence is suggestive of benefit against CAD and its complications (70). The Nurses Health Study of 90,000 women showed the benefits of vitamin E supplementation (71); in another study of 34,000 women without known CAD, vitamin E in the diet was associated with fewer coronary events (72). Ongoing prospective, controlled studies are examining the effects of vitamin E supplementation (400–600 IU/d) in 40,000 postmenopausal women and in 8000 women with known cardiovascular disease (70). Until the results of these studies are available, however, it is probably reasonable to recommend the use of 400 IU/d of vitamin E supplement in women with angina pectoris.

Hyperhomocysteinemia has also been shown to be a risk factor for CAD in women and men (73–76). In the Nurses Health Study, there were less nonfatal MIs and fatal CAD events during 14 years of follow-up in those nurses consuming multivitamins or a diet rich in folate and vitamin B_6 (75). Definitive prospective trials are anticipated. Meanwhile, folate supplementation, which lowers homocysteine levels, may be recommended.

Anti-Anginal Therapies

There is no justification for treating women and men with angina pectoris and CAD differently, and both sexes seem to accrue the same benefits from medical therapy and coronary artery revascularization. The three main classes of drugs are nitrates, beta-adrenergic blockers, and calcium-channel blockers. The aim of anti-anginal treatment is to reduce myocardial oxygen requirements and to increase myocardial perfusion.

Nitrates

Sublingual nitroglycerin is the only available treatment for rapid relief of angina episodes (77). Long-acting nitrates (e.g., isosorbide mononitrate and dinitrate) are available in multiple formulations for anti-anginal prophylaxis, using nitrate-free intervals to avoid tolerance. As yet, no studies have demonstrated a mortality benefit of nitrates in women with angina pectoris. Nitrates may also be metabolized differently in women than in men (*see* Table 15-6) (78,79).

Beta-Adrenergic Blockers

Beta-blockers are the cornerstone therapy for long-term anti-anginal prophylaxis (80). There is definitive evidence from studies performed in postinfarction patients that women received a mortality benefit. All available beta-blockers seem useful as anti-anginal treatments, and they can be used (albeit with caution) in patients with class II to III congestive heart failure (e.g., carvedilol) (64). Some gender differences in pharmacology have been noted. Women also have higher plasma blood levels of propranolol compared with men receiving the same daily dose. Women may also metabolize propranolol's enantiomers in a different fashion than men due to gender differences in the cytochrome P_{450} system in the liver (see Table 15-6) (77,81–83). Beta-blockers should be administered in doses high enough to achieve a reduction in heart rate both at rest and during exercise.

Calcium-Channel Blockers

Calcium-channel blockers are coronary and peripheral vasodilators that can lower blood pressure, heart rate, and myocardial contractility (84). They are divided into two groups: 1) dihydropyridines (e.g., nifedipine, amlodipine, nicardipine), which do not lower heart rate; and 2) L-channel rate-lowering agents (e.g., bepridil, diltiazem, verapamil).

Unlike beta-blockers, calcium-channel blockers have not been shown to reduce mortality after MI, although there is some evidence that verapamil and diltiazem may reduce the risk of reinfarction (84). Long-acting agents are preferred to avoid blood pressure fluctuations. Short-acting calcium-channel blockers are associated with higher rates of MI in case-controlled studies of both women and men (85). In the Nurses Health Study, nurses with hypertension who reported the use of calcium blockers in 1988 had a higher age-adjusted risk of MI and death over 6 years of follow-up than nurses on other antihypertensive agents (86); however, nurses on calcium-channel blockers were also more likely to be diagnosed with ischemic heart disease, diabetes, and pulmonary disease and to have more reported cardiovascular risk factors. Verapamil clearance is increased in women compared with men because of the greater activity in the cytochrome P_{450} system that is involved with verapamil metabolism (87,88). Amlodipine has been shown to have greater blood pressure–lowering effects in women than in men (*see* Table 15-6) (89).

Combination Therapy

Many studies have demonstrated additive anti-anginal effects when a beta-blocker is combined with a calcium-channel blocker or nitrate. Special care needs to be taken when beta-blockers are combined with diltiazem or verapamil in patients with myocardial conduction abnormalities or left ventricular dysfunction.

The additional benefit of combining different anti-anginal drugs is not always evident, and a recent study suggests that the improvement in anginal symptoms may be related to a clinical response to the new drug and not an additive action (90). Also, there is little evidence to suggest that triple therapy provides any additional benefit over one or two drugs. In severe, disabling, stable angina, bepridil may be combined with beta-blockers to achieve additional anti-anginal effects.

Choice of Agents

In women with stable angina pectoris, sublingual nitroglycerin and a beta-blocker should be used as first-line therapy. Calcium antagonists can be substituted for beta-blockers if the latter drugs are contraindicated or not well tolerated. Long-acting nitrates, calcium blockers, or both can be added to beta-blockers to achieve angina control if higher doses of beta-blockers cannot achieve maximal pain relief.

Other Anti-Anginal Treatments

In addition to their lipid-lowering actions, the HMG-CoA reductase inhibitors and estrogen may have effects on vascular endothelial function to improve coronary flow reserve in patients with angina (66,67). Studies are now investigating both treatments as potential anti-anginal treatments.

Invasive Procedures

Percutaneous transluminal coronary angioplasty with and without coronary artery stenting and coronary bypass surgery should be considered because of specific anatomy or poor control of symptoms despite aggressive medical management (2). After coronary angiography, there is less evidence for a gender bias in the observation that women undergo fewer bypass operations than men after having had coronary angiography (9). In the ACIP study, women with similar clinical presentations to men had less CAD and were therefore deemed better candidates for angioplasty than for bypass, whereas men with more CAD involvement were considered better candidates for bypass surgery (7).

The indications for performing an invasive intervention for CAD in women depend on the previous response to medical therapy and whether the patient is at a high risk of death because of specific anatomy. If a patient's symptoms are not controlled satisfactorily with medical treatment, the decision for angioplasty or bypass surgery is made according to the severity of coronary obstructive disease, the presence or absence of left main coronary disease, the underlying ventricular function, and concomitant diseases. Reperfusion not only relieves symptoms of angina but will often improve ventricular function as a consequence of augmented blood flow to the myocardium (91).

There has been limited direct comparison of medical and interventional therapy in patients eligible for both. In RITA-2 (Second Randomized Intervention Treatment of Angina), with an average follow up of 2.7 years, percutaneous transluminal coronary angioplasty was associated with a higher rate of nonfatal MI and death than medical treatment (6.3% vs. 3.3%) because of early procedure-related events and a similar rate of subsequent coronary artery bypass surgery. The greatest symptomatic benefit was with early angioplasty rather than initial medical therapy in those who at baseline developed angina when walking more than two blocks on level ground (Canadian Cardiovascular Society Grade 2) and an exercise stress test time of 9 minutes or less. Although multiple factors, including sex and age, did not affect outcomes, power for subgroup analysis by end point was inadequate (92).

Clinically, a patient's tolerance for chronic stable anginal symptoms varies. This has been substantiated in a study by Nease and colleagues (93). Patients with at least 3 months of chronic stable angina, without prior coronary artery bypass surgery or angioplasty, were interviewed about current functioning levels, the impact of angina, and personal preferences with several different qualitative techniques. Although those with more severe angina generally were bothered more by symptoms, there was a wide range of responses at each severity level. Therefore, when treatment options have an equal survival benefit, patient preference and functional class should impact on medical decisions.

Summary

Chest pain is a common complaint of women, and coronary disease as a cause may be underdiagnosed. Older women have a higher prevalence of CAD than younger women, the latter having a high false-positive rate from ECG stress testing. The choice of stress test should be individualized as discussed in several chapters.

Women with CAD and angina pectoris often have more risk factors for CAD, similar clinical presentations, and less anatomical disease than men. Women and men with angina pectoris benefit equally from aggressive lifestyle interventions and from pharmacologic therapies that target the atherosclerotic process and the clinical syndrome of angina pectoris. Women may metabolize various anti-anginal drugs differently than men, and their treatments should be titrated to achieve the desired clinical effect.

Women with chest pain who have positive noninvasive evaluations of ischemic heart disease do not seem to undergo fewer angiographic procedures; however, after angiography, the optimal treatment of angina pectoris in women and men may be different because anatomical disease in women and men with angina varies in severity.

REFERENCES

1. **Braunwald E.** The history. In: Braunwald E (ed). Heart Disease: A Textbook of Cardiovascular Medicine. 5th ed. Philadelphia: WB Saunders; 1997:1–14.
2. **Task Force of the European Society of Cardiology.** Management of stable angina pectoris. Eur Heart J. 1997;18:394–413.
3. **Goldman L, Hashimoto B, Cook EF, Loscalzo A.** Comparative reproducibility and validity of systems for assessing cardiovascular functional class: advantages of a new specific activity scale. Circulation. 1981;64:1227–34.
4. **Lerner DS, Kannel W.** Patterns of heart disease morbidity and mortality in the sexes: a 26-year follow-up of the Framingham population. Am Heart J. 1986;111:383–90.

5. **Nadelmann J, Frishman WH, Ooi WL, et al.** Prevalence, incidence, and prognosis of recognized and unrecognized myocardial infarction in persons aged 75 years or older: the Bronx Aging Study. Am J Cardiol. 1990;66:533–7.

6. **Mittelmark MB, Psaty BM, Rautaharju PM, et al.** Prevalence of cardiovascular diseases among older adults: the Cardiovascular Health Study. Am J Epidemiol. 1993;137:311–7.

7. **Frishman WH, Gomberg-Maitland M, Hirsch H, et al.** Differences between male and female patients with regard to baseline demographics and clinical outcomes in the Asymptomatic Cardiac Ischemia Pilot (ACIP) trial. Clin Cardiol. 1998;21:184–90.

8. **ACIP Investigators.** Asymptomatic Cardiac Ischemia Pilot (ACIP) study. Am J Cardiol. 1992;70:744–7.

9. **Weintraub WS, Kosinski AS, Wenger NK.** Is there a bias against performing coronary revascularization in women? Am J Cardiol. 1996;78:1154–60.

10. **Brunelli C, Cristofani R, L'Abbate A.** Long-term survival in medically treated patients with ischaemic heart disease and prognostic importance of clinical and echocardiographic data. Eur Heart J. 1989;10:292–303.

11. **Murabito JM, Evans JC, Larson MG, Levy D.** Prognosis after the onset of coronary heart disease: an investigation of differences in outcome between the sexes according to initial coronary disease presentation. Circulation. 1993;88:2548–55.

12. **Orencia A, Bailey K, Yawn BP, Kottke TE.** Effect of gender on long-term outcome of angina pectoris and myocardial infarction/sudden unexpected death. JAMA. 1993; 269:2392–7.

13. **Feild SK, Savard MA, Epstein KR.** The female patient. In: Douglas PS (ed). Cardiovascular Health and Disease in Women. Philadelphia: WB Saunders; 1993:4–20.

14. **Liao V, Copper RS, Ghali JK, Szocka A.** Survival rates with coronary artery disease for black women compared with black men. JAMA. 1992;268:1867–71.

15. **National Center for Health Statistics.** Vital Statistics of the United States, 1986. Volume II: Mortality, Part A. Washington, DC: U.S. Public Health Service DHHS Pub. No. (PHS) 89-1101; 1989.

16. **Weiner DA, Ryan TJ, McCabe CH, et al.** Correlations among history of angina, ST-segment response and prevalence of coronary artery disease in the Coronary Artery Surgery Study (CASS). N Engl J Med. 1979;301:230–5.

17. **Gibbons RF.** Exercise ECG testing with and without radionuclide studies. In: Wenger NK, Speroff L, Packard B (eds). Cardiovascular Health and Disease in Women. Greenwich: LeJacq Communications; 1993:73–90.

18. **Ellestad MH.** Stress testing in women. In: Ellestad MH (ed). Stress Testing: Principles and Practice. 4th ed. Philadelphia: FA Davis; 1996:361–3.

19. **Stone PH, Chaitman B, McMahon RP, et al.** Relationship between exercise-induced and ambulatory ischemia in patients with stable coronary disease: the Asymptomatic Cardiac Ischemia Pilot (ACIP) Study. Circulation. 1996; 94:1537–44.

20. **Friedman TD, Greene AC, Iskandrian AS, et al.** Exercise thallium-201 myocardial scintigraphy in women: correlation with coronary arteriography. Am J Cardiol. 1982; 49:1632–7.

21. **Meisner JS, Shirani J, Strom JA.** Use of pharmaceuticals in noninvasive cardiovascular diagnosis. In: Frishman WH, Sonnenblick EH. Cardiovascular Pharmacotherapeutics. New York: McGraw-Hill; 1997:975–88.

22. **Hung J, Chaitman BR, Lam J, et al.** Noninvasive diagnostic test choices for the evaluation of coronary artery disease in women: a multivariate comparison of cardiac fluoroscopy, exercise electrocardiography, and exercise thallium myocardial perfusion scintigraphy. J Am Coll Cardiol. 1984;4:8–16.

23. **Amanullah AM, Kiat H, Friedman JD, Berman DS.** Adenosine technetium-99m sestamibi myocardial perfusion SPECT in women: diagnostic efficacy in detection of coronary artery disease. J Am Coll Cardiol. 1996;27:803–9.

24. **Taillefer R, DePuey EG, Udelson JE, et al.** Comparative diagnostic accuracy of thallium-201 and technetium-99m sestamibi SPECT imaging (perfusion and ECG-gated SPECT) in detecting coronary artery disease in women. J Am Coll Cardiol. 1997;29:69–77.

25. **Amanullah AM, Berman DS, Hachamovitch R, et al.** Identification of severe or extensive coronary artery disease in women by adenosine technetium-99m sestamibi SPECT. Am J Cardiol. 1997;80:132–7.

26. **Iskandrian AE.** Gender differences in noninvasive testing [Editorial]. J Noninvasive Cardiol. 1997;14–16.

27. **Tobin JN, Wassertheil-Smoller S, Wexler JP, et al.** Sex bias in considering coronary bypass surgery. Ann Intern Med. 1987;107:19–25.

28. **Lauer MS, Pashkow FJ, Snader CE, et al.** Gender and referral for coronary angiography after treadmill thallium testing. Am J Cardiol. 1996;78:278–83.

29. **Shaw LJ, Miller DD, Romeis JC, et al.** Gender differences in the noninvasive evaluation and management of patients with suspected coronary artery disease. Ann Intern Med. 1994;120:559–66.

30. **Steingart RM, Packer M, Hamm P, et al.** Sex differences in the management of coronary artery disease. N Engl J Med. 1991;325:226–30.

31. **Lando HA, Gritz ER.** Smoking cessation techniques. JAMA. 1996;51:31–4.

32. **Sachs DP, Sawe U, Leischow SJ.** Effectiveness of a 16-hour transdermal nicotine patch in a medical practice setting, without intensive group counseling. Arch Intern Med. 1993;153:1881–90.

33a. **Frishman WH, Ismail A.** Tobacco smoking, nicotine, and nicotine replacement. In: Frishman WH, Sonnenblick EH (eds). Cardiovascular Pharmacotherapeutics. New York: McGraw-Hill; 1997:499–509.

33b. **Meier CR, Derby LE, Jick SS, et al.** Antibiotics and risk of subsequent first-time acute myocardial infarction. JAMA. 1999;281:427–31.

34. **DelVecchio A, Frishman WH, Fadel A, Ismail A.** Cardiovascular manifestations of substance abuse. In: Frishman WH, Sonnenblick EH (eds). Cardiovascular Pharmacotherapeutics. New York: McGraw-Hill; 1997:1115–49.

35. **Frishman WH, Weiser M, Michaelson MD, Abdeen MA.** The pharmacologic approach to the treatment of obesity. J Clin Pharmacol. 1997;37:453–73.

36. **Blair SN, Kampert JB, Kohl HW III, et al.** Influence of cardiorespiratory fitness and other precursors on cardiovascular disease and all-cause mortality in men and women. JAMA. 1996;276:205–10.

37. **Frishman WH, Nurenberg JR, Frishman E.** Cardiovascular considerations with use of psychoactive medications. In: Frishman WH, Sonnenblick EH (eds). Cardiovascular Pharmacotherapeutics. New York: McGraw-Hill; 1997:1039–52.

38. **Ridker PM, Manson JE, Gaziano JM, et al.** Low-dose aspirin therapy for chronic stable angina. Ann Intern Med. 1991;114:835–9.

39. **Antiplatelet Trialists' Collaboration.** Collaborative overview of randomised trials of antiplatelet therapy-1: prevention of death, myocardial infarction, and stroke by prolonged antiplatelet therapy in various categories of patients. BMJ. 1995;308:81–106.

40. **Aarons L, Hopkins K, Rowland M, et al.** Route of administration and sex differences in the pharmacokinetics of aspirin, administered as its lysine salt. Pharm Res. 1989;6:660–6.

41. **Ho PC, Triggs EJ, Bourne DWA, Heazlewood VJ.** The effects of age and sex on the disposition of acetylsalicylic acid and its metabolites. Br J Clin Pharm. 1985;19:675–84.

42. **Escolar G, Bastida E, Garrido M, et al.** Sex-related differences in the effects of aspirin on the interaction of platelets with subendothelium. Thromb Res. 1986;44:837–47.

43. **Spranger M, Aspey BS, Harrison MJC.** Sex differences in antithrombotic effect of aspirin. Stroke. 1989;20:34–7.

44. **Paganini-Hill A, Chao A, Ross RK, Henderson BE.** Aspirin use and chronic diseases: a cohort study of the elderly. BMJ. 1989;299:1247–50.

45. **Aspirin Myocardial Infarction Study Research Group.** The Aspirin Myocardial Infarction Study: final results. Circulation. 1980;62(Suppl V):V79–84.

46. **Manson JE, Stampfer MJ, Colditz GA, et al.** A prospective study of aspirin use and primary prevention of cardiovascular disease in women. JAMA. 1991;266:521–7.

47. **Second International Study of Infarct Survivors (ISIS-2) Collaborative Group.** Randomized trial of intravenous streptokinase, oral aspirin, both, or neither among 17,187 cases of suspected acute myocardial infarction: ISIS-2. Lancet. 1988;2:349–60.

48. **Harpaz D, Benderly M, Goldbourt U, et al.** Effect of aspirin on mortality in women with symptomatic or silent myocardial ischemia. Am J Cardiol. 1996;78:1215–19.

49. **Zimetbaum P, Frishman WH, Ooi WL, et al.** Plasma lipid and lipoproteins and the incidence of cardiovascular disease in the elderly: the Bronx Longitudinal Aging Study. Arterioscl Thromb Vasc Biol. 1992;12:416–23.

50. **Fetters JK, Peterson Ed, Shaw LS, et al.** Sex-specific difference in coronary artery disease risk factors, evaluation and treatment: have they been adequately evaluated? Am Heart J. 1996;131:796–813.

51. **LaRosa JC, Applegate W, Crouse JR III, et al.** Cholesterol lowering in the elderly: results of the Cholesterol Reduction in Seniors Program (CRISP) pilot study. Arch Intern Med. 1994;154:529–39.

52. **Scandinavian Simvastatin Survival Study Group.** Randomized trial of cholesterol lowering in 4444 patients with coronary heart disease: the Scandinavian Simvastatin Survival Study (4S). Lancet. 1994;344:1383–9.

53. **Frishman WH, Clark A, Johnson B.** Effects of cardiovascular drugs on plasma lipids and lipoproteins. In: Frishman WH, Sonnenblick EH (eds). Cardiovascular Pharmacotherapeutics. New York: McGraw-Hill; 1997:1515–59.

54. **D'Agostino RB, Kannel WB, Stepanians MN, et al.** Efficacy and tolerability of lovastatin in women. Clin Ther. 1992;14:390–5.

55. **Lewis SJ, Sacks FM, Mitchell JS, et al.** Effect of pravastatin on cardiovascular events in women after myocardial infarction: the Cholesterol and Recurrent Events (CARE) trial. J Am Coll Cardiol. 1998;32:140–6.

56. **Walsh JM, Grady D.** Treatment of hyperlipidemia in women. JAMA. 1995;274:1152–8.

57. **Adult Treatment Panel II.** Summary of the Second Report of the National Cholesterol Education Program (NCEP) Expert Panel on Detection, Evaluation, and Treatment of High Blood Cholesterol in Adults. JAMA 1993;269:3015–23.

58. **Saltzberg S, Stroh JA, Frishman WH.** Isolated systolic hypertension in the elderly: pathophysiology and treatment. Med Clin North Am. 1988;72:523–47.

59. **Kahn S, Frishman WH, Weissman S, et al.** Left ventricular hypertrophy on electro-cardiogram: prognostic implications from a 10-year cohort study of older subjects: a report from the Bronx Longitudinal Aging Study. J Am Geriat Soc. 1996;44:524–9.

60. **Frishman WH, Michaelson MD.** Use of calcium antagonists in patients with ischemic heart disease and systemic hypertension. Am J Cardiol. 1997;79:33–8.

61. **Davis BR, Cutler JA, Gordon DJ, Furberg CD, et al.** The ALLHAT Research Group: rationale and design for the Antihypertensive and Lipid Lowering Treatment to Prevent Heart Attack Trial (ALLHAT). Am J Hypertens 1996;9:342–60.

62. **Hansson L, Zanchetti A, Carruthers SG, et al.** Effects of intensive blood pressure lowering and low-dose aspirin in patients with hypertension: principal results of the Hypertension Optimal Treatment (HOT) randomised trial. Lancet. 1998;351:1755–62.

63. **Task Force of the Working Group on Heart Failure of the European Society of Cardiology.** The treatment of heart failure. Eur Heart J. 1997;18:736–53.

64. **Frishman WH.** Carvedilol. N Engl J Med. 1998;339:1759–65.

65. **Gomberg-Maitland M, Frishman WH, et al.** Hormones as cardiovascular drugs: estrogens, progestins, thyroxine, growth hormone, corticosteroids, and testosterone. In: Frishman WH, Sonnenblick EH (eds). Cardiovascular Pharmacotherapeutics. New York: McGraw-Hill; 1997:787–835.

66. **Holdright GR, Sullivan AK, Wright JL, et al.** Acute effect of oestrogen replacement therapy on treadmill performance in post-menopausal women with coronary artery disease. Eur Heart J. 1995;16:1566–70.

67. **Rosano GMC, Sarrel PM, Poole-Wilson PA, Collins P.** Beneficial effect of oestrogen on exercise-induced myocardial ischaemia in women with coronary artery disease. Lancet. 1993;342:133–6.

68. **Hulley S, Grady D, Bush T, et al.** The Heart and Estrogen/Progestin Replacement Study (HERS) Research Group: randomized trial of estrogen plus progestin for secondary prevention of coronary heart disease in postmenopausal women. JAMA. 1998;280:605–13.

69. **Egashira K, Inou T, Hirooka Y, et al.** Evidence of impaired endothelium-dependent coronary vasodilation in patients with angina pectoris and normal coronary angiograms. N Engl J Med. 1993;328:1659–64.

70. **Vakili BA, Frishman WH, Lin TS, et al.** Antioxidant vitamins and enzymatic and synthetic scavengers of oxygen-derived free radical scavengers in the prevention and treatment of cardiovascular diseases. In: Frishman WH, Sonnenblick EH (eds). Cardiovascular Pharmacotherapeutics. New York: McGraw-Hill; 1997:535–56.

71. **Stampfer MJ, Hennekens CH, Manson JE, et al.** Vitamin E consumption and the risk of coronary disease in women. N Engl J Med. 1993;328:1444–9.

72. **Kushi LH, Folsom AR, Prineas RJ, et al.** Dietary antioxidant vitamins and death from coronary heart disease in post menopausal women. N Engl J Med. 1996;334:1156–62.

73. **Schwartz SM, Siscovick DS, Malinow MR, et al.** Myocardial infarction in young women in relation to plasma total homocysteine, folate, and a common variant in the methylenetetrahydrofolate reductase gene. Circulation. 1997; 96:412–7.

74. **European Concerted Action Project.** Plasma homocysteine as a factor for vascular disease. JAMA. 1997;277:1775–81.

75. **Rimm EB, Willett WC, Hu FB, et al.** Folate and vitamin B_6 from diet and supplements in relation to risk of coronary heart disease among women. JAMA. 1998;279: 359–64.

76. **Stein JH, McBride PE.** Hyperhomocysteinemia and atherosclerotic vascular disease: pathophysiology, screening, and treatment. Arch Intern Med. 1998;158:1301–6.

77. **Abrams J.** The organic nitrates and nitroprusside. In: Frishman WH, Sonnenblick EH (eds). Cardiovascular Pharmacotherapeutics. New York: McGraw-Hill; 1997:253–65.

78. **Bennett BM, Twiddy DAS, Moffat JA, et al.** Sex-related difference in the metabolism of isosorbide dinitrate following incubation in human blood. Biochem Pharmacol. 1983;32:3729–34.

79. **Tam GS, Marks GS, Brien JF, Nakatsu K.** Sex and species related differences in the biotransformation of isosorbide dinitrate by various tissues of the rabbit and rat. Can J Physiol Pharmacol. 1987;65:1478–83.

80. **Frishman WH.** Alpha- and beta-adrenergic blocking drugs. In: Frishman WH, Sonnenblick EH (eds). Cardiovascular Pharmacotherapeutics Companion Handbook. New York: McGraw-Hill; 1998:23–64.

81. **Walle T, Walle UK, Cowart TD, Conradi EC.** Pathway selective sex differences in the metabolic clearance of propranolol in human subjects. Clin Pharmacol Ther. 1989;46:257–63.

82. **Gilmore DA, Gal J, Gerber JG, Nies AS.** Age and gender influence the stereo-selective pharmacokinetics of propranolol. J Pharm Exp Ther. 1992;261:1181–6.

83. **Walle T, Byington RP, Furberg CD, et al.** Biologic determinants of propranolol disposition: results from 1308 patients in Beta-Blocker Heart Attack Trial. Clin Pharm Ther. 1985;38:509–18.

84. **Frishman WH.** Calcium-channel blockers. In: Frishman WH, Sonnenblick EH (eds). Cardiovascular Pharmacotherapeutics. New York: McGraw-Hill; 1997:101–30.

85. **Psaty BM, Heckbert SR, Koepsell TD, et al.** The risk of myocardial infarction associated with antihypertensive drug therapies. JAMA. 1995;274:620–5.

86. **Michels KB, Rosner BA, Manson JE, et al.** Prospective study of calcium-channel blocker use, cardiovascular disease, and total mortality among hypertensive women: the Nurses Health Study. Circulation. 1998;97:1540–8.

87. **Schwartz J, Capili H, Daughery J.** Aging of women after S-verapamil pharmacokinetics and pharmacodynamics. Clin Pharm Ther. 1994;55:509–17.

88. **Gupta SK, Atkinson L, Tu T, Longstreth JA.** Age and gender related changes in stereoselection pharmacokinetics and pharmacodynamics of verapamil and norverapamil. Br J Clin Pharm. 1995;40:325–31.

89. **Kloner RA, Sowers JR, DiBona GF, et al.** Sex- and age-related antihypertensive effects of amlodipine: the Amlodipine Cardiovascular Community Trial Study Group. Am J Cardiol. 1996;77:713–22.

90. **Savonitto S, Ardissiono D, Egstrup K, et al.** Combination therapy with metoprolol and nifedipine versus monotherapy in patients with stable angina pectoris: results of the International Multicenter Angina Exercise (IMAGE) Study. J Am Coll Cardiol. 1996;27:311–6.

91. **LeJemtel TH, Sonnenblick EH, Frishman WH.** The diagnosis and management of heart failure. In: Alexander RW, Schlant RC, Fuster V (eds). Hurst's The Heart. 9th ed. New York: McGraw-Hill; 1998:745–81.

92. **RITA-2 Trial Participants.** Coronary angioplasty versus medical therapy for angina: the Second Randomized Intervention Treatment of Angina (RITA-2). Lancet. 1997; 350:461–8.

93. **Nease RF, Kneeland R, O'Connor GT, et al.** Variation in patient utilities for outcomes of the management of chronic stable angina: implications for clinical practice guidelines: Ischemic Heart Disease Patient Outcomes Research Team. JAMA. 1995;273: 1185–90.

CHAPTER 16

Acute Coronary Syndromes

LAURA J. COLLINS, MD
PAMELA S. DOUGLAS, MD

The myth that women are somehow protected from coronary artery disease (CAD) and all its complications has clearly been disproved; however, many public and professional attitudes remain unaffected. Slightly less than half of the 500,000 annual deaths from myocardial infarction (MI) occur in women (1). In contrast, annual mortality in women from breast and lung cancer combined does not exceed 100,000 deaths, yet more women and their physicians fear complications and death from cancer (1). One third of all deaths in women aged 25 to 64 are due to cardiovascular disease; thus younger women enjoy only relative protection from this condition (2). Although cardiovascular mortality has been steadily decreasing for men since the early 1980s, the same is not true for women and the reasons are uncertain (Fig. 16-1).

Myocardial infarction in women differs from that in men on many levels, including clinical presentation, in-hospital and late mortality, complications, eligibility and selection for treatment, response to treatment, and effects of risk factor modification. A fundamental dilemma is whether these discrepancies are primarily related to women's more advanced age and accordingly "older" cardiac status at the time of presentation, to their greater burden of comorbidities, or to other gender-related differences. Hormonal status in both pre- and postmenopausal women has been implicated in altering one's risk factor profile, and these issues must be more fully understood. This chapter focuses on the gender-related differences apparent in acute MI and unstable angina and highlights those areas lacking in information specific to gender-related issues.

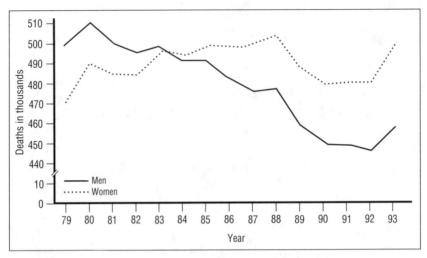

FIGURE 16-1 Cardiovascular disease mortality trends for U.S. men and women, 1979–93. Data are from the National Center for Health Statistics and the American Heart Association. (From 1997 Heart and Stroke Statistical Update. Dallas: American Heart Association; 1997; with permission.)

Clinical Presentation of Myocardial Infarction

Definitive data illustrating many of the differences in the clinical presentation of acute MI between men and women are lacking. For example, no conclusive data are available on whether gender-specific differences are present in the triggers of infarction, circadian variation of its occurrence, or risk of perioperative infarction during noncardiac surgery. However, the following observations have been made.

Women, compared with men, present a decade later in age with their first symptoms of coronary disease or with their first MI (3–7). A 26-year follow-up of the Framingham Heart Study (FHS) revealed that angina pectoris was the most likely initial presentation of coronary artery disease in women, occurring in 47% of women compared with 39% of men (6). Conversely, men were more likely than women to present with MI (43% versus 29%) (6). In the FHS, a significantly higher percentage of men presenting with angina subsequently had MI within 5 to 10 years of follow-up, which led many physicians to erroneously believe that anginal symptoms in women were less worrisome than in men (8,9). Two criticisms of this study are that no subjects over the age of 62 were included and that the diagnosis of CAD was based on symptoms, which in women are less reliable indicators of angiographic CAD (10–13).

Women with CAD/MI tend to have a greater number of individual cardiovascular risk factors than men (14). On average, women with MI are more likely to have a previous history of hypertension (3–5,15–19), congestive heart failure (3,15–17,20–22), unstable angina (6), diabetes (types I and II) (15–17,19–21,23–25), and a higher serum cholesterol level (5,19,26), and are less likely to have had a previous MI (3,16,18,20,24,27) or smoking history (4,5,8,16,18–20,24,26). The relative importance of each risk factor between genders remains controversial; it appears certain, however, that the presence of diabetes portends a greater increment in risk for women (see Early Mortality section). Women are also more likely to have concomitant obesity, valvular heart disease, cerebrovascular disease, and chronic dementia (25). Women typically present with a higher Killip class (20,24,25) and have a greater likelihood of rales and tachycardia on examination than men (20).

Women seek medical attention for symptoms of acute MI on average 1 hour later than men and have a longer time to treatment initiation (1.2 versus 1.0 hour, $p < 0.001$) (3,5,7,28,29), which may be partly accounted for by their more atypical symptoms, including a greater incidence of abdominal pain, dyspnea, nausea, and fatigue (3,12,30) in addition to or in the absence of a chest pain syndrome. However, despite women's more atypical presentation, acute EKG findings do not appreciably differ between the sexes (31,32a). Obviously, delay to presentation in the setting of an acute MI is dangerous and detrimental to myocardial salvage (32b). Although it is not fully understood why women persistently delay in seeking treatment, a recent study has made several observations that may explain this phenomenon. Dempsey and colleagues found that although women *immediately* perceive their pain as abnormal they tend to not acknowledge its serious nature until self-treatment and coping mechanisms fail to improve the situation (33). Other factors that may contribute to women's delay in presentation include the erroneous belief that acute MI is a male-dominated event, desire not to inconvenience others, and hesitation to involve others in personal health matters (33). In addition, the FHS revealed a higher incidence of silent (undetected) MI in women (6).

Not only do women having an acute MI tend to delay in their presentation to the hospital, but their treating physicians delay both the diagnosis and subsequent treatment. A study by Jackson and colleagues revealed that once a woman with acute MI arrives at the emergency room it takes 6 minutes longer before the first EKG is obtained and 23 minutes longer to the initiation of thrombolytic therapy than for a man (34a).

The pathophysiologic mechanism of an acute MI is usually complete thrombosis of a coronary artery (34b), often preceded by rupture of an atherosclerotic plaque (35). Gender-related differences in the pathology of acute MI have not been investigated; however, observational studies suggest that there are probably more similarities than differences (36). Owing to the higher incidence of non–Q-wave MI in women, one may infer that vasospasm may play a more significant role in the evolution of acute MI in women than in men (3,15,19,37–39). A recent study has found that fibrinogen, an essential cofactor for platelet aggregation and thus for acute thrombosis, is an equally important marker for CAD and clinical events in women and in men (36). In a group of young patients (< 45 years of age) studied 3 to 6 months after MI, there appeared to be greater platelet reactivity in young women compared with young men (40). It is unknown whether gender differences exist in atherosclerotic plaque composition and triggers of plaque rupture. The contribution of coronary vasospasm in the evolution of acute MI is unclear in both sexes. Clearly more investigation is warranted to determine if true gender differences exist in the pathophysiology of acute MI.

In several studies from the thrombolytic era (3,15,19,37,38), women have been shown to have a higher incidence of non-Q-wave (subendocardial) infarctions than men; Marmor and colleagues, however, found no significant difference between the sexes (41). Two studies revealed higher myocardial enzyme levels for men (16,19), whereas others reported no significant difference between the sexes when adjusted for body mass index (26). One study reported a higher frequency of inferior infarctions for women (42). Anterior infarctions in women have been reported to cover a larger territory than those in men, more often involving both the anteroseptal and anterolateral walls of the left ventricle (26). Women have also been shown to develop fewer collateral vessels after infarction, which may contribute to compromised systolic and diastolic function (38). Peri-infarct ventricular arrhythmias may be more common in men; however, they are independent of age and do not predict a worse prognosis in the setting of acute MI (26). Paradoxically, although women present at the time of their infarction with more comorbid conditions and a higher likelihood of congestive heart failure, there is little conclusive evidence that this is due to a greater extent of myocardial damage, because women tend to have better systolic left ventricular function after MI than men (15,18,38). The mechanisms underlying this mismatch are unknown.

Selected Risk Factors for Myocardial Infarction

Oral Contraceptives

The cardiovascular risk posed by oral contraceptives has been debated for several years and is hampered by the low incidence of ischemic heart disease in young women. Soon after oral contraceptives became available in 1960, multiple cases of thromboembolic events in young women were reported. It is now clear that the "early generation" of high-dose estrogen and progestin preparations increased thrombotic potential and thus cardiovascular risk in women, especially in those who smoked (relative risk for MI is markedly increased with smoking: RR = 20.8 for >15 cigarettes/day; RR = 3.5 for <15 cigarettes/day; RR = 0.9 for never smoked) (2). This increase in cardiovascular risk has been attributed to several factors, including detrimental effects on the lipid profile (increasing low-density lipoproteins [LDL] and triglycerides, decreasing high-density lipoproteins [HDL]), vasospasm, and an increase in thrombosis (43). Currently, it is believed that the increase in cardiovascular risk seen with contraceptives containing higher doses of estrogen was primarily due to an increase in the thrombotic potential and that this is the same mechanism probably responsible for the increased risk in stroke and MI in users of current oral contraceptive formulations who also smoke cigarettes.

A meta-analysis that analyzed 47 case-control and cohort studies found the relative risk for MI or stroke to be greater than one (1.6 and 1.8, respectively) for users of oral contraceptives. The investigators attributed this finding to methodologic flaws in study design rather than to drug toxicity. Flaws included difficulty in the accurate detection of cardiovascular events, uncertain accuracy when assessing past oral contraceptive use, and possible unequal susceptibilities to cardiovascular disease among patients in control and study groups. Taking these factors into account, the investigators found *no* increase in cardiovascular mortality rate for users of oral contraceptives (44).

There is no compelling evidence that the use of current oral contraceptive preparations (which contain significantly lower amounts of estrogen and progesterone) significantly increases one's cardiovascular risk in the absence of concomitant atherosclerotic risk factors. However, the relative risk of MI is increased at least four-fold in women with at least one other risk factor (45). Additionally, the long-term effects of these preparations in women older than age 35 are not known. Understanding the short- and long-term cardiovascular risks caused by current and past use of oral contraceptives is crucial and the topic demands further study.

Cocaine Abuse

Cocaine use among women is not uncommon and should always be considered in the differential diagnosis of a young women presenting with MI. A National Household Survey in 1991 revealed that 20% of women aged 26 to 34 years of age reported using cocaine at least once (46). There is a paucity of information as to whether there are gender-based differences for the risk of MI in users of cocaine, although it has been reported that cocaine-induced MI is most common in young men (47,48).

It is known that plasma levels of cocaine in women are lower than in men for any given dose of intranasal cocaine; however, the sexes have similar elevations in heart rates (49). This finding implies that women may have a heightened physiologic response to any given plasma level of cocaine; how this affects subsequent risk of MI is unknown. An autopsy study of cocaine users has shown that cocaine use appears to increase left ventricular mass and degree of coronary atherosclerosis in men but not in women (50).

Cocaine-associated myocardial ischemia/infarction is typically treated with aspirin, benzodiazepines, nitroglycerin, alpha-adrenergic antagonists, such as phentolamine, or calcium channel blockers. Beta-blockers should be avoided because of their ability to enhance coronary vasoconstriction in patients who have recently used cocaine (51). The use of thrombolytic therapy in cocaine-induced MI has not been well studied. A small retrospective analysis concluded that thrombolytic therapy for cocaine-induced MI was safe; however, creatinine kinase-MB (CK-MB) peak levels and the duration to peak CK-MB were similar in patients with and without thrombolytic therapy (52). Conversely, there are case reports of serious hemorrhagic complications, including hemorrhagic stroke, in this group of patients (53,54). Thus, until definitive studies are available, the routine use of thrombolytic therapy cannot be advocated in cocaine-induced MI and should be individualized to each case.

Menopause (and the Cardioprotective Effects of Estrogen)

It is well established that both natural and surgical menopause are associated with increased risk of MI in women. An overview of all prospective observational studies estimated that the reduction of relative risk of death from CAD is 0.50 for both current and past users of estrogen replacement therapy compared with never users (55). Data from the Nurses Health Study (NHS) suggest more than a 40% reduction in the risk of CAD and a 39% to 52% reduction in cardiovascular mortality in current users of estrogen replacement, whereas former users of hormone therapy have a 16% to 21% reduction (56). Additionally, the NHS ($n = 59,337$) demonstrated that the addition of progestin to hormonal therapy does not diminish estrogen's cardioprotective effects (57a). There is less evidence for the benefit of hormonal therapy in secondary prevention (57b). Evidence of the potential benefits of hormonal replacement must be weighed against cancer risks. (This is discussed in greater detail in Chapters 10 and 11.)

The manner in which estrogen conveys its cardioprotective effects is likely multifactorial, ranging from the improvement of lipid parameters to antiproliferative effects on smooth muscle cells and beneficial alterations in hemodynamics and the fibrinolytic system. Acute administration of estrogen has shown potentiation of endothelium-dependent vasodilatation in female atherosclerotic coronary arteries (58). Recently, the presence of the estrogen receptor on coronary artery endothelial cells has been described (59a). Future description of estrogen's interaction with its endothelial receptor on coronary arteries will provide additional insight into its cardioprotective effects (59b). Several nonendothelial-dependent mechanisms of vasodilatation have been proposed, including calcium channel blocker effect, inhibition of alpha-2 adrenergic response of vascular smooth muscle cells (60), and prostacyclin-mediated vasodilatation (61). The ability of estrogen to vasodilate atherosclerotic coronary arteries with minimal depression of systemic blood pressure may make it or its analogs an invaluable tool in the treatment of acute coronary syndromes in both women and men. (For a more extensive review, see Chapter 10.)

Complications of Myocardial Infarction

Many studies have reported higher in-hospital and 1-year mortality rates for women after MI (15,16,24–26,62–66b). These have been attributed in part to their more advanced age, more complications in the peri-infarct period, and women being more critically ill upon initial presentation. Congestive heart failure, cardiogenic shock (3,5,16,20–22,24,26), recurrent chest pain or angina (3,32), and unrecognized MI (67) have all been shown to occur more often in women, although these studies did not consistently adjust for age and other comorbid conditions. However, recent data from GUSTO and ISIS-3 reveal that, even after adjustment for age, a higher incidence of nonfatal complications was observed in women, including cardiogenic shock, peripheral bleeding, and congestive heart failure (7,66b). The incidence of recurrent angina and congestive heart failure in women is probably not due to the lack of collateral circulation, because the presence of angiographically visible collaterals was found to be equivalent for men and women post-MI (68). One study revealed that mechanical complications and atrioventricular block in the peri-infarction period were more age dependent than gender dependent (26).

The rate and predictors of reinfarction vary by gender. Reinfarction rates in GUSTO were higher in the over 10,000 women with acute MI than in men (5.1% versus 3.6%, $p < 0.001$). Previous trials revealed only a minimal increased risk of recurrent infarction in women compared with men in the thrombolytic era (7,25,69). This discrepancy may in part be explained by the larger number of women included in the GUSTO trial compared with earlier studies; however, this does not appear to translate to a higher long-term mortality rate for women (see section on Gender Issues in Mortality After Myocardial Infarction). Researchers from SPRINT (Secondary Prevention Israeli Reinfarction Nifedipine Trial) have shown that the clinical predictors of reinfarction differ for men and women (70). For example, even though peripheral vascular disease was a risk factor for predicting reinfarction for both sexes, a woman with peripheral vascular disease was twice as likely to have a reinfarction than a man with peripheral vascular disease. Whereas post-infarction angina, diabetes mellitus, cardiomegaly, and congestive heart failure were clinical predictors of reinfarction in women, they were not so in men (70).

The incidence of myocardial rupture is 1% to 3% after transmural MI. Whether myocardial rupture is more frequent in women is still controversial. An equal number of studies support each view; however, study numbers tend to be small and in most cases are not adjusted for baseline characteristics (71–75). For instance, MILIS (Multicenter Investigation of the Limitation of Infarct Study) (75) identified myocardial rupture in 1.7% of 845 patients and, in contrast to previous studies (73,74), there was not a higher incidence of rupture in women. Assessment of an unselected population of patients with acute MI found that myocardial rupture was found in 3.2% and accounted for 17% of overall deaths from MI. Women aged less than 70 years had the highest incidence of rupture, it being the cause of nearly half of the deaths in this group (73).

There are more complications seen post-MI in diabetic patients than in those who do not have diabetes. Diabetic men and women both have a higher incidence of cardiogenic shock, congestive heart failure, conduction disturbances, myocardial rupture, and recurrent MI than do nondiabetic patients (76–79). However, diabetic women appear to fare worse than diabetic men, the former having higher rates of recurrent MI (78), silent MI (80), and sudden death (78). Why diabetes in women compared with men portends a worse prognosis with respect to complications from MI and cardiovascular mortality is unclear. However, the explanation cannot be simply older age or a worse coronary risk factor profile (see the next section for further discussion).

Gender Issues in Mortality After Myocardial Infarction

Over the past decade, in-hospital and early mortality rates from acute MI have been decreasing in both sexes. For example, the Minnesota Heart Survey revealed that 28-day mortality rates between 1985 and 1990 declined from 15% to 12% in women and 13% to 10% in men (81). The gender difference in mortality has persisted from the prethrombolytic into the thrombolytic trials. Some authors have tried to more accurately assess the impact of gender by adjusting for observed gender differences such as age and comorbidities; their results have been inconsistent.

In the pre-thrombolytic era, most clinical trials presented assessments of early (in-hospital) and late mortality (unadjusted for age) rates that suggested that initial survival in men after MI was almost two-fold greater than in women (15,63,64). The Framingham Heart Study reported a 30-day mortality rate of 28% for women and 16% for men (63,64). A large multicenter study in Israel that included 1524 women revealed a persistently higher in-hospital mortality rate for women despite adjustment for age (23.1% versus 15.7%, p < 0.0005) and a 1-year, age-adjusted cumulative mortality rate of 31.8% for women and 23% for men (p < 0.0005) (16).

Most mortality data from the large thrombolytic trials—ISIS-2 (The Second International Study of Infarct Survival) (62), ASSET (Anglo-Scandinavian Study of Early Thrombolysis) (82), GUSTO (Global Utilization of Streptokinase and Tissue Plasminogen Activator for Occluded Coronary Arteries) (65), and GISSI-1 (Gruppo Italiano per lo Studio della Streptochinasi nell'Infarto Miocardico) (66)—support a gender difference in mortality prior to adjustment for age or other clinical variables. These trials consistently reveal a higher early mortality (21–35 days) rate for women (approximately two-fold) compared with men after thrombolysis (Table 16-1). However, both ASSET and ISIS-3 revealed little difference between the sexes, with only a 1.2- and 1.14-fold increase, respectively, in mortality rates for women and men (66b,82).

Only four of the thrombolysis trials addressed whether women have a higher mortality rate than men after MI after adjusting for critical baseline

Table 16-1 Unadjusted Mortality with Thrombolysis and Primary Angioplasty for Women and Men*

Trial	% Women	Treatment	Follow-up	Female Mortality	Male Mortality
				← % →	
GISSI-1 (66a,94)	20	SK	3 wk	18.5	8.8
(n = 11,806)			1 yr	28.3	14.5
ISIS-2 (62)	23	SK	5 wk	13.3	7.9
(n = 17, 187)		ASA		13.2	8.2
		Both		12.2	6.7
ASSET (82)	23	rt-PA	4 wk	8.6	6.8
(n = 5011)		Heparin			
GUSTO (107)	25	SK	4 wk	11.5	5.9
(n = 2431)	25	rt-PA		10.2	5.0
PAMI (84)					
(n = 395)	27	PTCA	In-hospital	4.0†	2.1

* SK = intravenous streptokinase, ASA = aspirin, rt-PA = recombinant tissue plasminogen activator, PTCA = primary percutaneous transluminal angioplasty, GISSI-1 = Gruppo Italiano per lo Studio della Streptochinasi nell'Infarto Miocardio, ASSET = Anglo-Scandinavian Study of Early Thrombolysis, GUSTO = Global Utilization of Streptokinase and Tissue Plasminogen Activator for Occluded Coronary Arteries, PAMI = Primary Angioplasty in Myocardial Infarction, ISIS-2 = Second International Study of Infarct Survival.
† p = not significant for mortality difference between men and women.

characteristics and age (Table 16-2). The International Tissue Plasminogen Activator/Streptokinase Mortality Study ($n = 1944$ women, 6317 men), which included 23% women, analyzed mortality with respect to gender, adjusting for age and baseline covariables including body mass index, weight, hours to treatment, Killip class, previous history of hypertension, diabetes, previous infarction, angina, and smoking (24). Women typically had "worse" baseline characteristics and received thrombolytic therapy an average of 18 minutes later than men. Although women treated with thrombolysis had higher unadjusted in-hospital (12% versus 7.2%, $p < 0.0001$) and 6-month (16.6% versus 10.4%, $p < 0.0001$) mortality rates than men, these differences were eliminated after correction for the above baseline variables with odds ratios of 1.11 and 1.02, respectively. Data from TAMI (Thrombolysis and Angioplasty in Myocardial Infarction) support the above findings ($n = 348$ women and 1271 men) (25). When adjusted for clinical variables, with or without correcting for the extent of CAD, men and women had similar mortalities, with a relative risk of 1.31 for women (95% CI, 0.83–2.06; $p =$ NS). In contrast, after 6 weeks of follow-up, TIMI-2 (Thrombolysis in Myocardial Infarction) found an increased mortality for women (RR = 1.54; 95% CI, 0.98–2.43; $p = 0.01$) even after controlling for age, clinical factors at time of presentation, and previous history of coronary risk factors (22). One analysis of the GUSTO-I Angiographic Trial has shown that after adjustment for clinical and angiographic variables women continue to have a higher 30-day mortality rate than men (odds ratio [OR] = 2.2) (Fig. 16-2) (68).

Table 16-2 Gender Comparison of Thrombolytic Trials with Adjusted Mortality (Odds Ratio, Women:Men)*

Trial	% Women	Treatment	Follow-up	Odds Ratio	p Value
International t-PA/SK‡ (24) ($n = 8261$)	23	rt-PA, SK, or both	In-hospital 6 month	1.11 1.02	NS NS
TAMI† (25) ($n = 1619$)	27	rt-PA, UK, or both	In-hospital	1.31	NS
TIMI-II† (22) ($n = 3339$)	18	rt-PA	6 week 1 year	1.54 1.39	0.01 NS

* Mortality adjusted for age, baseline clinical factors, demographics, and angiographic factors for each study; see individual references for detail.

UK = urokinase, rt-PA = recombinant tissue plasminogen activator, NS = not significant, SK = intravenous streptokinase, TAMI = Thrombolysis and Angioplasty in Myocardial Infarction, TIMI = Thrombolysis in Myocardial Infarction, International t-PA/SK = International Tissue Plasminogen Activator/Streptokinase Mortality Study.

† Multivariable logistic regression for age and other factors.

‡ Using Cox proportional hazards model.

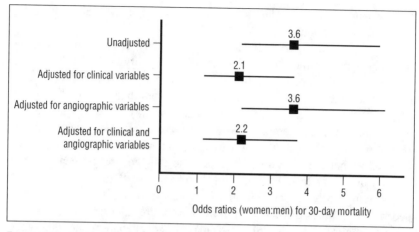

FIGURE 16-2 Effect of gender on 30-day mortality after myocardial infarction. The relative odds ratios (*squares*) and 95% confidence intervals (*horizontal lines*) for mortality are plotted for men versus women. A ratio greater than one denotes higher risk for mortality among women. Clinical variables included age, diabetes, history of previous MI, and initial heart rate and blood pressure. Angiographic variables included multivessel disease and 90-min TIMI flow grade. Data are from GUSTO-I. (From Woodfield SL, Lundergan CF, Reiner JS, et al. Gender and acute myocardial infarction: is there a different response to thrombolysis? J Am Coll Cardiol. 1997;29:35–42; with permission.)

Primary angioplasty in the treatment of acute MI has gained considerable favor over the past several years as an alternative to thrombolytic therapy and results in statistically similar mortality in men and women (83,84). The PAMI (Primary Angioplasty in Myocardial Infarction) Trial showed a trend toward higher early mortality in women than in men randomized to primary angioplasty (4.0% versus 2.1%, $p = 0.46$), although these results were not adjusted for age or other covariables (84).

Assessment of mortality data after MI is made difficult by the nonuniformity between studies in considering age and clinical variables, which may have a large effect on the final results and the methods involved in controlling for these specifics. The relatively small number of women included in these studies poses yet another difficulty. Owing to the rigorous entry criteria of clinical trials, these results may not be representative of actual MI patients treated in the community.

In an evaluation of elderly patients (≥75 years of age) with their first MI, Bueno and colleagues demonstrated that the early mortality rate was higher (40% versus 23%, $p = 0.01$) in women than men but was independent of sex and dependent on worsened left ventricular function post-infarction. The more complicated hospital course and worsened left ventricular systolic function were presumed secondary to a higher incidence of diabetes and hypertension in women patients (85).

Diabetic women after MI in the pre-thrombolytic era had an almost twofold higher in-hospital (86,87) and late (88) mortality rate. In GISSI-2 (n = 2332 women, 9335 men) insulin-dependent diabetic women having an acute MI treated with intravenous thrombolytic therapy had a two-fold increase (RR = 2.2; 95% CI, 1.4–3.5; 24% in-hospital mortality rate for insulin-dependent diabetic women compared with 13.9% for nondiabetic women) in the risk of in-hospital mortality compared with nondiabetic women and sevenfold higher mortality at 6 months (13.7% mortality for insulin-dependent diabetic women versus 4.3% for nondiabetic women) (Fig. 16-3) (76). There was a significantly higher mortality for diabetic women (especially insulin-dependent) compared with diabetic men even after adjustment for age and baseline clinical variables (76), which may be explained by gender differences in diabetic cardiovascular pathophysiology. Compared with diabetic men, diabetic women have been reported to have an altered fibrinolytic system with a lesser response to extrinsic thrombolysis (76), worsened left ventricular dysfunction in part due to diabetic cardiomyopathy (78,87,89), and a higher incidence of sudden-death post infarction (76).

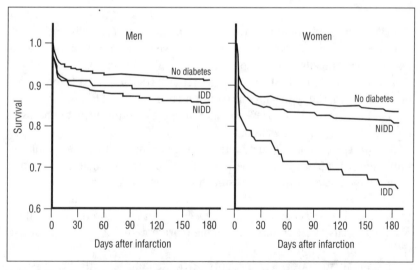

FIGURE 16-3 Survival curves showing gender difference after myocardial infarction at 6 months' follow-up for nondiabetic patients and for insulin-dependent (IDD) and non–insulin-dependent (NIDD) diabetic patients. Data are from GISSI-2 Study. (From Zuanetti G, Latini R, Maggioni AP, et al. Influence of diabetes on mortality in acute myocardial infarction: data from the GISSI-2 study. J Am Coll Cardiol. 1993;22:1788–94; with permission.)

An important recent review of sex differences in mortality after MI by Vaccarino and colleagues attempted to explore reported gender inconsistencies (90). They reviewed all studies available on sex differences in mortality after MI from 1966 through 1994 (pre- and post-thrombolysis) and included only those 27 studies that controlled at least for age and had 30 or more outcome events. In-hospital and early mortality rates were initially examined, followed by analysis of late mortality rates. The in-hospital or early mortality rate was greater in women by an average of 40% prior to adjustment for age, with the exception of one study (27) that was limited to black patients. When the data were adjusted for age, the sex difference in mortality declined to less than 20% and was statistically significant in only two studies (16,23). The six studies that adjusted for additional covariables found that, although the relative risk of mortality remained greater than one in all studies, fewer than half reached statistical significance (90). Vaccarino and colleagues concluded that women may have a survival disadvantage early after MI compared with men, but this can be largely explained by advanced age, worse clinical characteristics, and more comorbid conditions (90).Two analyses of the 30-day mortality rate in the GUSTO-I trial drew different conclusions as to the importance of gender as an independent predictor of mortality (see Thrombolysis section) (68,91). At this time, intrinsic gender differences cannot be fully excluded as contributors to higher early MI mortality in women.

Vaccarino's analysis of late mortality data following MI (90) showed similar variable results prior to age and other covariable adjustments, with four studies reporting a higher long-term mortality in women survivors (16,42,92,93), one showing a higher mortality for men (37), and seven studies showing similar mortality between the sexes or a trend toward better survival in women. When age adjustment was applied to mortality data, only one study (16) reported a higher mortality rate in women, although Vaccarino and colleagues thought this might be secondary to "incomplete age adjustment" (90). All other studies showed similar mortality rates for men and women or a trend toward lower late (>1 year) mortality for women. When additional covariables were taken into consideration, women appeared to have a higher long-term survival rate than men. Additionally, long-term follow-up (of 30-day survivors) of the GUSTO-I trial (n = 9117 women, 28,827 men) revealed similar mortality rates for age-matched men and women at 1 year post-MI (91).

Treatment of Myocardial Infarction

Primary and secondary risk factor modification are addressed in other chapters. Treatment issues discussed in this section include thrombolysis, primary angioplasty, cardiac catheterization, revascularization, and adjunctive medical therapy.

Thrombolysis

The introduction of thrombolytic therapy for the treatment of acute MI was a major advance, bringing the greatest improvement in mortality rates since the introduction of cardiopulmonary resuscitation and coronary intensive care units. The original thrombolysis placebo-controlled trials showed an overall 17% to 45% reduction in mortality (62,66,82) for both men and women (Table 16-3). ISIS-2 found that women treated with intravenous streptokinase and aspirin had a 31% reduction in mortality compared with placebo, whereas men had a 45% reduction (62). Other trials showed a more similar reduction in early mortality rates for men and women (66,82). The benefit for long-term mortality is less clear. GISSI-1 demonstrated a similar magnitude of mortality reduction with streptokinase for men and women, although this did not reach statistical significance in women because of the smaller number studied (94).

To date there is no evidence for a difference in the pharmacokinetics of thrombolytic agents between men and women in the setting of acute MI (95). Even though GUSTO-I demonstrated similar 90-minute patency rates for women and men (39% and 38%, respectively, for TIMI grade III flow); also similar patency rates (69.0% and 66.5%, respectively, for combined TIMI II and III grade flow) following thrombolysis, unadjusted 30-day mortality rates were

Table 16-3 Mortality Reduction by Gender for Thrombolysis or Primary Angioplasty Compared with Control Treatment*

Study	% Women	Treatment	Follow-up	Control	Female Mortality	Male Mortality
					<----------- % ----------->	
ISIS-2 (62) (n = 17,187)	23	SK + ASA	In-hospital	Placebo	31	45
GISSI-1 (66a) (n = 11,711)	20	SK	In-hospital	Standard care	19	17
GISSI-1 (94) (n = 11,696)	20	SK	1 yr	Standard care	10 (p = NS)	10 (p = 0.02)
ASSET (82) (n = 5011)	23	rt-PA + heparin	In-hospital	Placebo + heparin	21	28
PAMI (84) (n = 395)	27	PTCA	In-hospital	rt-PA	29 (p = 0.07)	6 (p = 0.46)

* For abbreviations see Table 16-1.

significantly worse for women than men (13% versus 4.8%) (68). As previously mentioned, it is unclear if a gender gap persists for the 30-day mortality in the GUSTO-I trial after adjustment for clinical and angiographic variables. After adjustment for age, diabetes, previous history of infarction, and initial heart rate and systolic blood pressure, Woodfield and colleagues concluded that gender remains an independent predictor of 30-day mortality (RR = 2.2, women:men) (68). In contrast, an analysis by Moen and colleagues of the GUSTO-I data revealed no significant influence of gender on 30-day mortality (RR = 1.06, women:men) after adjusting for similar clinical variables (91).

Elevated endogenous levels of tPA and PAI-1 have been associated with an increased incidence of coronary disease in both women and men (96–98). Despite similar efficacy rates between the genders with exogenous thrombolysis, some evidence suggests that gender-based differences in baseline levels of endogenous tPA and PAI-1 antigens and activity exist. Typically, women have been found to have lower levels of PAI-1 and tPA compared with age-matched men; however, this gender advantage disappears for postmenopausal women (99). Postmenopausal women have been found to have elevated levels of PAI-1 and tPA compared with premenopausal women; these levels may be decreased with estrogen replacement therapy (98,100). These findings present significant age- and gender-based differences in the endogenous fibrinolytic milieu that may not be reflected in the similar efficacy rates, since most women with MI are postmenopausal and not on hormone replacement therapy. How these endogenous factors may interact with exogenous thrombolysis and the development of coronary disease is unknown, and the subject merits further investigation.

Gender Bias in the Selection of Patients

In most trials, women deemed "eligible" received thrombolysis less often than men (3,21,101–107), but once women received thrombolysis they did well (5,25,106,108–110). This benefit may be less available to women, however, because many studies indicate that there is still a greater tendency not to proceed with thrombolysis in eligible women (102,105,111). This reluctance can be partially explained by older age, atypical presentation, more non–Q-wave MI, more comorbid medical conditions, and later time of presentation. However, there is evidence that some degree of selection bias may exist on the basis of sex (111). This must be examined more fully.

The MITI (Myocardial Infarction Triage and Intervention) registry revealed that men with acute MI were almost twice as likely to receive thrombolysis (14% versus 26%, $p < 0.0001$) as were women (3). However, it is uncertain if this discrepancy is caused by less frequent eligibility or gender bias. In comparison, the Western Washington Emergency Department rt-PA trial found women less likely to be eligible for thrombolysis but also demonstrated a gender bias because eligible men received thrombolytic therapy more often than did eligible women (78% versus 55%) (105). The U.S. Thrombolysis Study Investigators, addressing those factors accounting for gender bias in the utilization of thrombolytic therapy, found that women who were "strong" candidates for thrombolysis (i.e., short time to presentation, obvious EKG criteria, and without contraindications) received this therapy with the same frequency as the "strong" male candidates (102). However, if the decision to use thrombolysis became less clear, men were significantly more likely to receive thrombolysis than women. Their study did not address whether this was overuse in men or underuse in women.

Recent evidence suggests that age and gender bias present in the earlier days of thrombolytic therapy are on the decline but not yet abolished. A community analysis of patients with acute MI in Worcester, Massachusetts, revealed that between 1986 and 1991 there was an increase in the use of thrombolytics in both men (13.9% in 1986, 31.6% in 1991) and women (3.2% in 1986, 19.0% in 1991), with a greater relative increase seen in women (112). A national registry of patients with acute MI has shown a marked increase in the use of thrombolytics in the elderly, especially women, in the years between 1990 and 1994 (see Table 16-2) (113). However, analysis of patient records in Minnesota between 1992 and 1993 reveals a lower usage of thrombolytic agents among women patients (OR = 0.7; 95% CI, 0.6–1.0) with acute MI after adjusting for age and hospital type (114). A recent retrospective analysis by Krumholz and colleagues revealed that 56% of patients 65 years of age or older with acute MI who were eligible for thrombolysis did not receive it. Advanced age was among the strongest predictors of why thrombolysis was denied, and eligible women were less likely to receive thrombolysis than eligible men (40.1 % versus 48%, respectively) (115).

Overall, thrombolysis and primary angioplasty studies suggest that, given the best therapy in the current era and after controlling for clinical variables and age, gender differences in late post-infarction mortality can be reduced or eliminated (116). In clinical trials, all eligible patients receive the planned intervention. In the community, however, women are still less likely to receive thrombolytic therapy. Thus mortality after MI noted in clinical trials may underestimate mortality for women in the community (21).

Efficacy and Complications

The subgroup analyses comparing reperfusion rates after thrombolysis between women and men report similar pharmacokinetics and response to lytic therapy between the sexes (5,25,68,106,108–110). The TIMI Phase 1 Trial, a double-blinded randomized trial ($n = 290$ patients), revealed no gender difference in the rate of reperfusion (106). This was further supported by a review of all data from TAMI, which found no difference in infarct-related artery patency (74.3% for women versus 72.2% for men) (25). In addition, a smaller series by Becker and colleagues was in agreement with the TIMI and TAMI trials (95). As mentioned previously, the GUSTO-I Angiographic Trial, which enrolled 543 women (22.3% of total participants), demonstrated no significant gender difference in infarct-related artery patency at 90-minutes post-thrombolytic therapy (68). An assessment of noninvasive markers of reperfusion in GISSI-2 found that a decrease in ST-segment elevation was achieved less often in diabetic patients, particularly insulin-dependent diabetic women (76). This finding may suggest an altered physiologic response to thrombolysis in insulin-dependent diabetic women (see previous section on Gender Issues in Mortality After Myocardial Infarction).

Hemorrhagic complications in the setting of thrombolytic therapy, a major source of morbidity and mortality, are more common in women. Most studies show a two- to three-fold increase in the risk of hemorrhagic stroke in women, which is reduced but not fully eliminated by adjustment for age, body surface area or body weight less than 70 kg, and the use of anticoagulation before admission (24,25,76,93,117). Compared with previous trials, the PAMI (Primary Angioplasty in Myocardial Infarction) trial (a much smaller study than the previously stated trials: $n = 395$, 27% women) found an even higher risk of intracranial hemorrhage for women treated with t-PA compared with men (5.3% versus 0.7%) (83). In contrast, the GUSTO-I trial revealed that, after weight adjustment of the t-PA dose and adjustment for age and other baseline characteristics, there was no gender difference in the incidence of hemorrhagic stroke (7).

Aside from GUSTO-I, the other thrombolytic trials appear to show a consistently higher incidence of hemorrhagic stroke in women, especially older women, treated with thrombolytic therapy. Several large population studies are not in agreement as to whether there are gender-related differences in the general incidence of hemorrhagic strokes (118–121). It is important to remember that whereas blood pressure at the time of presentation is typically controlled for in final analyses, previous history is not, and a history of hypertension is typically more common in women who present with acute MI (3). Life-threatening noncerebral hemorrhagic complications appear to be more common in women as well, even after adjustment for age and baseline characteristics (7,122,123). Currently, the major thrombolytic trials support a gender difference in the risk of intracranial bleeding that is not solely attributable to advanced age or inappropriate dose for body size and may be partially explained by a higher incidence of hypertension in women presenting with MI. More detailed information concerning the absolute and relative contraindications for the use of thrombolytic therapy in acute MI can be found in the most recent ACC/AHA Guidelines for the Management of Patients with Acute Myocardial Infarction (124). An important exception to the usual contraindication of active bleeding is active menstrual bleeding. Although safety information is obviously limited for this small subgroup of patients, available data suggest that the use of thrombolytic therapy is safe, without significant bleeding, in actively menstruating women (124–127). Thus, younger women who have less risk of bleeding should be strongly considered for thrombolysis in the setting of acute MI. In older women, if primary angioplasty (discussed below) is available it avoids the small but real risk of hemorrhagic stroke.

Poor left ventricular function after MI portends a poor prognosis for both women and men (128–131). Review of the TAMI database found similar improvement in left ventricular function before discharge for both sexes (25). Preliminary animal data in rats (132) suggest that remodeling occurs differently post-MI in females compared with males, with less cavity dilation and less hypertrophy of the noninfarcted walls. Unfortunately, subgroup analysis on left ventricular function in women after thrombolysis is not available for the majority of the studies (see Chapter 19).

Primary Angioplasty versus Thrombolysis

The largest trial to date to address the issue of thrombolysis versus primary angioplasty in the treatment of acute MI is PAMI (Primary Angioplasty in Myocardial Infarction Study Group) (84). This multicenter trial randomized 395 patients, 27% of whom were women (without a separate randomization for each sex), who presented within 12 hours of the onset of the MI with either primary angioplasty or systemic thrombolysis with tPA (100 mg or 1.25 mg/kg for patients weighing less than 65 kg). The results revealed a lower in-hospital mortality rate for the angioplasty group and fewer complications, including fewer cases of early reinfarction and intracranial bleeding, with similar post-MI left ventricular function.

A separate analysis of the gender-specific outcome of the PAMI trial found a univariate trend toward reduced mortality among women treated with primary angioplasty compared with thrombolysis (4.0% versus 14.0%, $p = 0.07$) (83). The group of women responsible for the increased mortality in the t-PA treated patients were aged 65 years or older, whereas women less than 65 years of age had an in-hospital mortality rate similar to that for men, regardless of treatment modality. The incidence of intracranial bleeding was higher in women less than 65 years of age treated with tPA versus primary angioplasty (9.4% versus 0%, $p = 0.07$).

Cardiac Catheterization

The MIDAS (Myocardial Infarction Data Acquisitions System) (133), MITI (Myocardial Infarction Triage and Intervention) (3), and other trials

(14,19,134) revealed that women were less likely to undergo cardiac catheterization after MI. The MITI registry found that 58% of men in its population were referred for coronary angiography compared with 40% of women ($p < 0.0001$). These differences, and those in MIDAS, were not eliminated by controlling for age or multiple patient characteristics. In the SAVE trial fewer women than men (15.4% versus 27.3%, $p < 0.001$) were referred for cardiac catheterization after MI, despite greater functional disability from angina in women (14).

In contrast, other studies have found no difference in the use of cardiac catheterization between men and women in the post-infarction period, especially after controlling for age and extent of coronary disease (19,101,135). Funk and colleagues found that the characteristics of old age, black race, treatment by a woman physician, chronic dementia, cerebrovascular disease, and a neurologic complication accompanying MI were all associated with a decreased likelihood of cardiac catheterization in the immediate peri-infarction period (19).

Thus, it remains controversial as to whether women are truly referred less frequently than men for coronary angiography in the post-infarction period or whether this current referral pattern is justified by patient characteristics. Several factors may account for the differences in study results, including regional differences in aggressiveness of care or patient acceptance of catheterization. If future data do confirm a gender bias in the referral of patients for coronary angiography in the post-MI period, further study will be required to determine if this represents a pattern of overuse in men or underuse in women.

Coronary Revascularization

Most studies reveal lower overall use of PTCA (percutaneous transluminal coronary angioplasty) in women post-MI (3,19,133,134) but others have demonstrated no difference in PTCA rates (135,136). However, once a women undergoes a cardiac catheterization, data suggest that she has the same probability of having PTCA as does a man (3,19,133), which is in support of Healy's (137) frequently quoted contention that once women are shown to have CAD they are treated "as men would be."

Available data suggest that women who undergo PTCA for post-MI ischemia have procedural success rates similar to those for men (138,139). After PTCA, women's rates of coronary artery bypass grafting (CABG), repeat PTCA, recurrent infarction, and mortality are similar to men's after adjustment for age, severity of disease, and other clinical factors (138,139).

Surgical revascularization in women has been traditionally associated with a higher early mortality compared with men (140-143), which is also true after MI (3). This has been attributed to several factors: smaller vessel size, smaller body surface area (144), more comorbid conditions, advanced age, a more critical status at the time of surgery, and more advanced disease at the time of CABG, perhaps due to delayed referral (145–148). Although not specific to patients after MI, 6-year follow-up of the CASS (Coronary Artery Surgery Study) registry revealed no difference in survival rates for men and women after CABG (146). Longer follow-up (15 years) also revealed no gender differences in survival for surgical treatment of left main coronary disease (149).

Similar to the referral pattern for PTCA post-MI, several studies reveal equivalent rates of CABG for men and women once they have undergone coronary catheterization (3,129,133). However, others have shown a persistent difference even after adjusting for age, severity of CAD, and other clinical variables (134,135). Most data suggest that no specific gender discrepancy exists post-MI in referral of patients for catheter or surgical revascularization.

Adjunctive Medical Therapy

Gender Differences in Benefits

Although reperfusion therapy has afforded the greatest reduction in mortality from MI, adjunctive medical therapy remains important. Several studies have shown a significant mortality reduction for both women and men who receive beta-blockers after MI (150–154). (A detailed review of the efficacy of beta-blockers and other secondary pharmacotherapy can be found in Chapter 21.)

Although data are inconclusive, several studies suggest that women might experience greater benefit from beta-blockers than men (150–153). ISIS-I revealed a larger mortality rate reduction for women treated with atenolol compared with men (150). The Timolol Myocardial Infarction Trial revealed a 41% reduction in mortality rate for women, a reduction greater than for men (35%) (151). BHAT (Beta-Blocker Heart Attack Trial), which included 602 women, also showed a trend (nonsignificant) towards greater reduction in mortality for women (152,153). Accordingly, beta-blockers should be used after MI in almost all women.

Available data suggest that calcium channel blockers do not reduce the risk of recurrent infarction (155,156) or cardiovascular death, and in some studies they have been associated with an increase in mortality (156,157). In a case-controlled study short-acting calcium channel blockers increased the risk of MI in women and men.

Although it is widely recommended that angiotensin-converting enzyme (ACE) inhibitors be used post-MI in those patients with a left ventricular ejection fraction of 40% or less, the data available from individual treatment trials for women are far less convincing than the data for men. The SAVE (Survival and Ventricular Enlargement) trial demonstrated only a 2% (95% CI, 3–37) risk reduction in deaths for women from all causes compared with a 22% (95% CI, 6–36) risk reduction for men (158). Likewise, there was a large discrepancy in the risk reduction of cardiovascular death and morbidity, with a 28% (95% CI, 16–38) reduction in men compared with a 4% reduction (95% CI, 32–30) in women. The TRACE (Trandolapril Cardiac Evaluation) trial (<30% women) revealed a higher risk reduction for all-cause death in men taking the ACE inhibitor after MI (26%) compared with women (10%). In contrast, the AIRE (Acute Infarction Ramipril Efficacy) trial (<30% women) found no significant gender differences in the benefit received from ramipril. Although the authors of the SAVE trial addressed the more favorable results in men by using a proportional-hazards model to show that the benefits of captopril therapy were independent of sex (159), it is difficult to conclude that women and men receive equivalent benefit from this therapy based on available individual trial data. Why men should have more benefit from this treatment is unclear, although renin levels have been shown to be inversely related to estradiol levels (160a). These data accentuate the need for further clarification of gender differences in the renin angiotensin system and the use of ACE inhibitors post-MI and their optimal use in the female patient. At this time, the only meta-analysis data available on women and ACE inhibitors reveal similar benefit for women and men (160b). We currently advocate the use of ACE inhibitors in women after MI. Future trials or meta-analyses should more completely address this issue.

Two large randomized trials, ISIS-2 (62) and ISIS-2 Pilot Study (161), have demonstrated the benefit of aspirin in the setting of an acute MI. In ISIS-2 fewer than 25% of the patients were women and subgroup analyses were determined to be unreliable. A more recent trial ($n = 2418$ women) found that aspirin use in women with CAD reduced cardiovascular (RR = 0.61, 95% CI, 0.38–0.97) and all-cause mortality (RR = 0.66, 95% CI, 0.47–0.93) after adjustment for age, history of MI, systemic hypertension, diabetes, peripheral vascular disease, and current smoking. The women who benefited most from aspirin treatment were older, diabetic, symptomatic, or had previous MI history (162).

An overview of six trials found the use of intravenous nitrates given during the early period of an acute MI to reduce mortality rates by 45%, however; this overview did not achieve conventional statistical significance (163). Although these trials did not specifically analyze by gender, there are currently no data to suggest that women would receive less benefit from intravenous nitrates in this setting.

Gender Differences in Use
Based on the available data it is clear that following acute MI both beta-blockers and aspirin are indicated in women without obvious contraindications as adjuncts to reperfusion. Despite this knowledge, women and the

elderly (those greater than 70 years of age) are more frequently discharged after MI without prescription of these medications (22,164–168d). For example, a study by Wilkinson and colleagues (165) revealed that 23% of women compared with 41% of men ($p < 0.001$) were discharged on beta-blockers after their initial admission for MI. Beta-blockers are also less likely to be given to women than men during the initial presentation of acute MI (37% versus 43%, $p < 0.005$) (21). Prescribing patterns may be in flux, because some recent studies have shown similar prescribing patterns for women and men (169,170).

The Worcester Heart Attack Study reported that men were more likely to be treated with antiplatelet therapy than women (25% versus 19%, $p = 0.005$) in the acute phase of MI (21). There is also evidence that women are less likely to be discharged on aspirin therapy for secondary prevention after MI (75% versus 80%, $p < 0.01$) (166,170).

Women presenting with a non–Q-wave MI have also been shown to receive less anti-ischemic and antiplatelet therapy than men (171).

Several studies have reported the overuse of calcium channel blockers in the setting of an acute MI or in the peri-infarction period (168a,172), and at least one study showed a trend toward a higher usage in women compared with men (22).

Women were also more likely than men to receive digoxin or diuretic therapy in the setting of an acute MI and less likely to receive antiarrhythmic agents (21). Men are more likely to receive intravenous nitrates (21), which have been associated with a reduction in mortality (163,173). No gender-specific information is available concerning the pattern of use of ACE inhibitors in the post-MI period.

Whether these differential usage patterns in adjunctive medical therapy have any effect upon short- or long-term morbidity and mortality after MI in women is unclear. Data from an observational follow-up study of MI patients in London implicated the under-utilization of beta-blockers in women's relatively higher risk of recurrent ischemia in the post-infarction period; however, after adjustment for other clinical factors this difference became nonsignificant (165).

Unstable Angina

Defining gender differences in the clinical presentation, pathophysiology, treatment, and prognosis of unstable angina is a difficult task due to the heterogeneity of this entity. Unstable angina is typically defined as a significant change of a previously stable pattern of anginal symptoms. This may encompass an increase in the frequency and/or intensity of symptoms, rest symptoms, or occurrence of symptoms with less physical activity than was previously noted. Anginal symptoms in women may be misconstrued as unstable because women carrying a diagnosis of stable chronic angina have been found to have a higher incidence of rest angina, nocturnal angina, or angina provoked by mental stress than men with the same diagnosis (174). The gender differences in the clinical characteristics of patients presenting with unstable angina are similar to those previously noted for acute MI. Women were less likely than men to have a history of smoking but more likely to be older and have hypertension, diabetes mellitus, and a family history of premature coronary disease. Women were also less likely than men to have had a history of previous MI or previous coronary angiography or revascularization (171,175).

Studies have shown that the etiology of unstable angina is typically the subtotal occlusion of a coronary artery by a thrombus rich in platelets superimposed on a complicated plaque (176,177). Interestingly, TIMI IIIb found that up to 25% of women (compared with 16% of men) presenting with unstable angina or non–Q-wave MI have nonocclusive epicardial coronary disease, which suggests coronary vasospasm or small vessel coronary disease as other possible etiologies of myocardial ischemia in women or a higher proportion of women with noncardiac chest pain (175). Others have confirmed these findings with documentation of impaired angiographic coronary filling in one third of patients (male and female) with unstable angina/non–Q-wave MI and nonocclusive epicardial coronary disease, further implicating microvascular coronary dysfunction as a possible etiology (178).

Possible differences in mortality with unstable angina contrast with evidence for less severe CAD in women when diagnosis occurs after an acute event. Baseline characteristics, management, and 6-week outcomes after a non–Q-wave MI or with unstable angina were compared by gender, race, and age in the TIMI III Registry ($n = 3318$), which included substantial numbers of women (42%), blacks (28%), and elderly (25% with age >75). Women more often had hypertension, diabetes, and a family history of premature coronary disease and were less likely to smoke or to have had a previous MI (171). Compared with women, white men were more aggressively treated with anti-ischemic regimens and experienced more invasive procedures. Despite women undergoing less angiography and having less severe CAD, outcomes at 6 weeks were similar by gender and race (171). This implies that women may have a worse outcome with less severe disease. Whether more aggressive treatment in women (more intensive medical therapy and/or more diagnostic catheterizations) would have improved their outcome at 6 weeks is unknown. Older age may be the key, because in retrospective chart review older patients with unstable angina received fewer interventions (168d).

The mainstay of therapy has been directed towards antiplatelet agents and thrombin inhibitors. No gender subgroup analyses are available for the use of aspirin and heparin in the treatment of unstable angina. However, two studies (each including 27%–29% women) have shown that aspirin, heparin, or the combination of both decreases the incidence of MI in the treatment of women with unstable angina (179,180). Additionally, nitrates, beta-blockers, and calcium channel blockers have proven efficacious in treating this entity. Two studies (each including 26%–34% women) have found that women with unstable angina have platelets that are more aggregative than those in men (181,182); recent data suggest that this may be caused by more highly activated fibrinogen receptors (GpIIb/IIIa) on platelets (181). These findings suggest that women with unstable angina may require more aggressive platelet inhibition compared with men. A retrospective analysis that compared the use of a GpIIb/IIIa receptor inhibitor, Integrilin, with that of aspirin in women with unstable angina found that Integrilin was a better inhibitor of platelet aggregation and decreased Holter monitor–determined episodes of ischemia compared with the aspirin-treated group. Men treated with this same inhibitor of the platelet fibrinogen receptor did not fare better than those treated with aspirin alone (181). Ticlopidine, another antiplatelet agent, has been found effective at a dose of 250 mg bid, reducing the risk of fatal and nonfatal MI by 53% ($p < 0.006$) in both women (28% of study population, no subgroup analysis available) and men compared with conventional treatment with beta-blockers, calcium channel blockers, and nitrates (183). Direct comparisons between ticlopidine and aspirin in unstable angina have not been done.

The TIMI IIIb trial also found that the outcome of women with unstable angina or non–Q-MI was similar to that of men and dependent on the severity of illness rather than gender (175). Similarly, TIMI IIIa found that the subgroup of patients (both men and women) with unstable angina and nonocclusive coronary disease had a better short-term prognosis (2% incidence of MI and death) than did the subgroup with critical coronary obstruction (18% incidence of MI or death) (178).

Use of percutaneous revascularization in women with unstable angina has been shown to be similar in men with regard to initial success rate, mortality, and need for emergency CABG. At 4 years (mean) of follow-up there was no difference in survival or freedom from Q-wave MI, but more women than men had recurrence of severe anginal symptoms (52% versus 44%) and fewer women underwent subsequent CABG (184). TIMI IIIb found that women with unstable angina or non–Q-wave MI underwent CABG less frequently than men, but this was probably due to a higher incidence of multivessel disease in men. Mortality was higher in women than men (8.5% versus 2.2%) 42 days after CABG; however, owing to the small number of deaths a multivariate analysis was not possible to determine if this was independently related to gender.

In the BARI (Bypass Angioplasty Revascularization Investigation) trial, women and men with symptomatic multivessel disease were randomized to

PTCA or CABG (185). Women had more unstable angina (679 versus 619), were older, and were more likely to have congestive heart failure, diabetes, and hypertension. After adjustment for baseline variables, women had lower mortality rates than men but similar rates of recurrent MI at 5.4-year follow-up.

Clearly, better understanding of the pathophysiology of, and treatment options for, unstable angina in women will improve prognosis, including avoidance of future adverse cardiac events. Further research is required, especially in view of data supporting a higher level of platelet activation in women than is found in men.

Summary

Acute MI in women is associated with more atypical symptoms than present in men, which may lead to delays in presentation and treatment and less aggressive care. It is important for physicians to recognize these differences. Women appear to have an early survival disadvantage after MI that can be largely explained by more advanced age and other comorbid conditions. However, some population-based studies still suggest that women do worse than men. To determine whether gender is truly an independent risk factor in mortality from MI, any differences between the sexes in the aggressiveness of diagnosis and treatment of CAD must be eliminated. There appears to be no significant difference in long-term mortality and even a possibility that women may fare better.

Early reperfusion is an important predictor of early and late outcomes, and thrombolysis reduces mortality in women as well as men. To the extent that women are judged less eligible for thrombolysis, based on older age and concomitant disease, they are less likely to receive such therapy. Some studies have suggested an actual gender bias in the allocation of thrombolysis. Recent data suggest that primary angioplasty may be the preferred method of reperfusion, especially in elderly women; however, the availability of this therapy is limited.

Of all post-infarction medical therapies, beta-blockers have been the most carefully evaluated in women. Individual trial data regarding ACE inhibitors in women are not conclusive, but meta-analysis of individual patient data suggests equal benefit for women and men after MI. Although low-dose aspirin is effective after MI, results of primary prevention trials are awaited. The suggestion that women are still less likely to be prescribed proven therapy (e.g., beta-blockers) than are men needs further investigation.

In the presence of diabetes, the onset of CAD is not delayed in women. Diabetic women are more prone to complications and have a worse survival rate than men following acute MI. The etiologic mechanisms responsible for the poor prognosis for persons with diabetes are uncertain and probably multifactorial. Why diabetic women should fare considerably worse than diabetic men is also unknown.

Investigation into the gender-related similarities and differences of the pathophysiologic mechanisms of acute MI and unstable angina will be instrumental in optimizing both acute and chronic therapy for these conditions. Hormone replacement therapy in postmenopausal women appears to be a promising treatment for lipid abnormalities and reducing cardiovascular risk. Whether a role exists for the administration of estrogen in the setting of acute MI or unstable angina remains to be seen.

The clinical heterogeneity and more atypical presentation of unstable angina in women make this a challenging condition to diagnose and manage. Perhaps identification of the factors that make rest angina and mental stress angina more common in women with a history of chronic stable angina will provide insight into the pathophysiologic mechanisms of unstable angina in women as well as men.

Careful attention to clinical presentation, response to treatment, complications, and mortality of acute MI and unstable angina is necessary for understanding underlying pathophysiology and devising optimal treatment strategies for acute coronary syndromes in women.

REFERENCES

1. **American Heart Association.** Silent epidemic: the truth about women and heart disease. Dallas: American Heart Association; Publication No. 64-9702, 1995:1-3.

2. **Croft P, Hannaford PC.** Risk factors for acute myocardial infarction in women: evidence from the Royal College of General Practitioners' oral contraception study. BMJ. 1989;298:165-8.

3. **Maynard C, Litwin PE, Martin JS, Weaver WD.** Gender differences in the treatment and outcome of acute myocardial infarction: results from the Myocardial Infarction Triage and Intervention (MITI) Registry. Arch Intern Med. 1992;152:972-6.

4. **McCabe CH, Prior, MJ, Fraulini, T, et al.** Gender differences between patients with acute myocardial infarction, non–Q-wave myocardial infarction, and unstable angina-results from TIMI-II and T3B [Abstract]. J Am Coll Cardiol. 1993;21:271A.

5. **Jenkins JS, Flaker GC, Nolte B, et al.** Causes of higher in-hospital mortality in women than in men after acute myocardial infarction. Am J Cardiol. 1994;73:319-22.

6. **Lerner DJ, Kannel WB.** Patterns of coronary heart disease morbidity and mortality in the sexes: a 26-year follow-up of the Framingham population. Am Heart J. 1986; 111:383-90.

7. **Weaver WD, White HD, Wilcox RG, et al.** Comparisons of characteristics and outcomes among women and men with acute myocardial infarction treated with thrombolytic therapy. GUSTO-I Investigators. JAMA. 1996;275:777-82.

8. **Murabito JM, Evans JC, Larson MG, Levy D.** Prognosis after the onset of coronary heart disease: an investigation of differences in outcome between the sexes according to initial coronary disease presentation. Circulation. 1993;88:2548-55.

9. **Kannel WB, Feinlib, M.** Natural history of angina pectoris in the Framingham Heart Study. Am J Cardiol. 1972;29:154-63.

10. **Chaitman BR, Bourassa MG, Davis K, et al.** Angiographic prevalence of high-risk coronary artery disease in patient subsets (CASS). Circulation. 1981;64:360-7.

11. **Weiner DA, Ryan TJ, McCabe CH, et al.** Exercise stress testing: correlations among history of angina, ST-segment response and prevalence of coronary artery disease in the country artery surgery study (CASS). N Engl J Med. 1979;301:230-5.

12. **Welch CC, Proudfit WL, Sheldon WC.** Coronary arteriographic findings in 1,000 women under age 50. Am J Cardiol. 1975;35:211-5.

13. **Waters DD, Halphen C, Theroux P, et al.** Coronary artery disease in young women: clinical and angiographic features and correlation with risk factors. Am J Cardiol. 1978;42:41-7.

14. **Steingart RM, Packer M, Hamm P, et al.** Sex differences in the management of coronary artery disease. Survival and Ventricular Enlargement (SAVE) Investigators. N Engl J Med. 1991;325:226-30.

15. **Tofler GH, Stone PH, Muller JE, et al.** Effects of gender and race on prognosis after myocardial infarction: adverse prognosis for women, particularly black women. J Am Coll Cardiol. 1987;9:473-82.

16. **Greenland P, Reicher-Reiss H, Goldbourt U, Behar S.** In-hospital and 1-year mortality in 1,524 women after myocardial infarction: comparison with 4,315 men. Circulation. 1991;83:484-91.

17. **Henning R, Lundman T.** Swedish Co-operative CCU Study: a study of 2008 patients with acute myocardial infarction from 12 Swedish hospitals with coronary care unit. Part I. A description of the early stage. Part II. The short-term prognosis. Acta Medica Scand Suppl. 1975;586:1-64.

18. **Dittrich H, Gilpin E, Nicod P, et al.** Acute myocardial infarction in women: influence of gender on mortality and prognostic variables. Am J Cardiol. 1988;62:1-7.

19. **Funk M, Griffey KA.** Relation of gender to the use of cardiac procedures in acute myocardial infarction. Am J Cardiol. 1994;74:1170-3.

20. **Fiebach NH, Viscoli CM, Horwitz RI.** Differences between women and men in survival after myocardial infarction: biology or methodology? JAMA. 1990;263:1092-6.

21. **Goldberg RJ, Gorak EJ, Yarzebski J, et al.** A community-wide perspective of sex differences and temporal trends in the incidence and survival rates after acute myocardial infarction and out-of-hospital deaths caused by coronary heart disease. Circulation. 1993;87:1947-53.

22. **Becker RC, Terrin M, Ross R, et al.** Comparison of clinical outcomes for women and men after acute myocardial infarction. The Thrombolysis in Myocardial Infarction (TIMI-II) Investigators. Ann Intern Med. 1994;120:638-45.

23. **Puletti M, Sunseri L, Curione M, et al.** Acute myocardial infarction: sex-related differences in prognosis. Am Heart J. 1984;108:63-6.

24. **White HD, Barbash GI, Modan M, et al.** After correcting for worse baseline characteristics, women treated with thrombolytic therapy for acute myocardial infarction have the same mortality and morbidity as men except for a higher incidence of hemorrhagic stroke. The Investigators of the International Tissue Plasminogen Activator/Streptokinase Mortality Study. Circulation. 1993;88:2097-103.

25. **Lincoff AM, Califf RM, Ellis SG, et al.** Thrombolytic therapy for women with myocardial infarction: is there a gender gap? Thrombolysis and Angioplasty in Myocardial Infarction (TAMI) Study Group. J Am Coll Cardiol. 1993;22:1780-7.

26. **Robinson K, Conroy RM, Mulcahy R, Hickey N.** Risk factors and in-hospital course of first episode of myocardial infarction or acute coronary insufficiency in women. J Am Coll Cardiol. 1988;11:932-6.

27. **Liao Y, Cooper RS, Ghali JK, Szocka A.** Survival rates with coronary artery disease for black women compared with black men [published erratum appears in JAMA. 1993;269:870]. JAMA. 1992;268:1867-71.

28. **Franks PJ, Bulpitt PF, Hartley K, Bulpitt CJ.** Myocardial infarction and stroke during treatment of hypertensive patients with different diuretic regimes. J Hum Hypertens. 1991;5:45-7.

29. **Gurwitz JH, McLaughlin TJ, Willison DJ, et al.** Delayed hospital presentation in patients who have had acute myocardial infarction. Ann Intern Med. 1997;126:593-9.

30. **Willich SN, Lowel H, Lewis M.** Unexplained gender differences in clinical symptoms of acute myocardial infarction [Abstract]. J Am Coll Cardiol. 1993;21:238A.

31. **Raitt MH, Litwin PF, Martin JS, Weaver WD.** ECG findings in acute myocardial infarction: are there sex-related differences? J Electrocardiol. 1995;28:13-6.

32a. **Kudenchuk PJ, Maynard C, Martin JS, et al.** Comparison of presentation, treatment, and outcome of acute myocardial infarction in men versus women (The Myocardial Infarction Triage and Intervention Registry). Am J Cardiol. 1996;78:9-14.

32b. **Goldberg RJ, Modradd M, Gurwitz J, et al.** Impact of time to treatment with tissue plasminogen activator on mortality following acute myocardial infarction (The Second National Registry of Myocardial Infarction). Am J Cardiol. 1998;82:259-64.

33. **Dempsey SJ, Dracup K, Moser DK.** Women's decision to seek care for symptoms of acute myocardial infarction. Heart Lung. 1995;24:444-56.

34a. **Jackson RE, Anderson W, Peacock WT, et al.** Effect of a patient's sex on the timing of thrombolytic therapy. Ann Emerg Med. 1996;27:8-15.

34b. **Burke AP, Farb A. Malcolm GI, et al.** Effect of risk factors on the mechanism of acute thrombosis and sudden death in women. Circulation. 1998;97:2110-6.

35. **DeWood MA, Spores J, Notske R, et al.** Prevalence of total coronary occlusion during the early hours of transmural myocardial infarction. N Engl J Med. 1980;303:897-902.

36. **Eichner JE, Moore WE, McKee PA, et al.** Fibrinogen levels in women having coronary angiography. Am J Cardiol. 1996;78:15-8.

37. **Pohjola S, Siltanen P, Romo M.** Five-year survival of 728 patients after myocardial infarction: a community study. Br Heart J. 1980;43:176-83.

38. **Johansson S, Bergstrand R, Schlossman D, et al.** Sex differences in cardioangiographic findings after myocardial infarction. Eur Heart J. 1984;5:374-81.

39. **Legrand V, Deliege M, Henrard L, et al.** Patients with myocardial infarction and normal coronary arteriogram. Chest. 1982;82:678-85.

40. **Berglund U, Wallentin L, von Schenck H.** Platelet function and plasma fibrinogen and their relations to gender, smoking habits, obesity and beta-blocker treatment in young survivors of myocardial infarction. Thromb Haemost. 1988;60:21-4.

41. **Marmor A, Geltman EM, Schechtman K, et al.** Recurrent myocardial infarction: clinical predictors and prognostic implications. Circulation. 1982;66:415-21.

42. **Peter T, Harper R, Luxton M, et al.** Acute myocardial infarction in women: the influence of age on complications and mortality. Med J Aust. 1978;1:189-91.

43. **Stokes T, Wynn V.** Serum-lipids in women on oral contraceptives. Lancet. 1971;2:677-80.

44. **Katerndahl DA, Realini JP, Cohen PA.** Oral contraceptive use and cardiovascular disease: is the relationship real or due to study bias? J Fam Pract. 1992;35:147-57.

45. **D'Avanzo B, La Vecchia C, Negri E, et al.** Oral contraceptive use and risk of myocardial infarction: an Italian case-control study. J Epidemiol Community Health. 1994; 48:324-5.

46. **National Institute of Drug Abuse.** National Household Survey on Drug Abuse: Population Estimates—1991. Rev. ed. Washington, DC: Government Printing Office; 1992.

47. **Hollander JE, Hoffman RS.** Cocaine-induced myocardial infarction: an analysis and review of the literature. J Emerg Med. 1992;10:169-77.

48. **Minor R Jr., Scott BD, Brown DD, Winniford MD.** Cocaine-induced myocardial infarction in patients with normal coronary arteries. Ann Intern Med. 1991;115: 797-806.

49. **Lukas SE, Sholar M, Lundahl LH, et al.** Sex differences in plasma cocaine levels and subjective effects after acute cocaine administration in human volunteers. Psychopharmacology. 1996;125:346-54.

50. **Karch SB, Green GS, Young S.** Myocardial hypertrophy and coronary artery disease in male cocaine users. J Forensic Sci. 1995;40:591-5.

51. **Hollander JE.** The management of cocaine-associated myocardial ischemia. N Engl J Med. 1995;333:1267-72.

52. **Hollander JE, Burstein JL, Hoffman RS, et al.** Cocaine-associated myocardial infarction: clinical safety of thrombolytic therapy. Cocaine Associated Myocardial Infarction (CAMI) Study Group. Chest. 1995;107:1237-41.

53. **Hollander JE, Wilson LD, Leo PJ, Shih RD.** Complications from the use of thrombolytic agents in patients with cocaine associated chest pain. J Emerg Med. 1996; 14:731-6.

54. **LoVecchio F, Nelson L.** Intraventricular bleeding after the use of thrombolytics in a cocaine user. J Emerg Med. 1996;14:663-4.

55. **Stampfer MJ, Colditz GA.** Estrogen replacement therapy and coronary heart disease: a quantitative assessment of the epidemiologic evidence. Prev Med. 1991;20:47-63.

56. **Stampfer MJ, Colditz GA, Willett WC, et al.** Postmenopausal estrogen therapy and cardiovascular disease: ten-year follow-up from the Nurses' Health Study. N Engl J Med. 1991;325:756-62.

57a. **Grodstein F, Stampfer MJ, Manson JE, et al.** Postmenopausal estrogen and progestin use and the risk of cardiovascular disease. N Engl J Med. 1996;335:453-61.

57b. **Hulley S, Grady D, Bush T, et al.** Randomized trial of estrogen plus progestin for secondary prevention of coronary heart disease in postmenopausal women. JAMA. 1998;280:605-13.

58. **Gilligan DM, Quyyumi AA, Cannon RR.** Effects of physiological levels of estrogen on coronary vasomotor function in postmenopausal women. Circulation. 1994;89: 2545-51.

59a. **Kim-Schulze S, McGowan KA, Hubchak SC, et al.** Expression of an estrogen receptor by human coronary artery and umbilical vein endothelial cells. Circulation. 1996; 94:1402-7.

59b. **Vogel RA, Corretti MC.** Estrogens, progestins, and headache disease: can endothelial function define the benefits? Circulation. 1998;97:1223-6.

60. **Gisclard V, Flavahan NA, Vanhoutte PM.** Alpha adrenergic responses of blood vessels of rabbits after ovariectomy and administration of 17-beta-estradiol. J Pharmacol Exp Ther. 1987;240:466-70.

61. **Steinleitner A, Stanczyk FZ, Levin JH, et al.** Decreased in vitro production of 6-keto-prostaglandin F1-alpha by uterine arteries from postmenopausal women. Am J Obstet Gynecol. 1989;161:1677-81.

62. **ISIS-2 (Second International Study of Infarct Survival) Collaborative Group.** Randomised trial of intravenous streptokinase, oral aspirin, both or neither among 17,187 cases of suspected acute myocardial infarction. ISIS-2. Lancet. 1988;2: 349-60.

63. **Kannel WB, Sorlie P, McNamara PM.** Prognosis after initial myocardial infarction. The Framingham study. Am J Cardiol. 1979;44:53-9.

64. **Kannel WB, Thomas JT.** Incidence, prevalence and mortality of cardiovascular diseases in the heart, arteries, and veins. In: Hurst JW, ed. The Heart. New York: McGraw-Hill; 1986:557-65.

65. **GUSTO Angiographic Investigators.** The effects of tissue plasminogen activator, streptokinase or both on coronary-artery patency, ventricular function and survival after myocardial infarction. N Engl J Med. 1993;329:1615-22.

66a. **Gruppo Italiano per lo Studio della Streptochinasi nell'Infarto Miocardico (GISSI).** Effectiveness of intravenous thrombolytic treatment in acute myocardial infarction. Lancet. 1986;1:397-401.

66b. **Malacrida R, Genoni M, Maggioni AP, et al.** A comparison of the early outcome of acute myocardial infarction in women and men. N Engl J Med. 1998;338:8-14.

67. **Kannel WB, Abbott RD.** Incidence and prognosis of unrecognized myocardial infarction: an update on the Framingham study. N Engl J Med. 1984;311:1144-7.

68. **Woodfield SL, Lundergan CF, Reiner JS, et al.** Gender and acute myocardial infarction: is there a different response to thrombolysis? J Am Coll Cardiol. 1997;29:35-42.

69. **GISSI-2 Investigators, ANMCO and M Negri Institute, Italy.** Predictors of nonfatal reinfarction in survivors of myocardial infarction after thrombolysis: results from the GISSI-2 database. Circulation. 1993;88:I-490.

70. **Kornowski R, Goldbourt U, Boyko V, Behar S.** Clinical predictors of reinfarction among men and women after a first myocardial infarction. SPRINT (Secondary Prevention Israeli Reinfarction Nifedipine Trial) Study Group. Cardiology 1995;86:163-8.

71. **Held AC, Cole PL, Lipton B, et al.** Rupture of the interventricular septum complicating acute myocardial infarction: a multicenter analysis of clinical findings and outcome. Am Heart J. 1988; 116:1330-6.

72. **Naeim F, De la Maza LM, Robbins SL.** Cardiac rupture during myocardial infarction: a review of 44 cases. Circulation. 1972;45:1231-9.

73. **Dellborg M, Held P, Swedberg K, Vedin A.** Rupture of the myocardium: occurrence and risk factors. Br Heart J. 1985;54:11-6.

74. **Rasmussen S, Leth A, Kjoller E, Pedersen A.** Cardiac rupture in acute myocardial infarction: a review of 72 consecutive cases. Acta Med Scand. 1979;205:11-6.

75. **Radford MJ, Johnson RA, Daggett W Jr, et al.** Ventricular septal rupture: a review of clinical and physiologic features and an analysis of survival [Review]. Circulation. 1981;64:545-53.

76. **Zuanetti G, Latini R, Maggioni AP, et al.** Influence of diabetes on mortality in acute myocardial infarction: data from the GISSI-2 study. J Am Coll Cardiol. 1993;22:1788-94.

77. **Umachandran V, Ranjadayalan K, Kopelman PG.** Morbidity and mortality benefits in diabetics and the elderly [Abstract]. Eur Heart J. 1991;12:321.

78. **Abbott RD, Donahue RP, Kannel WB, Wilson PW.** The impact of diabetes on survival following myocardial infarction in men vs women: the Framingham Study [published erratum appears in JAMA. 1989;261:1884]. JAMA. 1988;260:3456-60.

79. **Singer DE, Moulton AW, Nathan DM.** Diabetic myocardial infarction: interaction of diabetes with other preinfarction risk factors. Diabetes. 1989;38:350-7.

80. **Margolis JR, Kannel WS, Feinleib M, et al.** Clinical features of unrecognized myocardial infarction–silent and symptomatic. Eighteen-year follow-up: the Framingham study. Am J Cardiol. 1973;32:1-7.

81. **McGovern PG, Pankow JS, Shahar E, et al.** Recent trends in acute coronary heart disease–mortality, morbidity, medical care, and risk factors. The Minnesota Heart Survey Investigators. N Engl J Med. 1996;334:884-90.

82. **Wilcox RG, von der Lippe G, Olsson CG, et al.** Trial of tissue plasminogen activator for mortality reduction in acute myocardial infarction. Anglo-Scandinavian Study of Early Thrombolysis (ASSET). Lancet. 1988;2:525-30.

83. **Stone GW, Grines CL, Browne KF, et al.** Comparison of in-hospital outcome in men versus women treated by either thrombolytic therapy or primary coronary angioplasty for acute myocardial infarction. Am J Cardiol. 1995;75:987-92.

84. **Grines CL, Browne KF, Marco J, et al.** A comparison of immediate angioplasty with thrombolytic therapy for acute myocardial infarction. The Primary Angioplasty in Myocardial Infarction Study Group. N Engl J Med. 1993;328:673-9.

85. **Bueno H, Vidan MT, Almazan A, et al.** Influence of sex on the short-term outcome of elderly patients with a first acute myocardial infarction. Circulation. 1995;92:1133-40.

86. **Stone PH, Muller JE, Hartwell T, et al.** The effect of diabetes mellitus on prognosis and serial left ventricular function after acute myocardial infarction: contribution of both coronary disease and diastolic left ventricular dysfunction to the adverse prognosis. The MILIS Study Group. J Am Coll Cardiol. 1989;14:49-57.

87. **Savage MP, Krolewski AS, Kenien GG, et al.** Acute myocardial infarction in diabetes mellitus and significance of congestive heart failure as a prognostic factor. Am J Cardiol. 1988;62:665-9.

88. **Smith JW, Marcus FI, Serokman R.** Prognosis of patients with diabetes mellitus after acute myocardial infarction. Am J Cardiol. 1984;54:718-21.

89. **Jacoby RM, Nesto RW.** Acute myocardial infarction in the diabetic patient: pathophysiology, clinical course, and prognosis. J Am Coll Cardiol. 1992;20:736-44.

90. **Vaccarino V, Krumholz HM, Berkman LF, Horwitz RI.** Sex differences in mortality after myocardial infarction: is there evidence for an increased risk for women? Circulation. 1995;91:1861-71.

91. **Moen EK, Asher CR, Miller DP, et al.** Long-term follow-up of gender-specific outcomes after thrombolytic therapy for acute myocardial infarction from the GUSTO-I Trial. J Women's Health. 1997;6:285-93.

92. **Pardaens J, Lesaffre E, Willems JL, De Geest H.** Multivariate survival analysis for the assessment of prognostic factors and risk categories after recovery from acute myocardial infarction: the Belgian situation. Am J Epidemiol. 1985;122:805-19.

93. **Maggioni AP, Franzosi MG, Santoro E, et al.** The risk of stroke in patients with acute myocardial infarction after thrombolytic and antithrombotic treatment. Gruppo Italiano per lo Studio della Sopravvivenza nell'Infarto Miocardico II (GISSI-2) and The International Study Group. N Engl J Med. 1992;327:1-6.

94. **Gruppo Italiano per lo Studio della Streptochinasi nell'Infarto Miocardico (GISSI).** Long term effect of intravenous thrombolysis in acute myocardial infarction: final report of the GISSI Study. Lancet. 1987;2:871-4.

95. **Becker RC.** Coronary thrombolysis in women. Cardiology. 1990;2:110-23.

96. **Ridker PM, Vaughan DE, Stampfer MJ, et al.** Endogenous tissue-type plasminogen activator and risk of myocardial infarction. Lancet. 1993;341:1165-8.

97. **Hamsten A, Wiman B, de Faire U, Blomback M.** Increased plasma levels of a rapid inhibitor of tissue plasminogen activator in young survivors of myocardial infarction. N Engl J Med. 1985;313:1557-63.

98. **Gebara OC, Mittleman MA, Sutherland P, et al.** Association between increased estrogen status and increased fibrinolytic potential in the Framingham Offspring Study. Circulation. 1995;91:1952-8.

99. **Koh SC, Yuen R, Viegas OA.** Plasminogen activators t-PA, u-PA and its inhibitor (PAI) in normal males and females. Thromb Haemost. 1993;66:581.

100. **Scarabin PY, Plu-Bureau G, Bara L, et al.** Haemostatic variables and menopausal status: influence of hormone replacement therapy. Thromb Haemost. 1993;70:584-7.

101. **Ridolfo B, Jamrozik KD, Hobbs MST.** Gender bias in management of myocardial infarction: prevalence and relevance to outcome [Abstract]. J Am Coll Cardiol. 1993;21:238A.

102. **Caro JJ, O'Brien JA, Holden-Wiltse J.** Why do women receive thrombolysis less often for acute myocardial infarction? [Abstract] Circulation. 1993;88:I-508.

103. **Pfeffer MA, Moye LA, Braunwald E, et al.** Selection bias in the use of thrombolytic therapy in acute myocardial infarction. The SAVE Investigators. JAMA. 1991;266:528-32.

104. **Varma VK, Murphy PL, Hood WP.** Are women with acute myocardial infarction managed differently from men? [Abstract]. J Am Coll Cardiol. 1992;19:20A.

105. **Maynard C, Althouse R, Cerqueira M, et al.** Underutilization of thrombolytic therapy in eligible women with acute myocardial infarction. Am J Cardiol. 1991;68:529-30.

106. **Chesebro JH, Knatterud G, Roberts R, et al.** Thrombolysis in Myocardial Infarction (TIMI) Trial. Phase I—A comparison between intravenous tissue plasminogen activator and intravenous streptokinase: clinical findings through hospital discharge. Circulation. 1987;76:142-54.

107. **Weaver WD, Wilcox RG, Morris D.** Women in GUSTO: baseline characteristics and effects of treatment regimen on mortality and complication rates [Abstract]. Circulation. 1993;88:I-508.

108. **Merx W, Dorr R, Rentrop P, et al.** Evaluation of the effectiveness of intracoronary streptokinase infusion in acute myocardial infarction: postprocedure management and hospital course in 204 patients. Am Heart J. 1981; 02:1181-7.

109. **Been M, de Bono DP, Muir AL, et al.** Coronary thrombolysis with intravenous anisoylated plasminogen-streptokinase complex BRL 26921. Br Heart J. 1985;53:253-9.

110. **Kasper W, Erbel R, Meinertz T, et al.** Intracoronary thrombolysis with an acylated streptokinase-plasminogen activator (BRL 26921) in patients with acute myocardial infarction. J Am Coll Cardiol. 1984;4:357-63.

111. **Kennedy JW, Martin GV, Davis KB, et al.** The Western Washington Intravenous Streptokinase in Acute Myocardial Infarction Randomized Trial [published erratum appears in Circulation. 1988;77:1037]. Circulation. 1988;77:345-52.

112. **Yarzebski J, Col N, Pagley P, et al.** Gender differences and factors associated with the receipt of thrombolytic therapy in patients with acute myocardial infarction: a community-wide perspective. Am Heart J. 1996;131:43-50.

113. **Gurwitz JH, Gore JM, Goldberg RJ, et al.** Recent age-related trends in the use of thrombolytic therapy in patients who have had acute myocardial infarction. National Registry of Myocardial Infarction. Ann Intern Med. 1996;124:283-91.

114. **McLaughlin TJ, Soumerai SB, Willison DJ, et al.** Adherence to national guidelines for drug treatment of suspected acute myocardial infarction: evidence for undertreatment in women and the elderly. Arch Intern Med. 1996;156:799-805.

115. **Krumholz HM, Murillo JE, Chen J, et al.** Thrombolytic therapy for eligible elderly patients with acute myocardial infarction. JAMA. 1997;277:1683-8.

116. **Kindwall KE.** Therapy for coronary heart disease in women. Cardiovasc Clinics. 1989;19:195-203.

117. **De Jaegere PP, Arnold AA, Balk AH, Simoons ML.** Intracranial hemorrhage in association with thrombolytic therapy: incidence and clinical predictive factors. J Am Coll Cardiol. 1992;19:289-94.

118. **Abu-Zeid HA, Choi NW, Nelson NA.** Epidemiologic features of cerebrovascular disease in Manitoba: incidence by age, sex and residence, with etiologic implications. Can Med Assoc J. 1975;113:379-84.

119. **Giroud M, Gras P, Chadan N, et al.** Cerebral haemorrhage in a French prospective population study. J Neurol Neurosurg Psychiatry. 1991;54:595-8.

120. **Bruno A, Carter S, Qualls C, Nolte KB.** Incidence of spontaneous intracerebral hemorrhage among Hispanics and non-Hispanic whites in New Mexico. Neurology. 1996;47:405-8.

121. **Nakayama T, Date C, Yokoyama T, et al.** A 15.5-year follow-up study of stroke in a Japanese provincial city. The Shibata Study. Stroke. 1997;28:45-52.

122. **Califf RM, Topol EJ, George BS, et al.** Hemorrhagic complications associated with the use of intravenous tissue plasminogen activator in treatment of acute myocardial infarction. Am J Med. 1988;85:353-9.

123. **Bovill EG, Terrin ML, Stump DC, et al.** Hemorrhagic events during therapy with recombinant tissue-type plasminogen activator, heparin, and aspirin for acute myocardial infarction: results of the Thrombolysis in Myocardial Infarction (TIMI), Phase II Trial. Ann Intern Med. 1991;115:256-65.

124. **Ryan TJ, Anderson JL, Antman EM, et al.** ACC/AHA guidelines for the management of patients with acute myocardial infarction: a report of the American College of Cardiology/American Heart Association Task Force on Practice Guidelines (Committee on Management of Acute Myocardial Infarction). J Am Coll Cardiol. 1996;28:1328-428.

125. **Lanter PL, Jennings CF, Roberts CS, Jesse RL.** Safety of thrombolytic therapy in normally menstruating women with acute myocardial infarction. Am J Cardiol. 1994;74:179-81.

126. **McCallister SH, Lips DL, Linnemeier TJ.** Thrombolytic therapy for acute myocardial infarction in actively menstruating women [Letter]. Ann Intern Med. 1993;119:955.

127. **Conti CR.** Is menstruation a contraindication to thrombolytic therapy? [Editorial]. Clin Cardiol. 1992;15:625-6.

128. **Kindwall KE.** Therapy for coronary heart disease in women. In: Douglas PS, ed. Heart Disease in Women. Philadelphia: FA Davis; 1989:195-202.

129. **Murdaugh CL, O'Rourke RA.** Coronary heart disease in women: special considerations [Review]. Curr Probl Cardiol. 1988;13:73-156.

130. **Hendel RC.** Myocardial infarction in women. Cardiology. 1990;2:41-57.

131. **Kannel WB, Abbott RD.** Incidence and prognosis of myocardial infarction in women: the Framingham study. In: Eaker ED, Packard B, Wenger NK, eds. Coronary Heart Disease in Women. New York: Haymarket Doymma; 1987:208-214.

132. **Litwin SE, Katz SE, Forman DE.** Gender differences in post-infarction left ventricular remodeling and function [Abstract]. J Am Coll Cardiol. 1995:130A.

133. **Kostis JB, Wilson AC, O'Dowd K, et al.** Sex differences in the management and long-term outcome of acute myocardial infarction: a statewide study. Myocardial Infarction Data Acquisition System (MIDAS) Study Group. Circulation. 1994;90: 1715-30.

134. **Ayanian JZ, Epstein AM.** Differences in the use of procedures between women and men hospitalized for coronary heart disease. N Engl J Med. 1991;325:221-5.

135. **Krumholz HM, Douglas PS, Lauer MS, Pasternak RC.** Selection of patients for coronary angiography and coronary revascularization early after myocardial infarction: is there evidence for a gender bias? Ann Intern Med. 1992;116:785-90.

136. **Behar S, Gottlieb S, Hod H, et al.** Influence of gender in the therapeutic management of patients with acute myocardial infarction in Israel. The Israeli Thrombolytic Survey Group. Am J Cardiol. 1994;73:438-43.

137. **Healy B.** The Yentl syndrome [Editorial]. N Engl J Med. 1991;325:274-6.

138. **Welty FK, Mittleman MA, Healy RW, et al.** Similar results of percutaneous transluminal coronary angioplasty for women and men with postmyocardial infarction ischemia. JAm Coll Cardiol. 1994;23:35-9.

139. **Khan JK, Rutherford BD, McConahay DR.** Why is the mortal risk of balloon coronary angioplasty increased in women [Abstract]? J Am Coll Cardiol. 1991;17:266A.

140. **Tyras DH, Barner HB, Kaiser GC, et al.** Myocardial revascularization in women. Ann Thorac Surg. 1978;25:449-53.

141. **Douglas JS, King SB, Jones EL, et al.** Reduced efficacy of coronary artery bypass in women. Circulation. 1981;64:11-6.

142. **Bolooki H, Vargas A, Green R, et al.** Results of direct coronary artery surgery in women. J Thorac Cardiovasc Surg. 1975;69:271-7.

143. **Loop FD, Golding LR, MacMillan JP, et al.** Coronary artery surgery in women compared with men: analyses of risks and long-term results. J Am Coll Cardiol. 1983; 1:383-90.

144. **James TN.** Anatomy of the coronary arteries in health and disease. Circulation. 1965;32:1020-33.

145. **Khan SS, Nessim S, Gray R, et al.** Increased mortality of women in coronary artery bypass surgery: evidence for referral bias. Ann Intern Med. 1990;112:561-7.

146. **Eaker ED, Kronmal R, Kennedy JW, Davis K.** Comparison of the long-term postsurgical survival of women and men in the Coronary Artery Surgery Study (CASS). Am Heart J. 1989;117:71-81.

147. **King KB, Clark PC, Hicks G Jr.** Patterns of referral and recovery in women and men undergoing coronary artery bypass grafting. Am J Cardiol. 1992;69:179-82.

148. **Rankin SH.** Differences in recovery from cardiac surgery: a profile of male and female patients. Heart Lung. 1990;19:481-5.

149. **Caracciolo EA, Davis KB, Sopko G, et al.** Comparison of surgical and medical group survival in patients with left main equivalent coronary artery disease: long-term CASS experience. Circulation. 1995;91:2335-44.

150. **ISIS-1 Collaborative Group.** Randomised trial of intravenous atenolol among 16,027 cases of suspected acute myocardial infarction. Lancet. 1986;2:57-67.

151. **Rodda BE.** The Timolol Myocardial Infarction Study: an evaluation of selected variables. Circulation. 1983;67:I101-6.

152. **Beta-Blocker Heart Trial Research Group.** A randomized trial of propanolol in patients with acute myocardial infarction. II. Morbidity results. JAMA. 1983;250: 2814-9.

153. **Beta-Blocker Heart Trial Research Group.** A randomized trial of propranolol in patients with acute myocardial infarction. I. Mortality results. JAMA. 1982;247:1707-14.

154. **Yusuf S, Peto R, Lewis J, et al.** Beta blockade during and after myocardial infarction: an overview of the randomized trials. Prog Cardiovasc Dis. 1985;27:335-71.

155. **Multicenter Diltiazem Post-Infarction Research Group.** The effect of diltiazem on mortality and reinfarction after acute myocardial infarction. N Engl J Med. 1988; 319:385-92.

156. **Held PH, Yusuf S, Furberg CD.** Calcium channel blockers in acute myocardial infarction and unstable angina: an overview. BMJ. 1989;299:1187-92.

157. **Koenig W, Lowel H, Lewis M, Hormann A.** Long-term survival after myocardial infarction: relationship with thrombolysis and discharge medication: results of the Augsburg Myocardial Infarction Follow-up Study 1985 to 1993. Eur Heart J. 1996; 17:1199-206.

158. **Pfeffer MA, Braunwald E, Moye LA, et al.** Effect of captopril on mortality and morbidity in patients with left ventricular dysfunction after myocardial infarction: results of the Survival and Ventricular Enlargement trial. The SAVE Investigators. N Engl J Med. 1992;327:669-77.

159. **Pfeffer MA, Braunwald E, Moye LA.** ACE inhibitors after myocardial infarction [Letter to the Editor]. N Engl J Med. 1993;328:968.

160a. **Schunkert H, Danser AH, Hense HW, et al.** Effects of estrogen replacement therapy on the renin-angiotensin system in postmenopausal women. Circulation. 1997;95: 39-45.

160b. **ACE Inhibitor Myocardial Infarction Collaborative Group.** Indications for ACE inhibitors in the early treatment of acute myocardial infarction: systemic overview of individual data from 100,000 patients in randomized trials. Circulation. 1998: 2202-12.

161. **ISIS-2 Collaborative Group.** Randomized factorial trial of high-dose intravenous streptokinase, of oral aspirin and of intravenous heparin in acute myocardial infarction. ISIS (International Studies of Infarct Survival) pilot study. Eur Heart J. 1987;8:634-42.

162. **Harpaz D, Benderly M, Goldbourt U, et al.** Effect of aspirin on mortality in women with symptomatic or silent myocardial ischemia. Israeli BIP Study Group. Am J Cardiol. 1996;78:1215-9.

163. **Yusuf S, Collins R, MacMahon S, Peto R.** Effect of intravenous nitrates on mortality in acute myocardial infarction: an overview of the randomised trials. Lancet. 1988;1: 1088-92.

164. **Tsuyuki RT, Teo KK, Ikuta RM, et al.** Mortality risk and patterns of practice in 2,070 patients with acute myocardial infarction, 1987-92: relative importance of age, sex, and medical therapy. Chest. 1994;105:1687-92.

165. **Wilkinson P, Laji K, Ranjadayalan K, et al.** Acute myocardial infarction in women: survival analysis in first six months. BMJ. 1994;309:566-9.

166. **Clarke KW, Gray D, Keating NA, Hampton JR.** Do women with acute myocardial infarction receive the same treatment as men? BMJ. 1994;309:563-6.

167. **Hannaford PC, Kay CR, Ferry S.** Agism as explanation for sexism in provision of thrombolysis. BMJ. 1994;309:573.

168a. **Antman EM, Lau J, Kupelnick B, et al.** A comparison of results of meta-analyses of randomized control trials and recommendations of clinical experts: treatments for myocardial infarction. JAMA. 1992;268:240-8.

168b. **Gottlieb SS, McCarter RJ, Vogel RA.** Effects of Beta-blockade on mortality among high risk and low risk patients after myocardial infarction. N Engl J Med. 1998; 339:489-97.

168c. **Krumholz HM, Radford MJ, Wang Y, et al.** National use and effectiveness of beta-blockers for the treatment of elderly patients after myocardial infarction. National cooperative cardiovascular project. JAMA. 1998;280:623-4.

168d. **Givgliano RP, Camargo CA, Lloyd-Jones DM, et al.** Elderly patients receive less aggressive medical and invasive management of unstable angina: potential impact of practice guidelines. Arch Intern Med. 1998;158:1113-20.

169. **Pagley PR, Yarzebski J, Goldberg R, et al.** Gender differences in the treatment of patients with acute myocardial infarction: a multihospital, community-based perspective. Arch Intern Med. 1993;153:625-9.

170. **Schwartz LM, Fisher ES, Tosteson ANA, et al.** Treatment and health outcomes of women and men in a cohort with coronary artery disease. Arch Intern Med. 1997; 157:1545-51.

171. **Stone PH, Thompson B, Anderson HV, et al.** Influence of race, sex, and age on management of unstable angina and non–Q-wave myocardial infarction. The TIMI III registry. JAMA. 1996;275:1104-12.

172. **Aronow WS.** Prevalence of use of beta-blockers and of calcium channel blockers in older patients with prior myocardial infarction at the time of admission to a nursing home. J Am Geriatr Soc. 1996;44:1075-7.

173. **Lau J, Antman EM, Jimenez-Silva J, et al.** Cumulative meta-analysis of therapeutic trials for myocardial infarction. N Engl J Med. 1992;327:248-54.

174. **Pepine CJ, Abrams J, Marks RG, et al.** Characteristics of a contemporary population with angina pectoris. TIDES Investigators. Am J Cardiol. 1994;74:226-31.

175. **Hochman JS, McCabe CH, Stone PH, et al.** Outcome and profile of women and men presenting with acute coronary syndromes: a report from TIMI IIIB. Thrombolysis in Myocardial Infarction (TIMI) Investigators. J Am Coll Cardiol. 1997;30:141-81.

176. **Sherman C, Litvak F, Grundfest W, et al.** Fiberoptic coronary angioscopy identifies thrombus in all patients with unstable angina [Abstract]. Circulation. 1985;72:III-12.

177. **Fuster V, Badimon L, Badimon JJ, Chesebro JH.** The pathogenesis of coronary artery disease and the acute coronary syndromes. N Engl J Med. 1992;326:310-8.

178. **Diver DJ, Bier JD, Ferreira PE, et al.** Clinical and arteriographic characterization of patients with unstable angina without critical coronary arterial narrowing (from the TIMI-IIIA Trial). Am J Cardiol.1994;74:531-7.

179. **Cairns JA, Gent M, Singer J, et al.** Aspirin, sulfinpyrazone, or both in unstable angina: results of a Canadian multicenter trial. N Engl J Med. 1985;313:1369-75.

180. **Theroux P, Ouimet H, McCans J, et al.** Aspirin, heparin, or both to treat acute unstable angina. N Engl J Med. 1988;319:1105-11.

181. **Goldschmidt-Clermont PJ, Schulman SP, Bray PF, et al.** Refining the treatment of women with unstable angina: a randomized, double-blind, comparative safety and efficacy evaluation of Integrelin versus aspirin in the management of unstable angina. Clin Cardiol. 1996;19:869-74.

182. **Swahn E, Wallentin L.** Platelet reactivity in unstable coronary artery disease. Thromb Haemost. 1987;57:302-5.

183. **Balsano F, Rizzon P, Violi F, et al.** Antiplatelet treatment with ticlopidine in unstable angina: a controlled multicenter clinical trial. The Studio della Ticlopidina nell'Angina Instabile Group. Circulation. 1990;82:17-26.

184. **Keelan ET, Nunez BD, Grill DE, et al.** Comparison of immediate and long-term outcome of coronary angioplasty performed for unstable angina and rest pain in men and women. Mayo Clinic Proc. 1997;72:5-12.

185. **Jacobs AK, Kelsey SF, Brooks MM, Faxan DP.** Better outcome for women compared with men undergoing coronary revascularization: a report from the Bypass Angioplasty Revascularization Investigation (BARI). Circulation. 1998;98:1279-85.

CHAPTER 17

Coronary Artery Bypass Grafting

Is It Worth the Risk?

RENEE S. HARTZ, MD

PAMELA CHARNEY, MD

In 1986, the Health Care Financing Administration (HCFA) released raw mortality data for coronary artery bypass grafting (CABG) by institution. Widespread misinterpretation of the data soon followed. Specifically, the conclusion that a "good CABG program should have a 2% operative mortality rate" became so prevalent that programs and individual surgeons with higher mortality rates were subjected to intense scrutiny. Some surgeons began to limit the number of very-high-risk patients offered CABG. Ironically, as is demonstrated in this chapter, for some high risk patients (many of whom are women), the benefit exceeds the operative risk. Although the HCFA data may have had a major impact on surgeons' practices, when assessed in a telephone survey of patients undergoing CABG in the past year, the effect of these reports on a patient's choice of surgeon was limited (1).

In response to the actions of the HCFA, the Society of Thoracic Surgeons (STS) developed a voluntary national database. Currently, data have been collected on almost a half-million surgical patients with isolated CABG without another simultaneous procedure (e.g., valve replacement). Analysis of outcomes in this large group of patients (2), coupled with numerous previous reports (3–8), leads to the conclusion that women have higher mortality rates and worse outcomes than do men, probably because the former are initially at higher risk. In this chapter, the indications and incidence of CABG are reviewed, followed by a discussion of risk factors affecting CABG performance and outcome.

Indications

Generally CABG provides a greater survival benefit than medical treatment in patients with proximal LAD (left anterior descending artery) disease (9–11) or in patients with three-vessel disease and decreased left ventricular (LV) systolic function (9,10). Either CABG or percutaneous transluminal coronary angioplasty (PTCA) provides similar survival benefit when diffuse coronary artery disease (CAD) and preserved LV systolic function are present (9).

Only in the past decade have gender patterns in referral for angiography and CABG been studied. Tobin and colleagues (12) noted in their follow-up of 390 consecutive patients referred for nuclear stress tests in 1982 and 1983 that only 4% of women with abnormal nuclear stress tests were referred for angiography compared with 40% of men with an abnormal nuclear stress tests. Khan and colleagues (6), in a retrospective review performed at a single teaching hospital from 1982 to 1987, found marked differences in the risk profiles of women and men with CABG. Women were significantly more likely to be ill with heart failure or unstable or post–myocardial infarction (MI) angina or to be symptomatic with less activity. In essence, these studies suggest that referral for revascularization in women is for severe and advanced symptomatology, whereas in men referral is more often because of an abnormal stress test. Although others have demonstrated similar findings (13), some studies of patients with established CAD have found conflicting results. For example, Krumholz and colleagues (14) found that after acute MI women underwent angiography and PTCA as often as men but CABG was performed significantly less frequently. After adjustment for patient age as well as disease severity, the differences in referral for CABG between women and men were of borderline significance only.

Incidence by Gender and Race

The percentage of women in most CABG series almost doubled in the early 1980s and then began to level off. Currently, in most data sets, one quarter of the patients having CABG is women. This figure may vary slightly depending on the referral base for the institution. The STS National Cardiac Database contained approximately 27% women in each year from 1991 to 1995 (15). Similarly, the University Hospital Consortium, a group of 26 teaching institutions, reported 26% women in their first CABG bench-marking project (16). In reports on CABG in elderly patients, however, the percentage of women is typically higher (46%) (17).

Race is another important predictor of the rate of CABG surgery. Although the overall 1986 Medicare national rate was 25.6 per 100,000 individuals, the rate was 27.1 per 100,000 for whites and 7.6 per 100,000 for blacks. Interestingly, gender differences in CABG surgery rates were more striking in whites than blacks. In whites, the rates for women and men were 16.2 and 40.4 per 100,000, respectively; in blacks, the rates were 6.4 and 9.3 per 100,000, respectively (18).

The association between race and CABG rates are greatest in the Southeast. Additionally, the number of practicing thoracic surgeons in the geographic area under study affects CABG surgery rates in whites but not in blacks (18).

Less information is available for other racial groups. When hospital discharge records from 1989 and 1990 were reviewed in the state of California, women of all ethnic groups received CABG less often than men and minority patients less often than whites (19). Even when controlled for age, diagnosis, and comorbidities, whites had 2.44 times the rate of CABG than that of blacks, 1.49 times than that of Latinos, and 1.09 times than that of Asians.

Unpublished STS data, made available for this chapter, include outcomes reported by gender and race for those patients entered in 1994 and 1995. Of the 201,365 patients with isolated CABG, 24.1% were white women, 64.8% were white men, 3.6% non-white women, and 7.5% non-white men (20).

Other Risk Factors

When comparing women and men, several factors have been examined in relation to CABG rates to postsurgical outcomes. The isolated importance of biologic age generally has been expanded to include review of comorbid conditions and functional status. The importance of body surface area and its relation to mature coronary artery size are discussed.

Age

In most reports, women undergoing CABG surgery are significantly older than men. This is expected because CAD generally presents 10 to 20 years later in women than in men (21). The mean age of patients in the STS database has been remarkably constant at 64.5 years from 1991 to 1995. Age and gender were available only for the 1994 to 1995 time period, during which women were significantly older than men (66.9 years and 63.6 years, respectively). At Emory University, the percentage of women older than 60 years of age in its CABG series increased from 45% in the mid-1970s to 77% in the late 1980s. A corresponding increase was seen in the men over 60 years of age from 29% to 60% (22). Similarly, in the Bypass Angioplasty Revascularization Investigation (BARI)—a randomized trial from 1988 to 1991 that compared

CABG and PTCA in symptomatic multivessel disease—the mean ages for women and men were 64 years and 60.5 years, respectively (23).

Comorbid Conditions

In analyzing survival of women and men in the Coronary Artery Surgery Study (CASS), Eaker and colleagues (3) reviewed 7384 patients operated on at 15 different surgical sites from 1975 to 1980 and followed them for an average of 6 years. When the baseline characteristics in women and men were compared, women were significantly more likely than men to be diabetic (15.0% vs. 10.6%), to be hypertensive (49.1% vs. 33.0%), and to have experienced heart failure (9.7% vs. 6.2%). Women were also more likely than men to have unstable angina and be in Canadian Class III (angina with minimal activity) or IV (angina at rest) (3). Similar findings were reported in a large series from Emory reported in 1993: 26% of women were diabetic, 61% were hypertensive, 10% were in heart failure, and 71% were in NYHA Class III or IV (22). These conditions were significantly more common in women than in men.

For patients entered into the STS database, patient characteristics significantly changed for both women and men from 1980 to 1990 when increasing numbers of women and elderly underwent CABG procedures (Table 17-1). When the data became available by gender (1994–95), it was seen that women

Table 17-1 Change in Profile of Society of Thoracic Surgeons Database: Patients (in Percent) Undergoing Coronary Artery Bypass Graft, 1980–90

Characteristic	1980	1990	p
Age (y)	58.50 ± 9.11	64.10 ± 10.20	< 0.001
Ejection fraction	0.62 ± 0.15	0.51 ± 0.14	< 0.001
Male	82.96	73.02	< 0.005
Female	17.04	26.98	< 0.005
Tobacco abuse	35.62	48.74	< 0.005
Diabetes mellitus	11.73	22.80	< 0.005
Hypertension	37.84	51.11	< 0.005
MI (< 21 d before CABG)	0.34	12.47	< 0.005
Cardiogenic shock	0.51	1.61	< 0.010
Unstable angina	28.51	47.84	< 0.005
Left main disease	6.93	11.70	< 0.005
First operation	98.12	92.99	< 0.005
Reoperation	1.88	7.01	< 0.005
Elective operation	95.89	81.78	< 0.005
Nonelective operation	4.11	18.22	< 0.005
Preoperative IABP	1.54	5.94	< 0.005

CABG = coronary artery bypass graft; IABP = intra-aortic balloon pump; MI = myocardial infarction.

Table 17-2 Society of Thoracic Surgeons National Cardiac Database, 1994–95: Characteristics of Patients (in Percent) by Gender

Characteristic	Male (72.2%)	Women (27.8%)	p
Preoperative renal failure	3.84	4.42	0.001
Preoperative hypertension	58.03	68.99	0.001
Elective status	64.33	59.11	0.001
Urgent status	26.47	29.46	0.001
Emergent status	8.20	9.98	0.001
Emergent/salvage	1.01	1.45	0.001
Use of internal mammary artery	76.43	65.05	0.001
Reoperative bleeding	2.23	2.24	0.867
Deep sternal infection	0.56	0.61	0.176
Permanent stroke	1.31	2.20	0.001
Prolonged ventilation	5.40	8.38	0.001
Postoperative renal failure	2.48	3.06	0.001
Postoperative dialysis dependency	0.77	1.07	0.001
Operative mortality	2.71	4.60	0.001
No. of distal anastomoses	3.49	3.21	0.001

were significantly more likely than men to have preoperative renal failure, diabetes, hypertension, and nonelective (i.e., urgent and emergency) operations (Table 17-2). However, compared with men, women who undergo CABG have had fewer previous myocardial infarcts and thus better LV function, fewer diseased arteries at the time of coronary angiography, and a lower incidence of significant left main stenosis until an advanced age (24).

Similarly, in BARI, women were not only older than men but also experienced more angina (67% vs. 61%) and had more comorbid medical conditions (29% vs. 23%). More women than men had congestive heart failure (14% vs. 7%), diabetes (31% vs. 15%), unstable angina (67% vs. 61%), hypertension (68% vs. 42%), and hypercholesterolemia (54% vs. 40%). Mean ejection fractions were higher in women than in men (59% vs. 57%), but women and men had a similar prevalence of ejection fractions less than 50% (21% vs. 23%) (23). Perhaps because of differences in patient selection, unlike with the STS data, the number of coronary arteries with significant disease (specifically left main disease) did not vary by gender.

Body Size and Coronary Artery Diameter

Women generally weigh less, are shorter, and have smaller body surface areas than do men; however, as illustrated in Figure 17-1, Christakis and colleagues (4) showed that women and men have similar body mass indices (body weight

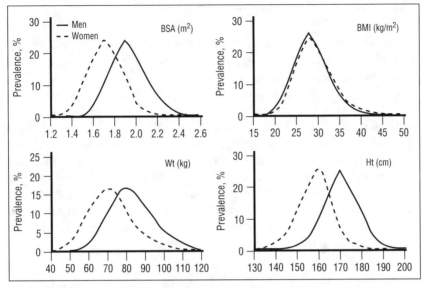

Figure 17-1 Weight, height, body surface area (BSA), and body mass index (BMI) for women and men. (From Christakis G, Weisel R, Buth K, et al. Is body size the cause for poor outcomes of coronary artery bypass operations in women? J Thorac Cardiovasc Surg, 1995;110:1344–58; with permission.)

in kilograms divided by height in meters). Although women have been found to have smaller coronary vessels than men (4,8,25), coronary artery lumen diameters generally have been related to body surface areas, not to body mass index.

One study showed strong correlation between probe-determined coronary diameter and median body surface area (5). These investigators measured coronary diameters in almost 1000 patients and found that all coronary artery diameters were smaller in women. The differences in size were significant for the mid-LAD, first diagonal, and obtuse marginal vessels, ranging from 2.3 to 1.66 mm diameter.

Technical Aspects

In this section, a discussion of preoperative conduit selection in women is followed by a review of the potential benefits of arterial rather than venous conduits, especially the use of the left internal mammary artery (IMA). Some preoperative issues are highlighted, followed by a discussion of minimally invasive CABG.

Preoperative Preparation

Preoperative preparation of any patient undergoing CABG should involve meticulous attention to the supply-to-demand ratio of the myocardium and a careful analysis of comorbid conditions and conduit selection. Women are more likely than men to be hypertensive and to exhibit diastolic dysfunction (4,6). Beta-blockers provide the greatest perioperative protection and should be used in the perioperative period whenever possible. Calcium-channel blockers may be useful for arterial spasm (26). Women are more likely than men to present with unstable angina, and every effort should be made to convert the angina to a more stable pattern by using intravenous nitrates and anticoagulants before surgery. Anxiolytic agents are probably underused in both women and men, although their use may contribute to lowering the blood pressure further, thus improving the supply-to-demand ratio.

Conduit Selection

Conduit selection is crucial in women and ideally planned preoperatively. The use of the IMA as a conduit (described later in this chapter) improves both short- and long-term outcomes. In the STS database (Tables 17-2 and 17-3), significantly fewer IMA grafts were performed in women than in men ($p = 0.001$). Non-white women received fewer IMA grafts than white women ($p = 0.001$). Women rarely receive arterial conduits, other than the IMA, as part of their revascularization. In most series of patients undergoing CABG, more women than men have diabetes, which essentially precludes the use of bilateral IMA grafts. The potential hazards include sternal wound complications (27).

Women have a higher incidence of varicose veins and previous vein stripping (25,28). In addition, women are more likely than men to have more peripheral vascular disease and, as noted previously, diabetes (2,25). All of these factors contribute to leg-vein wound complications. When required, duplex imaging of the entire saphenous system (greater and lesser) and of the inferior epigastric and radial arteries can be accomplished easily in the vascular laboratory or at bedside (Fig. 17-2). These conduit "maps" greatly assist the surgeon in planning the procedure, limiting incisions, and avoiding wound complications.

Minimally Invasive Technique

Recently, a new form of myocardial revascularization has emerged that occupies a position somewhere between PTCA and traditional CABG. Minimally

Table 17-3 Society of Thoracic Surgeons National Cardiac Database, 1994–95: Characteristics of Female Patients (in Percent) by Race

Characteristic	Non-White Women (3.6% of all patients)	White Women (24.1% of all patients)	p
Preoperative renal failure	48.37	34.55	0.001
Preoperative hypertension	78.34	68.14	0.001
Elective status	59.52	59.04	0.432
Urgent status	29.64	29.44	0.714
Emergent status	9.47	10.06	0.112
Emergent/salvage	1.37	1.46	0.514
Use of internal mammary artery	61.48	65.61	0.001
Reoperative bleeding	2.30	2.23	0.684
Deep sternal infection	0.78	0.58	0.044
Permanent stroke	2.35	2.18	0.323
Prolonged ventilation	9.98	8.13	0.001
Postoperative renal failure	3.56	2.98	0.006
Postoperative dialysis dependency	1.43	1.10	0.001
Operative mortality	5.13	4.51	0.017
No. of distal anastomoses	3.24	3.21	0.023

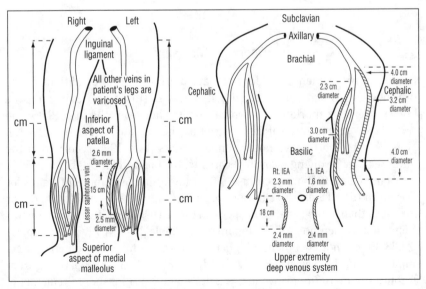

Figure 17-2 Lower and upper extremity deep venous systems.

invasive CABG is being performed in one of two ways: either with the intention of using cardiopulmonary bypass and endoaortic cross-clamping (port-access coronary artery bypass [PACAB]) or with the intention of avoiding cardiopulmonary bypass completely (minimally invasive coronary artery bypass [MIDCAB]). When these operations are successful, the recovery period is much shorter than with CABG. It is well known that a patent LAD or left IMA bypass to the LAD is a chief determinant of survival in patients with established CAD. The current goal of minimally invasive coronary artery surgery, as established by the Cardiovascular Surgery Council of the American Heart Association, is to achieve the same long-term results for IMA-LAD grafting as can be achieved with traditional methods. The Council feels that "the most likely future application of these newer procedures will be in patients with advanced coronary artery disease who are at high risk for surgery but who are known to have a survival benefit from the standard coronary bypass operation" (29).

No published data on women and MIDCAB exist. As has been reviewed in this chapter, the high risk patient is often female. A woman of tiny stature who is likely to die of low-output syndrome after traditional CABG or a woman who might not tolerate recuperation from a CABG may do well with an IMA to the LAD through a limited incision, because using an IMA graft will improve her survival. If necessary, symptoms can be reduced by PTCA of other stenoses.

Results

Operative Mortality

Because most women are older and have more comorbid conditions at the time of CABG, it is not unexpected that almost all surgical series document a higher operative mortality for women. In studies from the late 1970s and early 1980s, numerous authors arrived at the same conclusion (7,30–35). More recent reports have noted similar results. In a 1995 report from the CASS registry involving over 8000 patients, the operative mortality was 5.3% for women and 2.5% for men ($p = 0.001$) (36). Similarly, mortality rates for women in the STS database have been consistently higher than for men. For the more than 200,000 patients operated on in 1995, operative mortality was 4.60% for women and 2.71% for men (*see* Table 17-2). Only a few reports (23,28,36) did not document a higher operative mortality in women. For example, in an 11-year prospective study (1982–93) of 1487 patients from Toronto the mortality for women was 1.4% and 1.1% for men. Predictors of operative mortality in this series were urgent surgery, ejection fraction less than 40%, and age over 75 years (28). In the recent BARI trial, women and men after CABG had similar operative mortality (1.3% and 1.4%, respectively), postoperative MI (4.7% and 4.6%, respectively) as well as 5-year survival (87% and 88%, respectively) (23).

In the STS database population, 70 years of age seems to be the point at which there is a significant increase in operative mortality for all patients; 6.2% of these patients do not survive the operative period compared with only 2.4 % of patients younger than 70 years ($p < 0.005$) (37). Because older patients are more often women with comorbid conditions, the interaction of age and gender is especially important to explore. A group at Emory University analyzed the changing profile of patients undergoing CABG from 1974 to 1991 and concluded that the risk of death increased more in women than men because women were consistently older, had more emergency surgery and incidence of diabetes, and recently had more triple-vessel and left main CAD (22). According to Edwards and colleagues (37), who reviewed 10 years of STS data, each comorbid condition increases operative mortality significantly in univariate analysis (Table 17-4). Multivariate analysis is currently unavailable.

Complications of Surgery

Complications of surgery seem to be especially common in older, more afflicted women patients. After CABG, women reportedly have more strokes (5,22), postoperative hemorrhage (5,22), and heart failure (4,5,22). The STS database of the 1994 and 1995 data was analyzed by gender and demonstrated that both white and non-white women have more disabling strokes, prolonged mechanical ventilation, and postoperative renal failure than do men. The rates for prolonged ventilation and renal failure are greater in non-white women than in white women (see Table 17-3). In the BARI clinical trial, women after CABG were more likely than men to experience congestive heart failure or pulmonary edema (9.8% vs. 1.8%; $p < 0.001$).

The data relating to quality of life after surgery also reveal important gender differences in short-term recovery variables. Artinian and Duggan (38) demonstrated that within the first 6 weeks after surgery women had a slower recovery than men. Women reported more symptoms, including more difficulty with ambulation and depression in the immediate postoperative period. Similar findings were reported in a qualitative assessment by Moore (39), who described breast discomfort in female patients after CABG. Ayanian and colleagues (40) surveyed 454 CABG patients 6 months after surgery at one hospital. Before CABG, functional levels were more limited in women than in men; however, when scores were adjusted for age and severity of comorbid conditions, women reported similar or greater physical and psychosocial functioning than men after CABG (40).

Table 17-4   Univariate Analysis of the Effect of Preoperative Risk Factors on Operative Mortality After Coronary Artery Bypass Graft Surgery

Risk Factor	Mortality (%)		p
	With Risk Factor	Without Risk Factor	
Female gender	4.60	2.79	< 0.005
Smoking history	3.07	3.36	< 0.025
Diabetes mellitus	4.08	3.05	< 0.005
Hypertension	3.49	3.02	< 0.005
COPD	4.10	3.20	< 0.025
Previous CABG	7.14	2.94	< 0.005
MI (< 21 d before CABG)	7.26	2.52	< 0.005
Cardiogenic shock	23.07	2.97	< 0.005
Unstable angina	3.41	3.05	< 0.010
Intravenous nitrates	6.68	3.20	< 0.005
Elective operation	2.47	6.26	< 0.005
Nonelective operation	6.26	2.47	< 0.005
Single-vessel disease	2.65	3.20	< 0.050
Double-vessel disease	2.96	3.22	< 0.250
Triple-vessel disease	3.32	2.86	< 0.005
Left main disease	4.75	3.08	< 0.005
Preoperative IABP	9.53	2.84	< 0.005

CABG = coronary artery bypass graft; COPD = chronic obstructive pulmonary disease; IABP = intra-aortic balloon pump; MI = myocardial infarction.

Long-Term Outcomes

Although similar for women and men in clinical trials, long-term outcomes are generally worse for women in observational studies. In 1981, in a retrospective review at Emory University, women had a less thorough revascularization with fewer total grafts and no IMA grafts. Not surprisingly, it was demonstrated that women had less symptomatic relief from CABG (41). At a 21-month follow-up, only 53% of women were asymptomatic compared with 71% of the men ($p < 0.001$). Other authors have also reported women receiving fewer total grafts and fewer arterial conduits; women also have a shorter event-free survival time (8,42).

Gender-specific results are available from two clinical trials. Eaker and colleagues (3) reported on 6-year postoperative survival in the initial CASS report in 1989 and concluded that women and men had similar long-term survival rates. The authors hypothesized that older age, sedentary lifestyle, and the greater incidence of comorbid conditions in women were offset by the higher presurgical prevalence of previous MI and depressed LV function in men. In the BARI trial, mortality at 5.4 years of follow-up was similar in women and men regardless of whether they were randomly selected to receive CABG or PTCA (23). This is of particular interest because women had substantially more comorbid conditions and received less IMA grafts. In fact, when the Cox regression model was used to adjust for baseline differences between women and men, women who were randomly selected to receive an intervention (CABG or PTCA) had a significantly lower risk of mortality than men (relative risk, 0.6; 95% confidence interval 0.43–0.84; p = 0.003). No gender difference in the risk of death or MI was demonstrated.

Long-term quality of life after CABG surgery also has been examined recently. One year after CABG, women report postoperative depression more often than do men (43). Risk factors for depression included noncardiac chronic illness, postoperative fatigue, shortness of breath, and socioeconomic status. In a subgroup of BARI, post-CABG participants reported better ability to perform activities of daily living for the first 3 years than post-PTCA patients. However, no significant differences in functional ability at 4 and 5 years of follow-up were noted (44). Both physical and emotional function improved less in women than in men.

Special Considerations

The impact of diabetes on CABG outcome and the advantages of left internal mammary grafting are discussed in this section. The importance of body size and coronary artery size is then considered. Finally, historical data on estrogen therapy are reviewed.

Impact of Diabetes Mellitus on Outcome

Diabetes exerts a powerful independent effect on operative outcome in all age groups of both women and men, increasing operative mortality two- to fourfold (5,6,22). As noted earlier, women who require CABG are more likely to be diabetic. The perioperative mortality rate of nondiabetic patients in a prospective series of 3055 consecutive patients was 3.5%, 6.6% for diabetics on oral agents, and 10.8% for diabetics requiring insulin (45). Differences were significant even when adjusted for age, LV function, and other comorbid conditions. Diabetics in both the oral and insulin groups died most often of heart failure (45%), followed by arrhythmias, strokes, and pulmonary failure.

Review of two surgeons' clinical experience with a population in which 27% of the women had diabetes revealed that nondiabetic patients undergoing CABG had lower hospital mortality rates and greater probability of survival at 10 years (42). Female and male patients in this series were well matched for other attributes, except normal ejection fraction (55% and 44%, respectively). The overall mortality rates for women and men were 6.3% and 3.1%, respectively.

Although diabetic patients have higher mortality rates with CABG than do nondiabetics, those who require insulin therapy have improved long-term outcomes with CABG over PTCA. In a multicenter database, O'Keefe and colleagues (46) recently reviewed 15,809 patients, 12% of whom had diabetes. The two thirds of the diabetic patients who required insulin had a highly significant improvement in survival in both the PTCA and CABG arms of the study compared with those treated medically. Overall, CABG led to lower costs and longer life expectancy than did PTCA in diabetic patients (47,48). However, the 5-year survival difference between CABG and PTCA was not significant for diabetic women (83% and 72%, respectively; $p < 0.46$) but was for diabetic men (79% and 60%, respectively; $p < 0.001$) (23).

Diabetes is an important factor in the development of mediastinitis, sternal wound infection, and leg complications. Both sternitis and mediastinitis raise the operative mortality rate to at least 15% (15). In some hospital series, these two complications increase mortality rate in an extraordinary fashion. For example, the mortality rate of such patients is 60% at the Texas Heart Institute (49).

Impact of Left Internal Mammary–
Left Anterior Descending Artery Grafting on Outcome

Use of the left IMA as a bypass graft improves both short- and long-term results. This finding has been documented in several observational studies, including the CASS and STS databases. Review of IMA use in the CASS registry of over 5000 patients who were followed for over 15 years revealed that the 13% of patients who underwent an IMA graft to the LAD had both short- and long-term survival advantages (50). Results were similar in elderly patients, in those with impaired LV function, and in women and men. Long-term survival was consistently better for those with an IMA graft. A dramatic difference was observed at approximately 8 years after surgery, by which time venous grafts were more likely than IMA grafts to have occluded. Bergsma and colleagues (51) and Cooley (52) concluded that initial selection of conduit was an important predictor of survival. Figure 17-3 depicts the survival rates of patients with IMA grafts compared with those with vein grafts in this series. In a 10-year follow-up of patients with IMA grafts, 85% of patients were free of angina at 7 years (51).

More recently, short-term data have become available from the STS database. From 1987 to 1991 among the 38,586 patients entered in the STS database, operative mortality was 2.0% when the IMA was used and 4.5% when only saphenous veins were used ($p < 0.005$). Improved survival was seen in all patient subsets based on age, gender, ejection fraction, and operative priority.

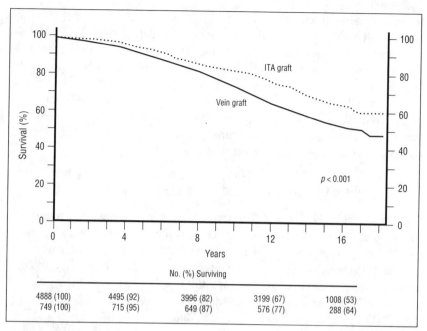

Figure 17-3 Estimated survival rates for patients with internal thoracic (internal mammary) artery bypass grafts and for those with vein grafts. (Reprinted with permission from Cameron A, Davis K, Green G, Schaff H. Coronary bypass surgery with internal thoracic artery grafts: effects on survival over a 15-year period. N Engl J Med. 1996;334:1–6.)

The only exception was in patients age 70 years and over who underwent a coronary reoperation (37).

In the CABG arm in the BARI randomized clinical trial, the rate of IMA graft was also lower in women than in men (72% and 85%, respectively) (23); however, CABG mortality outcome was similar (1.3% and 1.4%, respectively).

Several smaller studies have also observed benefit with IMA grafts usage in the elderly (53,54). At Johns Hopkins between 1980 to 1985, IMA grafts were used for only 11% of patients age 70 years or over. After 1985, IMA use in the elderly increased to 86%, with a decreased rate of hospital mortality, reduced surgical complication rates, and improved long-term survival (53). At Hahnemann University Hospital in Philadelphia, operative mortality and morbidity in octogenarians were similar regardless of the type of graft used; however, outcomes noted at 2 to 7 years of follow-up were better in the IMA group (54).

Despite these compelling indications for the use of arterial conduits, many surgeons still prefer to use only saphenous veins in older and sicker patients. In a retrospective review by Khan and colleagues (6), only 45% of women had IMA grafts compared with 64% of men ($p < 0.001$). Other authors have also noted fewer IMA grafts in women than in men (4,5). At Toronto General Hospital, Mickleborough (28) demonstrated that female gender is a predictor of IMA nonuse. The STS database also reveals that failure to use the IMA is significantly associated with both race and gender, with less use in women than in men and in non-white women than in white women (*see* Tables 17-2 and 17-3). Reasons implicated for IMA nonuse include "reluctance to dissect out the mammary artery in older women who had a soft, friable sternum at the time of sternotomy" (28), chronic steroid use (53), diabetes (28), and previous radiation (28).

Impact of Body Size and Coronary Artery Diameter

The impact of body size and coronary artery diameter has been frequently proposed as a reason for the worse outcomes noted in women (8,30,55); however, a causal relationship has never been established. Christakis and colleagues (4) attempted to answer the question in a prospective review of 7025 patients who underwent surgery from 1990 to 1994 and were then divided into quartiles based on height, weight, body surface area, and body mass index (BMI). Postoperative mortality did not differ between the highest and lowest quartiles in either gender. In every quartile, women had a higher incidence of mortality and low-output syndrome postoperatively. In men, the prevalence of low-output syndrome increased with decreasing body size. The same was not noted in women, but few women were in the highest quartile. The authors concluded that small body size may have contributed to low-output syndrome in both women and men. After adjustment for all other risk factors, female gender remained a significant predictor of operative mortality and low-output syndrome in this series. Interestingly, because IMA grafts were used less often in both genders when the body surface area was less than 1.79 m², this finding may have been a contributing factor to results in both women and men.

Obesity as a predictor of CABG outcome was evaluated prospectively in 11,101 consecutive patients undergoing CABG between 1992 and 1996 in Maine, New Hampshire, and Vermont. Patients were divided into nonobese (BMI ≤ 30), obese (BMI 31–36), and severely obese (BMI > 36). With increasing BMI, the percentage of women increased; women comprised 26% of the nonobese patients, 29% of the obese patients, and 41% of the severely obese patients. Although obesity was not associated with increased mortality, there was a substantially higher rate of serious sternal wound infections. There were also unexpectedly lower rates of re-exploration for bleeding in obese patients (55).

Coronary artery diameter may also contribute to operative technique and has been explored in several observational series. In a study of 220 patients undergoing arterial revascularization without another simultaneous procedure, Ramstrom and colleagues (25) explored reasons for use of arteries instead of venous grafts and found that the indication correlated with operative outcome. The number of arterial grafts used was similar across genders, but, for patients with "small vessel disease," operative mortality was significantly higher (7.8%) than for patients with "repeat CABG" (5.9%), "routine elective use" (0%), or "varicose/stripped saphenous veins" (0%). Small vessel disease (defined as "arteries smaller than 1 mm distal to a coronary probe, or smaller than 1.5 mm in conjunction with severe, diffuse disease distal to the anastomosis") was found in 30% of the study population. Women had a significantly higher incidence of small vessel disease in this series. At autopsy, all of the arterial grafts were patent but vein grafts were often closed, supporting the hypothesis that arterial grafts remain patent even with poor distal runoff. The authors concluded that small vessel disease or lack of venous grafts because of previous saphenous vein procedures represents special indications for multiple arterial bypass grafting.

O'Connor and colleagues (5) also observed that small arterial vessels increased the odds ratio for CABG operative mortality. For patients with a mid-LAD less than 2.5 mm, the odds ratio was 8.59 (confidence interval 95%, 1.16–63.81; $p = 0.036$). Even when adjusted for other risk variables, the odds ratio decreased to only 6.10. The increased risk of hospital mortality with a small LAD persisted, even when other variables (e.g., body surface area) were considered.

Impact of Estrogen Administration on Postoperative Outcome

Sullivan examined the relationship between postmenopausal estrogen therapy and survival in an observational study of 1091 women who underwent CABG. For the 92 women who received estrogens, the 5-year survival rate was 98.3% compared with 88.7% for nonusers. At 10 years, the difference was even more striking; 69.3% compared with 46.3%, respectively ($p < 0.001$) (56). There is a multicenter randomized trial in progress.

Discussion

The studies presented in this chapter confirm the long-standing clinical impression of the medical community that women undergoing CABG are at much higher operative risk than are men. They also clarify some of the reasons for this discrepancy.

Of the many risk stratification systems available for patients undergoing CABG, the STS database has been quoted often because it contains large numbers of patients and has the benefit of significant statistical power (57). Because it is composed largely of white male patients operated on in private practice settings (almost two thirds of the total number of patients), it contrasts with other studies from university centers where high-risk patients are routinely treated. Interestingly, the results from the latter seem to be more similar to STS data for female and non-white patients than to the white male group (*see* Table 17-2 and 17-3). These STS data demonstrate that white male patients are at lowest risk for mortality from CABG, non-white women are at highest risk, and the other two groups are somewhere in between. Examining the profiles of two typical patients undergoing CABG further emphasizes this point:

Mr. Jones, a white man aged 64 years with new onset angina pectoris, positive exercise stress test, triple-vessel CAD (70% proximal LAD, 75% circumflex, and 80% right coronary artery stenoses), and LV EF of 60% has a predicted operative mortality of 0.84%. Based on a recent Duke study designed to evaluate long-term survival benefits of CABG and PTCA compared with medical therapy, his chances of surviving 5 years are better with both CABG and PTCA than with medical therapy, but neither of the two interventional treatments has an advantage over the other in terms of long-term survival (11).

In comparison, Ms. Jackson, a black woman aged 73 years with hypertension, diabetes, unstable angina, pulmonary edema, two-vessel CAD (95% proximal LAD, 80% right coronary artery stenoses) and normal LV function has a predicted operative mortality three times that of Mr. Jones, but it is still only 2.57% (based on the older Bayesian method used by the STS database, into which priority of operation was not factored).

Since 1994, STS has begun to use a logistic model, in which priority of operation is part of the equation for operative outcome. The urgent nature of Ms. Jackson's surgery places her risk at 3.96%. If the operation were a true emergency (she must go immediately to the operating room from the catheterization laboratory or she would be likely to succumb), the risk is 6.76%. Ms. Jackson's chance of surviving 5 years is better with either form of interventional therapy than with medicine, but only with CABG is there an absolute survival advantage because her coronary artery lesions include a critical proximal LAD stenosis (11). In the recent BARI trial, survival was similar after CABG and PTCA for women with diabetes, although men with diabetes had lower mortality with PTCA (23).

The conclusion from the Duke data was that patients in all nine patient subgroups, with varying degrees of CAD severity, had better long-term outcome with interventional than with medical therapy (11). Patients with single-vessel disease, except for those with at least 95% proximal LAD stenosis, benefited from PTCA. Patients with three-vessel disease and those with two-vessel disease (including a 95% proximal LAD stenosis) benefited most from bypass surgery. Although the improvement in absolute survival was greatest for patients with three-vessel CAD who had CABG, the crucial distinctions in evaluating this information include 1) the definition of "severe" being a coronary stenosis greater than 75%, and 2) a 95% proximal LAD lesion representing a special situation in terms of prognosis.

> Mr. Jones presented in an early phase of his CAD. He has chronic stable angina but may desire CABG over PTCA because he cannot tolerate future limitations in lifestyle. He would do well with medical therapy or with PTCA but is considered an excellent candidate for CABG by the consulting surgeon.

> Ms. Jackson, who presented in an advanced state, has unstable angina and ischemic pulmonary edema. She and the surgeon really have little choice but to proceed with CABG because PTCA of the proximal LAD is risky and offers only short-term benefit in a patient with the type of anatomy she demonstrates.

One could argue, as many authors have in the past, that "age and acuity matching" negate the differences in operative mortality between the two genders. Mickleborough and colleagues' (28) study is an excellent example of gender matching and should serve as a benchmark. Unfortunately, this prospective series is relatively small (1487 patients) and, although there was a significant age difference in the genders, both women and men were young (62 years and 58 years, respectively) relative to the average age of patients in the U.S. population (67 years and 64 years, respectively). In addition, women in this study did not have the higher incidence of unstable angina and urgent operation usually seen in the United States but did have the advantages of better LV function and less severe CAD. Because the only predictors of operative mortality in the series studied by Mickelborough and colleagues were age greater than 75 years, depressed LV function, and need for urgent surgery, it is not surprising that there were no differences in operative mortality or complications of surgery between the two genders. Low mortality rates were achieved in women and men. When considering outcomes, the timing of the surgical procedure was critical.

Bickell and colleagues (58) determined in a historical cohort (1969–84) that women were less likely than men to be referred for CABG if the risk for operative mortality was low, but women were at least as likely as men to be referred if they had severe and advanced disease and a high operative mortality rate. In other words, among patients with little survival benefit from surgery, men are more likely to be referred and the reverse trend is observed in women. When the authors concluded that this "referral bias" actually may have resulted in a trend toward more appropriate treatment for women, they were echoing the sentiments of several earlier authors (6,12,13), all of whom felt that "perhaps men are referred too early and women too late."

Patterns of referral for CABG are not static, and temporal trends in CABG are being tracked. According to the STS database, the incidence of risk factors is increasing, whereas the observed operative mortality is remaining relatively constant at approximately 3% (57). Figure 17-4 graphically depicts the

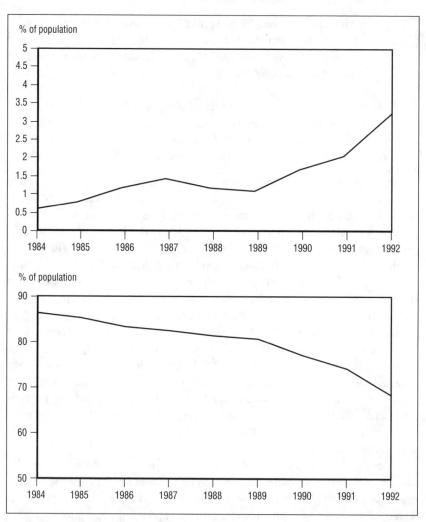

Figure 17-4 *Top,* Increasing trend of predicted high-risk (> 20%) coronary artery bypass graft patients in the Society of Thoracic Surgeons National Cardiac Database from 1984–92. *Bottom,* Decreasing trend of low-risk (0%–5%) coronary artery bypass graft patients in the Society of Thoracic Surgeons National Cardiac Database from 1984–92. (Reprinted with permission from Clark R. The Society of Thoracic Surgeons National Database Status Report. Ann Thor Surg. 1994;57:20–6.)

increasing incidence of high-risk patients and the decreasing incidence of low-risk patients entered into the STS database. However, Weintraub and colleagues (22), who reviewed 14,000 patients operated on at Emory University, demonstrated that "the population has changed and the prevalence correlates of in-hospital mortality have increased." At Emory, the overall mortality for women after CABG rate was 1.0% from 1974 to 1979 and 5.4% from 1988 to 1991 compared with the overall mortality for men (1.0% and 2.7%, respectively). The death rate in women could have increased to levels higher than that of men for several reasons. Perhaps women were older with more comorbid conditions (especially diabetes) or maybe they were often more ill and needed emergency surgery. Again, in contrast to those patients voluntarily entered into the STS database by private practice groups, this discrepancy undoubtedly reflects differences in referral patterns to Emory. However, in the BARI clinical trial, the unadjusted mortality rates for women and men were similar. After the Cox regression model was adjusted for baseline differences, women actually had better survival rates at 5 years (23).

Because it clearly has been determined that women are at greater risk for CABG complications, what factors in women are particularly worrisome to the cardiac surgeon? First is advanced age. Because women in the United States live at least 7 years longer than men (mean life expectancy of women is 80 years), the issue is increasingly relevant. By the year 2000, 6.2% of the population will be older than 80 and 40% of octogenarians will have cardiovascular disease (24). An observational CABG series of elderly patients documented advanced cardiac symptoms and multiple comorbid conditions but also an improvement in quantity and quality of life with surgery (53,54,59). However, more important than age is the patient's general health (including comorbid conditions) and whether the patient is being operated on for relief of symptoms or for prolongation of life. The point at which the chance of death or operative complications becomes too great is the real "cutoff age," whether that be 45 or 90 years. Octogenarians can be operated on at an acceptable risk, especially when the procedure is performed in an elective setting. Kaul and colleagues' (17) retrospective review of octogenarians at a single institution revealed a lower mortality rate in the 105 patients aged 80 years or over undergoing CABG (5.8%) compared with the 205 patients undergoing PTCA (8.6%). In very elderly patients, however, emergency CABG should be avoided because the operative mortality rate of such patients is 33% (59). Although nonstroke complications and a longer hospital stay were more prevalent after CABG, survival at 5 years was slightly better (66% CABG, 55% PTCA, $p < 0.01$).

The presence of multiple comorbid conditions is of particular concern to the surgeon. Commonly referred to as the "poor tissue" syndrome, especially when diabetes and peripheral vascular disease are present, it is predictive of poor outcome even in young patients. Both PTCA and CABG may have suboptimal results in patients with small vessels, diffuse disease, or both. Ramstrom and colleagues' (25) observation that diffuse CAD may represent a special indication for multi-arterial grafting deserves careful consideration. Recent reports of conduit use other than saphenous vein and IMA have appeared in the surgical literature. For example, the use of the radial artery as a conduit for CABG has resurfaced (60,61). Acar and colleagues (60) have demonstrated that pharmacologic dilation with calcium-channel blockers has resulted in a dramatic improvement in short- and long-term patency rates over those seen in the past. Finally, some patients should not undergo CABG at all but instead should be offered some other form of surgical therapy, such as transplantation, if there is associated congestive heart failure.

Summary

Although "risk stratification is the essence of the responsible cardiac surgeon" (57), it is also the referring physician's responsibility to inform the patient about the chances of surviving the procedure and how the patient might fare without CABG. Recent data provided by the STS database for this text confirm that, although gender and race are important in the risk-benefit equation for CABG, further efforts are required to clarify their impact.

Doctor John Kirklin has stated that "the greater the comparative benefit, the longer the duration of the comparative benefit, and the greater the absolute freedom from unfavorable events, the more compelling the indications for CABG" (9). His superb analysis of the natural history of ischemic heart disease, with and without CABG, is highly recommended. Similarly Davis and colleagues (36), in reviewing a group of patients with angiographically proven CAD in the CASS study, showed that "men and women with initial surgical treatment survived longer than those with medical treatment, although the benefits were clinically and statistically significant only in those at high risk." To paraphrase these authors, high-risk patients are those who need surgery the most, and CABG should not be denied when it offers improved long-term survival and can be accomplished at an acceptable mortality rate.

To answer the question posed in the title of this chapter, CABG is worth the risk for women who have appropriate indications (both anatomic and physiologic). Concern about potential surgical complications should not limit access to the benefits of CABG (62).

Newer therapeutic options, such as transmyocardial laser revascularization and minimally invasive coronary bypass surgery, may offer hope to those patients at extremely high risk for traditional bypass surgery performed with cardiopulmonary bypass and aortic cross-clamping. This group includes patients who are extremely small in stature and those who are very old with multiple comorbidities. Because both of these groups tend to be composed of women, we should rethink our traditional approach to revascularization but still keep in mind the fact that the risk-to-benefit ratio in these patients favors CABG more than for most patients undergoing the operation today.

REFERENCES

1. **Schneider EC, Epstein AM.** Use of public performance reports: a survey of patients undergoing cardiac surgery. JAMA. 1998;279:1638–42.

2. **Edwards FH, Carey JS, Grover FL, et al.** Impact of gender on coronary bypass operative mortality. Ann Thorac Surg. 1998;66:125–31.

3. **Eaker ED, Kronmal R, Kennedy JW, et al.** Comparison of the long-term, postsurgical survival of women and men in the CASS study. Am Heart J. 1989;117:71–81.

4. **Christakis G, Weisel R, Buth K, et al.** Is body size the cause for poor outcomes of coronary artery bypass operations in women? J Thorac Cardiovasc Surg, 1995;110:1344–58.

5. **O'Connor G, Morton J, Diehl M, et al.** Differences between men and women in hospital mortality associated with coronary artery bypass graft surgery. Circulation. 1993; 88:2104–10.

6. **Khan SS, Nessim S, Gary R, et al.** Increased mortality of women in coronary artery bypass surgery: evidence of referral bias. Ann Intern Med. 1990;112:561–7.

7. **Tyras DH, Barner HB, Kaiser GC, et al.** Myocardial revascularization in women. Ann Thorac Surg. 1978;25:449–53.

8. **Fisher LD, Kennedy JW, Davis KB, et al.** Association of sex, physical size, and operative mortality after coronary artery bypass in the Coronary Artery Surgery Study. J Thorac Cardiovasc Surg. 1982;84:334–41.

9. **Kirklin JW, Barratt-Boyes BG.** Stenotic arteriosclerotic coronary artery disease. In Cardiac Surgery. 2nd ed. New York: Churchill Livingstone; 1993:258–381.

10. **Yusuf S, Zucker D, Peduzzi P, et al.** Effect of coronary artery bypass graft surgery: overview of 10-year results from randomized trials by the Coronary Artery Bypass Graft Surgery Trialist Collaboration. Lancet. 1994;344:563–70.

11. **Jones R, Kesler K, Phillips H, et al.** Long-term survival benefits of coronary artery bypass grafting and percutaneous transluminal angioplasty in patients with coronary artery disease. J Thorac Cardiovasc Surg. 1996;111:1013–25.

12. **Tobin JN, Wassertheil-Smoller S, Wexler JP, et al.** Sex bias in considering coronary bypass surgery. Ann Intern Med. 1987;107:19–25.

13. **Ayanian JZ, Epstein AM.** Differences in the use of procedures between women and men hospitalized for coronary heart disease. N Engl J Med. 1991;325:221–5.

14. **Krumholz H, Douglas PS, Lauer MS, et al.** Selection of patients for coronary angiography and coronary revascularization early after myocardial infarction: is there evidence for a gender difference in the use of procedures? Ann Intern Med. 1992;116: 785–90.

15. **Society of Thoracic Surgeons Cardiac Surgery National Database Analysis.** Minneapolis: Summit Medical; 1996.

16. **University Hospital Consortium, Clinical Process Improvement.** CABG Clinical Benchmarking Database Project; 1996.

17. **Kaul T, Fields P, Wyatt D, et al.** Angioplasty versus coronary artery bypass in octogenarians. Ann Thorac Surg. 1994;58:1419–26.

18. **Goldberg KC, Hartz AJ, Jacobsen SJ, et al.** Racial and community factors influencing coronary artery bypass graft surgery rates for all 1986 Medicare patients. JAMA. 1992; 267:1473–7.

19. **Giacomini M.** Gender and ethnic differences in hospital-based procedure utilization in California. Arch Intern Med. 1996;156:1217–24.

20. **Society of Thoracic Surgeons National Cardiac Database, 1994–95.** Minneapolis: Summit Medical; 1996.

21. **Wenger NK.** Gender, coronary artery disease and coronary bypass surgery. Ann Intern Med. 1990;112:557–8.

22. **Weintraub WS, Wenger NK, Jones EL, et al.** Changing clinical characteristics of coronary surgery patients: Differences between men and women. Circulation. 1993;88:1179–86.

23. **Jacobs AK, Kelsey SF, Brooks MM, et al.** Better outcome for women compared with men undergoing coronary revascularization: a report from the Bypass Angioplasty Revascularization Investigation (BARI). Circulation. 1998;98:1279–85.

24. **Eaker E, Chesebro J, Sachs F, et al.** Cardiovascular disease in women. Circulation. 1988;88:1999–2009.

25. **Ramstrom J, Lund O, Cadavid E, et al.** Multiarterial coronary artery bypass grafting with special reference to small vessel disease and results in women. Eur Heart J. 1993; 14:634–9.

26. **Wenger NK.** Cardiovascular drugs: the urgent need for studies in women. JAMA. 1991; 46:117–20.

27. **Loop F, Lytle B, Cosgrove D, et al.** Sternal wound complications after isolated coronary artery bypass grafting: early and late mortality, morbidity, and cost of care. Ann Thorac Surg. 1990;47:179–87.

28. **Mickleborough L, Takagi Y, Murayama H, et al.** Is sex a factor in determining operative risk for aortocoronary bypass graft surgery? Circulation. 1995;90(Suppl II):80–4.

29. **Hartz R and the AHA Science Advisory and Coordinating Committee.** Minimally invasive heart surgery. Circulation. 1996;94:2669–70.

30. **Loop FD, Golding LR, Macmillan JP, et al.** Coronary artery surgery in women compared with men: analyses of risks and long-term results. J Am Coll Cardiol. 1983; 1:383–90.

31. **Bolooki H, Vargas A, Green R, et al.** Results of direct coronary artery surgery in women. J Thorac Cardiovasc Surg. 1975;69:271–7.

32. **Kennedy JW, Kaiser GC, Fisher LD, et al.** Clinical and angiographic predictors of operative mortality for the Collaborative Study in Coronary Artery Surgery (CASS). Circulation. 1981;63:793–802.

33. **Killen DA, Reed WA, Arnold M, et al.** Coronary artery bypass in women: long-term survival. Ann Thorac Surg. 1982;34:559–63.

34. **Hall RJ, Elayda MA, Gray A, et al.** Coronary artery bypass: long-term follow-up of 22,284 consecutive patients. Circulation. 1983;68(Suppl II):20–5.

35. **Gardner TJ, Hornefler PJ, Bott VL, et al.** Coronary artery bypass grafting in women. Ann Surg. 1985;201:780–4.

36. **Davis K, Chaitman B, Ryan T, et al.** Comparison of 15-year survival for men and women after initial medical or surgical treatment for coronary artery disease: a CASS registry study. J Am Coll Cardiol. 1995;25:1000–9.

37. **Edwards F, Clark R, Schwarz M.** Coronary artery bypass grafting: the Society of Thoracic Surgeons National Database experience. Ann Thor Surg. 1994;57:12–9.

38. **Artinian N, Duggan C.** Sex differences in patient recovery patterns after coronary artery bypass surgery. Heart Lung. 1995;24:483–94.

39. **Moore S.** A comparison of women's and men's symptoms during home recovery after coronary artery bypass surgery. Heart Lung. 1995;24:495–501.

40. **Ayanian JZ, Guadagnoli E, Cleary P.** Physical and psychosocial functioning of women and men after coronary artery bypass surgery. JAMA. 1995;274:1767–70.

41. **Douglas J, King S, Jones E, et al.** Reduced efficacy of coronary bypass surgery in women. Circulation. 1981;64(Suppl II):11–6.

42. **Carey J, Cukingnan R, Singer L.** Health status after myocardial revascularization: inferior results in women. Ann Thor Surg. 1995;59:112–7.

43. **Ai AL, Peterson C, Dunkle RE, et al.** How gender affects psychological adjustment one year after coronary artery bypass graft surgery. Women Health. 1997;26:45–65.

44. **Hlatky MA, Rogers WJ, Johnstone I, et al.** Medical care costs and quality of life after randomization to coronary angioplasty or coronary bypass surgery. N Engl J Med. 1997;336:92–9.

45. **James T, Quentin H, Birkmeyer J, et al.** Diabetes and coronary bypass graft surgery risk. Circulation 1996;94(Suppl I):2401A.

46. **O'Keefe J, McCallister E, Blackstone P, et al.** Is diabetes per se responsible for worse outcome after angioplasty than bypass surgery among diabetics? Am J Cardiol. 1997; 29(Suppl 2):181A.

47. **Bypass Angioplasty Revascularization Investigation (BARI).** Comparison of coronary bypass surgery with angioplasty in patients with multivessel disease. N Engl J Med. 1996;335:217–25.

48. **Bypass Angioplasty Revascularization Investigation (BARI).** Medical care costs and quality of life after randomization to coronary angioplasty or coronary bypass surgery. N Engl J Med. 1997;336:92–9.

49. **Wouters R, Wellens F, Venermen, et al.** Sternitis and mediastinitis after coronary artery bypass grafting: analysis of risk factors. Tex Heart Inst J. 1994;21:183–8.

50. **Cameron A, Davis K, Green G, Schaff H.** Coronary bypass surgery with internal thoracic artery grafts: effects on survival over a 15-year period. N Engl J Med. 1996;334: 1–6.

51. **Bergsma TM, Grandjean JG, Voors AV, et al.** Low recurrence of angina pectoris after coronary artery bypass graft surgery with bilateral internal thoracic and right gastroepiploic arteries. Circulation. 1998;97:2402–5.

52. **Cooley DA.** Coronary bypass grafting with bilateral internal thoracic arteries and the right gastroepiploic artery. Circulation. 1998;97:2384–5.

53. **Gardner TJ, Greene PS, Rykiel MF, et al.** Routine use of the left internal mammary artery graft in the elderly. Ann Thorac Surg. 1990;49:188–94.

54. **Morris R, Strong M, Grunewald K, et al.** Internal thoracic artery for coronary artery grafting in octogenarians. Ann Thorac Surg. 1996;62:16–22.

55. **Birkmeyer NJO, Charlesworth DC, et al.** Obesity and risk of adverse outcomes associated with coronary artery bypass surgery. Circulation. 1998;97:1690–4.

56. **Sullivan JM, El-Zeky F, Vander Zwaag R, Ramanathan KB.** Estrogen replacement therapy after coronary bypass surgery: effect on survival. J Am Coll Cardiol. 1994; 23:7A.

57. **Clark R.** The Society of Thoracic Surgeons National Database status report. Ann Thorac Surg. 1994;57:20–6.

58. **Bickell NA, Pieper KS, Lee KL, et al.** Referral patterns for coronary artery disease treatment: gender bias or good clinical judgment? Ann Intern Med. 1992;116:791–7.

59. **Williams D, Carrillo R, Traad E, et al.** Determinants of operative mortality in octogenarians undergoing coronary bypass. Ann Thorac Surg. 1995;60:1038–43.

60. **Acar C, Jebasa V, Carpentier A, et al.** Revival of the radial artery for coronary bypass grafting. Ann Thorac Surg. 1992;54:652–60.

61. **Dietl C, Benoit C.** Radial artery graft for coronary revascularization: technical considerations. Ann Thorac Surg. 1995;60:102–10.

62. **Hussain KM, Kogan A, Estrada AQ, et al.** Referral pattern and outcome in men and women undergoing coronary artery bypass surgery: a critical review. Angiology. 1998; 49:243–50.

CHAPTER 18

Percutaneous Transluminal Coronary Angioplasty

STEVE R. OMMEN, MD
DAVID R. HOLMES, JR., MD
MALCOLM R. BELL, MB, BS

Coronary artery disease (CAD) is the leading cause of death in women and men over 60 years of age (1). Sex-specific differences in the presentation of cardiac disease and possible differences in the outcome of coronary revascularization procedures have been noted (2). This has led to questions about the optimal application of current revascularization techniques in women. Early reports indicated higher complication rates and less success in women with respect to coronary artery bypass surgery (3,4). This trend was also observed for percutaneous transluminal coronary angioplasty (PTCA). Recent investigations have attempted to clarify whether this is caused by technical considerations, specific sex-related complications, or sex-bias in referral patterns. This chapter reviews referral patterns for angiography and angioplasty, safety and efficacy concerns in women (including early and late outcomes), and the use of angioplasty after acute myocardial infarction (MI).

Referral Patterns

A central question is whether women are as appropriately and aggressively referred for PTCA as men (Box 18-1). It is known that coronary artery disease is much less prevalent in women than in age-matched men (5-8); thus it would be expected that more diagnostic and therapeutic procedures are performed in men. It is also known that women present at an older age and have less

---

**Box 18-1 Characteristics of Women Referred for Percutaneous
Transluminal Coronary Angioplasty Compared with Men**

Older
Smaller coronary arteries
Higher prevalence of
    Congestive heart failure
    Hypertension
    Diabetes
    Hypercholesterolemia
    Comorbidity
    Severe angina
    Preserved left ventricular ejection fraction
Lower prevalence of
    Smoking
    Previous coronary artery bypass surgery
    Multivessel disease

---

multivessel disease despite more severe symptoms (5,9-14b). However, there is evidence that women are referred for coronary angiography and revascularization less frequently than men, even if the former have had a positive nuclear exercise test (15-17). Two studies showed that women hospitalized with CAD were less likely than men to have undergone previous diagnostic studies (15,16). Another study found that after adjusting for baseline characteristics and pretest probability of disease there was a similar referral pattern for both women and men (18). The evidence is conflicting with regards to referral for angiography and PTCA after acute MI (19,20a,20b). These observations may be the result of the patient's age, the physician's perceptions of the prevalence and severity of CAD in women, and questions about the reliability of diagnostic testing in women.

Once angiography has been performed and significant coronary artery disease is identified, the overall rate of referral for revascularization is similar for women and men. Data from 22,795 patients who underwent coronary angiography at Mayo Clinic showed that women were slightly more likely to have PTCA and men slightly more likely to have coronary artery bypass grafting (CABG) but that equal proportions of both sexes were referred for a revascularization procedure (9). Similar results were reported from two Canadian studies (21,22). The explanation for the differences in choice of revascularization method is not entirely clear but may be the result of the differing prevalence of multivessel disease, the perceived higher risk of CABG in women, differences in left ventricular function, a combination of the above, or some unknown factor.

There remain important differences between the men and women referred for PTCA. Women tend to have more severe angina but less extensive or severe obstructive coronary disease (5,9,10,12-14a). In the Bypass Angioplasty Revascularization Investigation (BARI) symptomatic patients with multivessel disease were randomized between CABG and angioplasty. Women and men participants undergoing angioplasty had similar numbers of lesions, but attempts of multilesion angioplasty occurred more in women and the success rate was higher for women than men (76% vs. 71%, $p < 0.01$) (23). Finally, women after initial PTCA required subsequent CABG less often than men.

Women undergoing PTCA generally are older and have more advanced cardiovascular risk profiles: a higher prevalence of hypertension, left ventricular hypertrophy, and diabetes mellitus. Women generally are smaller and have smaller coronary arteries (3,4,23). Other differences include more congestive heart failure despite better left ventricular systolic function in women. Women are also less likely to have had previous coronary revascularization.

One possible explanation for the increased severity of symptoms in women is that hypertension and left ventricular hypertrophy lead to small-vessel (nonepicardial) ischemia. Vascular reactivity is also known to be enhanced by estrogens and probably contributes to the delayed development of CAD in women (24a-25a). In a retrospective review of 428 postmenopausal women undergoing PTCA with an average of 22 months follow-up, estrogen users were younger, had slightly fewer diseased vessels, and had lower rates of MI and death, although the use of revascularization procedures was similar (25b).

Safety and Efficacy

A new area of concern was raised when the safety and efficacy of PTCA were found to be different for women compared with men. Data published from the initial National Heart, Lung, and Blood Institute's (NHBLI) PTCA registry revealed that PTCA was less successful technically and was associated with worse outcomes in women than in men (12). Several aspects of these findings need to be examined individually: technical success of the procedure, procedure-related complications, clinical improvement of symptoms, need for subsequent revascularization, and subsequent mortality.

Technical Success

There are multiple definitions of a successful PTCA, which increases the difficulty of comparing different studies. *Technical success* can be defined based on whether or not the angioplasty successfully reduced the degree of stenosis in the treated artery and by what magnitude. The success rate of PTCA has improved since the initial NHLBI report, which found technical success in less than 70% of cases, to a nearly 90% success rate in the more recent trials (10-14,26-28a). The statistically significant differences in success between the sexes reported in the NHLBI report have also been observed to vanish in later trials (Table 18-1). This can probably be attributed to increasing procedural experience and technical advances such as smaller, low-profile balloons and more responsive guidewires. These may be more beneficial in women and others with smaller arteries. At PTCA, the use of a bolus of Abciximab, a monoclonal antibody fragment against the platelet receptor α_{IIb}-β_3 integrin, improves outcomes initially and at three years of follow-up in women perhaps even more than in men (28b).

Early Outcome

In-hospital events and clinical success are also very important measures of the efficacy of PTCA (Table 18-2). Women who undergo PTCA have a significantly higher in-hospital mortality than men (10-12,14,26,27). The initial NHLBI report found that female sex, advanced age (> 60 years), and previous coronary bypass surgery were independent predictors of early mortality on multivariate analysis (12). The follow-up NHLBI series from 1985-86 also found female sex to be independently associated with mortality (26). Other studies have found that female sex is weakly independent or not independent after adjusting for age, body size (a surrogate estimation for coronary artery size), severity of symptoms, and/or multivessel disease (10,11,14,27). Conversely, a Northern New England regional study recently reported that even after adjusting for case-mix, women still had higher mortality after angio-

Table 18-1 Technical Success Rate of Coronary Angioplasty in Women Compared with Men

Author	N	Period	Success Rate (%)	
			Women	Men
Cowley et al (12)	3079	1977–81	60	66
McEniery et al (13)	3696	1980–86	93	94
Kahn et al (14)	9175	1992*	95	95
Kelsey et al (26)	2136	1985–86	84	87
Arnold et al (27)	5000	1980–88	94	93
Bell et al (11)	4071	1979–90	85	86
Weintraub et al (10)	10785	1980–91	91	90

*Year of publication.

Table 18-2   In-hospital Outcome After Percutaneous Transluminal Coronary Angioplasty

Author	Mortality (%)		Acute MI (%)		Urgent CABG (%)	
	F	M	F	M	F	M
Cowley et al (12)	1.8	0.7	5.7	5.5	6.5	6.6
Kahn et al (14)	1.4	0.8	1.7	1.4	1.6	1.6
Kelsey et al (26)	2.6	0.3	4.6	4.3	4.8	3.3
Arnold et al (27)	1.1	0.3	0.4	0.4	5.0	4.5
Bell et al (11)	2.0	1.0	1.1	2.0	4.6	3.6
Weintraub et al (10)	0.7	0.1	1.1	0.7	2.1	2.1

plasty than men (28a). This study was a very large, retrospective database of nearly all the PTCA procedures in the region (rather than the experience of a single institution). The investigators observed that, in addition to their own, only one other study had adequate statistical power to detect the differences in mortality observed in these trials (11,28a). Thus, there may be some small effect of sex on mortality, but this is poorly defined.

Neither the occurrence of acute MI after PTCA nor the need for urgent CABG has been found to have sex-specific differences. The Northern New England group did find more emergency (as opposed to urgent) bypass surgery in women (28a). The frequency of these outcomes appears to be decreasing for both sexes. In general, PTCA complications are more common in women (Table 18-3).

Complications specific to catheter-based coronary revascularization, such as coronary artery dissection, abrupt closure, spasm, and side-branch occlusions, also need to be considered when discussing the results of an intervention (28c). Two studies have reported significantly more coronary artery dissections in women, while a third showed a similar trend that was not statistically significant (12,13,26). There appears to be a trend of increased coronary occlusion, spasm, and side-branch compromise in women compared with men in these same reports.

The overall complication rate associated with PTCA appears to be unchanged or diminishing despite the procedure being used in higher risk patients as demonstrated in a comparison of the early and later NHLBI databases (26,29). Female sex was found to be an independent predictor of complication in this report (30). Noncardiac arterial complications (femoral artery pseudoaneurysm, peripheral emboli, retroperitoneal hemorrhage, etc.) are also more common in women (31-33). These complications may be related to the smaller arterial size in women, but this has not been formally investigated. The use of heparin in non–weight-adjusted doses in patients with acute MI appears to re-

Table 18-3 Complications of Percutaneous Transluminal Coronary Angioplasty

Author	Dissection (%)		Occlusion (%)		Spasm (%)		Branch Occlusion (%)	
	F	M	F	M	F	M	F	M
Cowley et al (12)	5.8	4.0	5.0	4.9	4.7	4.1	...	...
McEniery et al (13)	2.6	2.2	3.8	3.0	0.5	0.2	2.9	2.6
Kelsey et al (26)	6.8	4.5	6.0	4.3	1.5	1.0	1.8	1.8

sult in higher levels of anticoagulation in women and this may contribute to their increased vascular and bleeding complications (34).

Late Outcome

Factors that define the long-term success of angioplasty include survival, symptom improvement, the occurrence of restenosis, and the need for subsequent revascularization of the treated artery (Table 18-4). The report from the initial NHLBI cohort found that, once patients were discharged from the hospital, women had better survival than men (99.7% vs. 97.8%, $p < 0.05$) at a mean of 18 months after PTCA (12). A more recent study from the Cleveland Clinic with longer follow-up duration (48 months) also found male sex to be independently related to decreased long-term survival (27). The 1985-86 NHLBI registry (48-month follow-up) showed that late death was similar for men and women for the first couple of years but that the survival curves began to diverge near the end of the follow-up with higher cumulative mortality in women (10.8% vs. 6.6%, $p < 0.001$) (26). Two other studies found that sex was not independently associated with late survival (10,35).

Symptom improvement has varied but in general has been less in women. There was no sex-specific difference in the early NHLBI PTCA registry. Ninety percent of both men and women reported improvement at 18 months when need for subsequent revascularization was considered a symptom. However, men had a 10% higher frequency of repeat revascularization (CABG or PTCA); thus the nonrevascularization symptoms may have been more prevalent in women (12). Another study of similar follow-up duration (20 months) found that women, in comparison with men, had more chest discomfort before (82% vs. 77%) and after (42% vs. 28%) PTCA, less improvement in frequency (93% vs. 96%) or severity (89% vs. 94%) of symptoms, and more subsequent hospitalizations for chest pain (21% vs. 13%) (13).

Longer duration of follow-up revealed similar results with respect to symptom improvement. The 1985-86 NHLBI registry followed patients for 4 years and found that more men than women were free of anginal symptoms (81.8% vs. 70.3%) (26). Investigators at Emory University also showed more women

Table 18-4 Late Results After Percutaneous Transluminal Coronary Angioplasty

Author	Follow-up (mo)	Mortality (%)		Angina (%)		Restenosis (%)	
		F	M	F	M	F	M
Cowley et al (12)	18	0.3	2.2	10[†]	8	22	36
McEniery et al (13)	20	...	...	42	28	27	29
Kelsey et al (26)	48	11	7	30	18	...	...
Weintraub et al (10)	42	8[*]	5	40	27	...	...
Bell et al (35)	66	15	13	66	63	...	...

[*] 5-year estimate.
[†] Unimproved angina.

to have angina at 3.5 years of follow-up (40.2% vs. 26.7%) (10). A Mayo Clinic study with mean follow-up duration of 5.5 years confirmed more angina in women after PTCA (35). A subset of the Mayo Clinic data (611 patients followed for greater than 10 years) revealed no differences in the rates of recurrent severe angina (36).

The occurrence of MI was not different for women and men in any of these studies (10,12,13,26,35,36). Rates of subsequent revascularization procedures have been noted to be increased in men in some studies (10,12). The Mayo Clinic studies found that repeat PTCA was similar between the sexes but that subsequent CABG and overall revascularization occurred more often in men (35,36).

Restenosis rates have been reported from observational and subgroup analyses and generally show that there is either no difference or that women have less documented restenosis. Restenosis was more common in men in a subgroup follow-up angiographic study (22.4% vs. 36.2%, $p < 0.01$) (12). A subsequent study found no sex difference in restenosis rate (13). A Turkish study of risk factors for restenosis after successful PTCA found no sex-related differences in restenosis at 6 months, while hypertension and dyslipidemia were associated (37). Data from Belgium regarding the use of PTCA for restenosis found male sex to be predictive of second restenosis at 6 months (38).

There is also some retrospective evidence that estrogen replacement therapy in postmenopausal women may have a beneficial impact on events after PTCA. Estrogen therapy, compared with placebo, was associated with a lower frequency of death, nonfatal MI, or stroke (12% vs. 35%, $p = 0.001$) in a retrospective study of 337 women undergoing PTCA (39). Estrogen use remained independently associated with survival in multivariate analysis. Analysis of data from the Coronary Angioplasty Versus Excisional Atherectomy Trial (CAVEAT) revealed lack of estrogen use to be the strongest predictor of measure of restenosis in women undergoing atherectomy but not angioplasty (40).

Examination of combined endpoints generally shows that women fare better early after PTCA with increased difficulties with longer follow-up. Event-free, symptom-free survival (alive without angina, MI, or revascularization) was not different for men and women at 18 months but was better in men at 4 years (12,26). Event-free survival (alive without MI or revascularization but perhaps with symptoms) was better in women at 18 months (80% vs. 69%) but no different or slightly worse at more than 4 years (12,26,35). Analysis of rehospitalization rates after revascularization procedures among Medicare beneficiaries revealed that women had slightly more admissions for cardiac catheterization, subsequent revascularization, and other related events after index angioplasty (41).

Acute Myocardial Infarction

There is a known discrepancy in survival rates of men and women presenting with acute MI (42-45). Concerns that this difference may result from less aggressive application of therapy in women was raised by Krumholz et al, who reported that women were referred for diagnostic catheterization less frequently than men (22% vs. 36%) early after acute MI. However, this difference was not present after adjusting for age nor was there a difference in the rate of referral for angioplasty after diagnostic catheterization (20a). Similar results were observed in the Myocardial Infarction Triage and Intervention (MITI) registry (19) and two regional multicenter studies (46,47). Among patients undergoing direct PTCA for acute MI, women were older than men and less likely to have had previous revascularization (48).

The MITI data showed that survival was worse in women presenting with acute MI but no different than men once angioplasty (or thrombolysis) was performed (19). In a population-based analysis it was confirmed that survival after MI was not related to sex when patients were compared according to age (49). The Myocardial Infarction Data Acquisition System (MIDAS) study, based on discharge diagnoses in the state of New Jersey, found that cardiac catheterization was associated with lower mortality in both men and women. There was no significant difference between men and women once baseline variables and performance of catheterization were taken into account (47).

The efficacy of PTCA for acute MI was assessed in 670 patients. There were no sex-related differences in the need for repeat angiography, subsequent revascularization (PTCA and/or CABG) of the infarct-related artery, subsequent MI, or mortality over nearly 2 years of follow-up. Restenosis was less common in women (20% vs. 28%, $p < 0.05$) (48). Data from the Primary Angioplasty in Myocardial Infarction Study Group show that women receiving tPA (14% in-hospital mortality) did far worse than women treated with angioplasty (4% in-hospital mortality) and men treated by either means (2%–4% in-hospital mortality). However, tPA mortality in women occurred predominantly in those over 65 years old (50).

Newer Technology

Percutaneous catheter-based coronary revascularization has seen tremendous evolution in the past 20 years. With the introduction of newer technologies, the question of sex-related differences in success rates has again been raised. The risk of coronary artery perforation is increased with the newer devices, and women and the elderly appear to be at higher risk (51). One of the first reports on the newer devices found that women undergoing coronary atherectomy (directional, rotational, or extraction) tended to have more emergency surgical procedures and had a higher in-hospital mortality compared with men (52). Another group reported less technical success using atherectomy in women (53). Lower technical success rates (89% vs. 95%) and increased subsequent MI rates (5% vs. 0.4%) were found when directional atherectomy was investigated. Peripheral vascular complications also appear to occur more frequently in women (54,55). Multivariate analysis of another study of directional atherectomy found than when coronary artery size was entered into the model sex was no longer predictive of success (56). Restenosis was reported to be more common in men (57).

Coronary artery stents are used in a large number of clinical scenarios. Unfortunately, there are little data that provide insight to potential sex-related differences in their application and efficacy. Vessel size is a very important factor in determining which patients and/or lesions can be treated with coronary stents. Implantation of coronary artery stents was found to result in restenosis more often in men (36% vs. 7%), but subsequent experience has resulted in improved implantation and antiplatelet techniques since this report (58). Restenosis rates were similar, but technical success was lower (89% vs. 96%), while non–Q-wave MI and peripheral vascular complications were more common in women in a subsequent analysis (59).

Results from the Percutaneous Excimer Laser Coronary Angioplasty registry found that coronary perforation was more common in women and diabetic patients (60,61). The issue of arterial size is important for all the newer devices because they require larger peripheral access sites, larger guiding catheters, and larger delivery systems. These devices may cause more trauma to the peripheral and coronary vessels and thus may be the culprit in vascular complications.

In summary, catheter-based coronary artery revascularization procedures are performed at similar rates in women and men once obstructive lesions are identified. These procedures appear to carry slightly more risk in women, which may be related to differences in baseline characteristics such as age, comorbidity, and vessel size.

REFERENCES

1. Health, United States—1995 Chartbook. DHHS Pub. No. (PHS) 96-1232-1. Hyattsville, Maryland: U. S. Department of Health and Human Services, Public Health Service; 1996.

2. **Healy B.** The Yentyl syndrome. N Engl J Med. 1991;325:274-6.

3. **Fisher LD, Kennedy JW, Davis KB, et al.** Association of sex, physical size, and operative mortality after coronary artery bypass in the Coronary Artery Surgery Study (CASS). J Thorac Cardiovasc Surg. 1982;84:334-41.

4. **Loop FD, Golding LR, MacMillan JP, et al.** Coronary artery surgery in women compared with men: analysis of risks and long-term results. J Am Coll Cardiol 1983; 1:383-90.

5. **Chaitman BR, Bourassa MG, Davis K, et al.** Angiographic prevalence of high-risk coronary artery disease in patient subsets (CASS). Circulation. 1981;64:360-7.

6. **Janowitz WR, Agatston AS, Kaplan G, Viamonte M Jr.** Differences in prevalence and extent of coronary artery calcium detected by ultrafast computed tomography in asymptomatic men and women. Am J Cardiol. 1993;72(3):247-54.

7. **Kannel WB, Feinleib M.** Natural history of angina pectoris in the Framingham study: prognosis and survival. Am J Cardiol. 1972;29:154-63.

8. **Lerner DJ, Kannel WB.** Patterns of coronary heart disease morbidity and mortality in the sexes: a 26-year follow-up of the Framingham population. Am Heart J. 1986;111: 383-90.

9. **Bell MR, Berger PB, Holmes DR Jr., et al.** Referral for coronary artery revascularization procedures after diagnostic coronary angiography: evidence for gender bias? J Am Coll Cardiol. 1995;25:1650-5.

10. **Weintraub WS, Wenger NK, Kosinski AS, et al.** Percutaneous transluminal coronary angioplasty in women compared with men. J Am Coll Cardiol. 1994;24:81-90.

11. **Bell MR, Holmes DR Jr, Berger PB, et al.** The changing in-hospital mortality of women undergoing percutaneous transluminal coronary angioplasty. JAMA. 1993;269: 2091-5.

12. **Cowley MJ, Mullin SM, Kelsey SF, et al.** Sex differences in the early and long-term results of coronary angioplasty in the NHLBI PTCA registry. Circulation. 1985;71:90-7.

13. **McEnierny PT, Hollman J, Knezinek V, et al.** Comparative safety and efficacy of percutaneous transluminal coronary angioplasty in men and in women. Cathet Cardiovasc Diagn. 1987;13:364-71.

14a. **Kahn JK, Rutherford BD, McConahay DR, et al.** Comparison of procedural results and risks of coronary angioplasty in men and women for conditions other than acute myocardial infarction. Am J Cardiol. 1992;69:1241-2.

14b. **Jacobs AK, Kelsey SF, Brooks MM, et al.** Better outcome for women compared with men undergoing coronary revascularization: a report from the Bypass Angioplasty Revascularization (BARI). Circulation. 1998;98:1279-85.

15. **Steingart RM, Packer M, Hamm P, et al.** Sex differences in the management of coronary artery disease. N Engl J Med. 1991;325:226-30.

16. **Ayanian JZ, Epstein AM.** Differences in the use of procedures between women and men hospitalized for coronary artery disease. N Engl J Med. 1991;325:221-5.

17. **Tobin JN, Wassertheil-Smoller S, Wexler JP, et al.** Sex bias in considering coronary bypass surgery. Ann Intern Med. 1987;107:19-25.

18. **Mark DB, Shaw LK, DeLong ER, et al.** Absence of sex bias in the referral of patients for cardiac catheterization. N Engl J Med. 1994;330:1101-6.

19. **Maynard C, Litwin PE, Martin SJ, Weaver WD.** Gender differences in the treatment and outcome of acute myocardial infarction: results from the Myocardial Infarction Triage and Intervention (MITI) registry. Arch Intern Med. 1992;152:972-6.

20a. **Krumholz HM, Douglas PS, Lauer MS, Pasternak RC.** Selection of patients for coronary angiography and coronary revascularization early after myocardial infarction: is there evidence for a gender bias? Ann Intern Med. 1992;116:785-90.

20b. **Chandra NC, Ziegelstein RC, Rogers WJ, et al.** Observations of the treatment of women in the United States with myocardial infarction: a report from the National Registry of Myocardial Infarction-I. Arch Intern Med. 1998;158:981-8.

21. **Jaglal SB, Goel V, Naylor CD.** Sex differences in the use of invasive coronary procedures in Ontario. Can J Cardiol. 1994;10:239-44.

22. **Naylor CD, Levinton CM.** Sex differences in coronary revascularization practices: the perspective from a Canadian queue management project. Can Med Assoc J. 1993;149:965-73.

23. **Jacobs AK, Kelsey SF, Brooks MM, et al.** Better outcome for women compared with men undergoing coronary revascularization: a report from the Bypass Angioplasty Revascularization Investigation (BARI). Circulation. 1998;98:1279-85.

24a. **Reidel M, Rafflenbeul W, Lichtlen P.** Ovarian sex steroids and athersclerosis. Clin Invest Med. 1993;71:406-12.

24b. **Chester AH, Jiang C, Borland JA, et al.** Oestrogen relaxes human epicardial coronary arteries through non–endothelium-dependent mechanisms. Coron Artery Dis. 1995;6:417-22.

25a. **Gilligan DM, Badar DM, Panza JA, et al.** Effects of estrogen replacement therapy on peripheral vasomotor function in postmenopausal function in women. Am J Cardiol. 1995:75:264-8.

25b. **Abu-Halawa SA, Thompson K, Kirkeeide RL, et al.** Estrogen replacement therapy and outcome of coronary balloon angioplasty in postmenopausal women. Am J Cardiol. 1998;82:409-13.

26. **Kelsey SF, James M, Holubkov AL, et al.** Results of percutaneous transluminal coronary angioplasty in women: 1985-1986 National Heart, Lung, and Blood Institute's coronary angioplasty registry. Circulation. 1993;87:720-7.

27. **Arnold AM, Mick MJ, Piedmonte MR, Simpfendorfer C.** Gender differences for coronary angioplasty. Am J Cardiol. 1994;74:18-21.

28a. **Malenka DJ, GT OC, Quinton H, et al.** Differences in outcomes between women and men associated with percutaneous transluminal coronary angioplasty: a regional prospective study of 13,061 procedures. Northern New England Cardiovascular Disease Study Group. Circulation. 1996;94(9 Suppl):II–99-104.

28b. **Topol EJ, Ferguson JJ, Weisman HF, et al.** Long-term protection from myocardial ischemic events in a randomized trial of brief integrin beta-3 blockade with percutaneous coronary intervention. EPIC Investigator Group. Evaluation of Platelet IIb/IIIa Inhibition for Prevention of Ischemic Complication. JAMA. 1997;278:479-84.

28c. **OMeara JJ, Dehmer GJ.** Care of the patient and management of complications after percutaneous coronary artery interventions. Ann Intern Med. 1997;127:458-71.

29. **Detre K, Holubkov R, Kelsey S, et al.** Percutaneous transluminal coronary angioplasty in 1985-1986 and 1977-1981: the National Heart, Lung, and Blood Institute registry. N Engl J Med. 1988;318:265-70.

30. **Holmes DR Jr., Holubkov R, Vliestra RE, et al.** Comparison of complications during percutaneous transluminal coronary angioplasty from 1977 to 1981 and from 1985 to 1986: the National Heart, Lung and Blood Institute's Percutaneous Transluminal Coronary Angioplasty registry. J Am Coll Cardiol. 1988;12:1149-55.

31. **Omoigui NA, Califf RM, Pieper K, et al.** Peripheral vascular complications in the Coronary Angioplasty Versus Excisional Atherectomy Trial (CAVEAT-1). J Am Coll Cardiol. 1995;26:922-30.

32. **McCann RL, Schwartz LB, Pieper KS.** Vascular complications of cardiac catheterization. J Vasc Surg. 1991;14:375-81.

33. **Kent KC, Moscucci M, Mansour KA, et al.** Retroperitoneal hematoma after cardiac catheterization: prevalence, risk factors, and optimal management. J Vasc Surg. 1994;20:905-13.

34. **Granger CB, Hirsch J, Califf RM, et al.** Activated partial thromboplastin time and outcome after thrombolytic therapy for acute mycoardial infarction: results from the GUSTO-I trial. Circulation. 1996;93:870-8.

35. **Bell MR, Grill DE, Garratt KN, et al.** Long-term outcome of women compared with men after successful coronary angioplasty. Circulation. 1995;91:2876-81.

36. **Hasdai D, Bell MR, Grill DE, et al.** Outcome > 10 years after successful percutaneous transluminal coronary angioplasty. Am J Cardiol. 1997;79:1005-11.

37. **Gurlek A, Dagalp Z, Oral D, et al.** Restenosis after transluminal coronary angioplasty: a risk factor analysis. J Cardiovasc Risk. 1995;2:51-5.

38. **Piessens JH, Stammen F, Desmet W, et al.** Immediate and 6-month follow-up results of coronary angioplasty for restenosis: analysis of factors predicting recurrent clinical restenosis. Am Heart J. 1993;126:565-70.

39. **O'Keefe JH Jr, Kim SC, Hall RR, et al.** Estrogen replacement therapy after coronary angioplasty in women. J Am Coll Cardiol. 1997;29:1-5.

40. **O'Brien JE, Peterson ED, Keeler GP, et al.** Relation between estrogen replacement therapy and restensosis after percutaneous coronary interventions. J Am Coll Cardiol. 1997;28:1111-8.

41. **Lubitz JD, Gornick ME, Mentnech RM, Loop FD.** Rehospitalization after coronary revascularization among Medicare beneficiaries. Am J Cardiol. 1993;72:26-30.

42. **Kannel WB, Sorlie P, McNamara PM.** Prognosis after initial myocardial infarction: the Framingham study. Am J Cardiol. 1979;44:53-9.

43. **Puletti M, Sunseri L, Curione M, et al.** Acute myocardial infarction: sex-related differences in prognosis. Am Heart J. 1984;108:63-6.

44. **Tofler GH, Stone PH, Muller JE.** Effects of gender and race on prognosis after myocardial infarction: adverse prognosis for women, particularly black women. J Am Coll Cardiol. 1987;9:473-82.

45. **Greenland P, Reicher-Reiss H, Goldbourt U, et al.** In-hospital and 1-year mortality in 1,524 women after myocardial infarction. Circulation. 1991;83:484-91.

46. **Chiraboga DE, Yarzebski J, Goldberg RJ, et al.** A community-wide perspective of gender differences and temporal trends in the use of diagnostic and revascularization procedures for acute myocardial infarction. Am J Cardiol. 1993;71:268-73.

47. **Kostis JB, Wilson AC, O'Dowd K, et al.** Sex differences in the management and long-term outcome of acute myocardial infarction: a statewide study. Circulation. 1994;90:1715-30.

48. **Vacek JL, Rosamond TL, Kramer PH, et al.** Sex-related differences in patients undergoing direct angioplasty for acute myocardial infarction. Am Heart J. 1993;126:521-5.

49. **Orencia A, Bailey K, Yawn BP, Kottke TE.** Effect of gender on long-term outcome of angina pectoris and myocardial infarction/sudden unexpected death. JAMA. 1993;269:2392-7.

50. **Stone GW, Grines CL, Browne KF, et al.** Comparison on in-hospital outcome in men versus women treated by either thrombolytic therapy or primary coronary angioplasty for acute myocardial infarction. Am J Cardiol. 1995;75:987-92.

51. **Ellis SG, Ajluni S, Arnold AZ, et al.** Increased coronary perforation in the device era. Circulation. 1994;90:2725-30.

52. **Casale PN, Whitlow PL, Franco I, et al.** Comparison of major complication rates with new atherectomy devices for percutaneous coronary intervention in women versus men. Am J Cardiol. 1993;71:1221-3.

53. **Fishman RF, Friedrich SP, Gordon PC, et al.** Acute and long-term results of new coronary interventions in women and the elderly. Circulation. 1992;86(Suppl I):I-255.

54. **Bell MR, Garratt KN, Bresnahan JF, Holmes DR Jr.** Immediate and long-term outcome after directional coronary atherectomy: analysis of gender differences. Mayo Clin Proc. 1994;69:723-9.

55. **Moscucci M, Mansour KA, Kent KC, et al.** Peripheral vascular complications of directional coronary atherectomy and stenting: predictors, management, and outcome. Am J Cardiol. 1994;74:448-53.

56. **Movsowitz HD, Emmi RP, Manginas A, et al.** Directional coronary atherectomy in women compared to men. Clin Cardiol. 1994;17:597-602.

57. **Popma JJ, De Cesare NB, Pinkerton CA, et al.** Quantitative analysis of factors influencing late lumen loss and restenosis after directional atherectomy. Am J Cardiol. 1993;71:552-7.

58. **Foley JB, Penn IM, Brown RI, et al.** Safety, success, and restensosis after elective coronary implantation of the Palmaz-Schatz stent in 100 patients at a single center. Am Heart J. 1993;125:686-94.

59. **Fishman RF, Kuntz RE, Carrozza JP Jr, et al.** Acute and long-term results of coronary stents and atherectomy in women and the elderly. Coron Artery Dis. 1995;6:159-68.

60. **Bittl JA, Ryan TJ Jr., Keaney JF Jr., et al.** Coronary artery perforation during Excimer laser coronary angioplasty: the Percutaneous Excimer Laser Coronary Angioplasty Registry. J Am Coll Cardiol. 1993;21:1158-65.

61. **Baumbach A, Bittl JA, Fleck E, et al.** Acute complications of Excimer laser coronary angioplasty: a detailed analysis of multicenter results—coinvestigators of the U.S. and European Percutaneous Excimer Laser Coronary Angioplasty (PELCA) Registries. J Am Coll Cardiol. 1994;23:1305-13.

Chapter 19

Congestive Heart Failure

Ainat Beniaminovitz, MD
Donna M. Mancini, MD

Cardiac failure is the final common pathway for a variety of disease processes that affect the myocardium. Coronary artery disease and hypertension are the most common causes of heart failure; cardiomyopathy and valvular disease are less frequent causes. Diabetes predisposes to cardiac failure because of its association with accelerated coronary atherosclerosis and hypertension. Despite advances in treatments for the various causes that lead to heart failure, the incidence of congestive heart failure (CHF) is steadily increasing. Furthermore, because mortality from CHF remains high, CHF represents a significant cause of death for both women and men in the United States (1). Consequently, the possibility of gender differences in the incidence, etiology, prognosis, and therapeutic treatment of heart failure is important. Because coronary artery disease (CAD) constitutes the leading cause of CHF, most studies have focused on gender differences related to the development and treatment of ischemic heart disease. In this review, we not only summarize those findings but also address other data specifically related to heart failure.

Epidemiology

More than 2 million people in the United States are afflicted with heart failure; approximately 1 million are women. Approximately 400,000 new cases of CHF are diagnosed each year, with similar rates for women and men over 65 years of age. Congestive heart failure is a growing public health problem mainly because of the aging population and the increased incidence and prevalence of heart failure in the elderly. Furthermore, advances in the treatment of CAD (e.g., thrombolytic therapy) as well as improved hypertension and diabetes management have reduced mortality from coronary disease, thereby increasing the number of patients at risk for CHF. Over the past four decades, the incidence and prevalence of CHF have been increasing in both women and men (Fig. 19-1) (2,3).

The Framingham Study has provided much of the information on the natural history of the development of CHF in women and men (4). A 1993 report of this study included a 40-year follow-up from the serial examination of 9405 participants. During this period, heart failure developed in 321 women (6.4%) and 331 men (7.5%) (5). In subjects under 65 years of age, there was a slight male predominance, whereas in subjects over 75 years of age, there was a female predominance (Fig. 19-2). The Framingham investigators attributed this difference to the higher prevalence of CAD in men under 65 years of age. Even though the prevalence of coronary disease is higher in men, women are more likely to develop CHF after a myocardial infarction (MI) (4), which may explain the female predominance of CHF in the older age group.

Gender Differences in Prognosis

Once again, the Framingham Study has provided pivotal data about prognosis in patients with heart failure. In that cohort, the median survival time after

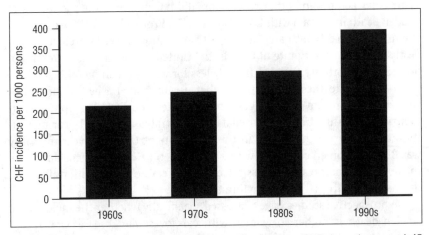

Figure 19-1 Estimated incidence of congestive heart failure (CHF) in patients aged 45 years and over by decade in the United States (1960s–90s).

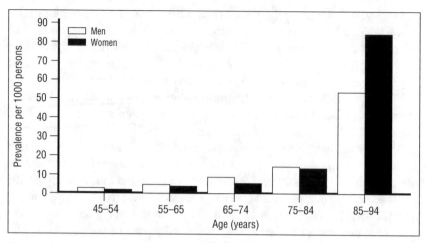

Figure 19-2 Prevalence of congestive heart failure in the United States by gender and age (Adapted from Kannel WB. Epidemiologic aspects of heart failure. Cardiol Clin. 1989;7: 1–9.)

the diagnosis of heart failure was better for women than men (3.2 years and 1.7 years, respectively). Five-year survival was also significantly better for women compared with men (38% and 25%, respectively) (5). The Framingham data suggested a gender-related difference in arrhythmogenic death. In this cohort, sudden death risk was higher in men with CHF; however, in women the sudden death risk associated with cardiac failure exceeded that associated with coronary disease without failure, whereas in men it did not. Adjustment for hypertension, electrocardiographic left ventricular hypertrophy, ventricular ectopy, and other risk factors did not diminish the excess risk of sudden death in women with CAD and CHF (1). From 1971 to 1975, data from the first National Health and Nutrition Examination Survey were used to investigate the mortality rate of CHF in the United States. In this data set, 10- and 15-year mortality was significantly less for women than men (6).

In contrast to these early studies that demonstrated a better survival in women, more recent data suggest the opposite. The SOLVD (Study of Left Ventricular Dysfunction) registry data demonstrated a higher 1-year mortality rate for women than men. In this 6271-patient cohort, 1-year mortality was 22% for women compared with 17% for men ($p < 0.001$). This difference in mortality was present across all causes of cardiovascular mortality, i.e., deaths from both CHF and arrhythmia (7).

No prospective studies have addressed specifically whether the incidence of sudden death is higher in women with cardiovascular disease. One recent large retrospective study of 355 consecutive survivors of out-of-hospital cardiac arrest (84 of whom were women; 271 were men) yielded important data about the sex differences in the epidemiology of sudden death and in the results of electrophysiologic testing in survivors of cardiac arrest (8). This study demonstrated that female survivors of cardiac arrest are less likely to have underlying CAD. The predictors of total and cardiac mortality also differed between female and male survivors. The most important predictor in women was CAD status, whereas the most important predictor in men was impaired left ventricular function. Furthermore, this and other studies have shown that female survivors of cardiac arrest with known CAD are less likely than men to have inducible ventricular tachycardia (9). Women are more likely than men to develop torsades de pointes during administration of antiarrhythmic drugs that prolong cardiac depolarization (10). These findings in conjunction with the Framingham and SOLVD data suggest an increased tendency towards arrhythmia and a greater risk for sudden death in women with cardiovascular disease. These findings in arrhythmogenesis also suggest that the biologic substrate between the sexes may be inherently different. Clearly, further studies are needed to elucidate these potential biologic differences.

In smaller single-investigator or single-center series, no difference in mortality between women and men with CHF could be detected (11,12). In our recent series of 467 ambulatory patients with CHF evaluated for heart transplantation, survival rates for women and men were similar (13). In a univariate analysis of the 268 patients (54 women, 214 men) at the Hospital of the University of Pennsylvania (HUP), women had a significantly increased survival by Kaplan–Meier analysis (log rank $\chi^2 = 5.48, p = 0.02$) This survival difference was not evident in our 199-patient cohort (37 women, 162 men) at Columbia Presbyterian Medical Center (CPMC). In a multivariate analysis with adjustment for ejection fraction, peak oxygen consumption (VO_2), presence of CAD, resting heart rate, mean arterial blood pressure, serum sodium, and presence of an intraventricular conduction delay (QRS > 20 ms), sex was no longer a significant prognostic variable at either institution (score $\chi^2 = 1.44, p = 0.23$ at HUP; score $\chi^2 = 2.18, p = 0.14$ at CPMC). The possibility that gender affects survival cannot be excluded completely by these data, given the overall small sample size. Over the past decade, another single-center study demonstrated that women with heart failure from nonischemic causes had significantly better survival rates than men with or without CAD (14).

Moreover, the United Network of Organ Sharing (UNOS) registry supports a similar finding of equivalent mortality rates among the sexes in heart failure. A compilation of the mortality data between 1996 for the UNOS 3564 wait-list candidates demonstrated an 18.8% mortality for the 831 women compared with a 21.6% mortality for the 2733 men on the list (UNOS Scientific Registry data as of April 8, 1997; UNOS transplantation information Web site).

Further evidence that overall prognosis in the modern era is worse for women with heart failure than for men comes from the National Hospital

Discharge Survey data from 1989. This report showed that the rate of hospital admissions with any discharge diagnosis of CHF was 8 in 1000 for women and 6.8 in 1000 for men (15). The diagnosis of CHF was made by general practitioners without any standard criteria; thus, the accuracy of the data is likely to be low compared with assessment by cardiologist or echocardiography. Nevertheless, these findings are concordant with findings from the SOLVD registry. Interestingly, among those participants in the Established Populations for Epidemiologic Studies of the Elderly (EPESE) cohort that were hospitalized with CHF, a lack of social support (as documented before admission) was an independent predictor of fatal and nonfatal cardiovascular events 1 year after discharge in women but not in men (16). Therefore, although earlier data suggested that mortality rates from heart failure were greater for men than for women, more recent data suggest similar or higher mortality rates for women.

Effects of Gender on Etiology

Coronary artery disease, hypertension, cardiomyopathy, and valvular heart disease are the most common causes of heart failure for both sexes. In the Framingham study, ischemic and hypertensive heart disease were the most common causes in women. Some current data reveal similar results (Table 19-1). The interventional SOLVD registry included 6271 patients (26% female). At entry, ischemic heart disease was the most common cause for both women and men followed by hypertensive heart disease. Interestingly, in SOLVD, women tended to have slightly less ischemic heart disease and more hypertensive heart disease than men (17).

Despite its lower prevalence in women, the fact that ischemic heart disease remains a major cause of CHF in women may be explained by the long-term prognosis data from the Framingham study. The data demonstrated that the incidence of CHF in the decade following a symptomatic acute MI was higher

Table 19-1 Heart Failure Etiology by Gender in the Framingham and SOLVD Registries

Etiology	Framingham (*n* = 652)		SOLVD (*n* = 6271)	
	Women (%)	Men (%)	Women (%)	Men (%)
Ischemic	27.0	46.0	51.0	65.0
Hypertensive	79.0	76.0	15.0	9.0
Valvular	3.2	2.4	7.5	6.2
Other	17.0	11.0	7.0	6.0

SOLVD = Study of Left Ventricular Dysfunction.

in women (4). Furthermore, numerous other epidemiologic and clinical studies have shown that short-term prognosis for women who have an acute MI is worse than for men (18–20). Despite the poor prognosis for women after an acute ischemic event, the rate of coronary angiography and revascularization after an acute MI is lower in women than men (21,22). Whether these gender-observed differences are caused by physician bias, referral bias, or complicating comorbidities (e.g., hypertension, diabetes, or CHF) at the time of acute MI presentation is unclear (23). Underdiagnosis of acute coronary syndromes (*see* Chapter 16) and underuse of effective therapies in women ultimately result in irreversible damage and development of CHF in this group.

Cardiomyopathy, another frequent cause of CHF, may result from a variety of factors, including hypertension; hypertrophy; and viral, alcoholic, and genetic causes. Sustained, increased afterload from hypertension increases the risk of cardiac failure threefold (24). In the Framingham study, hypertension was a frequent cause of CHF in women. A comparison of impacts of the various components of blood pressure on the incidence of cardiac failure once again delineates gender differences. Presence of systolic hypertension predicts future heart failure in women, whereas pulse pressure is more predictive in men (1).

Hypertrophic cardiomyopathy and diastolic dysfunction as causes of CHF are more prevalent in women than in men (25). Statistics from the National Center for Health reveal the incidence of hypertrophic cardiomyopathy to be 6% in women and 2% in men (26). The differential response of the female heart to pressure overload may account for the higher incidence of diastolic dysfunction in women. Using female and male rats, Malhotra and colleagues (27) described profound cardiac hypertrophy in female rats when subjected to renovascular hypertension and conditioning compared with the male rats. Other clinical data reveal an age-related increase in left ventricular mass in women but an age-related decrease in men (28).

Myocarditis as a cause of CHF occurs with similar frequency in both sexes. In a large multicenter trial of 214 biopsy-proven cases of myocarditis, the incidence of myocarditis in women and men was similar (29). In a smaller series of 27 patients with pathologic evidence of myocarditis, 12 patients were women (30). No differences in clinical features, histologic correlates, or clinical outcomes were observed between women and men. The incidence of autoimmune myocarditis, such as giant cell myocarditis, is also similar in women and men, with a fulminant course in young to middle-aged adults (31).

Chronic excessive consumption of alcohol can result in cardiomyopathy. Typically affected patients are men in the 30-to-55-year age group, who have a higher incidence of alcohol abuse than women (32). Excessive alcohol consumption is also associated with blood pressure elevation (*see* Chapter 9).

Postpartum cardiomyopathy (PPCM) is a cause of CHF that obviously occurs exclusively in women. Hormonal changes and volume overload are associated with pregnancy. (Later in this review we discuss the effect of sex hormones on cardiac function.) Postpartum cardiomyopathy has been theorized to be secondary to myocarditis, nutritional deficiencies, and hormonal and volume changes. The two leading suspected causes of myocarditis in PPCM are viral and immune factors (33,34). Hormonal alterations in pregnancy due to progesterone acting on T-cell expression may predispose certain pregnant women to myocarditis (35). Some investigators have reported enhanced maternal suppressor cell activity in human pregnancy (34).

Although familial cardiomyopathy generally tends to occur more frequently in men, several X-linked myopathies have been described, including Duchenne's and Becker's muscular dystrophies. X-linked myopathies that phenotypically affect both sexes may have distinct gender-specific clinical courses. In one such myopathy, described by Berko and Swift (36), affected men presented in their teens and early twenties with a rapidly progressive dilated cardiomyopathy that led to death within a year following symptom onset. In contrast, affected women developed clinical symptoms in their 40s, with a subsequent protracted clinical course that eventually lead to death. Recently, a variety of mitochondrial genetic defects involving respiratory chain enzymes have been described in patients with cardiomyopathy. These mitochondrial defects are maternally transmitted and are passed on equally to both genders (37).

Valvular heart disease represents a minor cause of heart failure in the general U.S. population. Whether acquired (rheumatic heart disease) or congenital, the prevalence of valvular disease and the incidence of progression to heart failure were found to be similar among women and men (38).

Women's Physiology and Gender Differences

Because muscular function is intimately associated with CHF, gender differences in muscle physiology may elucidate clinical gender differences in CHF. We examine the impact of estrogen and androgens on cardiac function, with special attention to factors that affect muscle function. Then some insights from exercise physiology are presented.

Impact of Sex Hormones on Cardiac Function

Differences in the natural history of some cardiovascular disorders in women and men may reflect inherent biology- or hormone-mediated gender differences (Fig. 19-3). Animal studies using hormone replacement have helped to

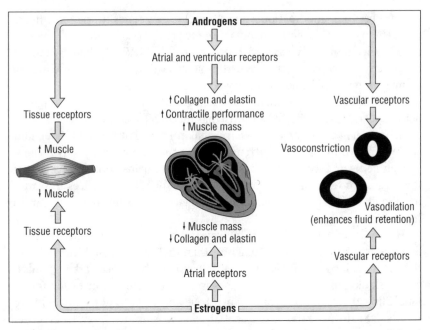

Figure 19-3 Different biological effects of androgens and estrogens on myocardial and vascular tissue.

delineate the effect of sex hormones. Direct and indirect effects on cardiac function result from sex hormones (39). Estrogen and androgen receptors located in blood vessels may contribute to the differences in vasoreactivity in women and men. These vascular hormone receptors may affect fluid status and blood pressure (40). Sex hormone receptors are also present in the heart. Androgen receptors are located in both atrial and ventricular tissue, whereas estradiol receptors are located only in atrial tissue. The rate of deposition of collagen and elastin in the myocardium is also influenced by sex hormones. Estradiol decreases the rate of collagen deposition, whereas androgens increase it (41,42). Myosin heavy chains and protein expression in the heart are also influenced by sex hormones. The differential effects of sex hormones on cardiac and vascular tissue may explain in part the gender differences in the incidence and sequelae of hypertension and CAD. It has been postulated that women are more prone to ventricular rupture after MI because of the decreased collagen deposition promoted by estrogens.

The effects of sex hormones on myocardial contractile performance have not been well studied. Myocardial contractile performances of female and male rats of the same age and similar left ventricular size have been compared. All indices of cardiac performance (i.e., stroke work, cardiac output, ejection fraction, and fractional shortening) were greater in the male hearts (43). The mechanical performance of the heart in gonadectomized and hormone-repleted animals has also been described (44,45). In both sexes, gonadectomy decreased contractile performance, with a greater decline in male animals. Interestingly, gonadectomy decreased heart weight in male animals only. Testosterone replacement increased cardiac mass and body weight in both genders. It also improved ventricular mechanical performance.

Echocardiographic analyses in normal men and women have demonstrated uniformly that left ventricular mass and chamber size are reduced in women compared with men. This relationship remains constant even when the data are normalized to body surface area (46,47). Differences in cardiac mass undoubtedly reflect differences in the effect of sex hormones on cardiac tissue.

The ability of the female heart to hypertrophy in response to increased cardiovascular loads may also be different than that of the male heart. Because the hypertrophic response is a key mechanism by which the heart responds to overwork or injury, gender differences in this response are critically important. Clinical data suggest that women have an exaggerated hypertrophic response (48). In patients with essential hypertension, the prevalence of left ventricular hypertrophy is greater in women than in men. Hypertrophic cardiomyopathy and diastolic dysfunction are more prevalent in women. Data also support an excessive hypertrophic response following pressure overload in female animals as compared with male animals. As discussed previously, cardiac mass increased by 46% in female rats compared with only 14% in their male counterparts when exposed to renovascular hypertension (39).

Gender Differences in Exercise Performance

The study of exercise physiology and performance has begun to define important gender differences. Peak Vo_2 is approximately 10% to 15% lower in women than in men, even when adjusted for age and body mass (49). Generally, this is attributed to the lower oxygen delivery of women because of their lower hemoglobin concentration and smaller blood volume. Differences between the genders in hemoglobin, blood volume, and muscle mass result largely from the effects of sex hormones.

Few studies have compared in detail the exercise performance of women and men. In studies using radionucleotide ventriculography, Sullivan and colleagues (50) demonstrated that though normal unconditioned men increased their ejection fraction significantly during upright bicycle exercise, female subjects had a flat response. Stroke volume increased to a similar degree in both sexes, but in women this was achieved through a 30% increase in end-diastolic volume. In contrast, men had no change in end-diastolic volume with exercise. Women are thus more reliant on the Frank–Starling mechanism to increase cardiac output during exercise, whereas men seem to have a greater contractile response.

Not unexpectedly, we and others have demonstrated that peak Vo_2 is lower in women than in men with heart failure. In 386 patients with heart failure referred for transplant evaluation, peak Vo_2 averaged 10.7 ml/kg/min for the 91 women and 12.9 mL/kg/min for the 295 men ($p < 0.01$) (51). In a recent multicenter study of 65 women and 238 men with dilated cardiomyopathy, exercise duration was found to be shorter in women than in men (7 ± 3 min vs. 10 ± 4 min; $p < 0.001$) (52). To our knowledge, no exercise hemodynamic studies specifically have compared women and men with CHF; however, during exercise, patients with CHF have only a minimal or no rise in ejection fraction. For women, exercise does not alter the ejection fraction, regardless of the absence or presence of CHF. In contrast, men without CHF increase their ejection fraction with exercise, whereas those with CHF cannot. This represents a real change in normal physiology in men, whereas in women it does not.

The exercise response also provides important prognostic information. We and others have consistently demonstrated that peak Vo_2 is an independent prognostic variable in heart failure (53). It is increasingly used as a key variable for therapeutic decisions, such as identification of cardiac transplant candidacy. The power of this variable may be diminished in women. Indeed, in an analysis of 272 patients, we demonstrated that absolute Vo_2 was less effective as a predictive parameter in women compared with men (54). For men, absolute or weight-normalized Vo_2 and percentage of predicted maximal Vo_2 were equally good predictors of survival (Cox model $\chi^2 = 18.725$ and 18.516, respectively). Among women, however, absolute Vo_2 did not achieve statistical significance as a predictor of survival; rather a percentage of predicted maximal Vo_2 was a better predictor (Cox model $\chi^2 = 4.876$; $p = 0.04$). This may be due to the fact that the difference between absolute and predicted Vo_2 is not as large in women as in men; therefore, using an absolute number may not have the same predictive value for women. Stelken and colleagues (55) similarly found that the percentage of predicted maximal Vo_2 had better predictive prognostic value than absolute peak Vo_2 in female patients with CHF.

Diagnostic Evaluation

Although represented in different proportions, the causes of heart failure are the same for both sexes; therefore, the diagnostic work-up for women and men is the same. The American College of Cardiology–American Heart Association Task Force recommended routine diagnostic studies for adult patients with chronic heart failure. These study recommendations include standard laboratory tests, thyroid function tests (in patients with atrial fibrillation and unexplained CHF), chest radiography, electrocardiography, and two-dimensional echocardiography. Noninvasive stress testing is recommended in patients with a high probability of CAD without angina who are revascularization candidates. Noninvasive testing to detect ischemia and viability or coronary arteriography should be undertaken in patients with a previous infarction without angina who are revascularization candidates. Finally, coronary arteriography is recommended for patients with angina or large areas of ischemic or chronically hypoperfused myocardium (56).

In the past, women have been at significant disadvantage in the work-up of CHF because physicians were less likely to rule out coronary disease. Furthermore, a lower specificity of exercise testing exists in women; therefore, when the resting electrocardiograph shows abnormality and the history suggests probable or atypical angina, thallium or other perfusion imaging is warranted (57).

Once etiology and correctable causes are identified (Fig. 19-4), the recommended therapeutic approach is identical in both sexes (58).

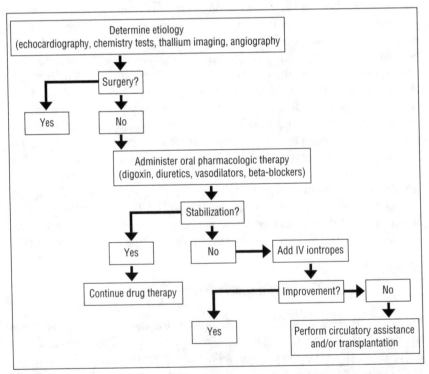

Figure 19-4 A therapeutic approach to the management of patients with congestive heart failure.

Therapeutic Modalities

Medical Therapy

Gender may affect the efficacy of medical therapy as well as the use of conventionally accepted therapy. As depicted in Table 19-2, of the 17,758 patients enrolled in the eight major heart failure mortality trials (i.e., Vasodilator–Heart Failure Trial I and II, Cooperative North Scandinavian Enalapril Survival Study [CONSENSUS], SOLVD, SOLVD prevention trial, Metoprolol in Dilated Cardiomyopathy study, Carvedilol study, and Digoxin study) only 17% were women (7).

In the clinical trials in which outcome by gender was analyzed, the beneficial effect of some therapies seemed to be reduced in women (*see* Chapter 21). This seems to be most striking in individual clinical trials of angiotensin-converting–enzyme (ACE) inhibitors. In CONSENSUS, men treated with enalapril had a 51% reduction in 6-month mortality ($p < 0.001$), whereas women had only a 6% mortality reduction (59). In CONSENSUS II, excess mortality was noted in the female group (13.5% of women treated with enalapril died compared with 11.2% of those treated with placebo) (60). Similarly, when morbidity and mortality were analyzed in the combined SOLVD trials, enalapril tended to produce a greater reduction in mortality, first heart failure hospitalization, and onset of new or worsening heart failure in men than in women (2). In the Survival and Ventricular Enlargement (SAVE) trial, a similar discrepancy in benefit of ACE after MI was seen in men compared with women. Using an analysis of proportional-hazards model, however, the benefits of captopril were independent of gender. Given the small number of women in the SAVE trial, conclusions about the similarity between the sexes in regard to mortality and morbidity may not be tenable (61); however, systemic overview

Table 19-2 Women (Percent) Enrolled in Heart Failure Treatment Mortality Trials

Trial	No. of Patients	Percent Women
V-HeFT I	642	0
CONSENSUS	253	30
V-HeFT II	804	0
SOLVD (treatment)	2569	20
SOLVD (prevention)	4228	13
MDC	380	27
Carvedilol	1094	23
Digoxin	7788	22

CONSENSUS = Cooperative North Scandinavian Enalapril Survival Study; MDC = Metoprolol in Dilated Cardiomyopathy; SOLVD = Study of Left Ventricular Dysfunction; V-HeFT = Vasodilator–Heart Failure Trial.

of individual data from 100,000 patients in randomized trials revealed similar proportional and absolute mortality for women and men (62).

Recently, carvedilol (a new combined α- and β-blocker with potent antioxidant effects) was shown to prolong survival in patients with heart failure. The reduction in mortality was similar with this drug in both women and men (63). Although powered to show a mortality effect, the Metoprolol in Dilated Cardiomyopathy (MDC) study did not demonstrate a mortality benefit of β-blockers in heart failure (64). Along with the bisoprolol (65) and bucindolol trials (66), the MDC trial was able to demonstrate a morbidity benefit (measured as a reduction in the number of CHF hospitalizations and improved functional status) and an improvement in ejection fraction. In all three studies, the benefits seen were not influenced by gender.

In contrast to β-blockers, a gender difference was noted on the morbidity effects of digitalis in heart failure. The recent National Institutes of Health–sponsored digoxin trial enrolled 7788 patients (67). In this trial, digitalis was found to be less effective in preventing recurrent hospitalization for CHF in women than in men (–2.4 [relative risk = 0.90] and –8.3 [relative risk = 0.71], respectively; $p < 0.05$).

Whether the beneficial effects of different medical therapies on mortality are equivalent in women and men remains unclear. This needs to be clarified because it has important clinical implications, e.g., β-blockers may be more beneficial than ACE inhibitors in women with CHF. Nevertheless, a mortality benefit probably exists in the use of ACE inhibitors and β-blockers for both women and men with CHF. Despite this fact, women are less likely to receive appropriate medical therapy (68,69). In a retrospective study of practice patterns in heart failure, records of 4606 hospitalized patients between 1992 and 1993 were reviewed. Hospitalized patients with CHF had a high all-cause mortality risk. In these patients, there was less-than-optimal use of proven therapy. This finding was particularly true among women and the elderly (67).

Mechanical Circulatory-Assist Devices

No specific studies have examined whether a gender difference exists with regard to use of and survivorship after ventricular mechanical circulatory support. However, an examination of the published literature on the experience with mechanical support reveals that significantly fewer women have undergone mechanical bridging to heart transplantation (70). This is partially explained by the fewer number of female transplant candidates. In addition, implantation of present-day assist devices requires a body surface area of greater than 1.5 m^2; thus, women are more likely to be disqualified on the basis of body size.

For those women who receive ventricular mechanical circulatory support, at least one published report notes survival rates to and from transplantation are similar to those in men. Pennington and colleagues (71) performed a multivariate analysis of 44 patients (9 women, 35 men) who had circulatory assist devices placed as a bridge to transplant. Thirty-one patients were supported with 32 Thoratec (18 left ventricular, 14 biventricular), 11 Novacor, and 2 Jarvik J-7-70 devices. The investigators concluded that hematologic profile, right ventricular status, and experience of the medical–surgical team were the significant variables affecting survivorship, not gender. As of July 1997, at Columbia Presbyterian Medical Center, 96 TCI LVAD devices have been used as a bridge to transplant. Survival for the 22 women on circulatory support awaiting transplant tended to be decreased early after implantation compared with the 74 men, but, overall, survival was not statistically significant between the groups ($p = 0.12$).

Transplantation

The overwhelming number of cardiac transplant recipients are men. Between 1990 and 1995, there were 2873 female compared with 9804 male transplant recipients (UNOS Scientific Registry data as of April 8, 1997; UNOS transplantation information Web site). Possible explanations for the under-representation of female candidates include the later age at which women develop heart failure, referral bias, selection bias, and less access to or acceptance of cardiac transplantation among women. In a study of 386 patients (91 women, 295 men) referred for transplantation evaluation over a 5-year period, the under-representation of female transplant candidates resulted from a gender difference in treatment preference rather than from physician selection bias (51).

The effect of gender on outcome after heart transplantation has been studied with conflicting results. In 1988, data from the Registry of the International Society for Heart Lung Transplantation (ISHLT) reported that women were at higher risk for death after heart transplantation; however, a more recent multivariate analysis of 13,695 patients by the ISHLT did not identify female gender as a risk factor. Interestingly, in this same analysis, use of a female donor organ was identified as a risk factor for decreased survival after transplant and may reflect immunologic differences in gender mismatch of recipient and donor. The UNOS registry supports similar survival after transplant. In 12,677 transplants performed between 1990 and 1995, female survivorship after transplant was similar to that of men (80.1% for women, 83.1% for men).

The results of single-center studies have been conflicting, with some demonstrating similar survival and others showing reduced survival rates after transplant. At the Columbia Presbyterian Medical Center, an early study examining 379 transplant recipients (75 women, 304 men) showed a significant reduction in 3-year actuarial survival in women after cardiac transplantation (72). This difference in survival was attributed to an increased risk of death from cytomegalovirus-related infection in women. More recent data on our female recipients, with subsequent implementation of CMV prophylaxis and without induction therapy, showed a similar survival rate to that observed in male recipients (Fig. 19-5). Other centers have reported an equivalent 85% 1-year survival in both women and men (73), despite an increased frequency of rejection and a decreased tolerance for corticosteroid-free maintenance immunosuppression in women (74,75).

After transplantation, heart transplant recipients achieve only 60% to 70% of predicted values for maximal exercise capacity. In an exercise capacity study after heart transplantation performed on 110 transplant recipients (21 women, 89 men), female recipients had a lower absolute exercise capacity but were able to achieve a greater proportion of their predicted capacity (76).

Summary

Congestive heart failure is the final common pathway for the multitude of diseases that affect the heart and is one of the leading causes of death in the

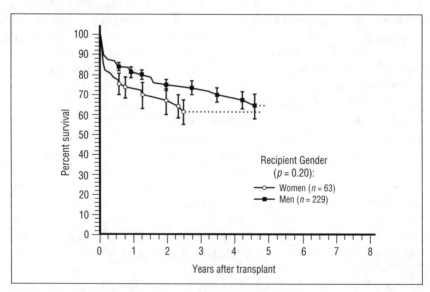

Figure 19-5 Kaplan–Meier survival curves for Columbia Presbyterian Medical Center post-transplantation patients, comparing men with women between January 1992 and December 1996.

United States for both men and women. Prevalence and incidence of the disease are similar between the sexes. The principal cause of CHF in both groups remains CAD. Despite this, many gender differences exist. The differential responses to cardiovascular stress and exercise performance may be attributed largely to the effects of sex hormones on cardiac and vascular tissues. Differences in current treatment and efficacy of medical therapy are beginning to be explored. All these factors may contribute to the observed differences in morbidity and mortality of CHF between the sexes.

Congestive heart failure represents the end result of numerous disease processes that affect the heart. Expanded research into how inherent biologic differences in cardiovascular function modify the disease state in men and women are needed. Epidemiologic evidence from the numerous survival studies in heart failure suggests that the mortality response to the different medical therapies varies between the sexes. Whether a "gender-tailored" medical therapy for CHF should be implemented deserves careful consideration. Clearly this question requires further investigation because, traditionally, therapy has been independent of gender. Psychologic, physiologic, morphologic, and true cardiovascular differences are clearly present between the sexes. Vive la difference!

REFERENCES

1. **Kannel WB.** Epidemiological aspects of heart failure. Cardiol Clin. 1989;7:1–9.

2. **Gillum RF.** Heart failure in the United States: 1970–1985. Am Heart J. 1987;1113: 1043–5.

3. **Smith WM.** Epidemiology of congestive heart failure. Am J Cardiol. 1985;55:3–8A.

4. **McKee PA, Castelli WP, McNamara PM, Kannel WB.** The natural history of congestive heart failure: the Framingham study. N Engl J Med. 1971;26:1441–6.

5. **Ho KKL, Pinsky JL, Kannel WB, Levy D.** The epidemiology of heart failure: the Framingham study. J Am Coll Cardiol. 1993;22(Suppl A):6–13A.

6. **Schocken DD, Arrieta MI, Leaverton PE, Ross EA.** Prevalence and mortality rate of congestive heart failure in the United States. J Am Coll Cardiol. 1992;2:301–6.

7. **Johnson M.** Heart failure in women: a special approach? J Heart Lung Transplant. 1993;S130–4.

8. **Albert CM, McGovern BA, Newell JB, Ruskin JN.** Sex differences in cardiac arrest survivors. Circulation. 1996;93:1170–6.

9. **Vaitkus PT, Kindwall E, Miller JM, et al.** Influence of gender on inducibility of ventricular arrhythmias in survivors of cardiac arrest with coronary artery disease. Am J Cardiol. 1991;67:537–9.

10. **Makkar RR, Fromm BS, Steinman RT, et al.** Female gender as a risk factor for torsades de pointes associated with cardiovascular drugs. JAMA. 1993;270:2590–7.

11. **Mancini DM, Eisen H, Kussmaul W, et al.** Value of peak exercise oxygen consumption for optimal timing of cardiac transplantation in ambulatory patients with heart failure. Circulation. 1992;83:778–86.

12. **Roul G, Moulichon M-E, Bareiss P, et al.** Prognostic factors of chronic heart failure in NYHA class II or III: value of invasive exercise hemodynamic data. Eur Heart J. 1995; 16:1387–98.

13. **Aaronson KD, Schwartz JS, Chen T, et al.** Development and prospective validation of a clinical index to predict survival in ambulatory patients referred for cardiac transplant evaluation. Circulation. 1997;95:2660–7.

14. **Adams KF, Dunlap SH, Sueta CA, et al.** Relation between gender, etiology, and survival in patients with symptomatic heart failure. J Am Coll Cardiol. 1996;7:1781–8.

15. **Graves EJ.** Detailed diagnoses and procedures: National Hospital Discharge Survey, 1989. Hyattsville, MD: National Center for Heath Statistics. DHHS Publication No. (PHS) 91-1769; 1991.

16. **Krumholz HM, Butler J, Miller T, et al.** Prognostic importance of emotional support for elderly patients hospitalized with heart failure. Circulation. 1998;97:958–64.

17. **Limacher MC, Yusef S.** Gender differences in presentation, morbidity, and mortality in the Studies of Left Ventricular Dysfunction (SOLVD): a preliminary report. In: Wenger NK, Speroff L, Packard B, eds. Cardiovascular Health and Disease in Women. Greenwich, CT: Le Jacq Communications; 1993:345–8.

18. **Pulleti M, Sunseri L, Curione M, et al.** Acute myocardial infarction: sex-related differences in prognosis. Am Heart J. 1984;108:63–6.

19. **Tofler GH, Stone PH, Muller JE, et al.** Effects on gender and race on prognosis after myocardial infarction: adverse prognosis for women, particularly black women. J Am Coll Cardiol. 1987;9:473–82.

20. **Dittrich H, Gilpin E, Nicod P, et al.** Acute myocardial infarction in women: influence on gender, mortality, and prognostic variables. Am J Cardiol. 1988;62:1–7

21. **Ayanian JZ, Epstein AM.** Differences in the use of procedures between women and men hospitalized for coronary heart disease. N Engl J Med. 1991;325:221–5.

22. **Steingart RM, Packer M, Hamm P, et al.** Sex differences in the management of coronary artery disease. N Engl J Med. 1991;325:226–30.

23. **Demirovic J, Blackburn H, McGovern PG, et al.** Sex differences in early mortality after acute myocardial infarction: the Minnesota Heart Survey. Am J Cardiol. 1995; 75:1096–101.

24. **Kannel WB.** Epidemiology of heart failure in the United States. In Poole P, Wilson P, Colucci W, Massie B, Chatterjee K, Coats A, eds. Heart Failure: Cardiac Function and Dysfunction. New York: Churchill Livingstone; 1997:279–88.

25. **Spirito P, Chiarella F, Carratino L, et al.** Clinical course and prognosis of hypertrophic cardiomyopathy in an outpatient population. N Engl J Med. 1989;320:749–55.

26. **Gillum RF.** Idiopathic cardiomyopathy in the United States: 1970–1982. Am Heart J. 1986;111:752–5.

27. **Malhotra A, Schaible TF, Capasso J, Scheuer J.** Correlation of myosin isoenzyme alterations with myocardial function in physiologic and pathophysiologic hypertrophy. Eur Heart J. 1984:5(Suppl F):61–7.

28. **Dannenberg AL, Levy D, Garrison RJ.** Impact of age on echocardiographic left ventricular mass in a healthy population (the Framingham study). Am J Cardiol. 1989;64:1066–8.

29. **Mason JW, O'Connell JB, Herskowitz A, et al.** A clinical trial of immunosuppressive therapy for myocarditis. N Engl J Med. 1995;333:269–75.

30. **Dec GW, Palacios IF, Fallon JT, et al.** Active myocarditis in the spectrum of acute dilated cardiomyopathies: clinical features, histologic correlates, and clinical outcome. N Engl J Med. 1985;312:885–90.

31. **Wilson MS, Bart RF, Baker PB, et al.** Giant cell myocarditis. Am J Med. 1985; 79:647–52.

32. **Regan TJ.** Alcoholic cardiomyopathy. In: Zipes DP, Rowlands DJ, eds. Progress in Cardiology. Philadelphia: Lea & Febiger; 1989:129.

33. **Yokoyama S, Kanda T, Suzuki T, Murata K.** Response of NK cell activity in postpartum myocarditis due to experimental virus infection. Circulation. 1991;84(Suppl II):634.

34. **Korithavongs T, Dossetor JB.** Suppressor cells in human pregnancy. Transplant Proc. 1978;10:911–3.

35. **Sanderson JE, Olsen EGJ, Gatei D.** Peripartum heart disease: an endomyocardial biopsy study. Br Heart J. 1986;56:285–91.

36. **Berko BA, Swift M.** X-linked dilated cardiomyopathy. N Engl J Med. 1987;316: 1186–91.

37. **McMinn TR, Ross J.** Hereditary dilated cardiomyopathy. Clin Cardiol. 1995;18:7–15.

38. **Collins JG.** Prevelance of selected chronic conditions: United States 1979–1981. Washington DC: U.S. Government Printing Office. DHHS Publ. No. (PHS) 86-1583; 1986.

39. **Malhotra A, Buttrick P, Scheuer J.** Effects of sex hormones on the development of physiologic and pathologic cardiac hypertrophy in male and female rats. Am J Physiol. 1990;259.

40. **Lieberman EH, Gerhard MD, Uehata A, et al.** Estrogen improves endothelium-dependent, flow-mediated vasodilation in postmenopausal women. Ann Intern Med. 1994; 121:936–49.

41. **Wolinsky H.** Effects of androgen treatment on the male rat aorta. J Clin Invest. 1972; 51:2552–6.

42. **Fischer GM, Swain ML.** Effects of sex hormones on blood pressure and vascular connective tissue in castrated and noncastrated male rats. Am J Physiol. 1977;232: H617–21.

43. **Schaible TF, Scheuer J.** Comparison of heart function in male and female rats. Basic Res Cardiol. 1984;79:402–12.

44. **Schaible TF, Malhotra A, Ciambrone G, Scheuer J.** The effect of gonadectomy on left ventricular function and cardiac contractile proteins in male and female rats. Circ Res. 1984;54:38–49.

45. **Scheuer J, Malhotra A, Schaible TF, Capasso J.** Effects of gonadectomy and hormonal replacement on rat hearts. Circ Res. 1987;61:12–9.

46. **Levy D, Savage DD, Garrison RJ, et al.** Echocardiographic criteria for left ventricular hypertrophy: the Framingham heart study. Am J Cardiol. 1987;59:956–60.

47. **Devereux RB, Reichek N.** Echocardiographic determination of left ventricular mass in man: anatomic validation of a method. Circulation. 1977;55:613–8.

48. **Topol EJ, Traill TA, Fortuin NJ.** Hypertensive hypertrophic cardiomyopathy of the elderly. N Engl J Med. 1985;312:277–83.

49. **Drinkwater BL.** Physiological responses of women to exercise. Exerc Sport Sci Rev. 1973;1:126–54.

50. **Sullivan MJ, Cobb FR, Higginbotham MB.** Stroke volume increases by similar mechanisms during upright exercise in normal men and women. Am J Cardiol. 1991;67: 1405–12.

51. **Aaronson KD, Schwartz JS, Goin JE, Mancini DM.** Sex differences in patient acceptance of cardiac transplant candidacy. Circulation. 1994;11:2753–61.

52. **De Maria R, Gavazzi A, Recalcati F, et al.** Comparison of clinical findings in idiopathic dilated cardiomyopathy in women versus men. Am J Cardiol. 1993;72:580–5.

53. **Mancini DM, Eisen H, Kussmaul W, et al.** Value of peak exercise oxygen consumption for optimal timing of cardiac transplantation in ambulatory patients with heart failure. Circulation. 1992;83:778–86.

54. **Aaronson K, Mancini DM.** Is percentage of predictive maximal exercise oxygen consumption a better predictor of survival than peak exercise oxygen consumption for patients with severe heart failure? J Heart Lung Transplant. 1995;5:981–9.

55. **Stelken AM, Younis LT, Jenninson SH, et al.** Improved risk stratification of ambulatory congestive heart failure patients using age and gender adjusted percent predicted peak exercise oxygen uptake. J Am Coll Cardiol. 1994;(Suppl):448A.

56. **Committee on Evaluation and Management of Heart Failure.** Guidelines for the evaluation and management of heart failure: report of the American College of Cardiology–American Heart Association Task Force on practice guidelines. J Am Coll Cardiol. 1995;26:1376–98.

57. **Parmley WW.** Pathophysiology and current therapy of congestive heart failure. J Am Coll Cardiol. 1989;13:771–85.

58. **Wenger NK, Speroff L, Packard B.** Cardiovascular health and disease in women. N Engl J Med. 1993;329:247–56.

59. **Kimmelstiel C, Holdberg RJ.** Congestive heart failure in women: focus on heart failure due to coronary artery disease and diabetes. Cardiology. 1990;77(Suppl 2):71–9.

60. **Swedberg K, Held P, Kjekshus J.** Effects of the early administration of enalapril on mortality in patients with acute myocardial infarction: results of the Cooperative New Scandinavian Enalapril Survival Study II (CONSENSUS II). N Engl J Med. 1992;327: 678–84.

61. **Pffefer MA, Braunwald E, Moye LA.** ACE inhibitors after myocardial infarction [Reply]. N Engl J Med. 1993;328:968.

62. **ACE Inhibitor Myocardial Infarction Collaborative Group.** Indications for ACE inhibitors in the early treatment of acute myocardial infarction: systemic overview of individual data from 100,000 patients in randomized trials. Circulation. 1998;97: 2202–12.

63. **Packer M, Bristow MR, Cohn JN, et al.** The effect of carvedilol on morbidity and mortality in patients with chronic heart failure. N Engl J Med. 1996;334:1349–55.

64. **Waagstein F, Bristow MR, Swedberg K, et al.** Beneficial effects of metoprolol in idiopathic dilated cardiomyopathy. Lancet. 1993;342:1441–6.

65. **CIBIS Investigators and Committees.** A randomized trial of beta-blockade in heart failure: the Cardiac Insufficiency Bisoprolol Study (CIBIS). Circulation. 994;90: 1765–73.

66. **Bristow MR, O'Connell JB, Gilbert EM, et al.** Dose-response of chronic beta-blocker treatment in heart failure from either idiopathic or ischemic cardiomyopathy. Circulation. 1994;89:1632–42 .

67. **Digitalis Investigation Group.** The effect of digoxin on mortality and morbidity in patients with heart failure. N Engl J Med. 1997;336:525–33.

68. **Stafford RS, Saglam D, Blumenthal D.** National patterns of angiotensin-converting–enzyme inhibitor use in congestive heart failure. Arch Intern Med. 1998;157: 2460–64.

69. **Clinical Quality Improvement Network Investigators.** Mortality risk and patterns of practice in 4606 acute care patients with congestive heart failure. Arch Intern Med. 1996;156:1669–73.

70. **McBride LR.** Bridging to cardiac transplantation with external ventricular assist devices. Semin Thorac Cardiovasc Surg. 1994;6:169–73.

71. **Pennington DG, McBride LR, Peigh PS, et al.** Eight years' experience with bridging to cardiac transplantation. J Thorac Cardiovasc Surg. 1994;107:472–81.

72. **Esmore D, Keogh A, Spratt P, et al.** Heart transplantation in females. J Heart Lung Transplant. 1991;10:335–41.

73. **Wechsler ME, Giardina EGV, Sciacca RR, et al.** Increased early mortality in women undergoing cardiac transplantation. Circulation. 1995;91:1029–35.

74. **Crandell BG, Renleund DG, O'Connell JB.** Increased cardiac allograft rejection in female heart transplant recipients. J Heart Lung Transplant. 1988;7:419–23.

75. **Kobashigawa J, Kirklin J, Naftel D, et al.** Pretransplantation risk factors for acute rejection after heart transplantation: a multi-institutional study: the Transplant Cardiologists Research Database Group. J Heart Lung Transplant. 1993;12:355–66.

76. **Renlund DG, Taylor DO, Ensley D, et al.** Exercise capacity after heart transplantation: influence of donor and recipient characteristics. J Heart Lung Transplant. 1996; 15:16–24.

CHAPTER 20

Psychosocial Issues

SUE C. JACOBS, PhD

PETER H. STONE, MD

Psychosocial factors have been linked to heart diseases for hundreds of years. In 1628, William Harvey, who discovered the circulatory system, noted that "a mental disturbance provoking pain, excessive joy, hope, or anxiety extends to the heart where it affects temper and rate" (1). The validity of this early observation has grown in the past half-century as our understanding of the mechanisms by which psychosocial factors may influence coronary artery disease (CAD) has increased (2).

Heart disease is the number one killer of women in the United States (3), with at least 25% of these deaths attributable to CAD (4). The known differences in the development and pathophysiology of CAD in women compared with men have been described aptly by Wenger and colleagues (5,6). In part, these differences may be related to gender and age differences in the incidence, expression, and impact of various psychosocial variables.

Contemporary cardiology and the biomedical model have greatly reduced deaths from CAD through advances in diagnosis and treatment with such technologies as percutaneous transluminal coronary angioplasty (PTCA), thrombolysis, coronary artery bypass graft (CABG) surgery and through managing life-threatening conditions such as acute myocardial infarction (MI) and unstable angina. In a 1996 *Science* editorial (7), two eminent biologists predicted the end of heart attacks by the year 2000 and diseases of the heart by the early twenty-first century because of such progress and the discovery of serum cholesterol–lowering drugs; however, this prediction is highly un-likely. The *Science* editorial viewpoint focused purely on biological processes that are pervasive in cardiovascular research and clinical practice, thus miss-ing important social, economic, environmental, and human (e.g., behavioral, emotional, cognitive) processes (8). Internists, cardiologists, and other health care providers need to attend to the day-to-day educational, psychosocial, and psychocultural factors that also may significantly affect the CAD patient's risk, prognosis, and quality of life.

The importance of a biopsychosocial approach to understanding health and disease has been documented extensively (9). The results of a number of studies highlight the significance of understanding, assessing, and treating psychosocial issues in both the primary and secondary prevention of CAD (10,11). Many authors have asserted that it is necessary to attend to psychoso-cial factors and their interaction with biologic factors in women's health issues, including CAD (12–15). Even the U.S. government, through the establishment in 1990 of an Office of Research on Women's Health by the National Institutes of Health (NIH), has acknowledged the importance of this biopsychosocial ap-proach and called for an integrated agenda for biomedical and biobehavioral research in women's health (16).

This chapter reviews various psychosocial factors and the ways they may affect cardiovascular health, CAD progression, and treatment outcome. Spe-cial attention is given to psychosocial issues in CAD in women (Box 20-1), al-though what is known is limited because until recently, as with other areas of medicine and psychology, most research had been with men. Psychosocial risk factors are described, followed by sections on the relationship of psy-chosocial issues to the detection, acute onset, treatment, rehabilitation, and prognosis of CAD. In each section, there is a brief overview of relevant litera-ture, with special attention given to what is or is not known about women and CAD. Recommendations are included for the health care provider in each do-main. The chapter concludes with some summary guidelines of psychosocial issues to address in women with or at risk for CAD.

Psychosocial Risk Factors for Coronary Artery Disease

Psychosocial factors that may affect the cause and prevention of CAD include socioeconomic status, race, hostility, anger, type A personality, depression, vi-tal exhaustion, perceived anxiety, stress (chronic and acute), social isolation, and social support. The impact of these factors on CAD may differ for women and men. Until recently most studies focusing on psychosocial factors in CAD excluded women or had sample sizes too small to detect gender differences (17). Other studies that have looked at gender differences in psychological

---

Box 20-1 Psychosocial Issues in Coronary Artery Disease in Women

---

Social factors
  Socioeconomic factors
    Lower class related to higher CAD risk
  Race
    Differences in socioeconomic factors confound many studies
Personality and role factors
  Hostility and anger
    May be related to increased cardiac reactivity
  Type A personality
    Possible predictor of angina
    May not predict risk of CAD
  Depression
    Risk factor in women and men but more common in women
  Vital exhaustion (Box 20-3)
  Stress (chronic and acute)
    In women, often related to events that occur to those they care for; acute
      myocardial infarction as a response to an acute trigger seems to occur less
      often than in men
  Isolation and social support
    Marriage has fewer positive mental and physical consequences for women
      than for men
    Women are less satisfied with post-MI support

---

factors and CAD also may be questionable because they were based on assumptions derived from research on men (18,19).

Coronary artery disease seems to be significantly more age related in women than in men; the Framingham study found a 40-fold increase in morbidity in women aged 75 to 84 years compared with those aged 35 to 44 years (20). After controlling for age, cigarette smoking status, systolic blood pressure, diabetes, cholesterol, and body mass index ($p < 0.05$ for all variables), a 20-year follow-up of 749 women in the Framingham study found that MI and CAD deaths were predicted by low educational level, tension, and lack of vacations. Among employed women, perceived financial status was also a factor. Among homemakers, loneliness during the day, difficulty falling asleep, housework affecting health, and a belief of being prone to heart disease were found to contribute to MI and CAD deaths (21). Box 20-2 profiles a woman at higher CAD risk, as suggested by a review of studies on women, psychosocial factors, and CAD conducted between 1980 and 1994 (22).

Box 20-2 Profile of a Woman with High Coronary Artery Disease Risk

---

Lower social class

Little formal education

Higher levels of perceived stress and physical tension

Typically a homemaker who feels unsupported socially

If works outside the home, still does all the home tasks

Seldom has a vacation

If a widow, at higher risk and may experience
    considerable loneliness and hopelessness

Smokes cigarettes

Consumes higher levels of dietary fat and cholesterol

Engages in little physical activity

Adapted from Brezinka V, Kittel F. Psychosocial factors of coronary heart disease in women: a review. Soc Sci Med. 1996;42:1351–65.

Socioeconomic Status and Race

As with gender, socioeconomic status (SES) and race are rarely addressed by psychological or medical researchers looking at CAD. Yet, the evidence is clear that SES is related to CAD risk and that lower SES and lower educational levels are risk factors for women (22). The 1995 Conference on SES and Cardiovascular Health and Disease summed up the strong relationships of SES to CAD, lifestyles, and major lifestyle biomedical CAD risk factors, with the most adverse patterns being for lower SES strata (23). Eaker (18), in her classic review of prospective studies of CAD that included women, noted that lower SES was related to CAD in women across various time periods and in different populations. More recently, the association between SES and overall health has been found to occur at all levels of SES (i.e., the higher a person moves up in SES, the healthier that person becomes) (24). This is also true for CAD. For example, Williams and colleagues (25), in a primarily white male sample, found that low SES and unmarried status increased the risk of CAD death. More specifically, those with an annual income of $40,000 or greater had an average 5-year survival rate of 0.91, whereas those with low income were almost twice as likely to die within 5 years. In another study, women with elementary school education were found to have the highest standard mortality ratios for CAD; these ratios decreased at each higher level of education (26). In the Nurses Health Study, Gliksman and colleagues (27) found that low SES in childhood was moderately related to an increased risk of nonfatal MI and total CAD in adulthood. For women from the most disadvantaged SES childhood backgrounds, the increased risk was not explained by other CAD risk factors, nutrition indices during gestation or childhood, or adult SES.

In a Glasgow study on the impact of SES on the incidence of and survival after MI and CAD death, Morrison and colleagues (28) found that 1) SES variation in rates of coronary events was greater for women than for men, 2) the largest social class gradient was in the proportion of deaths occurring outside the hospital, and 3) 68% of CAD deaths occurred before hospital admission (Fig. 20-1). The study authors recommended that 1) reduction in SES variation in mortality from CAD is best addressed by reducing the variation of event rates (i.e., by primary and secondary prevention), and 2) the allocation of resources for reduction of CAD mortality should take into account social class differences and the relative potential effect of hospital care and primary and secondary prevention.

Race is another important factor related to CAD. Total incidence of CAD was found to be higher in black women aged 25 to 54 years (relative risk [RR], 1.76; 95% confidence interval [CI], 1.36–2.29) than in white women of the same ages in the NHANES I Epidemiologic Follow-up Study (29). Age-adjusted risk, however, was lower for black men aged 25 to 75 years (RR, 0.78; 95% CI, 0.65–0.93) than for white men of the same ages. Significant independent risk factors for CAD in black women were age, systolic blood pressure, and smoking; for black men, independent risks factors were age, systolic

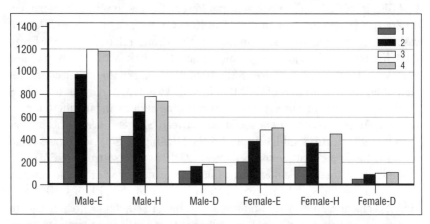

Figure 20-1 Socioeconomic status quartile, gender, and coronary events in the Glasgow study. 1–4 = socioeconomic status quartiles, with 1 being the most deprived group; D = number of people dying within 28 days of a coronary event among those who were alive upon arrival at hospital; E = number of coronary events; H = number of people with coronary events who were alive upon arrival at hospital. (Data from Morrison C, Woodward M, Leslie W, Tunstall-Pedoe H. Effect of socioeconomic group on incidence of, management of, and survival after myocardial infarction and coronary death: analysis of community coronary event register. BMJ. 1997; 314:541–6.)

blood pressure, serum cholesterol, low education, and low family income (30). Long-term survival of blacks in the Coronary Artery Surgery Study (CASS) found that blacks had higher mortality rates than whites over the long term, regardless of the type of initial treatment (31); however, 16 years after therapy, survival among nonsmoking blacks equaled that of whites.

Between 1960 and 1986, most U.S. SES groups showed gains in health; however, the least socioeconomically advantaged blacks seemed not to have gained at all (32). Escobedo and colleagues (33) looked at the relationship of SES, race, and CAD death in data from the 1986 National Mortality Follow-back Survey and the 1985 National Health Interview Survey (Table 20-1). Results suggested that younger blacks (both women and men) are more likely than younger whites to die of CAD (risk of premature death applies to sudden, nonsudden, and other coronary deaths). This study and others also found large differences in various CAD risk factors of obesity, diabetes, and hypertension between whites and blacks; however, the authors cautioned that environmental correlates of SES (e.g., family income, occupational status, educational attainment) may account for the large effect of low SES on the observed excess of black mortality:

> African Americans have less access to medical care, get lower quality of hospital care, and are less likely to receive diagnostic and therapeutic procedures for myocardial infarction after being admitted to hospitals than whites. Low socioeconomic status may be a marker for insufficient medical care. African Americans admitted to hospitals for acute myocardial infarction have higher case fatality rates than whites and are less likely than whites to survive symptomatic coronary heart disease. In the United States, social class explains a significant amount of coronary heart disease mortality among the general population.

It is also important to assess environmental factors related to SES and race as well as potential interactions between these variables. In the study by Escobedo and colleagues (33), 20% to 50% of the excess CAD mortality in younger blacks was not accounted for by the factors studied. The authors suggested that psychological factors, such as social factors and distress (which sometimes has been found to result in increased premature ventricular beat frequency, incidence of CAD, and hypertension in blacks), also may be responsible.

Interactions between race and income also seem to be operating in older adults. Although similar distributions of race, age, and gender were found among Medicare beneficiaries aged 65 years and over (34), the income of black beneficiaries was distributed unevenly, with only 6% in the highest income group and 73% in the lowest income group. Overall, in this study, which linked 1990 census data on median income with 1993 Medicare admin-

Table 20-1 Comparison of Risk Factors for Sudden and Nonsudden Coronary Deaths Among Whites and Blacks Aged 25 to 54 Years in 1986 in the United States

Risk Factor	Whites			Blacks		
	Sudden Death (%) (*n* = 281)	Nonsudden Death (%) (*n* = 271)	Controls (%) (*n* = 2015)	Sudden Death (%) (*n* = 92)	Nonsudden Death (%) (*n* = 62)	Controls (%) (*n* = 405)
Age (y)						
25–45	8	8	47	14	5	55
35–44	64*	51*	39	46*	62†	33
45–54‡	28§	41†	14	39¶	34¶	12
Gender						
Women	40	54	57	56	50	61
Men	60*	46*	43	44†	50†	39
Education						
> High school	26	25	45	14	15	33
High school	41	39	43	39	36	40
< High school	31	33	12	43	43	26
Family Income (thousands of dollars)						
> 25	34	38	56	14	11	35
15–25	22	18	20	12*	11	20
< 15	33*	31	14	57	55	34
Occupation						
White-collar	9	8	50	3	5	32
Blue-collar	15	12	33	16	25	46
Not in labor force	73¶	79§	17	81§	71†	22

* Odds ratio (95% CI) = 3.0–5.0. All odds ratios were adjusted for other coronary artery disease factors, age, gender, and number of physician visits in the past year.

† Odds ratio (95% CI) = 5.1–10.5.

‡ Women only in 45–54-year age group.

§ Odds ratio (95% CI) = 10.6–20.0.

¶ Odds ratio (95% CI) > 20.1.

Data from 1986 National Mortality Followback Survey and 1985 National Health Promotion and Disease Prevention Supplement.

istrative data, older black patients (both women and men) and low-income patients (both whites and blacks) had fewer physician visits, fewer mammograms, and fewer immunizations. For cardiac-related services, white patients had 33.8 per 1000 hospital discharges for ischemic heart disease in 1993 compared with 25.0 per 1000 for black patients (black-to-white ratio, 0.74; *p* <

0.001). The rates among white enrollees were higher for both PTCA and CABG (5.4 and 4.8 per 1000, respectively) than for black enrollees (2.5 and 1.9 per 1000, respectively). Black-to-white ratio for PTCA and CABG was 0.46 and 0.40, respectively ($p < 0.001$ for both). Mortality rates according to race, sex, and income are shown in Figure 20-2. The age-adjusted mortality rate was higher for black men than white men (black-to-white ratio, 1.19; $p < 0.001$) and also higher for black women than white women (black-to-white ratio, 1.16; $p < 0.001$). In all subgroups except African American women, the highest income group had the lowest mortality rates and the lowest income group had the highest mortality rates. The greatest difference in mortality based on income was found among white men (195 more deaths in the lowest income groups than in the highest income groups).

Many environmental correlates of SES were suggested in a longitudinal study of samples from England, Scotland, and Wales. Power and Mathews (35) observed that participants from lower SES had

1. Poorer growth in childhood

2. A greater likelihood of obesity in adulthood

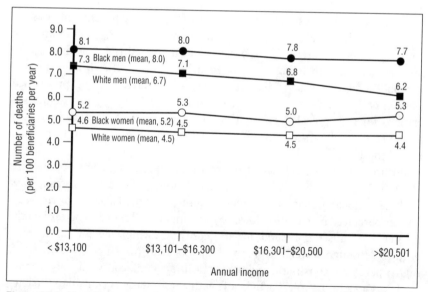

Figure 20-2 Mortality rates according to race, sex, and income among Medicare beneficiaries 65 years of age or over in 1993. Rates have been adjusted for age to the total Medicare population. Data were derived from the linked 1993 Medicare files and the 1990 U.S. Census information. (Adapted from Gornick ME, Eggers PW, Reilly TW, et al. Effects of race and income on mortality and use of services among Medicare beneficiaries. N Engl J Med. 1996;335:793.)

3. Poorer economic conditions in both childhood and adulthood

4. A less favorable cultural and behavioral environment in the parental home

5. Less social and emotional support and stimulation from their families of origin and, in turn, in their own families

6. Fewer educational qualifications

7. Less secure employment with greater job strain

A study on the impact of nutrition on the inequalities of health also points to correlates of SES and CAD risk (36). A number of recent studies provide possible clues into how environmental or other social psychologic factors may mediate or otherwise affect how race, SES, and gender influence health, CAD, and mortality. One study looked at neighborhood social context and racial differences in women's heart disease and found that women who live in communities with a high concentration of female-headed families are more likely to die of CAD, regardless of other demographic factors. In younger women, the effect was linked to low SES or poverty; in older women, however, the effect remained regardless of other census-track characteristics (37).

A second study investigated CAD and neighborhood environments in four U.S. communities that participated in the Atherosclerosis Risk in Community study (1987–89). Increased risk of CAD and increased levels of risk factors were associated with living in deprived neighborhoods. Black men in poor neighborhoods in Jackson, Mississippi, showed a decrease in CAD prevalence as neighborhood characteristics worsened. There were also inconsistent associations for CAD prevalence and serum cholesterol in black men. Increased serum cholesterol was associated with "richer neighborhoods" for black men in Jackson (38).

A third recent study looked at the relationship of two aspects of the sense of control (i.e., mastery and perceived constraints) and health to social class in three national probability samples of women and men aged 25 to 75 years. Higher perceived mastery and lower constraints were related to better health, greater life satisfaction, and lower depressive symptoms for all income groups. Although lower income participants had lower perceived mastery, higher perceived constraint, and poorer health overall, control beliefs seemed to play a moderating role. Participants with a high sense of control in the lowest income group showed levels of health and well-being similar to the higher income groups (39).

These three studies suggest that psychosocial variables (e.g., sense of control, social structure of neighborhood environment [in particular, living in a neighborhood with a high concentration of female-headed families]) may be useful in understanding SES differences in health and CAD.

Recommendations

In summary, higher rates of CAD are found generally in women and men with lower SES. Two broad pathways linking SES to CAD were proposed at the Conference on SES and Cardiovascular Disease and Health:

1. Less favorable patterns of established major lifestyle and biomedical risk factors (e.g., smoking, adverse diet, sedentary lifestyle, high serum cholesterol, high blood pressure, obesity, diabetes) are found more often in lower than in higher SES strata.

2. Less favorable patterns of psychosocial factors (e.g., hostility, depression, low social support, social isolation, racism, unemployment, and job instability, insecurity, strain, and powerlessness) are found more often in lower than in higher SES strata.

These have many implications for the health care provider working with lower SES women who may require special attention because they are less likely to avail themselves of health interventions and services. One suggestion is to allot more time to lower SES patients, who tend to rely on emergency rooms and clinics where less time is allotted per patient. Physicians need to be aware of the constraints that the lower SES patient may have on following preventive recommendations. For example, there may be many obstacles to the frequent recommendations for low-fat diets and exercise, including high costs, lack of access to health-food stores, lack of place and time to exercise, lack of control over time due to work and responsibilities to others, and lack of transportation or child care to come to a daytime appointment. Physicians may need to spend more time with their lower SES female patients to solve how to implement risk-reduction plans and to advocate community level solutions, such as increasing the availability of healthy food, exercise facilities, and screening and treatment clinics in poorer neighborhoods.

Hostility, Anger, and Type A Behaviors

The most researched relationship between the risk of CAD and psychosocial factors has been that of the relationship between hostility and the incidence of CAD (40–42). The link found between chronic hostility and CAD in men (43) also has been suggested in women, although only a few studies have included women (44,45). Type A behavior, a pattern of time urgency and free-floating hostility (46), was found to be an independent predictor of angina pectoris (but not of MI or fatal coronary events) in both women and men in the 20-year Framingham study follow-up report (47). Type A–related measures predicted neither angina pectoris nor MI in the community sample of 795 middle-aged urban Swedish women; low ratings of aggression, however, predicted electrocardiographic changes consistent with ischemic heart disease (48). One study compared two groups of women (one post-MI, the other physically sedentary) using several psychosocial measures, including the videotaped type A interview. The type A interview did not predict the recurrence of cardiac events (49). In fact, lower type A scorers tended to be at higher risk for cardiac events. This, as the authors point out, is a good example of the problems of using the type A interview or other diagnostic assessments with women that are based on men.

Self-reported hostility at a young age has been found to predict both CAD and all-cause mortality in men (50–52). Adams (53) looked at the relationship of hostility in Mills College women aged 24, 27, 43, and 52 years and the general health in approximately 105 women aged 52 years. Although interpretation is limited by the small, high-SES sample, hostility at each age was negatively correlated with general health at 52 years of age even after controlling for possible mediator variables such as cigarette smoking, body mass index, or negative life events.

One way hostility and anger may contribute to the development of CAD is through an exaggerated cardiovascular and hemostatic reactivity in response to behavioral stressors by people who are hostile compared with those who are not (54). Although most reactivity studies have been with men, studies with women also have supported the hypothesis that hostile people exhibit excessive cardiovascular reactivity to evoked anger-related emotional states (55–57). There seems, however, to be complex differences between the genders in reactivity to different kinds of stressors. Men have shown greater elevations in blood pressure, plasma norepinephrine, and low-density lipoprotein cholesterol levels and have been found to be to be "vascular reactors," responding with greater total peripheral resistance and systolic and diastolic blood pressure than women on a number of stressful laboratory tasks (58). Women, by contrast, have been found to be "cardiac reactors," responding with larger increases in heart rate than men in response to stressful tasks (58). Attitudinal hostility measures do not explain the significant gender differences in cardiovascular response to stress; however, one experimental study of white college women found that those with high cynical hostility showed greater increases in systolic blood pressure in an interpersonally stressful situation than those with low cynical hostility (59). Another study found that type A women who participated in an anger-recall interview manifested greater systolic reactivity when their anger was in response to frustration of autonomy needs, whereas type B women (those lacking the type A behavior pattern) showed greater blood pressure reactivity in response to affiliation needs. All women who suppressed their anger showed greater responses than those who expressed it assertively (60).

Saab and colleagues (61) found significant ethnicity by gender interactions for an active coping–speaking task. Black men responded to the active coping task with lower blood pressure, lower cardiac output (or heart rate), or both than black women, white men, and white women, who did not differ from each other. Relative to the other groups, black men also reported more inhibitory-passive coping, hostility, and less social support. White men and women also responded with greater systolic blood pressure increases during an inhibitory-passive coping task (mirror tracing). The authors point out that racial differences found in physiologic reactivity studies in men probably cannot be generalized to include women. They also suggest that social and environmental factors, rather than genetic factors, may play a role in the reactivity differences between blacks and whites.

High levels of expressed anger have been found to be a risk factor for CAD (RR, 2.66; 95% CI, 1.25–5.61) among older male veterans (62). Episodes of anger in the 2 hours before MI onset also have been found to increase the risk of MI in the ONSET study (63). Using two types of self-matched control data based on a case-crossover study design for the 1623 patients (501 women), the RR of MI following an episode of anger was 2.3 (95% CI, 1.7–3.2). The RR tended to be lower in men (1.9; 95% CI, 1.3–2.9) than in women (3.3; 95% CI, 2.1–5.3), but the difference was not significant ($p < 0.09$).

In women, research findings related to hostility, anger, or type A behavior and the risk of CAD have been summarized in a number of reviews (57,58,64). Even though the role of hostility–anger behavior in the development of CAD in women is not clear, it seems to work differently for women than men and differently for women in different situations. In general, reviews find that women do not differ from men in the emotional experience of anger and hostility as measured either by self-reports or behavioral observations rated by others. They have lower levels of attitudinal hostility than men on measures such as the Cook–Medley Hostility Inventory, and express feelings of anger more than men. They are less physically, and possibly verbally, aggressive than men (58).

Recommendations

On average, hostility and the type A behavior pattern seem like higher CAD risk factors for men than for women, although the evidence is contradictory and sparse. There is evidence, however, that the ways in which hostility and anger are expressed affect the risk of CAD in women. The pathways through which hostility and anger can affect CAD are numerous and complicated. For example, hostility is associated with higher consumption of caffeine, cigarette smoke, marijuana, alcohol, calories, and cholesterol. Additionally, for women only, higher animal fat and lower fiber consumption also are associated with hostility, anger, and CAD (14). Physicians should be aware of the relationship of hostility and anger to both CAD risk and preventive health behaviors. Behavioral treatment programs have been developed to reduce hostility and anger (65). Serious consideration should be given to the use of such treatment strategies in risk-reduction and cardiac rehabilitation programs either through referral to health care providers trained in cognitive–behavioral therapies or cardiac psychology or through the recommendation of appropriate self-help books (66,67).

Depression and Vital Exhaustion

Although most research on psychosocial factors and CAD has focused on the role of hostility and type A behavior in the etiology of CAD, recent studies point to the role of depression in the development of CAD for both women and men (11,68–70). Prospective data from the Baltimore Epidemiologic Catchment Area Study suggest that a history of dysphoria (RR, 2.07; 95% CI, 1.16–3.71) and a major depressive episode (RR, 4.54; 95% CI, 1.65–12.44) increase the risk of MI (11). Women are twice as likely to be depressed and to experience a comorbidity between depression and CAD as are men (70). In a community-based Swedish study, depressed women were five times more likely to develop angina in a 12-year interval than nondepressed women (45), and they had a sixfold increase in sudden cardiac death following the death of a significant other (71).

Research on vital exhaustion (defined in Box 20-3) also supports a link between depressive symptoms and CAD (72). In a prospective study of male Rotterdam city employees, vital exhaustion was found to have an age-adjusted RR of 2.28 for MI (73). In another study, 79 women hospitalized for first MI were

---

Box 20-3 Vital Exhaustion

Vital exhaustion, a debilitated emotional and physical state characterized by fatigue, increased irritability, and feelings of demoralization, is believed to be a precursor of myocardial infarction [69].

Vital exhaustion is measured by the Maastricht Questionnaire; questions include:

1. Do you often feel tired?
2. Do you have the feeling that you cannot cope with everyday problems as well as you used to?
3. Do little things irritate you more than they used to?
4. Would you want to be dead at times? (This question demonstrated the strongest association with age-adjusted relative risk of myocardial infarction over 4 years.)
5. Do you wake up with a feeling of exhaustion and fatigue? (This question has also been found to be a significant independent risk beyond the "vital exhaustion" total score based on 21 questions.)

compared with 90 women hospitalized in the general and orthopedic surgery wards at a Netherlands Hospital (74); after controlling for age, smoking, coffee consumption, diabetes, hypertension, nonanginal pain, and menopausal status, the RR for MI associated with vital exhaustion was 2.75 (95% CI, 1.28–5.81; $p < 0.01$). Long-lasting conflicts, unemployment, and financial problems in the family during childhood and adolescence were related to vital exhaustion. Unwanted childlessness, educational problems with children, financial problems, and prolonged marital problems were also related to vital exhaustion. Women who held jobs and took care of households with children showed higher vital exhaustion than working women without those responsibilities ($t = 4.25$; $p < 0.001$); this finding corresponds with the association between vital exhaustion and prolonged overtime in men (73).

Recommendations

Evidence is mounting to suggest a strong relationship between depression, vital exhaustion, and CAD in women and men as a risk factor for both CAD and for morbidity and mortality following cardiac events. It is important for physicians to recognize the symptoms of depression or a history of dysphoria for adults young and old. Some have suggested that primary care physicians administer a depression screening test to each patient at each visit (75) and that routine screening is particularly pertinent for patients who are at high risk for depression (Box 20-4). Box 20-5 lists the diagnostic criteria for a major depressive episode.

Box 20-4 Patients at High Risk for Depression

Recent loss or severe stress

Vague somatic symptoms

Any of the expected somatic or emotional symptoms of depression

Family history of depression, suicide, or mental illness

History of self-medicating behavior (e.g., including alcohol, stimulants [diet pills], nicotine)

History of self-destructive behavior

Currently on certain medications (particularly antihistamines, hormones, H_2-receptor blockers, anticonvulsants, and levodopa)

Major illness (e.g., stroke, CAD, cancer, diabetes)

Chronic pain

Postpartum

Adapted from Jacobs DG, Kopans BA, Meszler Reizes J. Re-evaluation of depression: what the general practitioner needs to know. Mind Body Med. 1995;1:20.

Box 20-5 Criteria for Major Depressive Episode

A. Five (or more) of the following symptoms have been present during the same 2-week period and represent a change from previous functioning and at least one of the symptoms is either depressed mood or loss of interest or pleasure.

Note: Do not include symptoms that are clearly due to a general medical condition or mood-incongruent delusions or hallucinations.

1. Depressed mood most of the day, nearly every day, as indicated by either subjective report (e.g., feels sad or empty) or observation (e.g., appears tearful) *Note: In children or adolescents, mood can be irritable.*

2. Markedly diminished interest or pleasure in all, or almost all, activities for most of the day, nearly every day (as indicated by either subjective account or observation made by others)

3. Significant weight loss or gain (e.g., change of more than 5% of body weight in a month when not dieting) or decrease or increase in appetite nearly every day *Note: In children, consider failure to make expected weight gains.*

4. Insomnia or hypersomnia nearly every day

5. Psychomotor agitation or retardation nearly every day (observable by others, not merely subjective feelings of restlessness or being slowed down)

6. Fatigue or loss of energy nearly every day

7. Feelings of worthlessness or excessive or inappropriate guilt (which may be delusional) nearly every day (not merely guilt or self-reproach about being sick)

8. Diminished ability to think or concentrate or indecisiveness nearly every day (either by subjective account or as observed by others)

9. Recurrent thoughts of death (not just fear of dying), recurrent suicidal ideation without a specific plan, or a suicide attempt or a specific plan for contemplating suicide

B. The symptoms do not meet criteria for a mixed episode (as defined in DSM-IV).

C. The symptoms cause clinically significant distress or impairment in social, occupational, or other important areas of functioning.

D. The symptoms are not due to the direct physiologic effects of a substance (e.g., a drug of abuse, a medication) or a general medical condition (e.g., hypothyroidism).

E. The symptoms are not better accounted for by bereavement (i.e., after the loss of a loved one), persist for more than 2 months, or are characterized by marked functional impairment, morbid preoccupation with worthlessness, suicidal ideation, psychosis, or psychomotor retardation.

Adapted from American Psychiatric Association. Diagnostic and Statistical Manual of Mental Disorders. 4th edition. Washington, DC: American Psychiatric Association; 1994.

An accurate diagnosis of depression requires ruling out a number of other diagnoses; an excellent aid to this is an algorithm showing the differential diagnoses of mood disorders in the *Diagnostic and Statistical Manual of Mental Disorders* of the American Psychiatric Association (76). It is important to consider the possible psychologic effects or contributions to depressive symptoms of cardiac drugs. Beta-blockers may cause fatigue, difficulty concentrating, loss of mental alertness, insomnia, nightmares, and sexual dysfunction. Certain calcium-channel blockers (e.g., nifedipine) can cause reflex tachycardia, which is often distressing to patients who report them as palpitations. Antilipid agents (statin drugs) may cause sleep disturbance. Finally, it is necessary to rule out other conditions that can mimic or contribute to depressive symptoms; Tabrizi and colleagues (77) provide a helpful mnemonic for this in Box 20-6.

If depression is identified, it is imperative to screen for suicidal thoughts. A nonjudgmental approach and open-ended questions encourage honesty from the patient. If a patient has a plan on how to commit suicide and the means to carry out that plan, psychological assessment for immediate inpatient management is essential.

The benefits from psychological and pharmacologic treatment of depression include a shorter duration of symptoms and a decrease in recurrence.

Box 20-6 Dementia: A Mnemonic for Remembering Those Conditions That Can Mimic or Contribute to Depressive Symptoms

---

Drugs (e.g., prescription medications, illicit substances, and, most importantly, alcohol) are one of the most common organic causes of depression; many medications can be associated with depression (especially certain antihypertensives, corticosteroids)

Endocrine conditions (especially hypothyroidism and hyperthyroidism, adrenal insufficiency, hyperparathyroidism)

Metabolic conditions (e.g., hyponatremia, hypokalemia)

Neurologic disorders (e.g., multiple sclerosis, Alzheimer disease)

Trauma (especially if a subdural hematoma or intracerebral bleeding is present; an ever-present danger in cardiac patients treated with thrombolytic agents, heparin, aspirin, and a variety of powerful antithrombin, anticoagulant, and antiplatelet medications)

Infections (particularly of the subacute central nervous system)

Avitaminosis (e.g., B_{12} deficiency)

From Tabrizi K, Littman A, Williams RB, Scheidt S. Psychopharmacology and cardiac disease. In: Allan R, Scheidt S (eds). Heart and Mind: The Practice of Cardiac Psychology. Washington, DC: The American Psychological Association; 1996:400; with permission.

Cognitive–behavioral and interpersonal psychotherapies have been found effective for depression. Psychotherapy is recommended for mild depression and, in combination with medication, for moderate-to-severe depression (78).

The management of depression can be accomplished by medical practitioners comfortable with providing care or by referral to psychologists, psychiatrists, or other mental health care providers. Some patients refuse referral for additional care despite the physician's efforts; these patients still require care. Bibliotherapy, a reading program, for depression has been found to be effective for older adults, with results maintained over a 2-year follow-up (79); physicians may want to recommend a behavioral approach (e.g., *Control Your Depression* [80]) or a cognitive approach (e.g., *The Feeling Good Handbook* [81]).

Increasingly, internists are prescribing newer antidepressants with or without consulting a more experienced colleague. It is important that physicians find safe and effective antidepressants for their patients, especially those who have had a previous MI. A recent study compared paroxetine (a selective serotonin-reuptake inhibitor) and nortriptyline hydrochloride (a tricyclic antidepressant) in depressed patients with ischemic heart disease (82). Treatment was considered effective, with a decline in the Hamilton Rating Scale for Depression of 50% and a final score of 8 or less. Monitoring included heart rate and rhythm, supine and sitting systolic and diastolic blood pressure, electrocardiographic conduction intervals, and indices of heart rate variability and rate of adverse events. Both paroxetine and nortriptyline were found to be effective treatments for depressed patients with ischemic heart disease; however, nortriptyline was associated with a slightly higher rate (18%; $p < 0.03$) of serious adverse cardiac events (predominantly in rate or rhythm disturbances) than paroxetine (2%).

For a brief overview of psychopharmacology for patients with CAD (including a summary of antidepressant commonly prescribed, their side effects, and potential drug interactions), see *Heart and Mind: The Practice of Cardiac Psychology* (77).

Anxiety and Panic Attacks

Anxiety and panic have been hypothesized to increase the risk of CAD, particularly sudden cardiac death (2). Panic disorder is characterized by recurrent panic attacks consisting of a sudden and intense fear or discomfort associated with a number of somatic symptoms (76). Approximately 1% to 5% of the overall population has panic disorder, with or without agoraphobia, and 50% to 75% of those afflicted are women (76). The prevalence of panic disorder is 16% to 25% in the emergency department; among noncardiac chest pain patients examined by a cardiologist, the prevalence of panic disorder increases to 31% to 56% (83). Because a number of the diagnostic symptoms of panic attack (e.g., chest pain, palpitations, shortness of breath, sweating, sensation of choking, paresthesia, hot flushes) are also signs of CAD, many patients consult physicians with a fear of dying of a heart attack. On medical examination, however, most patients do not have a serious cardiovascular condition.

Since the finding in a number of studies of what seems to be an increased risk of cardiovascular mortality among patients with panic-like anxiety, the belief of many panic disorder patients that they will die of a heart attack has been heightened. Fleet and Beitman (83) critically reviewed the six recent studies with such evidence to try to discover whether a patient with panic disorder can die from the cardiovascular consequences of a panic attack. Two of the most methodologically sound prospective studies were conducted by Kawachi and colleagues. In their first study of 39,999 men, self-reported symptoms of phobic anxiety were associated with an increased risk of fatal CAD (RR, 2.45; 95% CI, 1.00–5.96) and sudden cardiac death (RR, 6.08; 95% CI, 2.35–15.73) among the most anxious men over 2 years. The individual questions from the Crown–Crisp Experiential Index (used to measure phobic anxiety) that were associated with an elevated risk of fatal CAD were 1) "Always feeling panicky in crowds," 2) "Worrying unduly when relatives are late coming home," and 3) "Definitely feeling more relaxed indoors" (84).

Other studies have found similar results with men. In the Normotensive Aging Study, reduced heart rate variability was found in men with the highest anxiety scores, suggesting that phobic anxiety may increase risk of sudden cardiac death as a result of altered sympathovagal balance in the autonomic regulation of the heart (85). Frasure-Smith and colleagues (86) reported that increased anxiety was related to unstable angina admissions and recurrent fatal and nonfatal MI in their sample of 222 post-MI patients.

Fleet and Beitman (83) answered their question by indicating that, despite methodologic limitations, results from all of the studies suggest that panic-like anxiety is an independent risk factor for cardiovascular death, particularly sudden cardiac death. No one, however, has looked at the question based on thorough medical and psychiatric assessment in a prospective design. In addition, the associations, which had a low rate, were based primarily on studies of white men, who are two to four times less like likely to have panic attacks than women.

Recommendations

At this time, the risk of cardiovascular events in patients with panic disorder has not been adequately elucidated in the literature. It is recommended, however, that patients with panic disorder have thorough medical examinations and that they be referred to a mental health professional who is trained in the cognitive–behavioral therapies that are highly effective for this disorder. For patients with CAD and panic disorder, the studies may influence treatment to some extent, e.g., because laboratory mental stress can induce ischemia in patients with

CAD (87), it is possible that patients with both CAD and panic disorder could have ischemia associated with their panic attacks (83). One study of 10 healthy women with panic disorder found no evidence of ischemia during panic attacks with ambulatory monitoring (88). The possibility, however, is enough to question the use of the most widely used and studied drugs for panic disorder (i.e., tricyclic antidepressants and benzodiazepines) in patients with CAD and panic disorder. As noted above, tricyclic antidepressants have the potential for cardiac complications and interactions with many cardiac and antihypertensive drugs; they probably should be avoided by the patient with CAD. Although the benzodiazepines have no cardiotoxic side effects, there is the potential for dependence and abuse. In general, non-CAD patients with panic disorder should be reassured that there is a very low risk of heart attack from the panic attacks. Cognitive–behavioral interventions aimed at more realistic patient appraisal of panic symptoms should not be changed based on the existing research.

Psychological Stress

Psychological stress is a response composed of negative cognitive and emotional states that occur "when demands imposed by events exceed a person's ability to cope" (89). Research on psychological events and CAD has focused on stressful life events, job stress (or role strain), and reactivity to laboratory stressors. Newer studies have focused on adjustments to change.

McEwen (90) recently reviewed the long-term effects of physiologic response to stress, which he referred to as *allostatic load:*

> Allostasis, the ability to achieve stability through change, is critical to survival. Through allostasis, the autonomic nervous system, the hypothalamic–pituitary–adrenal axis, and the cardiovascular, metabolic, and immune systems protect the body by responding to internal and external stress. The price of this accommodation to stress can be allostatic load, which is the wear and tear that results from chronic overactivity or underactivity of allostatic systems.

He suggests an increasing importance of assessing allostatic load in the diagnosis and treatment of many illnesses. Allostatic load and its consequences (e.g., MIs triggered by surges in blood pressure, development of atherosclerosis accelerated by repeated blood pressure elevations over time) result from four type of situations:

1. Frequent stress
2. Prolonged exposure to stress hormones resulting from an inability to adapt to repeated stressors of the same type
3. Inability to recover after the termination of stress

4. Inadequate responses in one allostatic system (e.g., cortisol secretion) that trigger compensatory increases in another (e.g., inflammatory cytokines) (90)

According to McEwan, this means that physicians need to recognize and look at sources of stress in their patients' lives, including the stress of the illness itself, and to help patients reduce their allostatic load by "helping them learn coping skills, recognize their own limitations, and relax" (90).

Stressful Life Events
Stressful life events have been linked to the development (91) and acute onset (92,93) of MI; however, these studies did not look at gender differences. Other studies have found only a few gender differences in the number of stressful life events, the social desirability of those events, or the ability to control them: 1) single men experience more stressful events than single women or married men and women, 2) stressful events of married people are more positive, and 3) younger men seem to feel more in control of those events (94).

In secondary analyses of five epidemiologic surveys of the general population, women's vulnerability (increased psychological distress) to life events was found to be confined largely to "network" events (events that occur not to the women themselves but to people around them) (95). This demonstrates that the "emotional cost of caring" is responsible for a substantial part of the overall relationship between gender and distress. A 1998 study of elderly patients with CAD found that increased negative life events and lowered subjective social support were associated with the presence of major depression, even after accounting for age, gender, and race (96).

Triggers of Coronary Events
Even less attention has been given to possible gender differences in events or activities that trigger the acute onset of coronary events than has been given to gender differences in chronic risk factors. In the MILIS study, after taking age into account, Tofler and colleagues (97) found that men were more likely to report a precipitating factor for their MI than women (11.4% and 1.7%, respectively; $p < 0.02$). The most common precipitating factor reported by both women and men was emotional upset (20.7% and 17.5%, respectively). Men also had more external "triggers" for MI than women in an Israeli study (98). The apparent gender difference in susceptibility to triggers could be due to a number of factors, including 1) women's onset of MI is at an older age, 2) women are less likely to be exposed to triggers (e.g., heavy exertion), and 3) women are less susceptible to triggers (both physiologic and psychological).

Job Stress and Multiple Roles

Job stress has been considered a risk factor for CAD, especially job strain (the combination of contributions of low job-decision latitudes and high psychological job demands) and lack of social support at work (99). Women, however, have not been included in most studies of psychosocial job strain or job stress and CAD (18). A study of 242 middle-aged women in California revealed that those who were employed in managerial positions were healthier than unemployed women, with fewer CAD risk factors (100). The authors suggested that such employment could be associated with healthier lifestyles. They also suggested that psychosocial factors could be moderating the relationship between health and employment; these include the possibility that the managerial and professional women were working for job satisfaction more than financial need, had a more positive job attitude, and possibly an increased perception of control. A study of 1998 German women aged 25 to 64 years also found that employment may exert a beneficial influence on CAD risk in women as measured by high-density lipoprotein cholesterol (101). Among 13,778 Swedish workers, the highest prevalence of CAD was found in blue-collar men who had high job demands, low social support, and low work control (prevalence ratio, 7.22; 95% CI); the highest prevalence of CAD for women was in white-collar women with high job demands and low social support (prevalence ratio, 2.06; 95% CI) (102). In the Nurses Health Study, women doing shift work were found to have a increased risk of CAD incidents (i.e., nonfatal MI or fatal CAD) (RR, 1.51; 95% CI, 1.12–2.03) (103).

The multiple roles of caring for a family and working outside the home provide a possible explanation for gender differences in CAD risk. Theorell (104) hypothesized that the double roles (i.e., home and paid work) of Swedish women explained the finding that a moderate amount of overtime was associated with a decreased risk of MI in men but a corresponding increased risk in women. In a study of 202 professional women (105), the tension between career sacrifices and interpersonal commitments to spouses, children, and friends (interpersonal sacrifices) differentiated women with CAD from those without it ($p < 0.01$).

Recommendations

There are a variety of stressful life events that health care professionals should take into account when assessing the possible impact of stress on a woman's health and risk for CAD. It is especially important to ask women not only about what has been going on in their own lives but also about their multiple roles and about what has been going on in their social networks and in the lives of their loved ones. Unless asked, a woman may not tell you that she is worried about her daughter's alcohol abuse and having to care for her parents, her grandchildren, and her disabled husband while working part-time.

As noted in the previous discussion on SES, physicians need to consider a woman's financial resources when assessing her ability to adhere to risk-reduction programs or to take medications. If it seems her stress is greater than her resources, a referral to either social services or a stress management program may be especially beneficial.

Social Support and Isolation

The research on social support and isolation (a lack of social support) is somewhat unclear in terms of how social support functions in women and men and whether the impact on health is the same for women and men (106,107). For women, the role of social support is more complicated than for men. The consequences of social support are sometimes negative for women because, as noted above, they provide support as well as receive it; they often care for elderly relatives, are in supportive occupations (e.g., nursing or teaching), and care for children. Marriage has less positive mental and physical health consequences for women than for men. On the other hand, women recover more quickly from widowhood than men; this may be because women have many confidants, whereas men often have only their wives. There also may be gender differences in the types of support men and women provide, with women more likely to provide empathy or emotional support and men to provide advice. Both women and men prefer to self-disclose to women. Evaluative interactions, including advice giving, have been found to increase cardiovascular reactivity (108), whereas supportive interactions, including empathy, have been found to decrease reactivity (109).

The long-term mortality risk of CAD in women and men, however, is affected by social supports and social networks (110,111). Marital status and widowhood influence mortality risk differently in women and men, with men being at higher risk. In a sample consisting mainly of white men, Williams and colleagues (25) found that patients with either a spouse or a confidant had a 5-year survival rate of 0.82, whereas unmarried patients without a confidant had a 5-year survival rate of 0.52. Of all the SES variables, the presence or absence of a spouse or confidant was most prognostic. There was more than a threefold increase in the risk of death within 5 years for unmarried patients without a confidant compared with patients who were either married or had a close confidant. One study suggests that the loss of emotional support can precede death from CAD. Cottington and colleagues (71) found that 81 women aged 25 to 64 years who died suddenly from CAD were six times as likely to have experienced the death of a significant other within the past month compared with matched controls.

Berkman and colleagues (111) found that social networks or ties are related to CAD mortality risk factors and perhaps to CAD mortality but do not seem to account for gender differences in CAD risk. Social isolation and lack of emotional support seem to be important to both women and men.

Recommendations

The role of social supports and social networks, although complicated for women, clearly can have some buffering impact on health and CAD. It is important that physicians and other health care professionals assess their patients' social networks for the possibility of social isolation and the presence or absence of emotional support. They also need to assess for negative as well as positive supports. For example, physicians should not assume that a woman's husband will be a positive support; in fact, he may be the source of much stress and worry for her. If a woman is caring for a spouse, parent, or grandchild, she may have trouble complying with physician instructions either because of time constraints or a belief that her role is to care for others first.

If the woman is isolated, it is important to find interventions that reduce isolation and increase social support. Health care providers also should attend to gender differences in the type of support given or sought. Although receiving information and advice from a physician is important, for many female CAD patients it does not feel supportive. Women want and need emotional support and empathy, to know that they are heard and understood.

Psychosocial Issues in the Detection and Treatment of Coronary Events

There are numerous gender differences in the detection and treatment of CAD. Women present later and seek care more slowly for symptoms of acute disease (112–114). Women are referred less frequently for diagnostic tests (115–117) or invasive procedures (116,117) and are referred later and less often than men from community hospitals to university or other tertiary-care hospitals for cardiac dysfunction (118). Finally, women are included less often in clinical trials (116).

Many researchers have hypothesized that psychosocial and biologic factors may influence the detection and treatment of CAD in women. Although the extent of influence is not known and research is lacking in these areas, gender differences may be due to differences in the following factors:

1. Public's and physicians' beliefs about women's risks for heart disease (113,114,119,120)

2. Women's and physicians' perception of symptoms (120,121)

3. Physicians' decision-making processes (119)

4. Gender differences in attitudes (122)

Various psychosocial factors may work together to influence a woman's decision often to delay treatment. After adjusting for SES and clinical factors, Ayanian and Epstein (122) found that women and men presenting for exercise testing did not differ in their willingness to seek a second opinion, reduce physical activity, or take medication to avoid major cardiac surgery. Men, however, were more likely than women to describe themselves as risk takers (adjusted odds ratio, 2.5; 95% CI, 1.4–4.6).

The role of common sense models of heart disease in the attribution of cardiac-related symptoms was examined in a sample of young, healthy adults (123). Interestingly, participants were less likely to attribute symptoms portrayed in a brief fictional vignette about an individual experiencing symptoms to possible cardiac causes for female victims reporting stressful life events (M = 5.14) than for female victims without such stressors (M = 6.82) or for male victims with (M = 6.23) or without (M = 6.48) concurrent stressors. In an additional sample of undergraduate students, community-residing adults, and physicians, cardiac attributions to symptoms in the vignette remained lowest for female high-stress victims. Further exploration with undergraduate students indicated that stereotypes associating CAD with men may account for gender differences in attribution of cardiac-related symptoms. Figure 20-3 depicts the process of symptom perception and interpretation suggested by these studies (123).

Even with extensive educational campaigns by the American Heart Association and other organizations, CAD is still seen as a disease of men. The extent to which this perception prevails is what McKinlay and colleagues (121) refer to as the social construction of disease prevalence. The authors argue that the social context of decision making affects diagnosis; thus, for example, the rates of women with CAD are based somewhat on "real" CAD rates and somewhat on what researchers and physicians expect to find. These expectations and rates in turn affect the interpretation, diagnosis, and treatment of symptoms (121).

Gender differences in the treatment of acute coronary events are discussed in other chapters in this book. Psychosocial factors may play a role in several ways. Psychological stress during "acute treatment" for CAD, for example, has been found to be related to prognosis. Frasure-Smith (124) found that high levels of psychological stress in the hospital predicted a threefold increase in the risk of cardiac mortality over 5 years ($p < 0.0003$) and a 1.5-fold increase in the risk of reinfarction ($p = 0.09$) among men. Jenkinson and colleagues (125) found that social isolation and high life stress resulted in a fourfold increase in risk of mortality after acute MI. Although neither of these studies included women or reported gender differences, Toth (126) found no differences between women and men in stress scores nor did he identify stressful concerns when comparing levels of stress experienced at hospital discharge after acute MI.

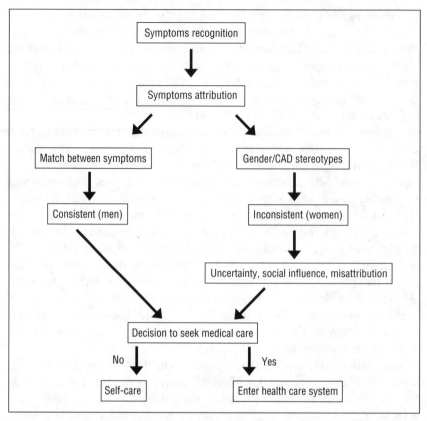

Figure 20-3 Algorithm demonstrating the influence of gender and coronary artery disease stereotypes on the interpretation of cardiac-related symptoms. (Adapted from Martin R, Gordon EEI, Lounsbury P. Gender disparities in the attribution of cardiac-related symptoms: contribution of common sense models of illness. Health Psychol. 1998;17:346–57.)

Frasure-Smith and colleagues (86) also examined the relationship of major depression, depressive symptoms, history of major depression, anxiety, anger-in and anger-out, and perceived social support measured in the hospital after an MI to the occurrence of cardiac events over the subsequent 12 months in 222 patients (49 women). Depressive symptoms, anxiety, and history of depression all predicted cardiac events, and the impact each had was independent of the others and other measures of cardiac disease severity. The only nonpsychological variable in the study to predict recurrent acute coronary syndromes was gender, although the impact was somewhat attenuated after controlling for history of depression and anxiety. In noting the limitations of this study, the authors cautiously suggested that women may be at increased risk for recurrent acute coronary syndromes after MI because of their greater tendency to express depression and anxiety.

Recommendations

More studies are needed to determine how and to what extent psychosocial factors (e.g., misinterpretation of symptoms and beliefs of women and their families about CAD, physician beliefs and attitudes about CAD, decision-making processes of both patients and physicians) influence the detection and management of CAD. Meanwhile, the medical and psychosocial research evidence suggests that consumer and physician education are needed to encourage early detection of CAD in women. Physicians can help by talking to their female patients about the risks of CAD and by emphasizing how women can reduce their risk by modifying behaviors such as smoking, obesity, and a sedentary or stressful lifestyle. Physicians also can explore with patients how controlling anger, hostility, or depression can decrease CAD risk.

In addition, physicians should educate their female patients, especially older women, about the signs and symptoms of CAD in women, encouraging them to seek care quickly and not to dismiss the symptoms as stress. Finally, physicians and other health care providers need to ask their own questions about CAD signs and to take seriously the concerns of their female patients about such symptoms, rather than minimize them.

The results of studies on the role of psychological stress and isolation during treatment suggest the need for interventions to reduce isolation, increase support, and reduce psychological stress during acute treatment. For example, one recommendation is the use of interventions that elicit the relaxation response before CABG surgery. This has been shown to reduce anxiety before and after cardiac surgery and improve a number of physical markers (127,128).

Prognosis, Rehabilitation, and Quality-of-Life Issues

Women with CAD have a higher rate of mortality than men (129), especially if they are of lower SES (130) and have a lower quality of life, poorer health, and reduced activity following an MI (131). More women (20%) have another MI during the first 4 years after MI than men (16%) (3) and in some studies are more likely to have restenosis after PTCA (132). Women may be more anxious, depressed, stressed, and unhappy with their social support following an acute MI (133). They are also more unlikely to enter cardiac rehabilitation programs and even after joining are more likely to drop out than men (134–136).

In the Cardiac Arrhythmia Suppression Trial, post-MI women were found to be limited more than men in their social functioning, to be less satisfied with their life situation, and to have had more emotional and physical stress symptoms, even after taking into account age and disease severity. Overall, women had a worse SES, psychosocial, and clinical profile than men (137). In the Swedish Follow-Up Chest study (138), 1 year after an MI women had significantly more psychological and psychosomatic complaints than men. These complaints included anxiety, feeling pressed for time, difficulty in relaxing, use of sleeping tablets, and headaches ($p < 0.01$) as well as depressive symptoms (e.g., waking up too early, waking up several times during the night [$p < 0.05$] and difficulty falling asleep).

Living alone after an MI also seems to create a risk for women (RR, 2.34; 95% CI, 1.17–4.66) and men (RR, 1.24; 95% CI, 0.75–2.03) for a recurrent cardiac event, although the difference in risk is not significant ($p = 0.14$) (139). This seems consistent with other research that found women and men with low social support (not married and without a confidant) and with low economic resources to be at increased risk for CAD-related deaths (25).

Powell and colleagues (140) found the following predictors of deaths among 83 female participants in the Recurrent Coronary Prevention Project: arrhythmias (RR = 4.01; $p = 0.004$), being divorced (interchangeable with "employed without a college degree"; RR = 3.43; $p = 0.01$), and the inverse of time urgency (interchangeable with "emotional arousability"; RR = 0.35; $p = 0.02$). Although these findings must be considered in terms of the study limitations, the authors suggest that many of the women in their sample had "unmet expectations" of living the wife and mother roles for which they opted in the 1940s and 1950s. They suggested that the combination of having to work, losing intimate supports, and the emotional byproducts of their "unmet expectations" of anger, resentment, loneliness, and dissatisfaction (especially if suppressed) was lethal for these women.

Cardiac rehabilitation exercise programs have been shown to reduce the risk of recurrent MIs by 25% (141), although fewer than 10% of all patients who could benefit from these programs participate (142). Women participate even less than men, but when they do they benefit as much or perhaps more than men (134,135,143). (These issues are discussed in more detail in Chapter 8.)

Recent evidence indicates that a stress management intervention program can offer benefits over and above the usual medical care and cardiac rehabilitation exercise programs in decreasing risks of a cardiac event in patients (10). In the study by Blumenthal and colleagues (10), as in other studies, patients who underwent stress management showed reductions in hostility and overall psychological distress. This is important because, as noted above, hostility has been associated with increased morbidity and risk for acute MI in some individuals. Hostility has also predicted restenosis after PTCA, although rates of restenosis were higher for women despite their hostility levels being lower (132). Also, clinical depression has been shown to be associated with increased mortality and morbidity after an MI (144); in the study by Blumenthal and colleagues (10), depression was reduced in the exercise group—a finding consistent with other studies.

Recommendations

The severe psychosocial problems that many women experience after acute CAD events and treatments decrease their daily functioning, productivity, and quality of life. Furthermore, for some women (especially those who are socially isolated, depressed, or both) these post-MI problems are associated with increased risk of recurrent events and death.

Health care providers need to assess for the possible difficulties confronting women with CAD and to do whatever possible to facilitate their recovery. Physicians need to attend to their female patients' world (i.e., their SES, psychosocial functioning [assessing especially for social isolation and depressive symptoms], risk behaviors, and clinical condition). This includes asking questions about their female patients' living situations and support. If a woman lives alone without adequate support, try to encourage relatives or friends to stay with her or arrange for home care visits. If the patient shows the aforementioned signs of depression, referral to an appropriate mental health professional for psychotherapeutic and psychopharmacologic treatment may be beneficial. The physician also may take steps to manage the depression.

It is also important to encourage women to attend cardiac rehabilitation and stress management programs. Physician recommendations have been found to be the most powerful predictor of participation in cardiac rehabilitation (143). When making the referrals to rehabilitation programs, assess the ability of the patient to attend; this may mean assistance with transportation, dependent care, and so on. If stress management is not an integral component of the local cardiac rehabilitation program, refer female patients to a stress management program or counseling that teaches relaxation techniques and cognitive–behavioral techniques for managing stress.

Health care providers also can play a role in decreasing social isolation and increasing social support, thus improving their patients' prognosis. Frasure-Smith (124) demonstrated how an intervention consisting of one brief contact with male patients recovering from an MI in the hospital followed by monthly 30-minute telephone interviews conducted by trained nursing aides reduced subsequent cardiac events.

Finally, physicians also may be able to improve prognosis and contribute to a better quality of life for their patients by attending to the often forgotten factors of religious faith and spirituality. Recent evidence suggests that spiritual concerns and issues of faith can play a potent role in helping patients make risk-reducing lifestyle changes, such as in Ornish and colleagues' (145) programs. Other studies found reduced death rates (2%–3%) in coronary surgery patients who reported gaining comfort from their religious beliefs and who regularly spent time with others in group activities compared with patients who did not (25% mortality rate) (146).

Based on their extensive experience leading post-MI groups of women and men, Bracke and Thoresen (147) suggested that health care providers can assist patients with CAD making lifestyle changes that reduce mortality and morbidity by helping them look at their unexplored and unresolved spiritual, religious, and existential issues.

Conclusion: Suggestions for Addressing Psychosocial Issues in Women

The evidence clearly indicates the significance of SES, health behaviors, and psychologic factors in the cause, prevention, detection, treatment, and recovery from CAD in women and men. It also suggests the importance of culture, race, environment, and neighborhood. Gender differences appear throughout the course of CAD.

Physicians play a key role in addressing psychosocial issues in their female patients who have or are at risk for CAD. This includes educating women about CAD symptoms and risks, advocating heart-healthy behavioral changes, listening carefully to the patient for symptoms, and emphasizing early detection and treatment. It also involves assessing for key psychosocial risks (e.g., low education and SES, depression and social isolation, anxiety and anger) and treating and referring accordingly. Treatments and referrals for female patients include not only treatment for clinical medical symptoms but also for social isolation (e.g., bringing in friends and family, referring to a support group), anxiety and depression (e.g., bibliotherapy, psychotherapy, drug management), stress management, and cardiac rehabilitation.

Below is a list of suggestions for physicians and other health care providers working with women with CAD or women seeking to reduce their risk of developing CAD or an acute coronary event:

1. Although heart disease is the number one killer of women in the United States, remember that both the cardiac and behavioral or psychosocial research on women still lag behind that of men. Relationships found in men may not hold true for women or may operate in a different way; for example, there is some evidence that the role of hostility and anger over the course of CAD may be different for men and women. Structured type A interviews do not consistently predict

recurrent cardiac events in women with CAD as they do for men with CAD. Another example is social support, which has a buffering effect on CAD in men but which may not always be positive for women, especially if it involves perceptions of obligations, caretaking, or role strain.

2. It is important for physicians to examine their own cultural or social assumptions for biases that could affect either the information obtained from patients or the delivery of care. For example, does your patient understand how to decrease fat from her diet, or does she believe she is able to do so financially? Does she have the money, transportation, or adequate child care to get to appointments or to attend cardiac rehabilitation programs? Although it may be difficult, it is essential to attend to the particulars of women's lives.

3. Women seem to experience more anxiety and depression after MI or cardiac surgery than men. Assess carefully the female patient's ability to work, social and familial interactions, sexual functioning, and level of emotional distress after MI or cardiac surgery.

4. Ask about the patient's social roles. Who are her supports? Whom does she support? What kind of role stresses does she have (e.g., work, being a single parent, caring for grandchildren or aging parents)?

5. Assess for history of psychiatric and mental health problems, especially history of depression. Look for current signs of depression or anxiety. Find out how often she expresses anger or cries. Research stress in her life, including role stresses, financial stresses, and "unmet expectations." Because there is a mind–body link, the comorbidity of CAD and mental illness or its symptoms can affect the course and treatment of both disorders.

6. Recent evidence suggests that spirituality and religious beliefs can play both positive and negative roles in changing CAD risk behaviors and in morbidity and mortality. Ask your patient about her spirituality and religious beliefs and what role she sees them playing in her health and coping. Although relatively new in modern medicine, this is not a new suggestion. Over 2500 years ago, Hippocrates noted that "You ought not to attempt to cure the body without the soul."

Whether assessing a patient's risk for developing CAD, taking steps to modify her risk factors, treating her acute onset of CAD, or assisting with her recovery or rehabilitation, listen to the woman with empathy and ask about her everyday life and relationships.

REFERENCES

1. **Harvey W.** Anatomical studies on the motion of the heart and blood. Springfield, IL: Charles C. Thomas; 1928:107.

2. **Allan R, Scheidt S.** Empirical basis for cardiac psychology. In: Allan R, Scheidt S, eds. Heart and Mind: The Practice of Cardiac Psychology. Washington, DC: The American Psychological Association; 1996:63–123.

3. **American Heart Association.** Heart and Stroke Facts: 1995 Statistical Supplement. Dallas, TX: American Heart Association; 1995.

4. **Higgins M, Thom T.** Cardiovascular disease in women as a public health threat. In: Wenger NK, Speroff L, Packard B, eds. Cardiovascular Health and Disease in Women. Greenwich, CT: Le Jacq Communications; 1993:15–9.

5. **Wenger NK, Speroff L, Packard B, eds.** Cardiovascular Health and Disease in Women. Greenwich, CT: Le Jacq Communications; 1993.

6. **Wenger NK.** The natural history of coronary artery disease in women. In: Charney P, ed. Coronary Artery Disease in Women: What All Physicians Need to Know. Philadelphia: American College of Physicians; 1999:3–35 [this publication].

7. **Brown MS, Goldstein JL.** Heart attacks: gone with the century? Science. 1996;272:629.

8. **Thoresen CE, Goldberg JH.** Coronary heart disease: a psychosocial perspective on assessment and intervention. In: Roth-Roemer S, Robinson Kurpius S, Carmin C, eds. The Emerging Role of Counseling Psychology in Health Care. New York: WW Norton; 1998:94–136.

9. **Engel GL.** The need for a new medical model: a challenge for biomedicine. Science. 1977; 196:129–36.

10. **Blumenthal JA, Jiang W, Babyak MA, et al.** Stress management and exercise training in cardiac patients with myocardial ischemia: effects on prognosis and evaluation of mechanisms. Arch Intern Med. 1997; 157:2213–23.

11. **Pratt LA, Ford DE, Crum RM, et al.** Depression, psychotropic medication, and risk of myocardial infarction: prospective data from the Baltimore ECA follow-up. Circulation. 1996;94:3123–9.

12. **Stanton AL.** Psychology of women's health: Barriers and pathways to knowledge. In Stanton AL, Gallant SJ, eds. The Psychology of Women's Health: Progress and Challenges in Research and Application. Washington, DC: American Psychological Association; 1995:3–21.

13. **Gallant SJ, Puryear Keita G, Royak-Schaler R (eds).** Health Care for Women: Psychological, Social, and Behavioral Influences. Washington, DC: American Psychological Association; 1997.

14. **Knox SS, Czajkowski S.** The influence of behavioral and psychosocial factors on cardiovascular health in women. In: Gallant SJ, Puryear Keita G, Royak-Schaler R, eds. Health Care for Women: Psychological, Social, and Behavioral Influences. Washington, DC: American Psychological Association; 1997:257–72.

15. **Jacobs SC, Sherwood JB.** The cardiac psychology of women and coronary heart disease. In: Allan R, Scheidt S, eds. Heart and Mind: The Practice of Cardiac Psychology. Washington, DC: American Psychological Association; 1996:197–218.

16. **Office of Research on Women's Health.** Opportunities for Research on Women's Health. Washington, DC: NIH publication no. 92-3457; 1992.

17. **Czajkowski SM, Hill DR, Clarkson TB, eds.** Women, Behavior, and Cardiovascular Disease. Proceedings of a conference sponsored by the National Heart, Lung, and Blood Institute, September 25–27, 1991. Washington, DC: NIH publication no. 94-3309; 1994.

18. **Eaker ED.** Psychosocial factors in the epidemiology of coronary heart disease in women. Psych Clin North Am. 1989;12:167–73.

19. **Chesney MA.** Social isolation, depression, and heart disease: research on women broadens the agenda [Editorial]. Psychosom Med. 1993;55:434–5.

20. **Lerner DJ, Kennel WB.** Patterns of coronary heart disease morbidity and mortality in the sexes: a 26-year follow-up of the Framingham population. Am Health J. 1986;111: 383–90.

21. **Eaker ED, Pinsky J, Castelli WP.** Myocardial infarction and coronary death among women: psychosocial predictors from a 20-year follow-up of women in the Framingham study. Am J Epidemiol. 1992;135:854–64.

22. **Brezinka V, Kittel F.** Psychosocial factors of coronary heart disease in women: a review. Soc Sci Med. 1996;42:1351–65.

23. **Lenfant C.** Conference on socioeconomic status and cardiovascular health and disease. Circulation. 1996;94:2041–4.

24. **Adler NE, Boyce T, Chesney MA, et al.** Socioeconomic inequalities in health: no easy solution. JAMA. 1993;269:3140–5.

25. **Williams RB, Barefoot JC, Califf RM, et al.** Prognostic importance of social and economic resources among medically treated patients with angiographically documented coronary artery disease. JAMA. 1992;267:520–4.

26. **Rogot E, Sorlie PD, Johnson NJ, Schmitt C.** A mortality study of 1.3 million persons. Washington, DC: National Heart, Lung, and Blood Institute; 1992.

27. **Gliksman MD, Kawachi I, Hunter D, et al.** Childhood socioeconomic status and risk of cardiovascular disease in middle aged US women: a prospective study. J Epidemiol Community Health. 1995;49:10–5.

28. **Morrison C, Woodward M, Leslie W, Tunstall-Pedoe H.** Effect of socioeconomic group on incidence of, management of, and survival after myocardial infarction and coronary death: analysis of community coronary event register. BMJ. 1997;314:541–6.

29. **Gilman RF, Mussolino ME, Madans JH.** Coronary heart disease incidence and survival in African American women and men: the NHANES I epidemiologic follow-up study. Ann Intern Med. 1997;127:111–8.

30. **Gilman RF, Mussolino ME, Madans JH.** Coronary heart disease risk factors and attributable risks in African American women and men: NHANES I epidemiologic follow-up study. Am J Public Health. 1998;88:913–7.

31. **Taylor HA, Mickel MC, Chaitman BR, et al.** Long-term survival of African Americans in the Coronary Artery Surgery Study (CASS). 1997;29:358–64.

32. **McCord C, Freeman HP.** Excess mortality in Harlem. N Engl J Med. 1990;322:173–7.

33. **Escobedo LG, Giles WH, Anda RF.** Socioeconomic status, race, and death from coronary heart disease. Am J Prev Med. 1997;13:123–30.

34. **Gornick ME, Eggers PW, Reilly TW, et al.** Effects of race and income on mortality and use of services among Medicare beneficiaries. N Engl J Med. 1996;335:791–9

35. **Power C, Mathews S.** Origins of health inequalities in a national population sample. Lancet. 1997;350:1584–9.

36. **James WPT, Nelson M, Ralph A, Leather S.** Socioeconomic determinants of health: the contribution of nutrition to inequalities in health. BMJ. 1997;314:1545–9.

37. **LcClere FB, Rogers RG, Peters K.** Neighborhood social context and racial differences in woman's heart disease mortality. J Health Soc Behav. 1998;39:91–107.

38. **Diez-Roux AV, Nieto FJ, Muntaner C, et al.** Neighborhood environments and coronary heart disease: a multilevel analysis. Am J Epidemiol. 1997;146:48–63.

39. **Lachman ME, Weaver SL.** The sense of control as a moderator of social class differences in health and well-being. J Pers Soc Psychol. 998;74:763–73.

40. **Friedman HS, ed.** Hostility, Coping, and Health. Washington, DC: American Psychological Association; 1982.

41. **Helmers KF, Posluszny DM, Krantz DS.** Associations of hostility and coronary artery disease: a review of studies. In: Siegman AW, Smith W, eds. Anger, Hostility, and the Heart. Hillsdale, NJ: Lawrence Erlbaum Associates; 1994:215–37.

42. **Smith TW.** Hostility and health: current status of a psychosomatic hypothesis. Health Psych. 1992;11:139–50.

43. **Dembroski TM, MacDougall JM, Costa PT, Grandits GA.** Components of hostility as predictors of sudden death and myocardial infarction in the Multiple Risk Factor Intervention Trial. Psychosom Med. 1989;51:514–22.

44. **Barefoot JC, Haney TL, Hershkowitz BD, William RB.** Hostility and coronary artery disease in women and men. Paper presented at the Twelfth Annual Meeting of the Society of Behavioral Medicine, Washington, DC; March 1991.

45. **Friedman M, Fleischmann N, Price VA.** Diagnosis of Type A Behavior Pattern. In: Allan R, Scheidt S, eds. Heart and Mind: The Practice of Cardiac Psychology. Washington, DC: The American Psychological Association; 1996:179–95.

46. **Thoresen CE, Low KG.** Women and the type A behavior pattern: review and commentary. J Soc Behav Pers. 1990;5:117–33.

47. **Eaker ED, Abbott RD, Kannel WB.** Frequency of uncomplicated angina pectoris in type A compared to type B persons (the Framingham study). Am J Cardiol. 1989;63:1042–5.

48. **Haellstroem T, Lapidus L, Bengtson C, Edstroem K.** Psychosocial factors and risk of ischemic heart disease and death in women: a 12-year follow-up of participants in the population study of women in Gothenburg, Sweden. J Psychosom Res. 1986;30:451–9.

49. **Graff-Low K, Thoresen CE, King A, Patillo J, Jenkins C.** Anxiety, depression, and heart disease in women. Int J Behav Med. 1995;1:305–19.

50. **Barefoot JC, Dahlstrom WG, Williams RB.** Hostility, coronary heart disease incidence, and total mortality: a 25-year follow-up study of 255 physicians. Psychosom Med. 1983;45:59–63.

51. **Barefoot JC, Dodge KA, Peterson BL, et al.** The Cook–Medley hostility scale: Item content and ability to predict survival. Psychosom Med. 1989;51:46–57.

52. **O'Connor NJ, Manson JE, O'Connor GT, Buring JE.** Psychosocial risk factors and nonfatal myocardial infarction. Circulation. 1995;92:1458–64.

53. **Adams SH.** Role of hostility in women's health during midlife: a longitudinal study. Health Psych. 1994;13:488–95.

54. **Blascovich J, Katkin ES, eds.** Cardiovascular Reactivity to Psychological Stress and Disease. Washington, DC: American Psychological Association; 1993.

55. **Suarez EC, Harlan E, Peoples MC, Williams RB.** Cardiovascular and emotional response in women: the role of hostility and harassment. Health Psych. 1993;12:459–68.

56. **Allen MT, Stoney CM, Owens JF, Matthews KA.** Hemodynamic adjustments to laboratory stress: the influence of gender and personality. Psychosom Med. 1993;55:505–17.

57. **Jacobs, SC, Kincs P, Northrup T, et al.** Reactivity Differences with Anger Recall Task: Communicative Versus Aggressive Expression. Poster presentation, Division 38, American Psychological Association Annual Convention in Chicago, Illinois; August 1997.

58. **Stoney CM, Engebretson TO.** Anger and hostility: potential mediators of the gender difference in coronary heart disease. In: Siegman AW, Smith TW, eds. Anger, Hostility, and the Heart. Hillsdale, NJ: Lawrence Erlbaum Associates; 1994:215–37.

59. **Powch IG, Houston BK.** Hostility, anger-in, and cardiovascular reactivity in white women. Health Psych. 1996;15:200–8.

60. **Anderson SF, Lawler KA.** The anger recall interview and cardiovascular reactivity in women: an examination of context and experience. J Psychosom Res. 1995;39:335–43.

61. **Saab PG, Llabre MM, Schneiderman N, et al.** Influence of ethnicity and gender on cardiovascular response to active coping and inhibitory-passive coping challenge. Psychosom Med. 1997;59:434–46.

62. **Kawachi I, Sparrow D, Spiro III A, et al.** A prospective study of anger and coronary heart disease. Circulation. 1996;94:2090–5.

63. **Mittleman MA, Maclure M, Sherwood JB, et al.** Triggering of acute myocardial infarction onset by episodes of anger. Circulation. 1995;92:1720–5.

64. **Weidner G.** The role of hostility and coronary-prone behaviors in the etiology of cardiovascular disease in women. In: Czajkowski SM, Hill DR, Clarkson TB, eds. Women, Behavior, and Cardiovascular Disease. Washington, DC; NIH publication no. 94-3309; 1994.

65. **Allan R, Scheidt S, eds.** Heart and Mind: The Practice of Cardiac Psychology. Washington, DC: American Psychological Association; 1996.

66. **Williams RB, Williams VP.** Anger Kills: Seventeen Strategies for Controlling the Hostility That Can Harm Your Health. New York: Times Books; 1993.

67. **Benson H, Stuart E, eds.** The Wellness Book: A Comprehensive Guide to Health and Treating Stress-Related Illness. New York: Fireside Books; 1993.

68. **Carney RM, Freedland KE, Smith LJ, et al.** Depression and anxiety as risk factors for coronary heart disease in women. In: Czajkowski SM, Hill DR, Clarkson TB, eds. Women, Behavior, and Cardiovascular Disease. Washington, DC, NIH publication no. 94-3309; 1994.

69. **Booth-Kewley S, Friedman H.** Psychological predictors of heart disease: a quantitative review. Psych Bull. 1987;101:110–2.

70. **Dimsdale JE.** Influences of personality and stress-induced biological processes on etiology and treatment of cardiovascular diseases in women. In: Wenger NK, Speroff L, Packard B, eds. Cardiovascular Health and Disease in Women. Greenwich, CT: Le Jacq Communications; 1993.

71. **Cottington EM, Matthews KA, Talbott E, Kuller LH.** Environmental events preceding sudden death in women. Psychosom Med. 1980;42:567–74.

72. **Appels A, Mulder P.** Fatigue and heart disease: The association between vital exhaustion and past, present, and future coronary heart disease. J Psychosom Res. 1989;33:727–38.

73. **Falger PRJ, Schouten EGW.** Exhaustion, psychological stressors in the work environment, and acute myocardial infarction in adult men. J Psychosom Res. 1992;36:777–86.

74. **Appels A, Falger PRJ, Schouten GW.** Vital exhaustion as risk indicator for myocardial infarction in women. J Psychosom Res. 1993;37:881–90.

75. **Jacobs DG, Kopans BS, Reizes JM.** Reevaluation of depression: what the general practitioner needs to know. Mind Body Med. 1995;1:17–22.

76. **American Psychiatric Association.** Diagnostic and Statistical Manual of Mental Disorders. 4th ed. Washington, DC: American Psychiatric Association; 1994.

77. **Tabrizi K, Littman A, Williams RB, Scheidt S.** Psychopharmacology and cardiac diseases. In: Allan R, Scheidt S, eds. Heart and Mind: The Practice of Cardiac Psychology. Washington, DC: American Psychological Association; 1996:397–419.

78. **Depression Guideline Panel.** Clinical Practice Guideline No. 5. Depression in Primary Care, Part 2: Treatment of Major Depression. Rockville, MD: US Department of Health and Human Services, Agency for Health Care Policy and Research. AHCPR Publication No. 93-0551; 1993.

79. **Scogin F, Jamison C, Davis N.** Two-year follow-up of bibliotherapy for depression in older adults. J Consult Clin Psychol. 1990;58:665–7.

80. **Lewinsohn P, Munoz R, Youngren M, Zeiss A.** Control Your Depression. Englewood Cliffs, NJ: Prentice-Hall; 1986.

81. **Burns D.** The Feeling Good Handbook. New York: Plume/Penguin; 1990.

82. **Roose SP, Laghrissi-Thode F, Kennedy JS, et al.** Comparison of paroxetine and nortriptyline in depressed patients with ischemic heart disease. JAMA. 1998;279:287–91.

83. **Fleet RP, Beitman BD.** Cardiovascular death from panic disorder and panic-like anxiety: a critical review of the literature. J Psychosom Res. 1998;44:71–80.

84. **Kawachi I, Coldwitz GA, Ascherio A, et al.** Prospective study of phobic anxiety and risk of coronary heart disease in men. Circulation. 1994;89:2225–9.

85. **Kawachi I, Sparrow D, Vokonas PS, Weiss ST.** Decreased heart rate variability in men with phobic anxiety. Am J Cardiol. 1995;75:882–5.

86. **Frasure-Smith N, Lespererance F, Talajic M.** The impact of negative emotions on prognosis following myocardial infarction: is it more than depression? Health Psych. 1995;14:388–98.

87. **Rosanski A, Bairey CN, Krantz DS, et al.** Mental stress and the induction of silent ischemia in patients with coronary artery disease. N Engl J Med. 1988;318:1005–12.

88. **Lint DW, Taylor CB, Freid-behar L, et al.** Does ischemia occur with panic attacks? Am J Psychiatry. 1995;154:1678–80.

89. **Cohen S, Tyrell DAJ, Smith AP.** Psychological stress and susceptibility to the common cold. N Eng J Med. 1991;325:606–12.

90. **McEwen BS.** Protective and damaging effects on stress mediators. N Engl J Med. 1998;338:171–9.

91. **Magni G, Corfini A, Berto F, et al.** Life events and myocardial infarction. Austr N Z J Med. 1983;13:257–60.

92. **Jacobs SC, Maclure M, Sherwood J, et al.** High frequency of positive or negative psychologically stressful events possibly trigger onset of myocardial infarction [Abstract]. Program Book, Society of Behavioral Medicine Annual Meeting; 1992.

93. **Jacobs SC, Friedman R, Mittleman M, et al.** Nine-fold increased risk of myocardial following psychological stress as assessed by a case-control study. Circulation. 1992; 86:789.

94. **Mulrey A, Dohrenwend BS.** The relation of stressful life events to gender. Issues Ment Health Nurs. 1983;5:219–37.

95. **Kessler RC, McLeod JD.** Sex differences in vulnerability to undesirable life events. Am Soc Rev. 1984;49:620–31.

96. **Krishnan KR, George LK, Pieper CF, et al.** Depression and social support in elderly patients with cardiac disease. Am Heart J. 1998;136:491–5.

97. **Tofler GH, Stone PH, Maclure M, et al.** Analysis of possible triggers of acute myocardial infarction (the MILIS study). Am J Cardiol. 1990;66:22–7.

98. **Behar S, Halabi M, Reicher-Reiss H, et al.** Circadian variation and possible external triggers of onset of myocardial infarction: SPRINT Study Group. Am J Med. 1993;94:395–400.

99. **Theorell T, Karasek RA.** Current issues relating to psychosocial job strain and cardiovascular disease. J Occup Health Psychol. 1996;1:9–26.

100. **Kritz-Silverstein D, Wingard DL, Barrett-Connor E.** Employment status and heart disease risk factors in middle-aged women: the Rancho Bernardo study. Am J Public Health. 1992; 82:215–9.

101. **Haertel U, Heiss G, Filipiak B, Doering A.** Cross-sectional and longitudinal associations between high density lipoprotein cholesterol and women's employment. Am J Epidemiol. 1992;135:68–78.

102. **Hall EM.** Multiple roles and caregiving stress in women. In: Czajkowski SM, Hill DR, Clarkson TB, eds. Women, Behavior, and Cardiovascular Disease. Washington, DC: NIH publication no. 94-3309; 1994.

103. **Kawachi I, Colditz GA, Stampfer MJ, et al.** Prospective study of shift work and risk of coronary heart disease in women. Circulation. 1995;92:3178–82.

104. **Theorell T.** Psychosocial cardiovascular risks on the double loads in women. Psychother Psychosom. 1991;55:81–9.

105. **Dixon JP, Dixon JK, Spinner JC.** Tensions between career and interpersonal commitments as a risk factor for cardiovascular disease among women. Women Health. 1991; 17:33–57.

106. **Shumaker SA, Hill DR.** Gender differences in social support and physical health. Health Psych. 1991;10:102–11.

107. **O'Leary A, Helgeson VS.** Psychosocial factors and women's health: integrating mind, heart, and body. In: Gallant SJ, Keita GP, Royak-Schaler R, eds. Health Care for Women: Psychological, Social, and Behavioral Influences. Washington, DC: American Psychological Association; 1997:25–40.

108. **Allen KM, Blascovich J, Tomaka J, Kelsey RM.** Presence of human friends and pet dogs as moderators of autonomic responses to stress in women. J Personality Soc Psych. 1991;61:582–9.

109. **Kamarck TW, Manuck SB, Jennings JR.** Social support reduces cardiovascular reactivity to psychological challenge: a laboratory model. Psychosom Med. 1990;52:42–58.

110. **Berkman LF.** Social support and cardiovascular disease morbidity and mortality in women. In: Czajkowski SM, Hill DR, Clarkson TB, eds. Women, Behavior and Cardiovascular Disease. Washington, DC; NIH publication no. 94-3309; 1994.

111. **Berkman LF, Vaccarino V, Seeman T.** Gender differences in cardiovascular morbidity and mortality: the contribution of social networks and support. In: Wenger NK, Sper-

off L, Packard B, eds. Cardiovascular Health and Disease in Women. Greenwich, CT: Le Jacq Communications; 1993.

112. **Fiebach NH.** Biobehavioral and psychosocial factors in the diagnosis and treatment of coronary heart disease in women. In: Czajkowski SM, Hill DR, Clarkson TB, eds. Women, Behavior and Cardiovascular Disease. Washington, DC: NIH publication no. 94-3309; 1994.

113. **Moser DK.** Gender differences in symptom recognition and health care seeking behaviors. In: Czajkowski SM, Hill DR, Clarkson TB, eds. Women, Behavior and Cardiovascular Disease. Washington, DC: NIH publication no. 94-3309; 1994.

114. **Wingard DL, Cohn BA, Cirillo PM, et al.** Gender differences in self-reported heart disease morbidity: are intervention opportunities missed for women? J Women Health. 1992;1:201–8.

115. **Shaw LJ, Miller DD, Romeis JC, et al.** Gender differences in the noninvasive evaluation and management of patients with suspected coronary artery disease. Ann Int Med. 1994;120:559–66.

116. **Detre KM, Stone PH.** Working group report: management of coronary heart disease in women. In: Wenger NK, Speroff L, Packard B, eds. Cardiovascular Health and Disease in Women. Greenwich, CT: Le Jacq Communications; 1993.

117. **Welty FK.** Gender differences in outcome after diagnosis and treatment of coronary artery disease. In: Czajkowski SM, Hill DR, Clarkson TB, eds. Women, Behavior and Cardiovascular Disease. Washington, DC: NIH publication no. 94-3309; 1994.

118. **Sherwood J, Maclure M, Goldberg RJ, et al.** Women are referred later than men for tertiary care following myocardial infarction. Circulation. 1992;86:39.

119. **Schulman KA, Escarce JJ, Eisenberg JM, et al.** Assessing physicians' estimates of the probability of coronary artery disease: the influence of patient characteristics. Med Decision Making. 1992;12:109–114.

120. **McKinlay JB, McKinlay SM, Crawford SL.** Does variability in physician behavior explain any of the gender difference in cardiovascular disease. In Czajkowski SM, Hill DR, Clarkson TB, eds. Women, Behavior, and Cardiovascular Disease. Washington, DC: NIH publication no. 94-3309; 1994.

121. **McKinlay JB, Crawford S, McKinley SM, Sellers DE.** On the reported gender differences in coronary heart disease: an illustration of the social construction of epidemiologic rates. Watertown, MA: New England Research Institute; 1993.

122. **Ayanian JZ, Epstein AM.** Attitudes about treatment of coronary heart disease among women and men presenting for exercise testing. J Gen Intern Med. 1997;12:311–4.

123. **Martin R, Gordon EEI, Lounsbury.** Gender disparities in the attribution of cardiac-related symptoms: contribution of common sense models of illness. Health Psych. 1998; 17:346–57.

124. **Frasure-Smith N.** In-hospital predictors of psychological stress as predictors of long-term outcome after acute myocardial infarction in men. Am J Cardiol. 1991;67:121–7.

125. **Jenkinson CM, Madeley RJ, Mitchell JR, Turner ID.** The influence of psychosocial factors on survival after myocardial infarction. Public Health. 1993;107:305–317.

126. **Toth JC.** Is stress at hospital discharge after acute myocardial infarction greater in women than in men? Am J Crit Care. 1993;2:35–40.

127. **Mandle CL, Domar AD, Harrington DP, et al.** Relaxation response in femoral angiography. Radiology. 1990;174:737–9.

128. **Mandle CL, Jacobs SC, Arcari PM, Domar AD.** The efficacy of relaxation response interventions with adult patients: a review of the literature. J Cardiovasc Nurs. 1996;10: 4–26.

129. **Tofler GH, Stone PH, Muller JE, et al.** Effects of gender and race on prognosis after myocardial infarction: adverse prognosis for women, particularly black women. J Am Coll Cardiol. 1987;9:473–482.

130. **Tofler GH, Muller JE, Stone PH, et al.** Multicenter Investigation of the Limitation of Infarct Size (MILIS): comparison of long-term outcome after acute myocardial infarction in patients never graduated from high school with that in more educated patients. Am J Cardiol. 1993; 71:1031–5.

131. **Conn VS, Taylor SG, Abele PB.** Myocardial infarction survivors: age and gender differences in physical health, psychosocial, state, and regimen adherence. J Adv Nursing. 1991;16:1026–34.

132. **Goodman M, Quigley J, Moran G, et al.** Hostility predicts restenosis after percutaneous transluminal coronary angioplasty. Mayo Clin Proc. 1996;71:729–34.

133. **Frank E, Taylor CB.** Psychosocial influences on diagnosis and treatment plans of women with coronary heart disease. In: Wenger NK, Speroff L, Packard B, eds. Cardiovascular Health and Disease in Women. Greenwich, CT: Le Jacq Communications. 1993:231–7.

134. **Haskell WL.** Cardiac rehabilitation and secondary prevention: issues of participation and benefit for women. In: Wenger NK, Speroff L, Packard B, eds. Cardiovascular Health and Disease in Women. Greenwich, CT: Le Jacq Communications; 1993.

135. **Downing J, Littman A.** Gender differences in response to cardiac rehabilitation. In: Czajkowski SM, Hill DR, Clarkson TB, eds. Women, Behavior and Cardiovascular Disease. Washington, DC: NIH publication no. 94-3309; 1994.

136. **Schron EB, Pawitan Y, Shumaker SA, Hale C.** Health quality of life differences between men and women in a postinfarction study. Circulation. 1991;84:245.

137. **Shumaker SA, Brooks MM, Schron EB, et al.** Gender differences in health-related quality of life among post-myocardial infarction patients: brief report from the Cardiac Arrhythmia Suppression Trials (CAST) investigators. Womens Health. 1997;3:53–60.

138. **Wiklund I, Herlitz JH, Johansson S, et al.** Subjective symptoms and well-being differ in women and men after myocardial infarction. Eur Heart J. 1993;14:1315–9.

139. **Case RB, Moss AJ, Case N, et al.** Living alone after myocardial infarction: impact on prognosis. JAMA. 1992;267:515–9.

140. **Powell LH, Shaker LA, Jones BA, et al.** Psychosocial predictors of mortality in 83 women with premature acute myocardial infarctions. Psychosom Med. 1993;55:426–33.

141. **Oldridge NB, Guyatt GH, Fischer ME, Rimm AA.** Cardiac rehabilitation after myocardial infarction: combined experience of randomized clinical trials. JAMA. 1988; 260:945–50.

142. **Wenger NK, Froelicher ES, Smith LK, et al.** Cardiac Rehabilitation. Rockville, MD: US Department of Health and Human Services. ACHPR publication no. 95-0672; 1995.

143. **Ades PA, Waldmann ML, Polk DM, Coflesky JT.** Referral patterns and exercise response in the rehabilitation of female coronary patients aged more than 62 years. Am J Cardiol. 1992;69:1422–5.

144. **Pennix WJH, Guralnik JM, Mendes de Leon CF, Pahor M, et al.** Cardiovascular events and mortality in newly and chronically depressed persons over 70 years of age. Am J Cardiol. 1998;81:988–94.

145. **Ornish D, Brown SE, Scherwitz LS, et al.** Can lifestyle changes reduce coronary artery disease? Lancet. 1990;336:129–33.

146. **Oxman TE, Freeman DH, Manheimer ED.** Lack of social participation or religious strength and comfort as risk factor for death after cardiac surgery in the elderly. Psychosom Med. 1995;57:5–15.

147. **Bracke PE, Thoresen CE.** Reducing Type A behavior patterns: a structured group approach. In: Allan R, Scheidt S, eds. Heart and Mind: The Practice of Cardiac Psychology. Washington, DC: The American Psychological Association; 1996:255–90.

CHAPTER 21

Pharmacologic Secondary Prevention

EVA M. LONN, MD

SALIM YUSUF, MBBS, DPHIL

Coronary artery disease (CAD) remains the leading cause of death and disability for both women and men in industrialized nations (1,2). Considerable progress has been made in the treatment of the acute phase of myocardial infarction (MI), which in turn has resulted in important improvements in short-term outcomes. Despite this progress, however, patients recovering from acute MI remain at increased risk for reinfarction and cardiac death, particularly during the first few months after acute MI but also over the long term. Comprehensive evaluation and aggressive intervention in survivors of MI are therefore essential. Women and men who have sustained a previous MI are targeted for secondary prevention, which is best described as the totality of therapeutic interventions aimed at reducing morbidity and mortality after a first event. Patients with other manifestations of cardiovascular disease and even asymptomatic patients with highly adverse risk factor profiles are also at considerable risk for adverse outcomes. It is therefore reasonable to apply many of the preventive therapeutic strategies evaluated best in MI survivors to a wider range of patients, those at high risk for morbidity and mortality caused by cardiovascular disease.

The determinants of outcomes for women after acute MI and for women in other high-risk categories are similar to those for men and include the degree of left ventricular dysfunction, the presence and extent of residual ischemia, and the degree of electrical instability of the myocardium. In addition, factors such as age, diabetes, hyperlipidemia, a history of smoking, and psychosocial factors may also greatly influence outcomes. It is important to evaluate these risk factors carefully to identify low-risk, intermediate-risk, and high-risk categories within this subgroup of patients, and, following such evaluation, to implement strategies proven to improve outcomes and quality of life. This chapter reviews the use of pharmacologic interventions in women with known CAD, emphasizing the management of women after acute MI. Lifestyle modifications, hormonal replacement therapy, emerging preventive strategies (e.g., the use of antioxidants), and the use of invasive therapies such as angioplasty and coronary artery bypass graft surgery are not reviewed in this chapter.

Women have been generally under-represented in studies of short- and long-term outcomes after MI as well as in epidemiologic investigations and clinical trials of coronary artery disease in general (3). Therefore, the evaluation of different cardiovascular therapies in women has been based generally on subgroup analyses within clinical trials. The frequent problems encountered in subgroup analyses apply (4). The results of such evaluations are subject to numerous potential sources of error and at times have been misleading. Often the sample size of the subgroups is inadequate. This is an important limitation in the study of cardiovascular therapies in women, particularly because women are under-represented in most cardiovascular trials. Also, there is too often a failure to specify *a priori* the subgroups of interest and the hypotheses to be tested. Finally, statistical methods may not reflect multiple comparisons (across various subgroups and for different outcomes). These limitations could lead to the chance findings of spurious subgroup effects or, conversely, to the failure to identify true subgroup findings.

It is essential, therefore, to analyze reports of potential gender-specific effects of various cardiovascular drugs while recognizing the difficulties and potential pitfalls of subgroup analyses. To minimize the potential for error, it is important to carefully evaluate the *totality of evidence* on the effects of each intervention studied, especially if there is only adequate statistical power prior to subgroup analysis. For this chapter, the overall study results (independent of gender) for each individual trial were assessed initially, followed by exploration of drug efficacy across various subgroups. Then, all methodologically sound clinical trials assessing the efficacy of the same intervention were compared. Finally, results were interpreted within the context of known biologic mechanisms and clinical plausibility.

This chapter focuses on the use of secondary pharmacologic interventions in women with known CAD, with an emphasis on the management of women after MI. For each class of medication, we briefly review the biologic rationale and mechanisms of action, the overall results of clinical trials, and potential gender-specific issues. We provide recommendations for the use of these interventions in women based on our current state of knowledge. Both the short-term preventive strategies to be implemented immediately following acute ischemic events and the long-term management of women with established CAD are reviewed.

Antithrombotic Therapies

The role of thrombosis in the pathophysiology of acute coronary syndromes is well established. Most acute coronary events are caused by spontaneous plaque fissuring and rupture, exposing the subendothelium and lipid pool, which are highly thrombogenic (5). This process leads to acute thrombus formation through the interaction of arterial wall elements, platelets, and the coagulation cascade. Formation of large, occlusive thrombi leads to acute MI or sudden cardiac death, whereas nonocclusive thrombi or spontaneous, rapid, partial lysis of the thrombus thus formed can cause unstable angina or small, non–Q-wave infarcts (6,7). Thrombosis is an important contributor to the progression of coronary artery lesions resulting from plaque rupture, with subsequent hemorrhage into the plaque, mural thrombosis, or both leading to stepwise plaque growth (8). Thrombus is also generated at sites of vessel wall damage following angioplasty and in coronary vein grafts (9,10). Therefore, antithrombotic interventions are key components of both acute management and the prevention of MI and unstable angina. Antiplatelet agents are reviewed, followed by a section on anticoagulants.

Antiplatelet Agents

Aspirin
Aspirin is the most widely used antiplatelet agent in CAD. It acts on the first step in the conversion of arachidonic acid to thromboxane A_2 (TXA_2), primarily by acetylation and permanent inhibition of cyclo-oxygenase TXA_2. Platelet aggregation and vasoconstriction are induced by TXA_2, resulting in platelet-rich thrombus formation. In addition to inhibition of platelet TXA_2 synthesis, aspirin has been reported to have effects on hemostasis that are unrelated to its ability to inactivate prostaglandin-H synthase, including inhibition of platelet function, enhancement of fibrinolysis, and suppression of plasma coagulation. These are likely to be much less important clinically than the inhibition of platelet TXA_2 synthesis (11).

The first Antiplatelet Trialists Collaboration (12) and the second International Study of Infarct Survival (ISIS-2) (13) firmly established aspirin as standard care for acute MI in both women and men. The ISIS-2 trial included approximately 4000 women randomly selected to receive streptokinase or placebo and aspirin or placebo, demonstrating a statistically significant 20% risk reduction in vascular deaths for women presenting with aspirin-treated acute MI. This was not significantly different from the 28% risk reduction in vascular mortality in men treated with aspirin in this study. The second Antiplatelet Trialists Collaboration clearly demonstrated the protective effects of aspirin in a wide range of high-risk women, including women with unstable angina, acute MI, and history of previous MI, stroke, or transient ischemic attack (TIA) (14). This overview of 145 randomized trials of "prolonged" antiplatelet therapy (≥ 1 month) included overall approximately 70,000 high-risk patients targeted for secondary prevention and approximately 30,000 low-risk individuals from trials of primary prevention. Its general results, referring to both women and men, demonstrate both statistically and clinically significant benefit derived from antiplatelet drugs (the most frequently used drug was aspirin) in a wide range of patients targeted for secondary prevention (Fig. 21-1). Individual patient data were obtained from 29 trials of high-risk patients, and separate analyses were planned *a priori* in several important subgroups, including women, the elderly, hypertensive patients, and people with diabetes. In most of these trials, the antiplatelet drug used was aspirin. Similar benefits were demonstrated in the pooled analysis of these secondary prevention trials for women and men (Fig. 21-2).

Thus, early concerns about a possible lack of benefit from aspirin in women are not confirmed by the prospectively planned subgroup analysis in this overview of approximately 10,000 high-risk women. Questions about the efficacy of aspirin in women were derived primarily from the Canadian Stroke Study of aspirin in patients with recent cerebrovascular events and from a number of other small trials in stroke prevention (15,16). In all these trials, conclusions were based on data-dependent subgroup analyses in relatively small patient groups. Based on the comprehensive data available at present, the use of aspirin is mandatory in secondary prevention in women with acute or previous MI, unstable angina pectoris, previous bypass graft surgery or angioplasty, chronic stable coronary artery disease, cerebrovascular disease, and peripheral vascular disease.

The Antiplatelet Trialists Collaboration also clearly demonstrated that the high-dose aspirin regimens (1000–1500 mg/d) that were widely studied in earlier trials are no more effective than medium doses of 75 to 325 mg/d, which are the current recommended doses. The optimal duration of treatment with aspirin following an acute ischemic event has not been established clearly in women or men, because most clinical trials have lasted only 1 to 3 years. In the second Antiplatelet Trialists Collaboration, continued benefit was noted 3 years after a vascular event, although there was a decrement in benefit with time. Unless data that suggest otherwise become available, it seems reasonable and prudent to continue aspirin indefinitely following acute MI and in all high-risk patients with established cardiovascular disease who can tolerate this intervention. (For further discussion of the role of aspirin, see Chapter 9.)

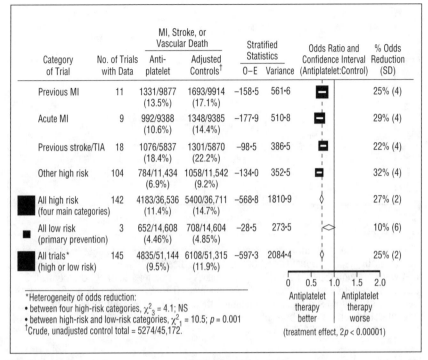

Category of Trial	No. of Trials with Data	MI, Stroke, or Vascular Death Antiplatelet	Adjusted Controls†	Stratified Statistics O–E	Variance	Odds Ratio and Confidence Interval (Antiplatelet:Control)	% Odds Reduction (SD)
Previous MI	11	1331/9877 (13.5%)	1693/9914 (17.1%)	−158·5	561·6		25% (4)
Acute MI	9	992/9388 (10.6%)	1348/9385 (14.4%)	−177·9	510·8		29% (4)
Previous stroke/TIA	18	1076/5837 (18.4%)	1301/5870 (22.2%)	−98·5	386·5		22% (4)
Other high risk	104	784/11,434 (6.9%)	1058/11,542 (9.2%)	−134·0	352·5		32% (4)
All high risk (four main categories)	142	4183/36,536 (11.4%)	5400/36,711 (14.7%)	−568·8	1810·9		27% (2)
All low risk (primary prevention)	3	652/14,608 (4.46%)	708/14,604 (4.85%)	−28·5	273·5		10% (6)
All trials* (high or low risk)	145	4835/51,144 (9.5%)	6108/51,315 (11.9%)	−597·3	2084·4		25% (2)

0   0.5   1.0   1.5   2.0

Antiplatelet therapy better | Antiplatelet therapy worse

(treatment effect, $2p < 0.00001$)

*Heterogeneity of odds reduction:
• between four high-risk categories, $\chi^2_3 = 4.1$; NS
• between high-risk and low-risk categories, $\chi^2_1 = 10.5$; $p = 0.001$
†Crude, unadjusted control total = 5274/45,172.

Figure 21-1 Major results of Antiplatelet Trialists Collaboration. Effects of antiplatelet therapy on overall major vascular events (e.g., myocardial infarction [MI], stroke, vascular death) in relevant high-risk patient groups and low-risk (primary prevention) groups are shown. SD = standard deviation; TIA = transient ischemic attack. (Adapted from Antiplatelet Trialists Collaboration. Collaborative overview of randomised trials of antiplatelet therapy. Part I: Prevention of death, myocardial infarction, and stroke by prolonged antiplatelet therapy in various categories of patients. BMJ. 1994;308:81–106.)

Ticlopidine, Clopidogrel, and Other Antiplatelet Agents

Aspirin inhibits only one of approximately 100 possible pathways that lead to platelet aggregation; therefore, several other antiplatelet agents with different mechanisms of action have been investigated alone and in combination with aspirin in different populations of patients with cardiovascular disease. Although specific analyses by gender have not been published, such trials demonstrated no clear overall benefit from certain agents such as dipyridamole, sulfinpyrazone, prostacycline, and iloprost; none of these agents is currently recommended in female MI survivors.

Several other antiplatelet agents, however, may be potentially useful. Ticlopidine has a wide range of effects, although the inhibition of ADP-induced platelet aggregation seems to be its most important action (11). Initial studies of ticlopidine focused on its use in secondary prevention after TIA or

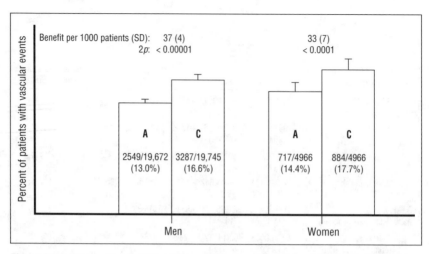

Figure 21-2 Effects of antiplatelet therapy on major vascular events in secondary prevention trials by gender. Benefit per 1000 patients indicates the number of vascular events that were prevented per 1000 patients treated. A = antiplatelet therapy; C = control; SD = standard deviation. (Adapted from Antiplatelet Trialists Collaboration. Collaborative overview of randomised trials of antiplatelet therapy. Part I: Prevention of death, myocardial infarction, and stroke by prolonged antiplatelet therapy in various categories of patients. BMJ. 1994;308:81–106.)

stroke. When compared with placebo, ticlopidine was effective in the prevention of recurrent stroke, MI, or vascular death in patients with recent stroke in the Canadian American Ticlopidine Study (CATS) (17). Important design features of this trial were the inclusion of a significant proportion of women (395 women comprising 48% of the total sample size) and predefined subgroup analyses for both sexes. The relative risk reduction with ticlopidine in the combined end point of stroke, MI, or vascular death was 34.2% for female ($p = 0.045$) and 28% for male patients ($p = 0.037$). The Ticlopidine Aspirin Stroke Study (TASS) of 3069 patients with recent TIA or stroke reported a small benefit in stroke prevention for ticlopidine compared with aspirin, although there were no significant differences in other end points (e.g., cardiovascular death and nonfatal cardiac events) (18). In this randomized study, there were close to 1100 women; subgroup analysis revealed a 3-year relative risk reduction for stroke of 27% in women and 19% in men. Ticlopidine also was effective in other clinical settings, such as in unstable angina in both women and men (19), although it has not been well studied in MI survivors.

Recently, the combination of aspirin and ticlopidine was found useful in the short-term prevention of stent thrombosis following intracoronary stent implantation (20). The importance of this finding in women has not been addressed specifically, and the potential additional benefit of ticlopidine and short-term aspirin over aspirin alone is not clear. Although promising, ticlopidine has not been shown to be superior to aspirin in secondary prevention in a wide range of patients with cardiovascular diseases (14). Meanwhile, this agent is being used increasingly in patients with contraindications to aspirin; however, frequent side effects (e.g., neutropenia, skin rashes, and diarrhea) have made the use of ticlopidine problematic.

Clopidogrel, a new thienopyridine derivative similar to ticlopidine also acts primarily by inhibiting ADP-induced platelet aggregation. The CAPRIE (Clopidogrel versus Aspirin in Patients at Risk of Ischemic Events) trial randomly selected 19,185 high-risk patients with clear evidence of coronary, cerebrovascular, or peripheral vascular disease to receive clopidogrel, 75 mg once daily, or aspirin, 325 mg once daily (21). Patients were followed for 1 to 3 years. Overall, the study demonstrated a small but statistically significant 8.7% (95% confidence interval [CI], 0.3–16.5; $p = 0.043$) relative risk (RR) reduction in favor of clopidogrel in the composite outcome cluster of ischemic stroke, MI, or vascular death. This study suggests that for a wide range of patients, such as those in the CAPRIE trial, treatment with aspirin prevents approximately 19 major clinical vascular events versus 24 such events prevented with clopidogrel. Importantly, there were no major differences in terms of safety. Severe neutropenia, reported in approximately 2.4% of all patients tested with ticlopidine, was extremely infrequent with clopidogrel, and severe gastrointestinal bleeding was less common than with aspirin. Over 5300 women were randomized in this trial, and the proportion of women was well balanced at baseline between the treatment groups. Clopidogrel was equally effective in women and men.[1] Recommendations regarding the role of clopidogrel in clinical practice will undoubtedly be influenced by its cost-effectiveness and further experience with this drug.

Another class of antiplatelet agents currently under active investigation is the GPIIb/IIIa receptor antagonists. These agents act by inhibiting the final common pathway leading to platelet aggregation and therefore offer theoretical advantages over other antiplatelet drugs. So far, GPIIb/IIIa inhibitors have been studied primarily as intravenous drugs in the prevention of acute complications in high-risk coronary angioplasty patients and in the management of unstable angina. Oral agents are also under development and will be tested in the near future in a wider range of patients.

Anticoagulants

The use of potent antithrombotic interventions including thrombolytic agents and intravenous heparin during the acute phases of MI and unstable angina is clearly established for both women and men. The efficacy and use of

---

[1]R. Roberts, personal communication.

thrombolytic agents for acute ischemia are reviewed in Chapter 16. Studies of the efficacy of oral anticoagulation in CAD are reviewed below.

Short-, intermediate-, and long-term anticoagulant strategies have been studied primarily in patients following MI and are reviewed here, with particular emphasis on data available for women. The most common anticoagulation regimens for intermediate- and long-term prevention after MI use coumarin drugs such as warfarin; these drugs act primarily by inhibiting γ-carboxylation of vitamin-K–dependent coagulation proteins (prothrombin and factors VII, IX, and X). In monitoring the intensity of warfarin treatment, the reporting of prothrombin time (PT) results as an international normalized ratio (INR) has gained wide acceptance and is recommended. The Fourth American College of Chest Physicians (ACPP) Consensus Conference on Antithrombotic Therapy recommends that INR be maintained at 2.0 to 3.0 for those survivors of acute MI for whom anticoagulation therapy is elected (22).

The benefit of short-term anticoagulation—up to 4 weeks after acute MI— was reported in several trials during the 1960s and 1970s. The three largest trials suggested overall improved outcomes for patients treated with anticoagulants, although a definite mortality benefit was demonstrated only in the Bronx Municipal Study conducted in 391 women and 745 men (23). In this study, there was a 61% odds reduction in all-cause mortality reported for women treated with anticoagulants during their hospital stay. The benefit in women appeared to exceed that in men, probably because women randomized in this trial had an overall higher risk profile than men as evidenced by hospital mortality rates that were twice as high (31% and 16%, respectively). The MRC Trial randomized patients (1096 men and 331 women) to receive a regimen of intravenous heparin followed by "therapeutic" oral anticoagulants versus no intravenous heparin and minimal-dose phenindione for 28 days and reported no overall benefit in mortality or infarction rates (24). Women were a predefined subgroup of interest. There were 163 deaths in women in the high-dosage anticoagulant group versus 168 deaths in the low-dosage group; reinfarction rates were also not significantly different. The third large trial of short-term anticoagulation after MI, the VA Study, did not include women and reported trends toward decreased mortality in men treated with oral anticoagulants for 4 weeks after MI (25). Overall, results of these early trials did not provide conclusive evidence for use of oral anticoagulants during the entire hospital stay following MI and up to 1 month post-infarction. These early studies had some methodologic problems; importantly, the sample sizes were not large enough to demonstrate potential clinically significant moderate-sized effects of oral anticoagulation. Aspirin was not widely used after infarct in these trials; therefore the impact of warfarin in addition to aspirin was not evaluated.

The question of short- and intermediate-term anticoagulation following acute MI should also consider the potential for left ventricular mural thrombus and the resultant risk of embolic stroke. A number of echocardiographic studies (generally small studies in patients of both sexes, with higher proportions of men) show that left ventricular mural thrombus develops in a significant proportion (up to 40%) of patients with acute anterior MI. This is much less frequent in patients with inferior infarcts (26–28). In-hospital anticoagulation with heparin followed by out-of-hospital treatment with warfarin reduces left ventricular mural thrombosis and the risk of embolic stroke (29,30). These conclusions are based generally on studies that do not allow gender-specific analyses. The biologic rationale for this approach is strong; therefore, for all patients, women and men, who have had Q-wave anterior MI, or who have echocardiographic evidence of left ventricular mural thrombus, severe left ventricular dysfunction, or post-MI atrial fibrillation, physicians generally recommend heparin soon after infarct, followed by warfarin for up to 3 months, with INR levels between 2.0 and 3.0. These recommendations, summarized in the Fourth ACPP Consensus Conference on Antithrombotic Therapy, have been widely incorporated into clinical practice (22).

Long-term oral anticoagulation following acute MI remains controversial. Studies conducted in the 1950s and 1960s had many methodologic limitations, creating inconsistencies in the reported results. In 1970, an International Anticoagulant Review Group attempted to overcome the problems of inadequate sample size that occurred in many early trials by pooling data from nine controlled trials of long-term anticoagulation following MI (31). The pooled data included 2205 men and 282 women and showed that mortality was reduced by 20% in men but that no clear benefit emerged for women. However, the small number of women, even in this pooled analysis, and other methodologic limitations did not allow definitive conclusions.

In the 1980s and 1990s, a number of studies have readdressed the role of long-term anticoagulation after MI. The Sixty-Plus Reinfarction Study randomly selected 747 men and 131 women over 60 years of age to receive either continued oral anticoagulation or placebo for 2 years after MI. The main study results were an overall mortality benefit for actively treated patients (RR = 43%; p = 0.017) and reduction in reinfarction rates (32). Bleeding complications, including intracranial hemorrhage, were more frequent in the anticoagulation group and occurred mostly when the level of anticoagulation was excessive. Subgroup analyses by gender were not reported. The Warfarin Reinfarction Study (WARIS) investigated 1214 patients, including 271 women (22%) who had sustained acute MI a mean of 27 days previously. The patients were randomized to receive warfarin, aiming for an INR of 2.8 to 4.8, or placebo; follow-up was extended for an average of 37 months, and patients were advised not to take aspirin (33). There was an overall decrease in total mortality with 24% relative risk reduction (RRR) (95% CI, 4%–44%; p = 0.027), reinfarctions with 34% RRR (95% CI, 19%–54%; p = 0.007) and strokes with 55% RRR (95% CI, 30%–77%; p = 0.0015). Serious bleeding complications were relatively rare (0.6%/year) for patients treated with warfarin. Subgroup analyses in women revealed that the benefits observed for the overall study results with regard to total mortality, risk of recurrent reinfarction, and risk of any major vascular events were present in women as well as men.[2] The number of events, particularly in women, were relatively small; thus, confidence intervals were wide. However, odds ratios for total mortality, reinfarction, and any vascular event were, respectively, 0.39, 0.65, and 0.45 for women and 0.82, 0.60, and 0.61 for men, favoring a treatment effect. Although these results suggest the possibility of higher benefits for women, statistical tests of homogeneity did not indicate significant differences in therapy response between women and men. The Anticoagulants in the Secondary Prevention of Events in Coronary Thrombosis (ASPECT) study of 3404 survivors of acute MI reported limited effects of long-term anticoagulation on mortality (RRR, 10%; 95% CI, 11%–27%; p = NS) but substantial benefit in reducing the risk of cerebrovascular events (RRR = 40%) and recurrent MI (RRR = 53%). Patients were not treated with aspirin (34). The study population consisted of 20% women; however, no assessment of possible gender-specific effects was reported.

Overall, patients treated with oral anticoagulants but not antiplatelet drugs had significant reductions in mortality and major vascular events (35). A meta-analysis of all the major long-term trials that compared oral anticoagulant therapy with placebo (without the use of antiplatelet drugs) is shown in Table 21-1. These trials included women and men, with much higher proportions of men. Insufficient individual patient data are available for analysis of specific effects in women. Based on the subgroup analyses in women in the WARIS study, the overall consistency of results across trials, and the strong

Table 21-1 Effect of Long-term Anticoagulants on Mortality, Reinfarction, and Stroke Following Myocardial Infarction*

	Mortality	Reinfarction	Stroke
14 trials[†]	0.79 (0.69, 0.90)	0.59 (0.51, 0.69)	0.46 (0.32, 0.66)
WARIS	0.72 (0.54, 0.97)	0.61 (0.45, 0.82)	0.51 (0.26, 0.99)
ASPECT	0.89 (0.72, 1.11)	0.43 (0.35, 0.55)	0.62 (0.41, 0.95)
Total	0.80 (0.72, 0.89)[‡]	0.55 (0.49, 0.62)[‡]	0.52 (0.35, 0.68)[‡]

* Results are expressed as odds ratio (95% confidence intervals) for total mortality, recurrent infarction, and stroke in patients assigned to active therapy versus placebo. Only trials that did not allow the use of aspirin are included.
[†] Generally small, older studies.
[‡] $p > 0.001$.
ASPECT = Anticoagulants in the Secondary Prevention of Events in Coronary Thrombosis; WARIS = Warfarin Reinfarction Study.

[2]W. Michealis, DuPont Merck Pharmaceutical Co., personal communication.

biologic rationale for the role of anticoagulants in the prevention of acute ischemic events, it is unlikely that effects would differ significantly by gender.

Significant benefit for oral anticoagulants over aspirin has not been demonstrated in the few randomized clinical trials that compared long-term anticoagulation with aspirin after MI and successful coronary thrombolysis. Few randomized clinical trials have directly compared these treatments after MI. The German–Austrian Aspirin Trial randomized 946 patients, including 203 women (21%), to receive phenprocoumon, aspirin (1.5 g/d), or placebo (36). Over 2 years of follow-up, the trend was toward worse outcomes for patients on phenprocoumon. In particular, aspirin was more effective in preventing deaths and coronary events in men, although the number of women was too small for subgroup analysis. The EPSIM (Enquète de Prévention Secondaire de l'Infarcte du Myocarde) trial of 1303 survivors of acute MI included women and men without analysis by gender. After a mean 29-month follow-up, all-cause mortality was 10.3% with anticoagulation and 11.1% with aspirin (37).

Trials comparing anticoagulation and aspirin after successful coronary thrombolysis had similar results. The multicentered Prevention of Reocclusion in Coronary Thrombolysis (APRICOT) study (38) compared the effects of coumadin and aspirin on infarct-related vessel patency (by coronary angiography) and on major clinical events. Patients were treated initially with intravenous thrombolytic therapy, then intravenous heparin. In those with angiographically demonstrated patent infarct-related arteries, patients were randomized to receive either 325 mg of aspirin daily or placebo (with heparin discontinued) or coumadin with continuation of heparin until oral anticoagulation was established. Approximately 20% of the 300 subjects were women. Angiographic reocclusion rates at 3 months were not significantly different. Overall mortality did not differ, although there were trends toward fewer reinfarctions in the aspirin-treated patients. An event-free clinical course was more likely in aspirin-treated patients versus placebo and versus coumadin.

The hypothesis that the combination of low-dose aspirin and fixed low-dose warfarin with minimal monitoring requirements might be more effective than aspirin alone in secondary prophylaxis after MI was evaluated recently in the Coumadin–Aspirin Reinfarction Study (CARS) in over 8800 patients (39). No benefit was demonstrated for two low doses of coumadin, 1 mg and 3 mg daily, in patients treated with aspirin. Similarly, the Post–Coronary Artery Bypass Graft Trial reported that low-dose warfarin did not reduce the progression of atherosclerosis in patients with aortocoronary saphenous vein bypass grafts (40). These trials included both women and men, although overall the proportion of men was much higher. No gender-specific differences in response to treatment were reported.

New anticoagulant strategies, such as the early initiation of oral anticoagulants in patients treated with intravenous antithrombotic agents in acute ischemic syndromes (aimed at preventing rebound phenomena), low-molecular-weight heparins, and even potentially more aggressive regimens (e.g., combinations of potent platelet inhibitors and potent inhibitors of thrombin generation) are currently under investigation.

In conclusion, there is overwhelming evidence that aspirin in intermediate doses of 80 to 325 mg/d should be administered in all patients, women and men, with acute MI and continued indefinitely in all those who can tolerate this therapy. Long-term oral anticoagulants after MI are recommended in the following patient groups:

1. Patients with anterior MI who are generally at high risk for left ventricular mural thrombus formation or those post-MI patients who have demonstrated left ventricular mural thrombus (treatment with oral anticoagulants should extend for the first 3–6 months after infarction)

2. Post-MI patients with persistent atrial fibrillation

3. Patients who do not tolerate aspirin or other antiplatelet agents such as ticlopidine and clopidogrel

These recommendations do not differ significantly for women and men.

Beta-Adrenergic Antagonists

The possibility of a beneficial effect of beta-adrenergic blockade after acute MI was proposed by Snow in 1965 (41). A number of mechanisms of action could account for the cardioprotective effects of beta-blockers in acute ischemic syndromes and in the long-term management of patients with coronary artery disease. These have been demonstrated in experimental and clinical studies (Box 21-1).

Clinical trials that assessed the use of these agents in the acute phases of MI and in long-term secondary prevention following acute ischemic events were conducted mostly in the 1970s and 1980s. The largest trial of early, short-term beta-blocker treatment in acute MI was the First International Study of Infarct Survival (ISIS-1) (42), in which 16,027 patients were assigned to treatment with intravenous atenolol followed by oral therapy or placebo. Treatment was initiated a mean of 5 hours after the onset of suspected acute MI. There was a 15% overall early survival benefit in the atenolol group, which was statistically and clinically significant. Benefits persisted at 1 year. Women were well represented in this study, comprising 23% of the total sample size (3696 female patients). Of the 1848 women treated with atenolol, 96 (5.2%) sustained vascular deaths, compared with 140 in the control group

---

Box 21-1 Beneficial Effects of Beta-blockers in Acute Evolving Myocardial Infarction and in Long-term Secondary Prevention After Myocardial Infarction

---

Reduction in myocardial oxygen demand as a result of increased heart rate, blood pressure, and myocardial contractility

Blockade of direct cardiotoxic effects of excessive catecholamines and counteraction of indirect effects of high levels of catecholamines (e.g., prevention of increased release and uptake of free fatty acids)

Redistribution of blood from epicardial areas to more ischemic subendocardial tissue

Anti-arrhythmic properties, with reduction in ventricular arrhythmia and elevation in ventricular fibrillation thresholds

Reduction in incidence of cardiac rupture

Reduction in frequency of recurrent ischemic episodes

Limitation of infarct size

(7.5%), resulting in a 31% RR reduction. For men, there was a 5% risk reduction in vascular mortality. Subgroup analyses did not identify statistically significant gender-specific differences in response to beta-blocker therapy. Although a quantitative gender-specific difference in response to beta-blockers cannot be excluded fully, the observed higher efficacy in women may be related to chance alone. It seems prudent to conclude that women benefit at least as much as men. After ISIS-1, a comprehensive overview was completed, because initial studies of early intravenous beta-blocker use in MI had demonstrated only general trends, with no conclusive evidence of early benefit. When results of ISIS-1, the Metaprolol in Acute Myocardial Infarction (MI-AMI) trial (43), and 27 smaller trials were pooled in this meta-analysis, an overall 13% risk reduction in mortality with early beta-blocker treatment was found (44).

The strategies of early intravenous administration of beta-blockers in acute MI versus delayed administration of these agents have been assessed in the thrombolytic era in the Thrombolysis in Myocardial Infarction (TIMI) IIB trial, in which 1434 patients were treated with recombinant-tissue plasminogen activator and aspirin (45). No overall mortality reduction was seen in patients receiving early intravenous metoprolol; however, the number of deaths was small and, therefore, the study lacked statistical power for the assessment of the effects of early beta-blocker therapy on mortality. There was a lower incidence of reinfarction and recurrent chest pain in the immediate intravenous beta-blocker group. Only approximately 15% of the study patients were women, and the numbers were obviously too small to assess potential differences based on gender. The American College of Cardiology and the American Heart Association jointly have included the use of intravenous beta-blockers as a Class I recommendation in both women and men with acute MI and no contraindication to these agents (46).

Whether beta-blockers are instituted early in the management of acute MI or not, these agents remain essential in long-term secondary prevention following acute ischemic events in most women and men. The long-term use of beta-blockers for secondary prevention after MI has been studied extensively. Over 23,000 patients recovering from MI have been evaluated in 26 randomized clinical trials. Many of these trials used long-term beta-blockers following oral or intravenous administration of these agents, whereas other studies instituted beta-blockade several days after the acute phase of a MI. Overall, these studies demonstrate a significant 23% reduction in mortality as well as significant reduction in reinfarctions (44,47). Early benefits derived from these agents seem to be maintained long-term, and detailed analyses of the results (based on various subgroups, including gender, age, site of MI, initial heart rate, risk category, and the presence or absence of ventricular arrhythmias on Holter monitoring) failed to reveal any preferential treatment effect in any category. Among the largest studies of long-term beta-blocker therapy following acute MI are the Norwegian Multicentre Trial (1488 men and 396 women) using timolol (48) and the Beta-blocker Heart Attack Trial (BHAT) (3,241 men and 596 women) using propranolol (49). Both revealed significant reductions in mortality rates up to 3 years after infarction and a subsequent report from the Norwegian Multicentre Study Group revealed continued benefits at least 6 years after infarction (50). Generally, women were under-represented in all these trials. The Beta-Blocker Pooling Project attempted to overcome the limitations related to sample size for important subgroups such as women (51a). Nine of the major trials of secondary long-term prevention with beta-blockers following acute MI were included in this overview, and subgroups of interest were defined *a priori*. This meta-analysis revealed an overall 24% lower mortality in the beta-blocker group compared with the placebo group. The odds ratios for total mortality were similar, 0.81 for women and 0.74 for men; thus, in this overview, the beneficial effect of beta-blockers on mortality seems similar in the two sexes. In general, the high-risk groups appeared to benefit more from therapy, both in terms of relative and absolute risk reduction in mortality, although lower-risk groups also benefited. Mortality benefits of beta-blocker therapy after MI in high-risk groups (e.g., older patients and those with low ejection fraction, chronic obstructive pulmonary disease, and diabetes) were shown recently in a large observational study of over 200,000 patients, including 92,559 women (51b). This conclusion is

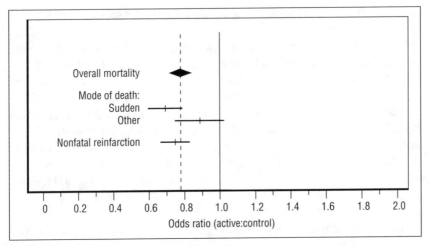

Figure 21-3 Meta-analysis of trials of long-term beta-blocker therapy following acute myocardial infarction. Odds ratios (active versus control) and 95% confidence intervals are shown. (Adapted from Yusuf Y, Peto R, Lewis J, et al. β-Blockade during and after myocardial infarction: an overview of the randomized trials. Prog Cardiovasc Dis. 1985;27:335–71.)

further strengthened by the biological rationale that clearly supports the role of beta-blockade and the consistency of the clinical evidence favoring these agents (benefits were demonstrated in most subgroups in different relevant end points, including total mortality, sudden death, and reinfarction) (Fig. 21-3).

An important practical question is the choice of a specific beta-blocker. Previous reviews have suggested a potential lack of benefit from beta-blockers with intrinsic sympathomimetic activity (ISA) (47). These conclusions were based on studies performed with pindolol and oxprenolol in which it was proposed that a lesser impact on heart rate with beta-blockers with ISA could account for their potential lower efficacy. However, studies performed with other β-blockers with ISA, such as alprenolol, practolol and more recently, acebutolol, did demonstrate significant mortality benefits. The APSI trial (Acebutolol et Prévention Secondaire de l'Infarcte) studied 607 patients (443 men and 164 women) and reported a very impressive 48% mortality reduction in high-risk post-MI patients treated with acebutolol, a β-blocker with moderate partial-agonist activity (52). Cardioselective compared with noncardioselective beta-blockers have not been demonstrated to be significantly different in this clinical setting. Obviously, in the patient with mild obstructive pulmonary disease, peripheral vascular disease, or diabetes use of a cardioselective beta-blocker such as metoprolol or atenolol is preferred. Also, whenever compliance is an issue, long-acting beta-blockers are preferred over short-acting agents.

Despite clear evidence of efficacy, low cost, acceptable side-effect profile, and extensive experience with these agents, only 30% to 42% of the 240,989 patients enrolled in the National Registry of Myocardial Infarction from 1990 to 1993 received long-term beta-blocker therapy in the United States (53a). Similar patterns of practice were documented elsewhere in the United States (53b,53c) and in other countries. A survey of five Canadian hospitals found that even after accounting for potential contraindications to beta-blockers, only 18% of those eligible for intravenous beta-blockade in acute MI received this treatment, and only 57% of those eligible received long-term oral therapy (54). In addition, women and men are prescribed beta-blocker treatment at different rates (see Chapter 16).

Beta-adrenergic antagonists should be given to all patients, women and men, for long-term secondary prevention following acute MI in the absence of clear contraindications, such as pulmonary edema, significant obstructive pulmonary disease, hypotension, bradycardia, or advanced conduction abnormalities. If tolerated, this treatment should be continued for at least 2 to 3 years and perhaps indefinitely.

Angiotensin-Converting Enzyme Inhibitors

Important prognostic factors for patients with coronary artery disease, especially after MI, are the extent of left ventricular dysfunction and the potential for future ischemic events. Angiotensin-converting enzyme (ACE) inhibitors are particularly useful in patients with previous MI and other high-risk categories of patients, because they can limit the progression of ventricular dysfunction and also may decrease the risk of future acute ischemic events. In experimental animal models and in humans, ACE inhibitors have been demonstrated to have numerous cardio- and vasculoprotective effects (Box 21-2) (55). These effects are mediated by blocking both circulating and tissue renin–angiotensin systems, leading to decreased angiotensin-II formation and by preventing breakdown of bradykinin. Angiotensin II has potent vasoconstrictive, proliferative, and prothrombotic effects, whereas bradykinin potentiation leads to accumulation of kinins, which act directly by increasing the release of endothelium-derived relaxing factor (EDRF) and prostaglandins, resulting in vasodilation, endothelial protection, and antithrombotic actions (Fig. 21-4).

The use of ACE inhibitors in acute phases of MI has been addressed in a number of large clinical trials that collectively reveal a modest but statistically significant 7% RR reduction in mortality, resulting in approximately five fewer deaths per 1000 patients treated (56). Generally, women are well repre-

Box 21-2 Beneficial Effects of Angiotensin-Converting–Enzyme
Inhibitors in Myocardial Infarction Survivors and Other
High-risk Patients

Cardioprotective effects
   Restoration of the balance between myocardial oxygen supply and demand
   Reduction in left ventricular afterload and preload
   Prevention or reduction in ventricular remodelling after myocardial infarction
   Reduction in left ventricular mass
   Reduction in sympathetic stimulation
   Reduction in the incidence of cardiac rupture after myocardial infarction
   Beneficial effect on reperfusion injury*
Vasculoprotective effects
   Direct anti-atherogenic effect*
   Antiproliferative and antimigratory effects on smooth muscle cells,
      neutrophils, and mononuclear cells
   Improvement and/or restoration of endothelial function
   Antioxidant properties*
   Protection from plaque rupture*
   Improvement in arterial compliance and tone
Antihypertensive effects
Antithrombotic effects
   Inhibition of platelet aggregation
   Enhancement of endogenous fibrinolysis

* Not demonstrated conclusively in humans

sented, particularly in the large studies; thus, 26% of the over 58,000 patients
in the Fourth International Study of Infarct Survival (ISIS-4) (57) and 22% of
the over 18,000 patients in the Gruppo Italiano per lo Studio della Sopravivenza nell'Infarto Miocardico (GISSI-3) trial were women (58). No definite
gender-related differential effects were shown, although benefits in women
were less obvious in ISIS-4 than in the GISSI-3 trial. It remains somewhat
controversial whether all patients with acute ST-segment elevation infarcts
should be treated early on with ACE inhibitors or whether the benefit observed in these trials was derived largely from high-risk patient groups (large
infarct, anterior location), and those alone should be targeted.

   The long-term use of ACE inhibitors after MI in patients with symptoms of
heart failure, asymptomatic left ventricular dysfunction, or both has been
well studied in large clinical trials and is clearly associated with reductions in
mortality, hospitalizations for heart failure and reinfarction rates. The Sur-

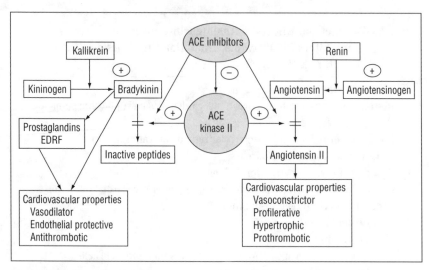

Figure 21-4 Overview of mechanisms of cardiovascular protective effects of angiotensin-converting enzyme (ACE) inhibitors. EDRF = endothelium-derived relaxing factor.

vival and Ventricular Enlargement (SAVE) study investigated 2231 patients (18% women) within 3 to 16 days after MI whose left ventricular ejection fraction was 40% or less. The patients were randomized to receive treatment with captopril or placebo for an average of 42 months (59). All-cause mortality was significantly reduced in the captopril group (RR = 19%; 95% CI, 3%–32%; p = 0.019), consistent with 42 lives saved for every 1000 patients treated for 42 months (or one life saved for every 23 patients treated for 42 months). In addition, statistically and clinically significant reductions in all predefined end points were shown, including cardiovascular death, heart failure, and recurrent MI. For women, benefits were less obvious, with risk reductions in total mortality of only 2% (95% CI, 53%–37%) and of only 4% (95% CI, 32%–30%) in the combined end point of cardiovascular mortality and major cardiovascular morbidity. However, it should be emphasized that the subgroup strata of women provided insufficient power for definitive conclusions, and a Cox proportional hazards model that examined the effects of captopril by gender revealed no gender-therapy interaction (60). The Acute Infarction Ramipril Efficacy (AIRE) study randomized 2006 patients with clinical evidence of heart failure within 3 to 10 days after an acute MI to receive ramipril or placebo (61). Women were well represented and comprised over 26% of the study population. Follow-up was continued for an average of 15 months. A highly significant 27% reduction in mortality was observed in patients treated with ramipril, consistent with 57 lives saved for every 1000 patients treated for 15 months. The benefit of ramipril was apparent earlier (within 30 days) and was of larger magnitude than in SAVE, which was consistent with the higher-risk patients enrolled in this study. Female patients seemed to benefit at least as much as men. The Trandolapril Cardiac Evaluation (TRACE) study randomized 1749 patients (28% women) with echocardiographic evidence of left ventricular dysfunction to begin trandolapril or placebo 2 to 6 days post-MI (62). Average follow-up was 26 months. The relative reduction in total mortality in the trandolapril group was 22% (95% CI, 9–23%; $p = 0.001$). Trandolapril also reduced the risk of death from cardiovascular causes, sudden death, and progression to severe heart failure. There was a trend toward a reduction in recurrent fatal or nonfatal MI in actively treated patients. Subgroup analyses in women revealed 101 deaths in 249 female patients treated with trandolapril compared with 113 deaths in 252 treated with placebo (RRR = 10%; 95% CI, 18%–31%). Overall, these results are less dramatic than for the entire study population; however, the number of women was small. Twelve subgroups were analyzed in this trial, and there was remarkable uniformity in benefits among the overwhelming majority of subgroups.

A meta-analysis of mortality results from these studies is shown in Table 21-2. When the trials of ACE inhibitors after *recent* MI are pooled (SAVE, AIRE, TRACE), the combined odds ratio of total mortality for treated women versus control is 0.79 (95% CI, 0.63–1.00; $p = 0.02$) and 0.72 for men (95% CI, 0.63–0.82; $p < 0.001$). Overall, these clinical trials of late administration of ACE inhibitors in patients with MI and overt heart failure or asymptomatic left ventricular dysfunction demonstrate significant mortality benefit. Possible gender-specific quantitative differences cannot be excluded fully.

Similar results emerged from the Studies of Left Ventricular Dysfunction (SOLVD) (63,64). Over 6500 patients with a left ventricular ejection fraction of 35% or less were randomly selected to receive enalapril or placebo; follow-up extended for an average of approximately 40 months. Patients with overt symptoms of heart failure entered the SOLVD treatment trial, whereas those with asymptomatic left ventricular dysfunction were included in the SOLVD prevention trial. In both SOLVD trials, left ventricular dysfunction most frequently resulted from ischemic causes and the majority of patients had a history of previous MI. Women were underrepresented in both the SOLVD prevention arm (representing less than 14% of asymptomatic patients) and treatment arm (representing approximately 20% of patients with overt heart failure). Significant overall benefits regarding total mortality, hospitalizations for heart failure, and risk of MI were documented for all subjects. The seemingly larger effects in men (*see* Table 21-2) could be related to chance and the limited number of women in SOLVD.

The consistency of results in multiple, large, well-conducted trials provides strong experimental evidence for the cardiovascular protective effects of

Table 21-2 Effect by Gender of Long-term Angiotensin-Converting–Enzyme Inhibitor Therapy on Total Mortality in Patients with Previous Myocardial Infarction and Significant Left Ventricular Dysfunction*

Trial	Women				Men			
	Deaths per No. of Patients (%)		Odds Ratio (95% CI)	p	Deaths per No. of Patients (%)		Odds Ratio (95% CI)	p
	ACE-I	Control			ACE-I	Control		
SAVE	37/186 (19.9)	41/204 (20.1)	0.99 (0.60, 1.62)	0.47	191/929 (20.6)	234/912 (25.7)	0.75 (0.60, 0.93)	0.004
AIRE	57/270 (21.1)	75/255 (29.4)	0.64 (0.43, 0.95)	0.01	113/734 (15.4)	147/727 (20.2)	0.72 (0.55, 0.94)	0.008
TRACE	101/249 (40.6)	113/252 (44.8)	0.84 (0.59, 1.20)	0.16	203/627 (32.4)	256/621 (41.2)	0.68 (0.54, 0.86)	0.006
SOLVD-P[†]	25/163 (15.3)	16/166 (9.61)	1.68 (0.88, 3.24)	0.94	199/1537 (12.9)	240/1516 (15.8)	0.79 (0.65, 0.97)	0.011
SOLVD-T[†]	47/145 (32.4)	50/138 (36.2)	0.99 (0.60, 1.62)	0.47	255/707 (36.1)	280/697 (40.2)	0.84 (0.68, 1.04)	0.056
Total[‡]	267/1013 (26.4)	295/1015 (29.1)	0.86 (0.70, 1.05)	0.07	961/4534 (21.2)	1157/4473 (25.9)	0.76 (0.69, 0.84)	< 0.001

* The test for interaction between women and men ($p = 0.26$) suggests no significant heterogeneity of results.

† Only patients with previous myocardial infarction in the SOLVD study are included.

‡ When only the trials of ACE-I in *recent* acute myocardial infarction (i.e., SAVE, AIRE, and TRACE) are pooled, the combined odds ratio for total mortality for women treated with ACE-I versus control is 0.79 (95% CI, 0.63–1.00; $p = 0.02$) and 0.72 for men (95% CI, 0.63–0.82; $p < 0.0001$).

ACE-I = Angiotensin-converting enzyme inhibitor(s); AIRE = Acute Infarction Ramipril Efficacy study; CI = confidence interval; SAVE = Survival and Ventricular Enlargement study; SOLVD-P = Studies of Left Ventricular Dysfunction Prevention trial; SOLVD-T = Studies of Left Ventricular Dysfunction Treatment trial; TRACE = Trandolapril Cardiac Evaluation study.

ACE inhibitors and supports their use in all patients with symptomatic or asymptomatic left ventricular dysfunction following acute MI.

Although ACE inhibitors are well tolerated generally, side effects of these drugs are reported more frequently in women. In the SOLVD trials, women experienced more frequent side effects of enalapril than did men, with higher incidence of symptomatic hypotension, altered taste, skin rash or pruritus, cough, gastrointestinal symptoms, and azotemia. Although women reported side effects more frequently, these did not result in higher rates of withdrawal from the study. Other investigations also reported higher rates of cough associated with ACE inhibitor therapy in women (65,66). ACE inhibitors can cause significant fetal and neonatal abnormalities, and the use of these drugs during pregnancy is strongly contraindicated (67a). (Gender-specific side effects of ACE inhibitors are reviewed also in Chapter 15.)

No strong data are available to support the preferential use of any specific ACE inhibitor. Theoretical considerations would favor ACE inhibitors with higher tissue affinity; practical considerations would favor long-acting agents. It seems prudent to use dosages similar to those tested in the large clinical trials or the highest tolerated dosage (i.e., captopril 50 mg tid, ramipril 5 mg bid, trandolapril 4 mg/d, or enalapril 10 mg bid as used in SAVE, AIRE, TRACE, and SOLVD, respectively) in the absence of side effects and to continue therapy indefinitely (67b).

The relevant potential benefit of ACE inhibitors in patients with small infarcts and overall preserved left ventricular systolic function and in individuals in other high-risk categories is currently under investigation in several large clinical trials (68). (ACE inhibitors are discussed further in Chapters 16 and 19.)

Lipid Lowering

Based on a wealth of experimental data, the central role of lipids and particularly low-density lipoprotein (LDL) cholesterol in the genesis and progression of the atherosclerotic process is well established (69). Epidemiologic studies also clearly and uniformly establish a strong association between hypercholesterolemia and the risk of subsequent development of CAD (70,71). These studies have focused largely on men. In general, such epidemiologic investigations indicate a 2% to 3% difference in risk for CAD for each 1% difference in LDL cholesterol levels. Although fewer longitudinal studies on cholesterol included women, in most such studies, a clear association between increased cholesterol levels and cardiovascular risk is demonstrated in women as well (70,72).

Randomized controlled clinical studies provide the most conclusive evidence that hypercholesterolemia and, in particular, a high level of LDL cholesterol are causally related to 1) the development of CAD and 2) increased mortality and morbidity in individuals with established disease. Until recently, such trials have concentrated almost exclusively on men; however, recent clinical trials have clearly and firmly established the importance of aggressive lipid lowering in secondary prevention of coronary events in women with established cardiovascular disease.

By using angiographic techniques, a large number of clinical trials have evaluated the effects of cholesterol-lowering therapies (e.g., drugs, lifestyle interventions) on the progression of coronary atherosclerosis. At least five such studies (73–77) have evaluated the progression of atherosclerotic disease by qualitative angiography and at least 12 trials have used quantitative angiography in evaluating the effect of cholesterol-lowering on atherosclerosis progression (40,78–88). Entry criteria for these trials differed significantly with regard to the clinical characteristics of the patients as well as to cholesterol levels. Overall, with the exception of the Harvard Atherosclerosis Reversibility Project (HARP) study (82), which included a small number of subjects with a mean baseline LDL cholesterol of 138 mg/dL (lower than most other studies), all of the treated groups showed a decrease in the percent mean stenosis, in the minimal lumen diameter, or in both compared with control subjects. Most of these trials included exclusively men or randomized only small proportions of women.

Reviewing several specific trials is illustrative. Women were well represented in the San Francisco Arteriosclerosis Specialized Center for Research (SCOR) Intervention trial, a small but interesting study of heterozygous familial hypercholesterolemic patients treated with diet and combined drug regimens (80). Of a total of 72 patients completing the trial, 41 (56.9%) were women. Aggressive lowering of LDL cholesterol (> 38%) was achieved in both sexes. After 2 years of treatment, there was an overall slight regression in mean percent area stenosis for coronary lesions in treated patients and a significant progression of disease in controls. The changes appeared more dramatic for women than for men, although in this small study the intergroup difference was not significant. The authors of this investigation concluded that the reduction of LDL cholesterol levels can induce regression of coronary atherosclerotic lesions in women and men with familial hypercholesterolemia. Two angiographic studies with 3-hydroxy-3-methylglutaryl (HMG) co-enzyme A reductase inhibitors (statins) included gender analysis. Women constituted 18.1% (n = 54) of 299 participants in the Canadian Coronary Atherosclerosis Intervention Trial (CCAIT) (86). Treatment with lovastatin for a mean of 2 years resulted in a 29% decrease in LDL cholesterol levels, which translated into retardation in the angiographic progression of existent coronary lesions and the prevention of new lesions. Results in women appeared to be of the same magnitude as those in men, and on multivariate analysis gender did not emerge as a significant determinant of the efficacy of the study intervention. Also, women were well represented in the Pravastatin Limitation of Atherosclerosis in the Coronary Arteries (PLAC 1) study (88); 136 of the total of 408 patients randomized (33%) were women. In this study of patients with mild-to-moderate hyperlipidemia, there was an overall reduction in angiographically assessed minimal coronary artery diameter in patients treated with pravastatin compared with placebo. Importantly, there were also trends toward a reduction in clinical adverse events. No specific gender-related differences were reported.

Although studies such as the NHLBI Coronary Intervention Study (73), the Program on the Surgical Control of the Hyperlipidemias (POSCH) (76), the Multicentre Anti-Atheroma Study (MAAS) (84), and the recent Post Coronary Artery Bypass Graft Trial (40) did not systematically exclude women, only approximately 10% or less of the participants were women. No specific gender-related differential effects of lipid lowering on atherosclerosis progression in native or saphenous vein grafts were reported in these studies. In addition to retardation of progression of CAD angiographically, results of POSCH showed a decrease in total mortality and fatality due to CAD in patients who underwent partial ileal bypass following a first MI, with a mean follow-up of 9.7 years. Mortality among the 78 women in the trial (9.3% of the 838 patients studied) was similar to that of men.

Although data derived from the coronary atherosclerosis "regression" trials are limited for women, it seems likely that overall beneficial effects observed in these studies apply to women as well as men; however, it is unclear whether the magnitude of these effects is similar for both genders. Overall, fewer data are available for women.

The coronary atherosclerosis "regression" trials demonstrate that aggressive cholesterol-lowering therapies are effective in retarding the progression of CAD and may even induce regression of this process in certain patients. These studies are of short duration (approximately 2 years for most trials) and generally demonstrate statistically significant but small 1% to 2% improvements in the percentage diameter stenosis or minimal luminal diameter of stenotic lesions. However, despite the modest absolute changes in the anatomic extent of coronary atherosclerosis, some individual studies have demonstrated reductions in angina, exercise-induced myocardial ischemia, and, even more importantly, reductions in major clinical cardiovascular events (e.g., MI, the need for revascularization). When pooled, the coronary angiographic studies, which total approximately 8000 patient-years of follow-up, reveal a 24% reduction in total mortality and a 47% reduction in nonfatal MI with active lipid-lowering treatment (89).

Several explanations have been proposed for the apparent discrepancy between the degree of angiographic change and the reduction in coronary events in these studies. It has been suggested that aggressive lipid lowering is associated with a reduction in the lipid core of coronary lesions, decreasing the propensity of these lesions to rupture, and thereby resulting in a lower risk for acute coronary events. Lipid lowering also has been shown to improve endothelial function in the coronary arteries in both experimental models and in humans (90,91). This results in normalization of vasoreactive responses and enhanced myocardial perfusion, which may contribute to lesser activation of thrombotic mechanisms and less plaque fissuring.

Randomized trials that evaluate the impact of lipid-lowering interventions on major clinical events (e.g., total mortality, cardiovascular mortality, risk for MI) provide the most conclusive evidence for the efficacy of treatment. The first generation of large pharmacologic lipid-lowering trials in primary prevention (e.g., World Health Organization cooperative trial [92], Lipid Research Clinics Coronary Primary Prevention trial [93], Helsinki Heart Study [94]) concentrated almost exclusively on men. Secondary prevention after MI was the focus in the Coronary Drug Project (CDP) (95) and, in the only study to include women (20% of patients), the Stockholm Ischemic Heart Disease Secondary Prevention study (96a). (*Note*: Two even earlier trials of clofibrate included women and reported a reduction in clinical end points, but these trials were methodologically limited [96b,96c].) Because these first-generation trials lowered cholesterol only modestly (approximately 10%) and frequent drug side effects limited compliance, they had inadequate power to provide reliable estimates of lipid-lowering on total mortality, particularly in women. Overall, however, these early secondary prevention trials did demonstrate reductions in the risk for MI and death (97).

The magnitude of these effects is consistent with predictions derived from epidemiologic data on hypercholesterolemia as a coronary risk factor (70,98). The early studies could not, however, adequately address the role of lipid lowering in secondary or primary prevention in women.

More recently, women have been better represented in lipid-lowering trials of secondary prevention with more effective agents. Statins lower total cholesterol approximately 25% and LDL cholesterol approximately 30%, which is approximately 2.5 times more effect than seen with first-generation agents such as cholestyramine or fibrates. This large effect, combined with increased duration of treatment in trials of high-risk populations, resulted in much greater reductions in coronary events.

The landmark Scandinavian Simvastatin Survival Study (4S) trial enrolled 4444 patients, including 827 (18.6%) women with angina pectoris or previous MI (99a). These patients had significant hypercholesterolemia at baseline (on average, total cholesterol was 261 mg/dL [6.75 mmol/L] and LDL was 188.32 mg/dL [4.87 mmol/L]). Patients were randomized to receive simvastatin or placebo, and follow-up extended for a median of 5.4 years. A highly significant 30% reduction in all-cause mortality was documented in the simvastatin group. In addition, there was a 42% reduction in the risk of coronary death, a 34% reduction in the risk of major coronary events, a 37% reduction in revascularization procedures, and an overall 26% increase in the event-free survival of actively treated patients. Women were a predefined subgroup in this trial. Only 52 of 827 women died during this trial—25 (6%) in the placebo group and 27 (7%) in the simvastatin group; therefore, there was insufficient power to analyze the effects of simvastatin on all-cause mortality in women. However, women treated with simvastatin had a risk reduction of 14% for coronary mortality ($p = 0.67$), 34% for major coronary events ($p = 0.012$), 36% for nonfatal MI ($p = 0.011$), 49% for revascularization procedures ($p = 0.012$), and 31% for any atherosclerosis-related end point ($p =$

0.006). These benefits were similar in magnitude to those in men (99b). The risk of cancer and other noncardiovascular deaths was similar with treatment or placebo.

Further important evidence for the role of aggressive lipid lowering in women following MI is provided by the Cholesterol and Recurrent Events (CARE) trial (100a). In this study, 4159 patients (3583 men and 576 women) with recent MI and only mild elevation in total and LDL cholesterol levels (mean baseline total cholesterol level was 209 mg/dL [5.4 mmol/L]; mean baseline LDL was 139 mg/dL [3.59 mmol/L]) were randomized to pravastatin, 40 mg, or placebo; follow-up extended for a median of 5.4 years. There was an overall reduction of 24% in the primary end point, fatal coronary events, or nonfatal MI. In addition, the need for coronary bypass graft surgery or angioplasty was reduced by approximately 25%, and the frequency of stroke was reduced by 31%. Among those who showed the greatest and earliest response to pravastatin were female MI survivors enrolled in this trial.

Women treated with pravastatin in the CARE trial had a risk reduction of 43% for CAD death or nonfatal MI (the primary study end points) ($p = 0.035$), 46% for combined coronary events ($p = 0.001$), 48% for coronary angioplasty ($p = 0.025$), 40% for coronary artery bypass graft surgery ($p = 0.14$), and 56% for stroke ($p = 0.01$) (100b). Men in the CARE trial also showed a reduction in risk, but the magnitude tended to be less than in women. Although direct comparisons of the effects of lipid lowering with statins between women and men cannot be derived from this study, it is prudent to conclude that cholesterol lowering is important in secondary prevention in women and is at least as effective as in men.

Statins are the most effective pharmacologic agents in attaining lipid lowering; their efficacy and safety have been proven in large clinical trials. Statins are therefore the drugs of choice for management of hypercholesterolemia in post-MI patients and in other high-risk individuals. The use of statins in secondary prevention in women and men also has been proven to be a cost-effective intervention (101a). At present, there is no clear indication as to which statin should be prescribed; the magnitude of cholesterol-lowering effect and individual tolerance seem to be the best therapeutic guides.

In summary, these recent trials have demonstrated clearly that aggressive lipid lowering represents a potent intervention in modifying the natural history of CAD in women and men. Lipid lowering results in the retardation of the anatomic progression of CAD. It can lead to plaque stabilization and improvement in endothelial function and, most importantly, results in significant reductions in the risk for MI and cardiac death. Therefore, all women and men with existing cardiovascular disease should be counselled with regard to aggressive hygienic measures, diet, and exercise. If hypercholesterolemia persists with even modest elevations in total and LDL cholesterol, aggressive lipid-lowering therapy with statins should be prescribed.

Despite overwhelming evidence for the benefits and safety of cholesterol lowering in secondary prevention and the publication and wide dissemination of guidelines for the management of hyperlipidemia, the majority of hypercholesterolemic women with CAD remain untreated or suboptimally treated (101b).

From our perspective, several aspects regarding lipid-lowering drug therapy in women require further exploration:

1. The role of cholesterol lowering in primary prevention in women (although the recent AFCAPS/TEXCAPS trial demonstrated reduced coronary events in middle-aged women without their CAD being treated with lovastatin [101c])

2. The importance of lowering triglycerides and directing therapy toward raising HDL cholesterol levels

3. The magnitude of LDL cholesterol levels to be targeted (although it seems reasonable to aim for 2.6 mmol/L [100mg/dL] as suggested by the National Cholesterol Education Program guidelines [102a])

4. The potential interaction between hormone replacement and pharmacologic lipid-lowering therapies in postmenopausal women (although this has been addressed in small studies [102b,102c])

Many of these issues are discussed further in Chapters 4 and 10.

Drug Interventions with No Proven Efficacy and with Potential for Harm in the Long-term Management of Coronary Artery Disease

Calcium-Channel Blockers

Calcium-channel blockers have anti-anginal, vasodilatory, and antihypertensive properties. They have been used widely in CAD as anti-anginal agents, in acute ischemic syndromes, and in the long-term management of patients after MI. In general, individual trials and meta-analyses have failed to demonstrate a survival benefit for patients treated with calcium-channel blockers in the acute phases of MI or in the prophylactic, long-term care thereafter. Furthermore, some trials revealed increased mortality in patients treated with short-acting nifedipine preparations in the setting of acute ischemic syndrome (103). Overall, calcium-channel blockers are not recommended for routine treatment or secondary prevention after acute MI (46). In general, these agents should be reserved for the treatment of a subset of patients with angina or hypertension that is inadequately controlled by other agents. These recommendations extend to both female and male patients because no gender-specific differences have been demonstrated in response to these agents.

The impact of calcium-channel blocker administration after MI depends, in part, on left ventricular function. In women and men with preserved left ventricular function, verapamil was shown to have no significant adverse effect on mortality, either during or after acute MI in several clinical trials. The DAVIT-II (Danish Verapamil Infarction Trial) demonstrated a 20% reduction in major cardiovascular events in the verapamil group (104). Diltiazem is also a calcium-channel blocker that slows heart rate. When administered short-term in selected patients without manifestations of heart failure following MI, it has been associated with a reduction in cardiovascular events; however, patients with evidence of pulmonary congestion assigned to receive diltiazem had an increase in adverse cardiac events, including reinfarction or cardiac death (105,106). These studies included both women and men, with a preponderance of male patients.

The overall evidence regarding the use of calcium-channel blockers in acute ischemic syndromes and in the long-term secondary prevention following MI identifies no definite role for the widespread use of these agents. If beta-adrenoreceptor blockers are contraindicated or poorly tolerated, calcium antagonists that slow heart rate (e.g., verapamil or diltiazem) may be an appropriate alternative for secondary prevention in individuals with preserved left ventricular function. Despite general lack of benefit in randomized trials, these drugs have been prescribed widely for patients with acute MI and for women and men with a history of previous infarction and a variety of other ischemic syndromes.

Antiarrhythmic Drugs

Sudden cardiac deaths account for 30% to 60% of all mortality during the first year after MI, and 75% of such deaths are due to ventricular tachycardia or fibrillation. These considerations and the fact that the mortality rate of patients with frequent ventricular premature depolarizations after MI is increased led to the hypothesis that long-term supression of asymptomatic ventricular premature beats with anti-arrhythmic drugs after MI infarction would decrease mortality. This hypothesis was tested in the Cardiac Arrhythmia Suppression Trial (CAST) in 2309 survivors of MI, 20% of whom were women who received placebo or an anti-arrhythmic drug (107). The specific anti-arrhythmic drugs used were flecainide, encainide, and moricizine. This study was terminated long before its anticipated end due to a significant increase in mortality in patients randomized to receive active anti-arrhythmic therapy. The same results were suggested by a previous meta-analysis of 18 long-term trials of 6300 patients after MI, which revealed a significant 21% increase in mortality among those assigned to Class I anti-arrhythmic drugs (44). Therefore, the prophylactic long-term use of Class I anti-arrhythmic drugs in women and men with asymptomatic ventricular arrhythmias after MI is strongly contraindicated.

Amiodarone, a Class III anti-arrhythmic drug, has shown promise in several small studies. More recently the results of two moderately sized, randomized, placebo-controlled trials in survivors of acute MI were reported. The Canadian Amiodarone Myocardial Infarction Arrhythmia Trial (CAMIAT) evaluated the use of amiodarone in 213 women (18% of patients) and 989 men with recent MI and frequent ventricular premature depolarizations (108). The European Myocardial Infarction Amiodarone Trial (EMIAT) studied 232 women (16% of patients) and 1254 men with recent MI and left ventricular ejection fraction of 40% or less (109a). Both trials reported a decrease in arrhythmic deaths but no definite impact on total or cardiac mortality in amiodarone-treated patients. Patients receiving amiodarone experienced relatively frequent side effects and had high drug-discontinuation rates. Gender-specific analyses were not reported. Two comprehensive meta-analyses demonstrated a small, statistically significant reduction in total mortality rates of approximately 15% and a more significant 30% reduction in the risk for sudden death in high-risk women and men after MI or with heart failure who were treated with amiodarone (109b,109c). The benefits of amiodarone were similar in women and in men. These studies do not support the systematic prophylactic use of amiodarone in all women and men after MI but suggest a role for this drug in the treatment of patients with symptomatic ventricular arrhythmias and those at particularly high risk for sudden cardiac death following myocardial infarction.

Summary

Women with previous MI or other manifestations of CAD are at particularly high risk for future adverse cardiac events. Aggressive risk-factor modification through lifestyle changes and consistent use of pharmacologic interventions with proven benefit should be incorporated into the routine management of these women (Table 21-3). In general, the same classes of drugs have been shown to be effective or to lack efficacy in both women and men. This should be the major determinant influencing the application of secondary prevention strategies for women; the possibility of quantitative gender-specific differences in side effects or speculation about relative efficacy should not limit use of these agents. Guidelines for the comprehensive management of women and men with coronary and other vascular disease have been summarized in the

Table 21-3 Guide to Comprehensive Risk Reduction for Patients with Coronary and Other Vascular Diseases

Risk Intervention	Recommendations
Smoking Goal: complete cessation	Strongly encourage patient and family to stop smoking Provide counselling, nicotine replacement, and formal cessation programs as appropriate
Lipid management Primary goal: LDL < 100 mg/dL Secondary goals: HDL > 35 mg/dL; TG < 200 mg/dL	Start AHA Step II Diet in all patients (≤ 30% fat, < 7% saturated fat, < 200 mg/dL cholesterol) Assess fasting lipid profile (in post-MI patients, lipid profile may take 4–6 weeks to stabilize) Add drug therapy according to the following guide: If LDL < 100 mg/dL, no drug therapy If LDL = 100–130 mg/dL, consider adding drug therapy to diet* If LDL > 130 mg/dL, add drug therapy to diet* If HDL < 35 mg/dL, emphasize weight management and physical activity
Physical activity Minimum goal: 30 minutes 3–4 times per week	Assess risk, preferably with exercise test, to guide prescription Encourage minimum of 30–60 minutes of moderate-intensity activity three or four times per week, supplemented by an increase in daily lifestyle activities Advise medically supervised programs for moderate- to high-risk patients.
Weight management	Start intensive diet and appropriate physical activity intervention as outlined above in patients > 120% of ideal weight for height; particularly emphasize need for weight loss in patients with hypertension, elevated triglycerides, or elevated glucose levels
Antiplatelet agents/ anticoagulants	Start aspirin, 80–325 mg/d, if not contraindicated Manage warfarin to international normalized ratio: 2–3.5 for post-MI patients not able to take aspirin
ACE inhibitors after MI	Start early after MI in stable high-risk patients (anterior MI, previous MI, Killip class II or higher [S_3 gallop, rales, radiographic CHF]) Continue indefinitely for all with LV dysfunction (EF ≤ 40) or symptoms of failure Use as needed to manage blood pressure or symptoms in all other patients
Beta-blockers	Start in high-risk post-MI patients (arrhythmia, LV dysfunction, inducible ischemia) at 5–28 days[†] Observe usual contraindications Use as needed to manage angina rhythm or blood pressure in all other patients
Estrogens	Consider estrogen replacement in postmenopausal women[‡] Individualize recommendation consistent with other health risks
Blood pressure control Goal: ≤ 140/90 mm Hg	Initiate lifestyle modification (e.g., weight control, physical activity, alcohol moderation, and moderate sodium restriction) in all patients with blood pressure > 140 mm Hg systolic or 90 mm Hg diastolic Add blood pressure medication, individualized to patient's other requirements and characteristics (e.g., age, race, need for drugs with specific benefits), if blood pressure is not less than 140 mm Hg systolic or 90 mm Hg diastolic in 3 months or if *initial* blood pressure is > 160 mm Hg systolic or 100 mm Hg diastolic

* Suggested drug therapy is dependent on TG levels: if TG < 200 mg/dL, then administer statin, resin, or niacin; if TG = 200–400 mg/dL, then statin or niacin; if TG > 400 mg/dL, then consider combined drug therapy of niacin, fibrate, and statin. If LDL goal is not achieved, consider combination therapy.

† The available evidence also can be interpreted as use of beta-blockers in all patients after MI without contraindication.

‡ No definitive proof is available to support this intervention. (see Chapter 10).

ACE = angiotensin-converting enzyme; AHA = American Heart Association; CHF = congestive heart failure; EF = ejection fraction; HDL = high-density lipoprotein; LDL = low-density lipoprotein; LV = left ventricular; MI = myocardial infarction; TG = triglycerides.

Adapted from Smith SC, Blair SN, Criqui MH, et al. Preventing heart attack and death in patients with coronary disease. Circulation. 1995;92:2–4.

27th Bethesda Conference Report endorsed by the American College of Cardiology and the American Heart Association (110). Similar guidelines have been issued by the European Society of Cardiology (111).

Although the guidelines have been stated clearly and have been widely publicized, pharmacologic interventions that clearly benefit CAD patients who are targeted for secondary prevention remain grossly underused. Such concerns emerged from studies conducted in the United States, Europe, and Canada (112–114). Several investigations suggest that suboptimal preventive care is a particular problem in the current management of women and the elderly (115). Adequate implementation of risk-reduction strategies in all women and men with cardiovascular disease is mandatory and should be a high priority for everyone involved in the care of these patients.

REFERENCES

1. Morbidity and Mortality: Chartbook on Cardiovascular, Lung, and Blood Diseases. Bethesda, MD: National Heart, Lung, and Blood Institute, US Department of Health and Human Services; 1992.

2. Heart and Stroke Facts: 1995 Statistical Supplement. Dallas: American Heart Association; 1995.

3. **Gurwitz JH, Nananda F, Avorn J.** The exclusion of the elderly and women from clinical trials in acute myocardial infarction. JAMA. 1992;268:1417–22.

4. **Yusuf S, Wittes J, Probstfield J, Tyroler HA.** Analysis and interpretation of treatment effects in subgroups of patients in randomized clinical trials. JAMA. 1991;266: 93–8.

5. **Chesebro JH, Badiman JJ, Ortiz AF, et al.** Conjunctive antithrombotic therapy for thrombolysis in myocardal infarction. Am J Cardiol. 1993;72:66–74G.

6. **Fuster V, Badimon J, Chesebro JH.** The pathogenesis of coronary artery disease and the acute coronary syndromes. N Engl J Med. 1992;326:242–318.

7. **Falk E, Fernandez-Ortiz A.** Role of thrombosis in atherosclerosis and its complications. Am J Cardiol. 1995;75:5B–11B.

8. **Brushke AVG, Kramer JR, Bal ET, et al.** The dynamics of progression of coronary atherosclerosis studied in 168 medically treated patients who underwent coronary arteriography three times. Am Heart J. 1989;117:296–305.

9. **Ip J, Fuster V, Badimon L, et al.** Syndromes of accelerated atherosclerosis: role of vascular injury and smooth muscle cell proliferation. J Am Coll Cardiol. 1990;15: 1667–87.

10. **Solymoss BC, Nadeau P, Millenne D, Campeau L.** Late thrombosis of saphenous vein coronary bypass grafts related to risk factors. Circulation. 1988;78(Suppl I):140–3.

11. **Hirsh J, Dalen JE, Fuster V, et al.** Aspirin and other platelet-active drugs: the relationship among dose, effectivenes, and side effects. Chest. 1995;108:247–57S.

12. **Antiplatelet Trialists Collaboration.** Secondary prevention of vascular disease by prolonged antiplatelet treatment. Br Med J. 1988;296:320–31.

13. **ISIS-2 Collaborative Group.** Randomised trial of intravenous streptokinase, oral aspirin, both, or neither among 17,187 cases of suspected acute myocardal infarction: ISIS-2. Lancet. 1988;II:349–60.

14. **Antiplatelet Trialists Collaboration.** Collaborative overview of randomised trials of antiplatelet therapy. Part I: Prevention of death, myocardial infarction, and stroke by prolonged antiplatelet therapy in various categories of patients. BMJ. 1994;308: 81–106.

15. **Canadian Cooperative Study Group.** A randomized trial of aspirin and sulfinpyrazone in threatened stroke. N Engl J Med. 1978;299:53.

16. **Gent M, Barnett HJM, Sackett DL, Taylor DW.** A randomized trial of aspirin and sulfinpyrazone in patients with threatened stroke: results and methodologic issues. Circulation. 1980;62(Suppl V):97–105.

17. **Gent M, Easton JD, Hachinski VC, et al.** The Canadian–American Ticlopidine Study (CATS) in thromboembolic stroke. Lancet. 1989;I:1215–1220.

18. **Hass WK, Easton JD, Adams HP, et al.** A randomized trial comparing ticlopidine hydrochloride with aspirin for the prevention of stroke in high-risk patients. N Engl J Med. 1989;321:501–7.

19. **Balsano F, Rizzon P, Violo F, et al.** Antiplatelet treatment with ticlopidine in unstable angina: a controlled multicenter clinical trial. Circulation. 1990;82:17–26.

20. **Hall P, Nakamura S, Maiello L, et al.** A randomized comparison of combined ticlopidine and aspirin therapy versus aspirin therapy alone after successful intravascular ultrasound-guided stent implantation. Circulation. 1996;93:215–22.

21. **CAPRIE Steering Committee.** A randomised, blinded, trial of clopidogrel versus aspirin in patients at risk of ischaemic events (CAPRIE). Lancet. 1996;348:1329–39.

22. **Hirsch J, Dalen JE, Deykin D, et al.** Oral anticoagulants: mechanism of action, clinical effectiveness, and optimal therapeutic range. Chest. 1995;108(Suppl): 231–46S.

23. **Drapkin A, Merskey C.** Anticoagulant therapy after acute myocardial infarction: relation of therapeutic benefit to patient's age, sex, and severity of infarction. JAMA. 1972;222:541–8.

24. Assessment of short-term anticoagulant administration after cardiac infarction: report of the Working Party on Anticoagulant Therapy in Coronary Thrombosis to the Medical Research Council. BMJ. 1969;1:335–42.

25. **Veterans Administration Cooperative Study.** Anticoagulants in acute myocardial infarction: results of a cooperative clinical trial. JAMA. 1973;225:724–9.

26. **Weinreich DJ, Burke JF, Pauletto FJ.** Left ventricular mural thrombi complicating acute myocardial infarction: long-term follow-up with serial echocardiography. Ann Intern Med. 1984;100:789–94.

27. **Johannessen KA, Nordrehaug JE, von der Lippe G.** Left ventricular thrombosis and cerebrovascular accident in acute myocardial infarction. Br Heart J. 1984;51:553–6.

28. **Keating EC, Gross SA, Schlamowitz RA, et al.** Mural thrombi in myocardial infarctions: prospective evaluation of two-dimensional echocardiography. Am J Med. 1983;74:989–95.

29. **Turpie AGG, Robinson JG, Doyle DJ, et al.** Comparison of high-dose with low-dose subcutaneous heparin to prevent left ventricular mural thrombosis in patients with acute transmural anterior myocardial infarction. N Engl J Med. 1989;320:352–7.

30. **Vaitkus PT, Barnathau ES.** Embolic potential, prevention, and management of mural thrombus complicating anterior myocardial infarction: a meta-analysis. J Am Coll Cardiol. 1993;22:100–9.

31. **International Anticoagulant Review Group.** Collaborative analysis of long-term anticoagulant administration after acute myocardial infarction. Lancet. 1970;1:203–9.

32. Report of the Sixty-Plus Reinfarction Study Research Group: a double-blind trial to assess long-term anticoagulant therapy in elderly patients after myocardial infarction. Lancet. 1980;2:989–94.

33. **Smith P, Arnesen H, Holme I.** The effect of warfarin on mortality and reinfarction after myocardial infarction. N Engl J Med. 1990;323:147–52.

34. **ASPECT Research Group.** Effect of long-term oral anticoagulant treatment on mortality and cardiovascular morbidity after myocardial infarction. Lancet. 1994;343:499–503.

35. **Yusuf S, Michaelis W, Hua A, et al.** Effects of oral antocoagulants on mortality, reinfarction, and stroke after myocardial infarction. Circulation. 1995;8(Suppl I):343.

36. **Breddin D, Loew D, Lechner K, et al.** The German–Austrian Aspirin Trial: a comparison of acetylsalicylic acid, placebo and phenprocoumon in secondary prevention of myocardial infarction. Circulation. 1980;62(Suppl 5):63–72.

37. **EPSIM Research Group.** A controlled comparison of aspirin and oral anticoagulants in prevention of death after myocardial infarction. N Engl J Med. 1982;307:701–8.

38. **Meijer A, Verheugt FWA, Werter CJPJ, et al.** Aspirin versus coumadin in the prevention of reocclusion and recurrent ischemia after successful thrombolysis: a prospective placebo-controlled angiographic study. Results of the APRICOT study. Circulation. 1993;87:1524–30.

39. **Coumadin-Aspirin Reinfarction Study (CARS) Investigators.** Randomised double-blind trial of fixed low-dose warfarin with aspirin after myocardial infarction. Lancet. 1997;350:389–96.

40. **Post-Coronary Artery Bypass Graft Trial Investigators.** The effect of aggressive lowering of low-density lipoprotein cholesterol levels and low-dose anticoagulation on obstructive changes in saphenous-vein coronary-artery bypass grafts. N Engl J Med. 1997;336:153–62.

41. **Snow PJD.** Effect of propranolol in myocardial infarction. Lancet. 1965;2:551–3.

42. **ISIS-1 Collaborative Group.** Randomised trial of intravenous atenolol among 16,027 cases of suspected acute myocardial infarction: ISIS-1. Lancet. 1986;2:57–66.

43. **MIAMI Trial Research Group.** Metoprolol in acute myocardial infarction (MIAMI): a randomized placebo-controlled international trial. Eur Heart J. 1985;6:199–226.

44. **Teo KK, Yusuf S, Furberg CD.** Effects of prophylactic antiarrhythmic drug therapy in acute myocardial infarction: an overview of results from randomized controlled trials. JAMA. 1993;270:1589–95.

45. **Roberts R, Rogers WJ, Mueller HS, et al.** Immediate versus deferred β-blockade following thrombolytic therapy in patients with acute myocardial infarction: results of the Thrombolysis in Myocardial Infarction (TIMI) II-B study. Circulation. 1991;83:422–37.

46. **Ryan TJ, Anderson JL, Antman EM, et al.** ACC/AHA guidelines for the management of patients with acute myocardial infarction: a report of the American College of Cardiology/American Heart Association Task Force on Practice Guidelines (Committee

on Management of Acute Myocardial Infarction). J Am Coll Cardiol. 1996;28: 1328–1428.

47. **Yusuf Y, Peto R, Lewis J, et al.** β-Blockade during and after myocardial infarction: an overview of the ranndomized trials. Prog Cardiovasc Dis. 1985;27:335–71.

48. **Norwegian Multicenter Study Group.** Timolol-induced reduction in mortality and reinfarction in patients surviving acute myocardial infarction. N Engl J Med. 1981;304:801–7.

49. **Beta-Blocker Heart Attack Trial Research Group.** A randomized trial of propranolol in patients with acute myocardial infarction. Part I: Mortality results. JAMA. 1982; 247:1707–14.

50. **Pedersen TR.** Six-year follow-up of the Norwegian Multicenter Study on timolol after acute myocardial infarction. N Engl J Med. 1985;313:1055–8.

51a. **Beta-Blocker Pooling Project Research Group.** The Beta-Blocker Pooling Project (BBPP): subgroup findings from randomized trials in post-infarction patients. Eur Heart J. 1998;9:8–16.

51b. **Gottlieb SS, McCarter RJ, Vogel RA.** Effect of β-blockade on mortality among high-risk and low-risk patients after myocardial infarction. N Engl J Med. 1998;339: 489–96.

52. **Boissel J-P, Leizorovicz A, Picolet H, Peyrieux J-C.** Secondary prevention after high-risk acute myocardial infarction with low-dose acebutolol. Am J Cardiol. 1990; 66:251–60.

53a. **Rogers WJ, Bowlby LJ, Chandra NC, et al.** Treatment of myocardial infarction in the United States (1990–1993): observations from the National Registry of Myocardial Infarction. Circulation. 1994;90:2103–14.

53b. **Chandra NC, Ziegelstein RC, Rogers WJ, et al.** Observations of the treatment of women in the United States with myocardial infarction. Arch Intern Med. 1998; 158:981–8.

53c. **Krumholz HM, Radford MJ, Wang Y, et al.** National use and effectiveness of β-blockers for treatment of elderly patients after acute myocardial infarction: National Cooperative Cardiovascular Project. JAMA. 1998;280:623–9.

54. **Tsuyuki RT, Gill S, Hilton JD.** Patterns of practice analysis for acute myocardial infarction. Can J Cardiol. 1994;10:891–896.

55. **Lonn EM, Yusuf S, Jha P, et al.** Emerging role of angiotensin-converting enzyme inhibitors in cardiac and vascular protection. Circulation. 1994;90:2056–69.

56. **Latini R, Maggioni AP, Flather M, et al.** ACE inhibitor use in patients with myocardial infarction: summary of evidence from clinical trials. Circulation. 1995;92: 3132–7.

57. **ISIS-4 Collaborative Group.** ISIS-4: a randomized factorial trial assessing early oral captopril, oral mononitrate, and intravenous magnesium sulphate in 58,050 patients with suspected acute myocardial infarction. Lancet. 1995;345:669–85.

58. **Gruppo Italiano per lo Studio della Sopravivenza nell'Infarto Miocardico.** GISSI-3: effects of lisinopril and transdermal glyceryl trinitrate singly and together on 6-week mortality and ventricular function after acute myocardial infarction. Lancet. 1994; 434:1115–22.

59. **Pfeffer MA, Braunwald E, Moyé LA, et al.** Effect of captopril on mortality and morbidity in patients with left ventricular dysfunction after myocardial infarction: results

of the Survival and Ventricular Enlargement Trial (SAVE). N Engl J Med. 1992;327: 669–77.

60. **Moyé LA, Pfeffer MA, Wun CC, et al.** Uniformity of captopril benefit in the SAVE study: subgroup analysis. Eur Heart J. 1994;15(Suppl B):2–8.

61. **Acute Infarction Ramipril Efficacy (AIRE) Study Investigators.** Effect of ramipril on mortality and morbidity of survivors of acute myocardial infarction with clinical evidence of heart failure. Lancet. 1993;342:821–8.

62. **TRACE Study Group.** The trandolapril cardiac evaluation (TRACE) study: rationale, design, and baseline characteristics of the screened population. Am J Cardiol. 1994;73:44–50C.

63. **SOLVD Investigators.** Effect of enalapril on survival in patients with reduced left ventricular ejection fractions and congestive heart failure. N Engl J Med. 1991;325: 293–302.

64. **SOLVD Investigators.** Effect of enalapril on mortality and the development of heart failure in asymptomatic patients with reduced left ventricular ejection fractions. N Engl J Med. 1992;327:685–91.

65. **Kostis JB, Shelton B, Gosselin G, et al.** Adverse effects of enalapril in the Studies of Left Ventricular Dysfunction (SOLVD). Am Heart J. 1996;131:350–5.

66. **Alderman CP.** Adverse effects of angiotensin converting enzyme inhibitors. Ann Pharmacokin. 1996;30:55–61.

67a. **Hausseus M, Keirse MYNC, Vankelcom F, Van Assche FA.** Fetal and neonatal effects of treatment angiotensin-converting enzyme inhibitors. Obstet Gynecol. 1991;78: 128–135.

67b. **Luzier AB, Forrest A, Adelman M, et al.** Impact of angiotensin-converting–enzyme inhibitor underdosing on rehospitalization rates in congestive heart failure. Am J Cardiol. 1998;82:465–9.

68. **Pepine CJ.** Ongoing clinical trials of angiotensin-converting enzyme inhibitors for treatment of coronary artery disease in patients with preserved left ventricular function. J Am Coll Cardiol. 1996;27:1048–1052.

69. **Fuster V, Gotto AM, Libby P, et al.** Pathogenesis of coronary disease: the biologic role of risk factors. J Am Coll Cardiol. 1996;27:964–1047.

70. **Law MR, Wald NJ, Thompson SG.** By how much and how quickly does reduction in serum cholesterol concentration lower risk of ischaemic heart disease? BMJ. 1994; 308:367–72.

71. Summary of the second report of the National Cholesterol Education Program (NCEP) Expert Panel on Detection, Evaluation, and Treatment of High Blood Cholesterol in Adults (Adult Treatment Panel II). JAMA. 1993;269:3015–23.

72. **Moreno GT, Manson JE.** Cholesterol and coronary heart disease in women: an overview of primary and secondary prevention. Coron Artery Dis. 1993; 4:580–7.

73. **Brensike JF, Levy RI, Kelsey SF, et al.** Effects of therapy with cholestyramine on progression of coronary arteriosclerosis: results of the NHLBI Type II Coronary Intervention Study. Circulation. 1984;69:313–24.

74. **Blankenhorn DH, Nessim SA, Johnson RL, et al.** Beneficial effects of combined colestipol-niacin therapy on coronary atherosclerosis and coronary venous bypass grafts. JAMA. 1987;257:3233–40. [Published erratum. JAMA. 1988;259: 2698.]

75. **Cashin-Hemphill L, Mack WJ, Pogoda JM, et al.** Beneficial effects of colestipol-niacin on coronary atherosclerosis: a 4-year follow-up. JAMA. 1990;264:3013–7.

76. **Buchwald H, Varco RL, Matts JP, et al.** Effect of partial ileal bypass surgery on mortality and morbidity from coronary heart disease in patients with hypercholesterolemia: report of the Program on the Surgical Control of the Hyperlipidemias (POSCH). N Engl J Med. 1990;323:946–55.

77. **Schuler G, Hambrecht R, Schlierf G, et al.** Regular physical exercise and low-fat diet: effects on progression of coronary artery disease. Circulation. 1992;86:1–11.

78. **Ornish D, Brown SE, Scherwitz LW, et al.** Can lifestyle changes reverse coronary heart disease? The Lifestyle Heart Trial. Lancet. 1990;336:129–33.

79. **Brown G, Albers JJ, Fisher LD, et al.** Regression of coronary artery disease as a result of intensive lipid-lowering therapy in men with high levels of apolipoprotein B. N Engl J Med. 1990;323:1289–98.

80. **Kane JP, Malloy MJ, Ports TA, et al.** Regression of coronary atherosclerosis during treatment of familial hypercholesterolemia with combined drug regimens. JAMA. 1990;264:3007–12.

81. **Blankenhorn D, Azen SP, Kramsch DM, et al.** Coronary angiographic changes with lovastatin therapy: Monitored Atherosclerosis Regression Study (MARS), MARS Research Group. Ann Intern Med. 1993;119:969–76.

82. **Sacks FM, Pasternak RC, Gibson CM, et al.** Effect on coronary atherosclerosis of decrease in plasma cholesterol concentrations in normocholesterolaemic patients. Lancet. 1994;344:1182–6.

83. **Watts GF, Mandalia S, Brunt JN, et al.** Independent associations between plasma lipoprotein subfraction levels and the course of coronary artery disease in the St. Thomas Atherosclerosis Regression Study. (STARS). Metabolism. 1993;42:1461–7.

84. Effect of simvastatin on coronary atheroma: the Mulicentre Anti-Atheroma Study (MAAS). Lancet. 1994;344:633–8.

85. **Haskell WL, Alderman EL, Fair JM, et al.** Effects of intensive multiple risk factor reduction on coronary atherosclerosis and clinical cardiac events in men and women with coronary artery disease: the Stanford Coronary Risk Intervention Project (SCRIP). Circulation. 1994;89:975–90.

86. **Walters D, Higginson L, Gladstone P, et al.** Effects of monotherapy with an HMG-CoA reductase inhibitor on the progression of coronary atherosclerosis as assessed by serial quantitative arteriography: the Canadian Coronary Atherosclerosis Intervention Trial. Circulation. 1994;89:959–68.

87. **Jukema JW, Burschke AV, van Boven AJ, et al.** Effects of lipid lowering by pravastatin on progression and regression of coronary artery disease in symptomatic men with normal to moderately elevated serum cholesterol levels: the Regression Growth Evaluation Statin Study (REGRESS). Circulation. 1995;91:2528–40.

88. **Pitt B, Mancini GBJ, Ellis SG, et al.** Pravastatin limitation of atherosclerosis in the coronary arteries (PLAC 1): reduction in atherosclerosis progression and clinical events. J Am Coll Cardiol. 1995;26:1133–9.

89. **Waters D.** Lessons from coronary atherosclerosis "regression" trials. Cardiol Clin. 1996;14:31–50.

90. **Anderson TJ, Meredith IT, Yeung AC, et al.** The effect of cholesterol lowering and antioxidant therapy on endothelium-dependent coronary vasomotion. N Engl J Med. 1995;332:488–93.

91. **Treasure CB, Klein JL, Weintraub WS, et al.** Beneficial effects of cholesterol-lowering therapy on the coronary endothelium in patients with coronary artery disease. N Engl J Med. 1995;332:481–7.

92. **Committee of Principal Investigators.** WHO cooperative trial on primary prevention of ischemic heart disease with clofibrate to lower serum cholesterol: final mortality follow-up. Lancet. 1984;2:600–4.

93. **Lipid Research Clinics Program.** The Lipid Research Clinics Coronary Primary Prevention Trial results. Part 1: Reduction in incidence of coronary heart disease. JAMA. 1984;251:351–64.

94. **Frick MH, Elo O, Haapa K, et al.** Helsinki Heart Study. Primary-prevention trial with gemfibrozil in middle-aged men with dyslipidemia: safety of treatment, changes in risk factors and incidence of coronary heart disease. N Engl J Med. 1987;317: 1237–45.

95. **Coronary Drug Project Research Group.** Clofibrate and niacin in coronary heart disease. JAMA. 1975;231:360–81.

96a. **Carlson LA, Rosenhamer G.** Reduction of mortality in the Stockholm Ischemic Heart Disease Secondary Prevention Study by combined treatment with clofibrate and nicotinic acid. Acta Med Scand. 1988;223:405–18.

96b. **Research Committee of the Scottish Society of Physicians.** Ischaemic heart disease: a secondary prevention trial using clofibrate. BMJ. 1971;4:775–84.

96c. **Physicians of Newcastle-upon-Tyne Region.** Trial of clofibrate in the treatment of ischaemic heart disease. BMJ. 1971;4:767–775.

97. **Canner PL, Berge KG, Wenger NK, et al.** Fifteen-year mortality in Coronary Drug Project patients: long-term benefit with niacin. J Am Coll Cardiol. 1986;1245–55.

98. **Gould AL, Rossouw JE, Santanello NC, et al.** Cholesterol reduction yields clinical benefit: a new look at old data. Circulation. 1995;91:2274–82.

99a. **The Scandinavian Simvastatin Survival Study Group.** Randomised trial of cholesterol lowering in 4444 patients with coronary heart disease: the Scandinavian Simvastatin Survival Study (4S). Lancet. 1994;344:1383–89.

99b. **Miettinen TA, Pyorala K, Olsson AG, et al.** Cholesterol-lowering therapy in women and elderly patients with myocardial infarction on angina pectoris. Circulation. 1997;96:4211–8.

100a. **Sacks FM, Pfeffer MA, Move LA, et al.** The effect of pravastatin on coronary events after myocardial infarction in patients with average cholesterol levels. N Engl J Med. 1996;335:1001–9.

100b. **Lewis SJ, Sacks FM, Mitchell JS, et al.** Effect of pravastatin on cardiovascular events in women after myocardial infarction: the Cholesterol and Recurrent Events (CARE) trial. J Am Coll Cardiol. 1998;32:140–6.

101a. **Johannesson M, Jonsson B, Kjekshus J, et al.** Cost effectiveness of simvastatin treatment to lower cholesterol levels in patients with coronary heart disease. N Engl J Med. 1997;336:332–6.

101b. **Schrott HG, Bittner V, Vittinghoff E, et al.** Adherence to national cholesterol education program treatment goals in postmenopausal women with heart disease: the Heart and Estrogen/Progestin Replacement Study (HERS). JAMA. 1997;277:1281–6.

101c. **Downs JR, Clearfield M, Weis S, et al.** Primary prevention of acute coronary events with lovastatin in men and women with average cholesterol levels: results of AFCAPS/TEXCAPS. JAMA. 1998;279:1615–22.

102a. **Grundy SM, Bilheimer D, Chait A, et al.** National Cholesterol Education Program: second report of the expert panel on detection, evaluation and treatment of high blood cholesterol in adults (Adult treatment panel II). Washington, DC; US Department of Health and Human Services. [National Institutes of Health Publication No 93-3095; 1993].

102b. **Davidson MH, Testolin LM, Maki KC, et al.** A comparison of estrogen replacement, pravastatin, and combined treatment for the management of hypercholesterolemia in postmenopausal women. Arch Intern Med. 1997;157:1186–92.

102c. **Darling GM, Johns JA, McCloud PI, Davis SR.** Estrogen and progestin compared wth simvastatin for hypercholesterolemia in postmenopausal women. N Engl J Med. 1997;337:595–601.

103. **Yusuf S, Held P, Furberg C.** Update of effects of calcium antagonists in myocardial infarction or angina in light of the second Danish Verapamil Infarction Trial (DAVIT-II) and other recent studies. Am J Cardiol. 1991;67:1295–7.

104. **Danish Study Group on Verapamil in Myocardial Infarction.** Effect of verapamil on mortality and major events after acute myocardial infarction (DAVIT-II). Am J Cardiol. 1990;66:779–85.

105. **Mulicenter Diltiazem Postinfarction Trial Research Group.** The effect of diltiazem on mortality and reinfarction after myocardial infarction. N Engl J Med. 1988;319: 385–92.

106. **Gibson RS, Boden WE, Theroux P, et al.** Diltiazem and reinfarction in patients with non–Q-wave myocardial infarction: results of a double-blind, randomized, multicenter trial. N Engl J Med. 1986;315:423–9.

107. **Epstein AE, Hallstrom AP, Rogers WJ, et al.** Mortality following ventricular arrhythmia suppression by encainide, flecainide, and moricizine after myocardial infarction: the original design concept of the Cardiac Arrhythmia Suppression Trial (CAST). JAMA. 1993;270:2451–5.

108. **Cairns JA, Connolly SJ, Roberts R, Gent M.** Randomised trial of outcome after myocardial infarction in patients with frequent or repetitive ventricular premature depolarisations: CAMIAT. Lancet. 1997;349:675–82.

109a. **Julian DG, Camm AJ, Frangin G, et al.** Randomised trial of effect of amiodarone on mortality in patients with left-ventricular dysfunction after recent myocardal infarction: EMIAT. Lancet. 1997;349:667–74.

109b. **Amiodarone Trials Meta-Analysis Investigators.** Effect of prophylactic amiodarone on mortality after acute myocardial infarction and in congestive heart failure: meta-analysis of individual data from 6500 patients in randomised trials. Lancet. 1997;350:1417–24.

109c. **Sim I, McDonald KM, Lavori PW, et al.** Quantitative overview of randomized trials of amiodarone to prevent sudden cardiac death. Circulation. 1997;96:2823–9.

110. 27th Bethesda Conference. Matching the intensity of risk factor management with the hazard for coronary events. J Am Coll Cardiol. 1996;27:957–1047.

111. **Pyorala K, De Backer G, Graham I, et al.** Prevention of coronary heart disease in clinical practice: recommendations of the Task Force of the European Society of Cardiology, European Atherosclerosis Society, and European Society of Hypertension. Eur Heart J. 1994;15:1300–31.

112. **Fox R.** Meeting highlights: 18th Congress of the European Society of Cardiology, August 25-29, 1996. Circulation. 1996;94:3052–3.

113. **Rogers WJ, Bowlby LJ, Chandra NC, et al.** Treatment of myocardial infarction in the United States (1990–1993): observations from the National Registry of Myocardial Infarction. Circulation. 1994;90:2103–14.

114. **Herholz H, Goff DC, Ramsey DJ, et al.** Women and Mexican Americans receive fewer cardiovascular drugs following myocardial infarction than men and non-Hispanic whites: the Corpus Christi Heart Project, 1988–1990. J Clin Epidemiol. 1996; 49:279–87.

115. **Clinical Quality Improvement Network (CQIN) Investigators.** Low incidence of assessment and modification of risk factors in acute care patients at high risk for cardiovascular events, particularly among females and the elderly. Am J Cardiol. 1995;76:570–3

Conclusion

Chapter 22

Future Directions

For decades, coronary artery disease (CAD) was not perceived as a major contributor of morbidity and mortality in women. This misperception developed in part because men, especially middle-aged men, have a dramatically higher rate of diagnosis. With increasing age, however, the incidence of CAD in women dramatically increases to rates similar to those of men (Fig. 22-1). Furthermore, the first presentation of CAD in women is typically angina, whereas in men it is myocardial infarction (MI). Thus, when the early Framingham data seemed to indicate that the natural history of angina was substantially more benign in women than in men (1), it was yet another reason to consider CAD a male-specific disease. After 30 years of follow-up, however, the Framingham Heart Study revealed that CAD mortality was 23% in women and 34% in men (2).

In middle-aged populations around the world, there is a consistent ratio of male-to-female CAD deaths, varying from 2.5 to 4.5 (3). The cause of this excess CAD mortality in men has not been determined, although the variable differences between countries suggest that "sex is not destiny with regard to coronary heart disease" (3). Studies have been performed only recently among the elderly, in whom the sex ratio is smaller.

Neither public nor physician acceptance of the importance of CAD in women has yet to evolve adequately. In a national telephone survey of U.S. women, 58% "believed they were as likely or more likely to die of breast cancer than coronary artery disease" (4); however, between the ages of 40 and 60 years as many women die of heart disease as of breast cancer (4). Although

575

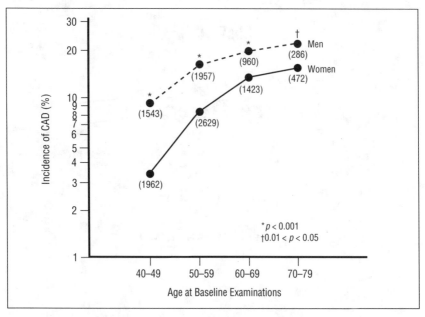

Figure 22-1 Ten-year incidence of coronary artery disease (e.g., angina, myocardial infarction, coronary insufficiency, or death) among women and men by age. Data are from the Framingham Heart Study. (From Eaker ED, Castelli WP. Coronary heart disease and its risk factors among women in the Framingham study. In: Eaker ED, Packard B, Wenger NK, et al, eds. Coronary Heart Disease in Women: Proceedings of an NIH Workshop. New York: Haymark Doyma; 1987:122–130; with permission.)

86% of the women surveyed saw a doctor regularly, 47% of women 45 to 59 years of age and 44% of women over 59 years of age reported that their physicians had "never talked to them about heart disease" (4).

In this chapter, several evolving areas within CAD are reviewed. First, the importance of personal characteristics beyond gender is considered. Although the importance of age, race, and socioeconomic status has been explored in the past decade, these issues require further study. Second, the ways in which CAD presents in asymptomatic and symptomatic women are explored. Newer models that assess CAD risk with attention to gender are reviewed, as are gender issues in angina, MI, and sudden death.

Specific Patient Characteristics: Age, Race, and Socioeconomic Factors

As specific patient characteristics receive increasing scrutiny, age, race, and socioeconomic status are being explored as predictors of CAD.

Age

As reviewed elsewhere in this book, rates of CAD increase with advancing age. More recent clinical trials have included older subjects, and this elderly population (both with and without CAD) is predominantly female.

Younger women have substantially lower rates of CAD, yet identifying high-risk young women for possible primary prevention is important. Young women with CAD mortality and morbidity are more likely to have a history of tobacco exposure (5), obesity (5), diabetes (5), hypertension (5), early menopause, and (less often) cocaine abuse (*see* Chapter 16). Race and socioeconomic status impact on the prevalence of many of these risk factors. For example, black women have higher rates of obesity and early-onset diabetes.

Race

When race was first considered as a prognostic variable in CAD outcome studies, some authors suggested that black women had a poorer prognosis after MI. However, the number of black women on which this analysis was based was small (6). In addition, results were confounded by differences in socioeconomic status. Social class at birth has been associated with morbidity at 33 years of age (7). As studies considering both factors are made available, the importance of considering race and socioeconomic status simultaneously has become more obvious.

Differences in CAD mortality rates among blacks and whites have been studied to a limited extent (6,8). Analysis of data from the 1986 National Mortality Feedback Survey, the 1985 National Health Interview Survey, and the U.S. Bureau of Census revealed that young black women (< 55 years of age) had more than twice the rate of CAD mortality (sudden and nonsudden) than young white women (8). With 11.3 CAD deaths per 100,000, young black women exceed the rates for young men 45 years of age or under (9.2 deaths per 100,000 black men and 5.9 deaths per 100,000 white men) as well as white women under 55 years of age (4.8 deaths per 100,000). Importantly, family income, occupational status, and educational level account for more of this observed difference than traditional coronary risk factors (8). Similarly, black women in the Multicenter Investigation of the Limitation of Infarct Size study (n = 63 of 985 randomized subjects) had a higher cumulative 4-year mortality after MI than other sex/race groups (6).

Birthplace was found to be more important than race for blacks studied in the New York City area. Among the New York City black population, 54% were born in the northeastern United States, approximately 20% were born in the southern United States, and 17% were born in the Caribbean. The comparison group was the northeastern-born white population. Age-adjusted CAD death rates in New York City were higher for black women (593.7 per 100,00) than white women (393.1 per 100,000). Mortality rates were lower in women than in men; however, consideration of birthplace greatly altered risk assessment for some populations. For example, the risk for Caribbean black women was lower than that of white women or the other black women studied (Table 22-1) (9). Initial studies tended to use race as a surrogate marker for socioeconomic class, whereas more recent studies have assessed each domain, revealing more complex relationships.

Possible physiologic racial differences are just beginning to be explored further. In 1998, electrocardiographic differences among healthy blacks and whites were described (10). Differences in tobacco metabolism also have been documented in U.S. blacks and whites (11). Slower cotinine clearance and higher serum cotinine levels are seen in black smokers (11). Similarly, higher cotinine levels were found in subjects in the National Health and Nutrition Study when black smokers were compared with both white and Hispanic populations (12).

Few studies of other racial groups have been published. Although the Hispanic population has been rapidly increasing in the United States, there is a lag in studies comparing Hispanic with black and white populations. Many of the published studies that include Hispanics have recruited predominantly Mexican Americans. Potential differences between Mexican Americans and Hispanic immigrants originating from the Caribbean have been studied even less. Similar limitations exist for other racial groups. The British literature has documented some health differences in East Indian immigrants who are at increased risk of advanced CAD at diagnosis and who experience more events after immigration to Britain (13).

Table 22-1 Age-Adjusted Death Rates from Coronary Artery Disease Among Non-Hispanic Blacks and Whites Living in New York City, 1988 to 1992*

Age (y)	Blacks from Southern U.S.		Blacks from Northeast U.S.		People from Caribbean		Whites from Northeast U.S.	
	Women	Men	Women	Men	Women	Men	Women	Men
25–44	12.4	30.1	10.1	23.1	3.2	7.4	5.1	16.8
45–64	223.8	406.5	151.5	318.9	105.3	165.2	133.1	339.8
≥ 65	1815.0	2117.5	981.0	1467.5	1409.2	2149.1	1620.8	2429.8

* Mortality per 100,000 adjusted for age in 5-year age groups.
Adapted from Fang J, Madhavan S, Alderman MH. The association between birthplace and mortality from cardiovascular causes among black and white residents of New York City. N Engl J Med. 1996;335:1545–51.

Socioeconomic Factors

Morbidity and mortality from CAD are higher in individuals with lower socioeconomic status (*see* Chapter 20). Standards for the assessment of socioeconomic status have included years of formal education (14), owning a car (15), absolute (16) or relative (17) income, and parental status (15). More recently, exploration of the strength of the association of socioeconomic status and outcome has become more sophisticated. The importance of economic status also was found in the Duke catheterization population (consecutive patients with ≥ 75% stenosis of at least one coronary artery at catheterization). With a 9-year median follow-up, the most important prognostic factor was extent of CAD and ejection fraction at catheterization regardless of gender. Economic status and social support factors, however, were independent of clinical indicators of disease severity and catheterization, which explained approximately 12% of the prognoses of individual women and men. By 5 years of follow-up, those with incomes less than $10,000 were almost twice as likely to die as those with incomes of $40,000 or more (16).

When coronary events (MI and coronary death) recorded from a community register from Glasgow were compared with socioeconomic status (defined by postal address) during 1985 through 1991, women and men were found to have increasing coronary event rates with decreasing socioeconomic status. Review of the community registry revealed that women had substantially fewer coronary events ($n = 1551$) than men ($n = 3991$), reflecting the age range of 25 to 64 years. Women and men of lower socioeconomic class were at increased risk for MI and death before hospitalization compared with those of a higher socioeconomic class from the same economically depressed city (1). Lower socioeconomic status also has been related to higher rates of tobacco use and higher inpatient mortality after MI (1). Differences in event rates were greater between classes for women than men.

Exploration of the relationship between CAD, socioeconomic class, and work environment was taken a step further by the Whitehall studies, which for decades have considered the risk of development of CAD in British civil service workers. The first study, begun in 1967, found men at less prestigious and lower-income positions had nearly triple the mortality from CAD than men at higher positions. Traditional CAD risk factors explained less than 50% of the difference in CAD mortality rates. In the 1980s, a follow-up study that included both female and male civil servants (initially aged 35 to 55 years) assessed employment factors with potential impact on the incidence of CAD. Women were at lower employment grades substantially more often than men (e.g., secretarial rather than executive) and had more angina (6.7% and 3.5%, respectively) but less ischemia diagnosed by a physician (1.9% and 2.4%, respectively). For both women and men, lower position in the hierarchy and lack of job control (defined personally by the civil servant and supervisor) generally were found to be significant predictors of coronary events (i.e., angina, severe chest pain episode lasting > 30 min, or physician-diagnosed CAD) (18,19).

Recently, the importance of the size of the gap between lower and higher socioeconomic classes within a country has been explored. Physicians favoring relative differences between incomes note that nations with low absolute incomes (and usually limited differences in relative income) often have low coronary event rates. It has been suggested that relative income differences lead to social divisions and this lack of cohesion results in "social exclusion," which causes psychologic distress described as "low control, insecurity, and loss of self-esteem similar to racism or sexism" (17). Research in this area has been hampered by variable response rates, especially by those at the highest and lowest incomes.

The relative importance of socioeconomic status in different times through the life span has been a controversial factor (15,20). Studies that explore the importance of birth weight, parental status, and first employment to current employment have focused predominantly on men. In these studies, coronary events were predicted equally by current and parental socioeconomic status (15). In the Nurses Health Study, increasing birth weight was associated with decreased risk of nonfatal MI as well as decreased rates of diabetes, adult hypertension, and self-reported elevated cholesterol (21a).

There are other limitations of the completed studies focusing on socioeconomic status. Many of the earlier studies defined family social status by the head of household's income. Yet, increasingly, family income is more accurately defined by including the contributions from all employed family members. Additional important confounders of family income require further investigation; for example, child care costs compared with estimates of the unpaid labor provided by parents providing child care at home. Patient characteristics that might change over time, such as functional status (21b) and education (22), are now receiving more attention. Other areas that require future study, including psychosocial issues related to secondary prevention, are discussed in Chapter 20.

Asymptomatic Women

When considering CAD prevention, each risk factor should be assessed for its prevalence, its prognostic value, and evidence for effective intervention. Patient-specific characteristics play a role in each of these. Individual risk factors for CAD in women have been reviewed in other chapters. Further information is required in at least three areas. First, tobacco use and cessation in women demand urgent attention (*see* Chapter 2). Second, although it is well documented that diabetic women have higher rates of coronary events, the study of what interventions are most effective has been limited (*see* Chapter 3). Finally, further understanding of the relationship between CAD outcomes and the use of hormonal therapy awaits completion of the Women's Health Initiative (*see* Chapters 10 and 11).

Increasingly, national prevention guidelines also have been acknowledging issues related to gender within published recommendations (23). Because women generally have fewer coronary events than men, individual risk factors may predict adverse events more accurately in women than in men. Important risk factors for both women and men include tobacco use, hypertension, physical activity, diabetes, obesity, and lipid levels (24a,24b).

One of the essential future directions is to consider the relationships between risk factors. Cohort studies provide models to consider the effect of the combination of multiple risk factors on the risk of CAD events (23,25,26). When more individual risk factors are present, the risk of coronary events is higher, and the cumulative risk is greater than the sum of its parts (23,25,27). This is reviewed with data from the Third National Health and Nutrition Examination Survey, the Framingham Heart Study, and the Chicago Heart Association Detection Project in Industry.

Although race and socioeconomic status have been discussed in a previous section, the Third National Health and Nutrition Examination Survey, 1988 to 1994, also considered the intersection between race and socioeconomic status and the prevalence of cardiovascular risk factors (25). Systolic blood pressure, tobacco use, body mass index, leisure-time activity, non–high-density lipoprotein cholesterol levels, and the presence of non–insulin-dependent diabetes were assessed in black ($n = 1762$), Mexican American ($n = 1481$), and white women ($n = 2023$) aged 25 to 64 years. All women participated in both a home questionnaire and physical examination in a mobile examination center. Socioeconomic status was determined by the highest educational level attained and a poverty-to-income ratio based on family income and size. This sample included more white women of low socioeconomic class than previous studies attempting comparison.

Results stress the importance of race when socioeconomic class is included in the model. As expected, increasing age was associated with greater prevalence for all risk factors; however, there were substantial variations in other associations. Race comparisons found that black and Mexican American women had higher body mass index, higher systolic blood pressure, higher incidence of diabetes, more leisure-time activity, and lower tobacco use than white women of similar socioeconomic status (Table 22-2). Both race and education level are important variables for leisure-time activity and current smoking status. With increasing age, black and Mexican American women

Table 22-2 Cardiovascular Risk Factors by Level of Education for Black, Mexican-American, and White Women Aged 25 to 64 Years (NHANES III, 1988–1994)*

	Sample Size	BMI, Mean (SD) (kg/m²)	Systolic BP, Mean (SD) (mm Hg)	NIDDM (%)	No Leisure-Time Activity (%)	Current Smoker (%)	Non–HDL-C† Mean (SD) mmol/L	mg/dL
Race or ethnicity								
Black	1762	29.2 (7.3)	120.9 (21.0)	7.4	39.7	33.1	3.7 (1.1)	143.1 (42.6)
Mexican-American	1481	28.6 (6.3)	114.7 (17.1)	8.4	43.5	15.7	3.8 (1.1)	148.2 (42.1)
White	2023	26.3 (6.4)	114.0 (15.8)	4.3	20.5	30.0	3.8 (1.1)	148.8 (43.8)
Education level, y								
<9	934	27.6 (6.1)	118.9 (20.3)	8.7	52.9	34.6	4.3 (1.2)	165.3 (44.7)
9–11	850	28.2 (7.2)	118.2 (18.7)	9.5	33.4	49.2	4.0 (1.2)	156.6 (45.1)
12	1896	27.4 (7.0)	115.9 (16.4)	4.7	27.0	32.9	3.9 (1.1)	150.5 (44.4)
>12	1586	25.7 (6.0)	112.4 (15.5)	3.2	14.0	20.4	3.6 (1.1)	140.5 (40.7)
Education and race or ethnicity								
<9 y								
Black	171	29.5 (7.0)	130.8 (24.9)	20.0	64.5	32.6	4.2 (1.3)	162.3 (50.8)
Mexican-American	643	29.1 (5.7)	117.5 (19.4)	11.5	60.8	16.0	3.9 (1.1)	151.9 (41.6)
White	120	26.3 (5.8)	116.6 (18.3)	4.5	45.8	44.8	4.5 (1.1)	172.8 (42.8)
9–11 y								
Black	362	30.1 (8.1)	123.6 (21.5)	11.3	47.0	49.2	3.7 (1.0)	143.5 (39.9)
Mexican-American	249	29.0 (6.6)	112.8 (14.1)	6.8	47.1	18.3	3.8 (1.1)	148.4 (43.4)
White	239	27.6 (6.9)	117.3 (18.0)	9.3	28.3	52.8	4.2 (1.2)	160.8 (45.8)

12 y								
Black	714	29.4 (7.3)	120.8 (20.4)	5.1	40.7	34.6	3.7 (1.0)	141.6 (42.5)
Mexican-American	353	28.4 (7.0)	113.5 (15.6)	6.1	29.7	17.0	3.7 (1.0)	144.7 (40.5)
White	829	27.0 (6.8)	115.2 (15.6)	4.6	24.6	33.2	3.9 (1.2)	152.2 (44.7)
>12 y								
Black	515	28.3 (6.8)	117.0 (19.3)	5.4	27.8	23.5	3.6 (1.0)	139.8 (40.4)
Mexican-American	236	27.5 (6.0)	111.2 (14.3)	6.4	18.0	10.8	3.7 (1.1)	143.9 (43.6)
White	835	25.4 (5.8)	111.9 (15.0)	2.9	12.3	20.3	3.6 (1.0)	140.5 (40.6)

* Means, standard deviations (SD), and percentages were calculated with normalized sample weights. NHANES III = Third National Health and Nutrition Examination Survey; BMI = body mass index; BP = blood pressure; NIDDM = non-insulin-dependent diabetes mellitus.

† Non–HDL-C indicates non–high-density lipoprotein cholesterol. Non–HDL-C values were highly correlated with NHANES III low-density lipoprotein cholesterol values ($r = 0.95$) and were on average 0.65 mmol/L (25 mg/dL) higher than low-density lipoprotein cholesterol.

Adapted from Winkleby M, Kraemer HC, Ahn DK, Varady AN. Ethnic and socioeconomic differences in cardiovascular disease risk factors: findings for women from the Third National Health and Nutrition Examination Survey, 1988 to 1994. JAMA. 1998;280:356–62.

had greater increases in the prevalence of hypertension than white women. In contrast, smoking rates were more stable with increasing age for black and Mexican American women; they decreased for white women. This diverse cohort may provide important information with further follow-up.

In contrast, the cardiac risk profile for asymptomatic subjects aged 50 years in the Framingham cohort was used to predict who would be alive at age 75. This cohort was white and had less socioeconomic variation. For women, longer survival was associated with lower daily cigarette use, lower systolic blood pressure, higher forced vital capacity, and parental survival to age 75 (27).

The prevalence and relative importance of smoking status, hypertension, and hyperlipidemia have been explored in the Chicago Heart Association Detection Project in Industry (23). Among those employed in the Chicago area and enrolled, 8686 female and 10,503 male participants (almost all of whom were white and aged 40–64 years) were followed for 22 years. At the time of enrollment, history of current tobacco use was obtained, a single blood pressure measurement was recorded, and cholesterol levels were determined. Current tobacco use was reported by 35% of women (40% of men), hypertension (blood pressure ≥ 140/90) was noted in 53% of women (64% of men), and hypercholesterolemia (cholesterol levels ≥ 240 mg/dL) was present in 30% of women (22% of men).

Approximately 80% of participants in the Chicago Heart Association Detection Project in Industry initially had at least one of these risk factors. Two risk factors were found in approximately 34% of women (38% of men). Fewer than 7% of all patients had all three risk factors. When CAD mortality was considered, those with the most risk factors were at the greatest risk of death. Tobacco use was a more important predictor of mortality in women than in men (relative risk of 2.85 and 1.68, respectively ; $p < 0.001$ when current smokers were compared with current abstainers). In a subsequent analysis, the number of risk factors present at screening also directly correlated with the eventual size of Medicare reimbursements (27). Those without risk factors had the lowest number of Medicare claims.

In a model derived from data from the Lipid Research Clinics program, an estimate of the benefits of modifying lipid intake, hypertension, and tobacco use was developed (28). Low-risk subjects were defined in this model as nonsmokers whose blood pressure was 120/80 and whose ratio of low-density lipoprotein (149 mg/dL) to high-density lipoprotein (43 mg/dL) cholesterol levels was 3.5. In this model, as in others, low-risk women benefited less from intervention than low-risk men. High-risk women and men and those with previous coronary events benefited substantially from intervention.

In summation, these studies indicate that women without traditional cardiovascular risk factors (e.g., tobacco, hypertension, high cholesterol levels, diabetes, physical inactivity, family history, older age) are at low risk for coronary events. As the number of risk factors increase, so does the risk of a cardiac event. The largest benefit is derived from aggressive preventive measures in women with multiple risk factors or previous coronary events (29,30).

The potential importance of timing of a preventive intervention still has not been explored. Because women often present with CAD a decade later than men, there may be a larger window for initiating prevention. For example, when is the optimum time to initiate hormonal replacement therapy? Beginning treatment at menopause (average age of 52 years) may not be as effective or as well tolerated as prescribing therapy a decade later to prevent diseases that occur later in life. The Women's Health Initiative will address this issue.

The definition of new risk factors for CAD also depends on the evolving pathophysiology of CAD (3,31–33). The role of plaque disruption has been an increasing focus of research (31), and inflammation may play a previously underemphasized role. The specific pathways leading to inflammation, such as chronic infections from *Chlamydiae* (3) to *Helicobacter pylori* (2), have been explored. The role of hormones has been expanded to include consideration of adrenal androgens such as dehydroepiandrosterone sulfate (3).

Angina

Generally, women visit physicians more often than men and report more symptoms, including chest pain. The diagnosis of angina can be challenging. (The appropriate history is described in detail in Chapter 15; other potential reasons for chest pain can be found in Chapter 12.) Assessing a woman's risk for CAD can be affected by the physician's preconceived biases. In a study in which an actress portrayed the same script with different clothes and affect, physicians who reviewed the actress describing chest pain in an "exaggerated, emotional presentation style" predicted less CAD than physicians exposed to the same scripted chest pain portrayed in a "businesslike affect" (34).

As reviewed in other chapters, anginal symptoms in women are less predictive of abnormal coronary anatomy than in men. In the Coronary Artery Surgery Study, CAD was diagnosed in 63% of women with definitive angina, in 40% of women with probable angina, and in 4% of women with non-ischemic pain (35). The management of women with angina requires both prevention of MI and symptom management. (The noninvasive evaluation of women with chest pain is discussed in Chapters 13, 14, and 15.)

Generally, physicians have not appreciated some of the gender differences in presentation and management of CAD. In a Gallup Poll taken in 1996 in Washington, DC, "nearly two thirds of the primary care physicians surveyed (256 internists and family practitioners) said that there is no difference between men and women in the symptoms, signs, or diagnosis of heart disease"

(4). Meanwhile, researchers in angina, as in other aspects of CAD, explore and extend our understanding of significant gender differences. When patients with a history of chest pain and angiography that indicate no more than slight coronary artery abnormalities received acetylcholine by intracoronary infusion, substantial gender differences were noted (36). Of the 117 patients studied, large-artery spasm (n = 63) occurred predominantly in men (23 women, 40 men), whereas microvascular spasm (n = 29) occurred more often in women (20 women, 9 men). Patients with microvascular spasm had less coronary artery constriction after acetylcholine infusion, although angina (93%) and ischemic changes on electrocardiographic examination (83%) were often noted. Lactate levels in the coronary sinus were higher after acetylcholine infusion in patients with microvascular spasm (82%) than in patients with large-artery spasm (53%).

Acute Myocardial Infarction

Myocardial infarction results in serious mortality and morbidity in both women and men. Presently, it seems that the early prognosis of acute MI in women is worse than in men; however, with longer follow-up, prognosis may be similar (*see* Chapter 16). Sudden death is discussed in a separate section, but a high percentage of first MIs are lethal in women. In the Framingham Heart Study, at 30 years of follow-up, the first presentation of MI resulted in death in 39% of women and in 31% of men (2).

There are substantial gender differences in the presentation and natural history of MI. Some may be physiologic and others may be related to differences in management, as discussed in many chapters of this book. Although women with MI are older and have more comorbid conditions (*see* Chapter 16), increasing attention to the interaction of age and gender has led to exploration of their relationship. Evaluation of data from the MI Project II found an overall early mortality rate of 14% in women after hospitalization for MI compared with 10% in men. On further analysis, women under 80 years of age had substantially greater mortality than men the same age, whereas women over 80 had a lower mortality than did men (Fig. 22-2) (37).

Differences in the natural history of female MI are undergoing increasing scrutiny (38–40). In a recent review of data from the National Registry of Myocardial Infarction I trial, women had a higher mortality during hospitalization (38). As in earlier studies, women arrived for evaluation longer after symptoms began and received less thrombolytic treatment, aspirin, beta-blockers, and invasive interventions (i.e., catheterization, percutaneous transluminal coronary angioplasty, and coronary artery bypass graft). Women had higher mortality rates than men, even at similar ages or after similar interven-

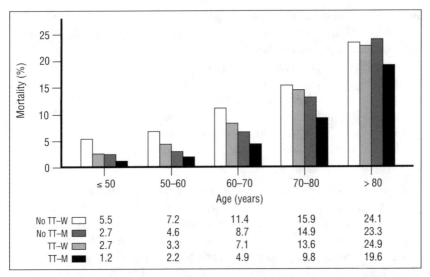

No TT-W ▢	5.5	7.2	11.4	15.9	24.1
No TT-M ▧	2.7	4.6	8.7	14.9	23.3
TT-W ▧	2.7	3.3	7.1	13.6	24.9
TT-M ■	1.2	2.2	4.9	9.8	19.6

Figure 22-2 Mortality rates by age in women (W) and men (M) treated with (TT) and without (No TT) thrombotic therapy. Absolute mortality in each category is also displayed. Mortality figures were not adjusted for other confounding variables, including hypertension, diabetes, tobacco use, and hyperlipidemia. (From Vaccarino V, Horowitz RI, Meehan TP, et al. Sex differences in mortality after myocardial infarction: evidence for a sex-age interaction. Arch Intern Med. 1998;158:2054–62; with permission.)

tions (*see* Fig. 22-2). Death resulted from cardiogenic shock, followed by sudden death, arrhythmias, and then myocardial rupture and electromechanical dissociation. Similar results were noted in a Spanish registry of patients under 80 years of age who experienced their first MI (40). In addition to a later presentation for care, women had higher mortality rates during hospitalization and the first 6 months after diagnosis. Women developed acute pulmonary edema or cardiogenic shock more often than men (25% and 11%), but women developed severe arrhythmias (defined as at least one episode of ventricular fibrillation or sustained ventricular tachycardia requiring immediate medical care) less often than men (15% vs. 24%). Whether more aggressive treatment in women will improve mortality and morbidity has yet to be determined.

Silent MI in the Framingham study was common, representing 25% of MIs when diagnosed on the basis of new Q waves on a screening electrocardiographic examination. Despite obtaining further history, almost one half of subjects had no symptoms. Silent MIs are more common in women than in men (35% and 28%) (2). The prognosis of silent MI has not been adequately studied; however, sudden death is one possible sequelae (41,42).

In long-term follow-up, women have more symptoms than men, although long-term mortality may be similar (*see* Chapter 16). Women tend to have more angina and congestive heart failure despite better systolic left ventricular function. (Important gender differences in the pathophysiology of congestive heart failure are reviewed in Chapter 19.)

Clinical treatment trials usually are conducted on populations that are at higher risk for a event; thus, it is easier to test the hypothesis that treatment will improve outcome. Historically, interventions for MI have been tested predominantly in middle-aged men. With few female subjects, information available on gender has tended to depend on post-hoc analysis. The inherent problems of subgroup analysis have been articulated by Lonn and Yusuf (*see* Chapter 21):

> Essentially, post-hoc subgroup analysis often lacks the power to test the hypothesis, and the dangers of depending on subgroup analysis include both an overestimation and underestimation of treatment effect. Aspirin as secondary prevention for women is a recent example of the potential hazards of subgroup analysis. Initial subgroup analysis raised the possibility of harm. Yet further trials have demonstrated that women as well as men benefit from aspirin preventive therapy.

Meanwhile, there has been a lag in translating results of treatment trials into practice. For example, in some studies women are prescribed aspirin less often than men (38,43). The important lesson is to use subgroup analysis as a hypothesis-generating tool whenever possible, rather than as a conclusion. Because MI is being studied increasingly in older patients, more prospective information about women will become available.

Sudden Death and Arrhythmias

Historically, limited attention has been focused on sudden death in women. In an early epidemiologic case-controlled study, risk factors for sudden death in white and black women were similar to the cardiac risk factors for MI (44). By the 30-year follow-up in the Framingham study, more information about sudden death became available (2). Sudden death is common in both women and men and accounts for 37% of the coronary deaths in women (46% of coronary deaths in men). After MI, men experienced sudden death more often than women (12% and 5%, respectively). The proportion of sudden deaths occurring in someone without previously documented CAD was 67% of women and 55% of men. In fact, in those women under 65 of years age, 90% of the sudden deaths occurred in women without a previous history of CAD.

Insights into the pathophysiology of sudden death are available by reviewing a recent study that compared autopsy results of female hearts after sudden death (n = 51) or trauma (n = 15) (41). The women who had experienced sudden death and had significant coronary artery pathology (n = 41) often experienced a witnessed death (n = 36; 71%). Reported symptoms included chest pain (n = 8), dizziness (n = 3), back pain (n = 2), tingling in the left shoulder (n = 1), shortness of breath (n = 1), malaise (n = 1), fatigue (n = 1), nausea and vomiting (n = 1), stomach distention (n = 1), and fever and chills (n = 1). The medical histories of the women who experienced sudden death included hypertension (n = 11), history of heart disease (n = 9), and medication for diabetes (n = 5). Tobacco use was noted in 58% compared with 50% of the controls. Healed MIs were found in 35% of cases.

Pathologic examination revealed eroded plaque with acute thrombus (n = 18), stable plaque with healed infarct (n = 18), ruptured plaque with acute thrombus (n = 8), and stable plaque without infarction (n = 7). The acute thrombus associated with plaque erosion occurred more often in younger female smokers without obesity or elevated cholesterol or glycohemoglobin levels. Lesions of this type have also been noted in early atherosclerosis (42). By comparison, plaque rupture was found more often in older women with elevated cholesterol. Further assessment of women dying with stable plaque without infarction revealed no association with known cardiac risk factors. Although sudden death is rare, tobacco use is an important risk factor in young women. (Gender differences in tobacco use and cessation are discussed in detail in Chapter 2.) Although only two patients had a previously documented MI, 35% of the sample had evidence of a previous MI. The relationship between sudden death and previous silent MI requires further elucidation. A possible pathway after silent MI is the development of significant arrhythmias.

Gender differences in arrhythmia identification, natural history, and management are just beginning to be explored. Generally, it is known that torsades de pointes occurs more commonly in women than in men (45). Preliminary small studies have considered heart rate variability (46) and QT duration (47). Heart rate variability is different in younger women and men (33 ± 4 years of age) but similar in older women and men (67 ± 3 years of age) (46).

In a Norway population survey, palpitations were reported more commonly by women (17%) than by men (12%) (48). In patients presenting to an emergency room with palpitations, men were more likely than women to have irregular beats (57% and 40%, respectively) and symptoms that lasted more than 5 minutes (77% and 61%, respectively) (49). Although cardiac causes of palpitations were most common, psychiatric diagnoses (predominantly panic attacks) were a close second (43% and 31%, respectively) (49). After MI, women die less often of arrhythmia than men (38). Finally, in a retrospective review of 31,913 entries in a German pacemaker registry, when pacemakers are implanted, women are more likely to receive a single-chamber pacer, whereas men are more likely to receive a dual-chamber pacer (50).

Conclusion

Further clarification of the similarities and differences between patients may improve the care each one receives. As is obvious from not only this chapter but from the entire book, attention to sex, age, race, and social factors will provide additional important insights into the pathophysiology, natural history, and treatment of CAD. This frontier is just beginning to open.

REFERENCES

1. **Morrison C, Woodward M, Leslie W, Turnstall-Pedoe H.** Effect of socioeconomic group on incidence of, management of, and survival after myocardial infarction and coronary death: analysis of community coronary event register. BMJ. 1997;314: 541–6.

2. **Kannel WB, Abbott RD.** Incidence and prognosis of myocardial infarction in women: the Framingham study. In: Eaker ED, Packard B, Wenger NK, et al. (eds). Coronary Heart Disease in Women: Proceedings of an NIH Workshop. New York: Haymark Doyma; 1987:208–214.

3. **Barrett-Connor E.** Sex differences in coronary heart disease: why are women so superior? The 1995 Ancel Keys Lecture. Circulation. 1997;95:252–64.

4. **Legato MJ, Padus E, Slaughter E.** Women's perceptions of their general health, with special reference of their risk of coronary artery disease: results of a national telephone survey. J Womens Health. 1997;6:189–98.

5. **Kreuger DE, Ellenberg SS, Bloom S, et al.** Risk factors for fatal heart attack in young women. Am J Epidemiol. 1981:113:357–70.

6. **Toiler GO, Stone PH, Muller JE, et al.** Effects of gender and race on prognosis after myocardial infarction: adverse prognosis for women, particularly black women. J Am Coll Cardiol. 1987;9:473–82.

7. **Power C, Matthews S.** Origins of health inequalities in a national population sample. Lancet. 1997;350:1584–9.

8. **Escobedo LG, Giles WH, Anda RF.** Socioeconomic status, race, and death from coronary heart disease. Am J Prev Med. 1997;13:123–30.

9. **Fang J, Madhavan S, Alderman MH.** The association between birthplace and mortality from cardiovascular causes among black and white residents of New York City. N Engl J Med. 1996;335:1545–51.

10. **Vitelli LL, Crow RS, Shahar E, et al.** Electrocardiographic findings in a healthy biracial population. Am J Cardiol. 1998;81:453–9.

11. **Perez-Stable EJ, Herrera B, Jacob P, Benowitz NL.** Nicotine metabolism and intake in black and white smokers. JAMA. 1998;280:152–6.

12. **Caraballo RS, Giovino GA, Pechacek TF, et al.** Racial and ethnic differences in serum cotinine levels of cigarette smokers: Third National Health and Nutrition Examination Survey, 1998 to 1991. JAMA. 1998;280:135–9.

13. **Shaukat N, Lear J, Lowy A, et al.** First myocardial infarction in patients of Indian subcontinent and European origin: comparison of risk factors, management, and long-term outcome. BMJ. 1997;314:639–42.

14. **Case RB, Moss AJ, Case N, et al.** Living alone after myocardial infarction: impact on prognosis. JAMA. 267:515–9.

15. **Smith GD, Hart C, Blane D, et al.** Lifetime socioeconomic position and mortality: prospective observational study. BMJ. 1997:314;547–52.

16. **Williams RB, Barefoot JC, Califf RM, et al.** Prognostic importance of social and economic resources among medically treated patients with angiographically documented coronary artery disease. JAMA. 1992; 267:520–4.

17. **Wilkinson RG.** Socioeconomic determinants of health. Health inequalities: relative or absolute material standards? BMJ. 1997;314:591–5.

18. **Bosma H, Marmot MG, Hemingway H, et al.** Low job control and risk of coronary heart disease in Whitehall II (prospective cohort) study. BMJ. 1997;314:558–5.

19. **Marmot MG, Bosma H, Hemingway H, et al.** Contribution of job control and other risk factors to social variations in coronary heart disease incidence. Lancet. 1997;350: 235–9.

20. **Power C, Matthews S, Manor O.** Inequalities in self-rated health: explanations from different stages of life. Lancet. 1998;351:1009–14.

21a. **Rich-Edwards JW, Stampfer MJ, Manson JE, et al.** Birth weight and risk of cardiovascular disease in a cohort of women followed up since 1976. BMJ. 1997;315:396–400.

21b. **Sullivan M, LaCroix A, Baum C, et al.** Coronary disease severity and functional impairment: how strong is the relationship? J Am Geriatr Soc. 1996;44:1461–5.

22. **Pincus T, Esther R, DeWalt DA, Callahan LF.** Social conditions and self-management are more powerful determinants of health than access to care. Ann Intern Med. 1998; 129:406–11.

23. **Lowe LP, Greenland P, Ruth RJ, Dyer AR, et al.** Impact of major cardiovascular disease risk factors, particularly in combination, on 22-year mortality in women and men. Arch Intern Med. 1988;158:2007–14.

24a. **Turnstall-Pedoe H, Woodward M, Tavendale R, et al.** Comparison of the prediction by 27 different factors of coronary heart disease and death in men and women of the Scottish heart health study: a cohort study. BMJ. 1997;315:722–9.

24b. **Njolstad I, Arnesen E.** Preinfarction blood pressure and smoking are determinants for a fatal outcome of myocardial infarction: a prospective analysis from the Finnmark Study. Arch Intern Med. 1998;158:1326–32.

25. **Winkleby M, Kraemer HC, Ahn DK, Varady AN.** Ethnic and socioeconomic differences in cardiovascular disease risk factors: findings for women from the Third National Health and Nutrition Examination Survey, 1988-1994. JAMA. 1998;280:356–62.

26. **Goldberg RJ, Larson M, Levy D.** Factors associated with survival to 75 years of age in middle-aged men and women. Arch Intern Med. 1996;156:505–9.

27. **Daviglus ML, Kiang L, Greenland P, et al.** Benefit of a favorable cardiovascular risk-factor profile in middle age with respect to Medicare costs. N Engl J Med. 1998;339:1122–9.

28. **Grover SA, Paquet S, Levinton C, et al.** Estimating the benefits of modifying risk factors of cardiovascular disease: a comparison of primary versus secondary prevention. Arch Intern Med. 1998;158:655–62.

29. **Newnham HH, Silberberg J.** Coronary heart disease: women's hearts are hard to break. Lancet. 1997;349:sI3–6.

30. **Perlman JA, Wolf PH, Ray R, Lieberknecht G.** Cardiovascular risk factors, premature heart disease, and all-cause mortality in a cohort of Northern California women. Am J Obstet Gynecol. 1988;158:1568–74.

31. **O'Keefe JH, Conn RD, Lavie CJ, Bateman TM.** The new paradigm for coronary artery disease: altering risk factors, atherosclerotic plaques, and clinical prognosis. Mayo Clin Proc. 1996;71:957–65.

32. **Gurfinkel E, Bozovich G, Darcoa A, et al.** Randomised trial of roxithromycin for non–Q-wave coronary syndromes: ROXIS pilot study. Lancet. 1997;350:404–7.

33. **Danesh J, Collins R, Peto R.** Chronic infections and coronary artery disease: is there a link? Lancet. 1997;350:430–6.

34. **Birdwell BG, Herbers JE, Kroenke K.** Evaluating chest pain: the patient's presentation style alters the physician's diagnostic approach. Arch Intern Med. 1993;153: 1991–5.

35. **Weiner DA, Ryan TJ, McCabe CH, et al.** Exercise stress testing: correlations among history of angina, ST-segment response and prevalence of coronary artery disease in the Coronary Artery Surgery Study (CASS). N Engl J Med. 1979;301:230–5.

36. **Mohri M, Koyanagi M, Egashira K, et al.** Angina pectoris caused by coronary microvascular spasm. Lancet. 1998;351:1165–9.

37. **Vaccarino V, Horowitz RI, Meehan TP, et al.** Sex differences in mortality after myocardial infarction: evidence for a sex-age interaction. Arch Intern Med. 1998;158: 2054–62.

38. **Chandra NC, Ziegelstein RC, Rogers WJ, et al.** Observations of the treatment of women in the United States with myocardial infarction: a report from the National Registry of Myocardial Infarction-I. Arch Intern Med. 1998;158:981–8.

39. **Gillum RF, Mussolino ME, Madans JH.** Coronary heart disease incidence and survival in African-American women and men: the NHANES I Epidemiologic Follow-Up study. Ann Intern Med. 1997;127:111–8.

40. **Marrugat JM, Sala J, Masia R, Pavesi M, et al.** Mortality differences between men and women following first myocardial infarction. JAMA. 1998;280:1405–9.

41. **Burke AP, Farb A, Malcolm GT, et al.** Effect of risk factors on the mechanism of acute thrombosis and sudden death in women. Circulation. 1998;97:2110–6.

42. **Oparil S.** Pathophysiology of sudden coronary death in women: implications for prevention. Circulation. 1998;97:2103–4.

43. **Goldberg RJ, Gorak EJ, Yarzebski J, et al.** A community-wide perspective of sex differences and temporal trends in the incidence and survival rates after myocardial infarction and out-of-hospital deaths caused by coronary heart disease. Circulation. 1993;87:1947–53.

44. **Krueger DE, Ellenberg SS, Bloom S, et al.** Risk factors for fatal heart attack in young women. Am J Epidemiol. 1981;113:357–70.

45. **Makkar RR, Fromm BS, Steinman RT, et al.** Female gender as a risk factor for torsades de pointes associated with cardiovascular drugs. JAMA. 1993;270:2590–7.

46. **Stein PK, Kleiger RE, Rottman JN.** Differing effects of age on heart rate variability in men and women. Am J Cardiol. 1997;80:302–5.

47. **Burke JH, Ehlert FA, Kruse JT, et al.** Gender-specific differences in the QT interval and the effect of autonomic tone and menstrual cycle in healthy adults. Am J Cardiol. 1997;79:178–81.

48. **Lochen ML, Snaprud T, Zhang W, Rasmussen K.** Arrhythmias in subjects with and without a history of palpitations: the Tromso study. Eur Heart J. 1994;15:345–9.

49. **Weber BE, Kapoor WN.** Evaluation and outcomes of patient with palpitations. Am J Med. 1996;100:138–48.

50. **Schuppel R, Buchele G, Batz L, Koenig W.** Sex differences in selection of pacemakers: retrospective observation study. BMJ. 1988;316:492–5.

Index